PRACTICE OF MEDICINE

EDITED BY

FREDERICK TICE, M.D., F.A.C.P.

CLINICAL PROFESSOR OF MEDICINE, UNIVERSITY OF CHICAGO,
RUSH MEDICAL COLLEGE; FORMERLY PROFESSOR OF MEDI-
CINE AND CLINICAL MEDICINE AND HEAD OF THE
DEPARTMENT OF MEDICINE, UNIVERSITY OF
ILLINOIS COLLEGE OF MEDICINE;
ATTENDING STAFF (MEDICINE),
COOK COUNTY HOSPITAL
CHICAGO, ILL.

VOLUME IV

HAGERSTOWN, MARYLAND

W. F. PRIOR COMPANY, INC.

1941

PRINTED IN THE UNITED STATES OF AMERICA

CONTENTS

VOLUME IV

INFECTIOUS DISEASES (*Continued*)

iv   CONTENTS

PRACTICE OF MEDICINE

VOLUME IV

INFECTIOUS DISEASES (CONTINUED)

YELLOW FEVER

By CHARLES F. CRAIG, M.D., M.A. (HON.), F.A.C.P., F.A.C.S., COLONEL, U. S. ARMY MEDICAL CORPS (RET.), D.S.M.

Synonyms.—Typhus icteroides, yellow jack, black vomit, febris flava, typhus amarillo, vomito prieto, vomito negro.

Definition.—Yellow fever is an acute, febrile, infectious and, under certain conditions, contagious disease caused by a filtrable virus and transmitted from man to man by mosquitoes, usually by *Aedes aegypti*. Clinically, in typical cases, it is characterized by a sudden onset, fever of variable duration, a slow pulse as compared with the temperature, albuminuria, jaundice, hematemesis, hemorrhages and anuria. Many latent infections occur in which the symptoms are so slight as not to be recognized, as well as mild infections in which the symptoms are atypical.

Etiology.—The cause of yellow fever is a filtrable virus. As noted in the discussion of the history of this infection, numerous organisms have been described, from time to time, as the cause of this disease, but in 1900 the United States Army Yellow Fever Commission, composed of Drs. Reed, Carroll, Lazear and Agramonte, demonstrated that the true cause was a filtrable virus. This discovery has been confirmed and amplified by numerous investigators, especially by the West African Yellow Fever Commission of the Rockefeller Foundation and by other workers connected with that Foundation, to whom we owe most of our more recent knowledge regarding the etiology and epidemiology of this infection.

Stokes and his coworkers proved that the yellow fever virus may pass the Berkefeld V and N filter candles and the Seitz (EK) asbestos disk filter at a negative pressure of 400 mm. of mercury, but the Berkefeld W candle was able to retain the virus. The presence of blood serum increases the filtrability of the virus. Later, Bauer and Mahaffy passed the virus through the Berkefeld V, N and W candles and the Pasteur-Chamberland L_2 bougie.

The yellow fever virus is ultramicroscopic in size, and Findlay and Broom (1933) and Bauer and Hudson (1935), by passing it through collodion filters of known porosity, determined that it measures between 17 and 28 millimicrons in diameter. The size of the virus is not altered by repeated passage through experimental animals.

The virus can pass through the unbroken skin, as demonstrated by experiments upon susceptible animals, and many accidental laboratory

1

infections have shown that man may become infected through the blood of infected experimental animals, thus proving that yellow fever is contagious under certain conditions. A laboratory infection has occurred in man in taking a specimen of blood for a microscopic examination, and another, in making a routine biochemical examination of a yellow fever patient's blood.

The virus is present in the infected individual's blood during the first three or four days after the appearance of clinical symptoms and probably during the latter portion of the incubation period. It is possible for man to become infected by the contamination of the skin or mucous membranes with the blood of yellow fever patients during this period and in performing autopsies upon patients dying of the disease during the first four days after the appearance of clinical symptoms. The reason why so few infections have occurred from autopsies is that in most instances the patients die after the fourth day of the disease, at which time the virus has disappeared from the blood. The virus is a most powerful one, a dilution of one part in one billion being sufficient to kill a Macacus monkey when injected subcutaneously.

The virus is usually killed after an exposure to a temperature of 60° C. (140° F.) for 10 minutes, but may be preserved and will retain its virulence for 154 days if dried *in vacuo* and kept in a sealed tube at low temperatures. It will remain virulent when mixed with 50 per cent glycerol for 100 days. Sawyer, Kitchen and Lloyd (1929) found that a specimen of the virus which had been dried and sealed in glass was still virulent for monkeys after 9¼ years in storage at temperatures a little over 0° C.

The yellow fever virus is destroyed by many chemicals. Exposure for 30 minutes at 30° C. (86° F.) to 0.3 per cent phenol, 16.7 per cent alcohol and 6.7 per cent formalin inactivates this virus. Findlay (1934) determined that a 1 to 100,000 dilution of methylene blue and subsequent exposure to a pointolite source of light killed the virus, while Hindle and Findlay (1930) found that it was destroyed in acid media of pH 3.0 to 4.0. Bauer (1931) found that the virus remained active in the tissues of infected monkeys dead for so long that their organs were decomposed.

Under natural conditions the yellow fever virus is both viscerotropic and neurotropic in its action, but when the virus is passed through mice by intracerebral injection, it practically loses its power to attack the viscera but its power to attack the nervous system is increased, as first shown by Theiler in 1930. After continued culture in tissues, as in the chick embryo, the naturally pantropic virus, i.e., capable of attacking both the viscera and the nervous system, loses almost all of its viscerotropic and neurotropic properties but is still very active as an antigen in the production of immunity.

Like most viruses, the yellow fever virus can be cultivated only in living tissue cultures. Lloyd, Theiler and Ricci (1936) cultivated this virus in tissue cultures, employing whole mouse embryos for the culture medium, while Theiler and Smith (1937) obtained excellent results by cultivation of the virus in chick embryos, and this is the method employed at present for obtaining the living virus for vaccination purposes. Cultivated in this manner the virus loses its viscerotropic properties and is only feebly neurotropic.

For many years our knowledge of yellow fever was hindered by the lack of any laboratory animal apparently susceptible to this infection. However, in 1927 Stokes and Bauer demonstrated that the Indian monkey, *Macacus sinicus,* was susceptible to infection, the injection of yellow fever blood into this animal being followed by a fatal infection showing the pathologic lesions of the disease. It was afterward determined that the common *Macacus rhesus* is also susceptible, as well as *Macacus cynomolgus* and *Macacus nemestrinus.* From an epidemiological standpoint, the interesting fact that monkeys living in endemic yellow fever regions are immune to infection, apparently due to infections acquired in early life, explained why native monkeys in such regions had never been experimentally infected. Although the discovery that certain monkeys could be infected with yellow fever resulted in many advances in our knowledge of this infection, the great cost of these animals prohibited extended research, and a great advance in this respect was made by the discovery by Theiler (1930) that intracerebral injection of the yellow fever virus into white mice was followed by a specific form of encephalitis, the virus multiplying in the brain, while the viscera, as the lungs and liver, were not affected. This discovery has made possible many advances in the diagnosis of yellow fever and in the elucidation of immunologic problems regarding this infection.

Immunology.—It has been known for many generations that one attack of yellow fever is followed by an immunity to later infection, an immunity that was usually regarded as persisting throughout life. The more recent observations upon both natural and experimental yellow fever, in both man and susceptible animals, have confirmed this belief and it is probable that second attacks of this disease never occur, although some are recorded in the older literature upon this subject. Sawyer (1931) examined the blood serum of numerous individuals, employing the mouse protection test, and found that the sera of individuals who had suffered from yellow fever years before, were still protective to mice, thus demonstrating that immune substances were still present in such sera. In eight individuals who had suffered from the disease thirty-one to thirty-three years previously, six were still protective for mice, and in one individual who had suffered from yellow fever seventy-five years previously, the blood serum neutralized the virus. These findings prove that immunity to yellow fever is, in all probability, a lifelong immunity, and have made possible yellow fever surveys and the determination of past infection in a population. (See Diagnosis.)

A *passive immunity* to yellow fever, of uncertain duration, may be produced by the injection of sufficient amounts of convalescent yellow fever serum, and this method of protection was formerly used by the Rockefeller Foundation for the protection of its workers in the laboratory and in the field. However, the occurrence of infections following the use of this method showed that it was not efficient and it was succeeded by the method of vaccination elaborated by Sawyer, Kitchen and Lloyd (1932). This method consisted in the subcutaneous injections of enough immune human serum to produce a passive immunity, followed by a single injection of living yellow fever virus rendered practically harmless by continued passage intracerebrally through mice. The employment of this method caused a cessation of the laboratory infections but it was not applicable to general immunization, as the amount of convalescent serum required would have been prohibitive and there was some danger that the virus might revert to its pantropic nature and thus prove dangerous. Further observations have resulted in the use of a vaccine prepared from culture of the virus on chick embryos, the strain of the virus used by the Rockefeller Foundation being that known as "17 D," derived from the Asibi strain. This strain, originally very virulent, has lost most of its virulence by prolonged tissue culture and has been developed in the Laboratories of the Foundation, in New York. This vaccine has been employed in Brazil since 1937, with excellent results, and Sawyer (1939) states that in 1938 no less than 1,059,252 persons were vaccinated with it in Brazil and that over 90 per cent of the vaccinated individuals showed protective antibodies in their blood after vaccination. It has not yet been determined how long protection lasts after vaccination with the cultured virus, but since its use no accidental infections have occurred among laboratory personnel, some of whom have been vaccinated for as long as three years. Up to the time of writing (1940) no serious complications have been reported following vaccination with this virus.

As this method of vaccination introduces a living yellow fever virus into the body, it has been suggested that the virus might multiply to such an extent as to be present in the blood in sufficient amounts to infect *Aedes* mosquitoes. However, Whitman (1939) has shown that the "17 D" strain of the virus after culture upon tissues cannot be transmitted by *Aedes* mosquitoes and that the quantity of virus present in the circulating blood of vaccinated individuals is too small, at any time, to infect mosquitoes.

For a further discussion of yellow fever vaccination, as regards its application, dosage and reactions, see under the heading "Prophylaxis."

Valuable contributions to our knowledge of the immunology of yellow fever, and various methods of immunization by means of sera and vaccines, have been made by Sawyer, Lloyd, Theiler, Finlay, Findlay and MacCallum, H. H. Smith, Soper, Sorel, James and others, but the literature is now so great that it is impossible to review it in the space allotted this contribution. Suffice it to say, that at the present time we possess safe and reliable methods for the protection of individuals from this infection and that, of the methods employed, vaccination with the "17 D" strain, mentioned above, when cultured on chick embryo tissue, is apparently most efficient, safe, and has stood the test of experience.

Both complement-fixing and precipitin bodies can be demonstrated in the blood serum of individuals who have recovered from an attack of yellow fever and, for a while, it was hoped that tests based upon this fact would be found useful in diagnosis, but such tests, while important from theoretical and research standpoints, have not proved of much value in practice.

Epidemiology.—Two decades ago it was believed by many that our knowledge of the epidemiology of yellow fever was practically complete, following the demonstration by the Army Yellow Fever Commission, of the transmission of the disease by the mosquito, *Aedes aegypti*, and the disappearance of the disease in epidemic form after the application of methods resulting in the destruction of the transmitting mosquitoes. However, it was soon determined that isolated cases of the disease were occurring continually and that it was impossible to eliminate the disease from the Western Hemisphere, which had been the dream of the Rockefeller Commission. Continued research by members of the International Health Division of this Foundation furnished the explanation, for by the use of the viscerotome and surveys made with the aid of the mouse protection test, it was determined that the disease was endemic in the Amazon valley in Brazil and elsewhere. The examination of sections of the liver removed by the viscerotome, in all patients dying of febrile conditions in Brazil, proved that many of them had perished from yellow fever, while the results of the mouse protection test demonstrated that the disease had been prevalent in many localities where its past or present occurrence had not been suspected. The mouse protection test showed that immunity to yellow fever was widespread in Brazil and that individuals living in localities, usually near the jungle, where *Aedes* mosquitoes were not found, had suffered from the disease and were immune, while the viscerotome demonstrated that cases were occurring in such localities. Thus, in discussing the epidemiology of yellow fever it is necessary to consider that of the form of the fever occurring in cities and towns, or *urban yellow fever*, and that form occurring in the jungle, known as *jungle yellow fever*, remembering that etiologically and pathologically these forms are identical, as is the yellow fever of Africa and that of South America.

Urban yellow fever, occurring in cities, towns and villages, usually in epidemic form if a sufficient nonimmune population is present, is transmitted by the mosquito, *Aedes aegypti*, for while many other mosquitoes have been experimentally incriminated, none other has been found to transmit the infection under natural conditions in such localities. In regions where the disease is endemic it becomes epidemic whenever a large nonimmune population is introduced, as was well illustrated in Havana, Cuba, when an epidemic of yellow fever occurred whenever a large number of immigrants arrived from Spain. In the endemic areas most of the inhabitants are immune, having suffered from the infection in childhood. There is some evidence that this acquired immunity is not always complete but is augmented by mild, unrecognized attacks of the disease occurring in later life.

From the endemic regions the infection may be spread through the agency of ships, automobiles, trains and airplanes carrying infected mosquitoes or individuals in the incubation stage of the disease. Unless *Aedes* mosquitoes are present no spread of the infection can occur even though infected mosquitoes or individuals are introduced into a new locality. Epidemics of yellow fever always occur during the seasons when *Aedes aegypti* mosquitoes are most numerous, and in temperate regions the occurrence of frost will end an epidemic because such temperatures kill the adult *Aedes* and prevent the breeding of these mosquitoes.

Jungle yellow fever was first described by Soper, Penna, Cardoso, Serafim, Frobisher and Pinheiro (1933), and differs from urban yellow fever epidemiologically in that it is not transmitted by *Aedes aegypti*, is contracted by individuals living near the forest or jungle and after entering such localities, and affects children over four years of age and adults, i.e., those who are old enough to enter the jungle or forests in the endemic regions. Jungle yellow fever does not often occur in epidemic form, for obvious reasons, but Sawyer (1939) states that it did occur in epidemics in certain regions in Brazil from 1934 to 1938. Usually it

40102

occurs only in workers in, or near, the jungle, and those affected are usually adult males, women and children escaping because the infection is not spread in the home, *Aedes aegypti* being absent.

The transmitting agent, or agents, of jungle yellow fever are still unknown, but Shannon, Whitman and Franca (1938) have found two species of wild mosquitoes caught in the jungle to be naturally infected with the virus. It is evident that some reservoir host must be present in the jungle in order that the infection be perpetuated and the evidence is in favor of monkeys being such a reservoir host, for many of these animals, caught in the jungle, have been shown to have antibodies present in their blood serum. However, it is also true that yellow fever occurs in regions in the jungle where monkeys are very few in number, so that it appears as though there must be some other animal, or animals, which act as reservoirs of the virus. Intensive research is now being devoted to this phase of yellow fever and it is only a question of time until this mystery will be solved.

The usual *method of transmission* of yellow fever in *urban communities* is through the bites of infected *Aedes* mosquitoes. The virus of yellow fever, as already stated, is present in the blood of infected individuals during the incubation stage of the disease and for three or four days after the appearance of symptoms. If an *Aedes aegypti* mosquito bites the infected individual during this period it will become infected but will not be able to transmit the infection to man until an interval of from eight to fourteen days, usually twelve days, has elapsed from the time of the infective feeding. After becoming infective, the mosquito remains so until its death, and such mosquitoes have lived in captivity for as long as 160 days. Agramonte states that, in his own experience, a mosquito that had bitten a yellow fever patient fifty-six days previously, produced an infection in a volunteer, and was still infective seventy-six days after biting the patient, while others have shown that the mosquito may remain infective for as long as 120 days. It is very doubtful that individual mosquitoes live for so long a time in nature because of their numerous natural enemies, exposure to extremes of temperature and other biologic conditions, as well as to accidents of various kinds. The incubation period of the virus in the mosquito is not due to any cyclical development of the virus but is the time necessary for the virus to multiply sufficiently to reach the salivary glands, and at this time the virus may be demonstrated in all parts of the insect.

Mechanical transmission of the yellow fever virus by mosquitoes and other arthropods is possible, if the arthropod be interrupted in feeding upon a yellow fever patient and then bites a normal individual within a short time. Just how important mechanical transmission may be during an epidemic has not been ascertained but that it may be quite important in rapidly spreading the infection is not beyond the realm of possibility.

Aedes aegypti is a domestic mosquito, breeding in almost any collection of water near human habitations or even within the habitations. Rain barrels, empty bottles or cans, clogged gutters, cisterns, fire buckets, water closet tanks, flower vases, tree stumps, tree holes, fountains and any other receptacle which will contain water for the period of time necessary for the evolution of this species, are favorite breeding places. The average period of time between the deposition of the fertilized egg and the emergence of the adult mosquito is usually from twelve to sixteen

TABLE I

MOSQUITOES OTHER THAN AEDES AEGYPTI INCRIMINATED IN YELLOW FEVER,
BASED ON EXPERIMENTAL EVIDENCE

(From Craig and Faust's "Clinical Parasitology," Lea and Febiger, Philadelphia.)

SPECIES	DISTRIBUTION	BREEDING PLACES
*†*Aëdes africanus*	Ethiopian	Tree holes, stumps; also semidomestic.
A. luteocephalus	W. Ethiopian	Tree holes, cut bamboo.
†A. simpsoni	Ethiopian	Tree holes, leaf axils.
A. stokesi	W. Ethiopian	Tree holes, banana and bamboo stumps.
†A. vittatus	Ethiopian and Oriental	Rock pools, cement drains, gutters.
†A. irritans	W. Ethiopian	Crab holes.
†A. nigricephalus	W. Ethiopian	Crab holes.
†A. punctocostalis	W. Ethiopian	Crab holes.
*†A. fluviatilis	Neotropical	Rock pools along rivers.
*†A. scapularis	Neotropical	Rain pools.
†A. serratus	Neotropical	Rain pools.
†A. leucocelænus	Neotropical	Uncleared land.
*†A. nubilus	Neotropical	
*†A. triseriatus	Nearctic	Tree holes.
*†A. geniculatus	Palæarctic	Tree holes.
†A. terrens	Neotropical	Tree holes.
†A. fulvithorax	Neotropical	Tree holes.
*†A. albopictus	Oriental and E. Nearctic	Domestic, similar to *A. ægypti*.
†A. variegatus (?) (syn. A. scutellaris?)	Australasian	Tree holes, cocoanut shells, tins, etc., in bush.
*†Eretmopodites chrysogaster	Ethiopian	Tree holes, stumps; also semidomestic.
*†Culex fatigans	Tropical	Domestic.
C. nigripalpus	Neotropical	
*†C. thalassius	W. Ethiopian	Crab holes.
*†Mansonia africana	Ethiopian, Oriental, Australasian	Aquatic plants.
*†M. uniformis	W. Ethiopian	Coastal swamps and marshes.
†M. fasciolata	Neotropical	Attached to sedges and *Equisetum*.
†M. juxtamansonia	Neotropical	
†M. chrysonotum	Neotropical (Brazil only)	Attached to sedges and *Equisetum*.
†M. albicosta	Neotropical (Brazil only)	Attached to sedges and *Equisetum*.
†M. titillans	Neotropical	Attached to floating water plants.
†Psorophora cingula	Neotropical	In wooded areas and semidomestic.
†P. ferox	Neotropical	Wild, in wooded areas.
†Wyeomia bromeliarum	Neotropical	Bamboo joints.
†W. oblita	Neotropical	Water-holding plants.
†Limatus durhami	Neotropical	In natural and artificial containers.
†Hæmagogus janthinomys	Neotropical	Forests.
†H. uriartei	Neotropical	Forests.
†H. capricorni	Neotropical	Forests.

* Efficient transmitters.
† Good incubators.

days when conditions are most favorable, but this period may be much prolonged if conditions are unfavorable.

Aedes aegypti is a readily recognized species because of its black legs, banded with white, and the markings in white upon the thorax, in front of the wings, consisting of silvery lines against a black background, forming an appearance suggesting a lyre, the outer, or curved lines, being thick, forming the frame of the instrument, while the inner straight lines are thin, forming the strings of the lyre.

While *Aedes aegypti* is the usual transmitting agent of yellow fever in urban regions it has no part in the transmission of the jungle type, as already stated. Many other species of mosquito, as well as other arthropods, have been found to be experimentally capable of transmitting yellow fever, so that the statement formerly accepted, that *Aedes aegypti* is the only insect capable of transmitting this infection, is no longer tenable.

In addition to *Aedes aegypti* the species of mosquitoes which have been found by experiment to be efficient transmitters and good incubators of the yellow fever virus are given in Table I.

Besides the mosquitoes tabulated in Table I, the following arthropods have been found capable of transmitting the yellow fever virus experimentally: *Stomoxys calcitrans, Stenocephalus canis, Cimex lectularius, Cimex hemipterus, Panstrongylus megistus, Ornithodorus moubata, Ornithodorus rostrata* and *Amblyomma cajennense*. In these arthropods transmission is purely mechanical in type and it will be observed that flies, fleas, bedbugs, triatomata and ticks are all represented in this list. Whether or not any of these arthropoda have anything to do with the transmission of yellow fever in nature is unknown. In the instance of the bedbugs, the feces are infective when deposited upon the skin of the experimental animal.

The virus of the jungle type of yellow fever has been found to be present in naturally infected mosquitoes of the species *Aedes leucocelaenus* and *Haemagogus capricorni*.

RACE.—The *influence of race* upon the epidemiology of yellow fever is of little importance provided previous exposure to the infection is eliminated. All races of mankind are susceptible to the infection but in endemic areas the natives are less apt to suffer from the clinical disease because of an immunity that has been acquired in early life. Thus, the adult negro in endemic regions in Africa seldom suffers from yellow fever but usually the blood of such negroes is found to contain immune bodies, proving that they had been infected in infancy or childhood. In nonendemic regions yellow fever is as common in negroes as in the white man, although in the former the attacks are usually less severe, thus showing a partial immunity to the disease. At the present time there is no evidence available that any race is naturally immune to yellow fever and the oft-repeated statement that the Chinese are less susceptible to the virus than other races has not been proved and is not true, in all probability.

SEX exercises no influence upon the epidemiology of this infection save insofar as it conduces to infection. Females and males are equally susceptible, although some authorities state that during epidemics more infections are observed among males than among females. The writer believes that this statement does not rest upon sufficient evidence and the fact that *Aedes aegypti* is a house mosquito would lead one to believe the opposite, as females, who are more constantly in the house, would apparently be more often bitten by such mosquitoes.

AGE is of great importance in the epidemiology of yellow fever as surveys have shown that the disease is most commonly observed in infants and young children in endemic regions. In these, yellow fever is often a very mild disease and is frequently unrecognized clinically, thus accounting for the inaccuracy of our knowledge of the distribution of yellow fever before the employment of the viscerotome and the mouse protection test in making surveys for this infection. During epidemics it has been noted that most of the infections occur between the ages of fifteen and forty-five years.

Symptomatology.—The *period of incubation* of yellow fever varies from three to seven days but may be shortened or prolonged in rare instances. Agramonte states that it may be only a few hours, while Sawyer states that it may be as long as ten days. Prodromal symptoms are not observed either in natural or experimental infections.

The *onset* is almost always sudden, seldom with a definite chill, though chilly sensations may be present. Muscular pains, especially in the back and legs, and marked headache quickly develop; the skin and mucous membranes are greatly congested; the face is flushed and swollen; the conjunctivae are greatly congested, while the eyes appear brilliant and have a frightened or anxious expression. Sore throat may be present, especially in children. There is marked nervousness and the patient is frequently much worried or scared over his condition. The skin is hot and dry and constipation is usually present, although diarrhea, accompanied by hemorrhages, may develop rapidly in very malignant infections.

The temperature rapidly ascends to 39 or 40° C. (102.2 to 104° F.) and the pulse is rapid and of increased tension. In the average case the temperature continues high for from two to three days, during which time the conjunctivae may become jaundiced and albumin appears in the urine. The tongue is coated with a yellowish-white fur, the breath is foul, and bleeding may occur from the mucous membranes of the nose or gums. Nausea or vomiting may be present and there is usually marked tenderness and pain in the epigastrium.

Usually, in a typical case, the temperature recedes on the second, third or fourth day of the disease, accompanied by relief in the severity of the acute symptoms. This recession of the fever is only temporary, for in typical cases there is a secondary rise in the fever, with a recurrence of the muscular pains, headache, nausea, epigastric pain and general discomfort, while the jaundice increases and also the amount of albumin in the urine.

The pulse, instead of rising in frequency with the secondary temperature rise, continues to fall and patients are observed at this time having a temperature of 39° C. (102.2° F.) with a pulse rate of 60 to 65 beats per minute, or even less. This lack of corelation between the temperature and pulse in yellow fever is known as *Faget's sign* and is of great importance in the diagnosis of the disease.

The stage of the disease that has just been described is sometimes called the "stage of acute congestion," while that initiated by the secondary rise in the temperature is known as the "stage of stasis."

40102

The *"stage of stasis,"* which usually begins upon the third or fourth day of the disease, is especially characterized by the occurrence of hemorrhages. The temperature may remain elevated but usually slowly declines in infections having a favorable prognosis, but jaundice becomes more marked and the urine may contain a very large amount of albumin. Hemorrhages may occur from the nose, gums and mucous membranes, and the patient may vomit material containing black specks or the vomitus may be black in color, due to hemorrhage from the stomach, the so-called "black vomit" of yellow fever. Petechiae may appear upon the skin and in very severe cases hemorrhage may occur from the intestine. In fatal cases black vomit, intestinal hemorrhage, hemorrhages from the nose and mouth, delirium and coma usually precede death. In yellow fever, death usually occurs between the sixth and ninth days from the onset of symptoms, but in virulent infections it may occur in from forty-eight to seventy-two hours, the symptoms present being intense headache, chills, high fever, delirium, marked prostration, large amounts of albumin in the urine, anuria, and rapid development of convulsions or coma, followed by death.

A well-marked leukopenia is present in yellow fever, the lowest leukocyte count being present between the fifth and sixth days after symptoms occur.

ANALYSIS OF SYMPTOMS.—*The Fever.*—The fever in this infection usually begins with chilly sensations or a chill and rises gradually, reaching its maximum in from twelve to twenty-four hours after the onset. In very mild cases it may not go above 39° C. (102.2° F.) but in severe infections it may reach 41° C. (105.8° F.), although it rarely rises above 39.5° C. (103.1° F.). After from thirty-six to forty-eight hours, in most typical cases, there is a distinct remission in the temperature but it seldom falls to normal. The duration of this first stage varies from thirty-three to sixty hours, the average duration being about forty-three hours in ten experimental cases observed by Agramonte.

The remission in the temperature usually lasts from three to twenty-six hours, after which it gradually rises again reaching its maximum within a few hours and fluctuating slightly for another period of from two to five days, and then falls to normal or below and convalescence begins. In cases of average severity the permanent fall in the temperature occurs between the fifth and ninth days after the onset of the symptoms.

Hyperpyrexia is extremely rare in yellow fever and is usually caused by some complication, such as the malarial fevers. A long-continued fever does not occur unless caused by some complication.

In very mild symptomatic cases the remission in the temperature is permanent and recovery occurs without a secondary rise in the fever.

The Pulse.—The yellow fever virus has a marked effect upon the heart muscle and the character of the pulse is of great importance in the diagnosis and prognosis of this infection. At the outset, the pulse corresponds with the temperature, the beats increasing in frequency with the rise in the fever, the pulse at the height of the temperature being from 90 to 120 beats per minute, and usually full and bounding in character. This rate is maintained until the temperature remits, when the pulse rate recedes with the fall in the temperature, at the end of the remission it being from 65 to 75 beats per minute. With the secondary rise in the fever the pulse does not increase in frequency but continues to decrease until, with a temperature of 39° C. (102.2° F.), there may be a pulse rate varying from 40 to 65 beats per minute. This falling pulse rate with a rising temperature was first called attention to by Faget, and is known as "Faget's sign." It is present not only in cases of average severity and in fatal cases, but is also noted in the mildest clinical infections with the yellow fever virus. In cases having a bad prognosis the slowing of the pulse during the secondary rise in the fever is accompanied by shallow breathing, cyanosis and other signs of cardiac failure, and death usually results in such cases and is caused by cardiac failure. Thus, the slowing of the pulse cannot be regarded as a favorable prognostic sign unless it is unaccompanied by symptoms and signs of cardiac insufficiency.

Circulatory System.—Aside from the effect upon the heart, as shown by the marked bradycardia, the yellow fever virus apparently has a marked effect upon the integrity of the capillaries. During the early stage of the disease there is intense capillary congestion and hemorrhages occur during this time but are more severe in the later stage of the infection after the secondary rise in the temperature. During the first three days there may be epistaxis and the gums may be swollen and bleed easily upon pressure. Later, the mucous membranes of the nose, mouth and throat bleed easily and the gums are covered with a bloody mucus. Hemorrhage into the stomach may occur as well as into the intestine.

The *heart*, even in mild or moderate attacks of yellow fever, is markedly affected. At first the muscle is stimulated but soon the blood pressure begins to fall, the beats become lessened in number and diminished in force, and collapse may occur ending in death. Dilatation of the heart sometimes occurs and the profound effect of the virus upon the heart muscle is demonstrated by the fall in blood pressure, the lessening in the force of the apical pulsations, and the disappearance or lessening of the heart sounds, as well as the cardiographic changes. Berry and Kitchen (1931) have studied the electrocardiograms in cases of accidental infection with yellow fever in laboratories and have noted that the T waves in all the leads show increased height on the third, as compared with the second, day of the infection, and that this change was progressive for about a week, when daily fluctuations occurred and changes in contour were noted. The reduction in the frequency of the pulse they found to be due to a sinus bradycardia. Chagas and de Freitas (1929), in a study of fatal cases of yellow fever, found in some cases the electrocardiographic changes were limited to alterations of the terminal wave of the ventricular complex, while in others nodal rhythm, inversion of the P wave, variations in conduction time and intraventricular block were noted.

Digestive System.—Symptoms connected with the digestive system are prominent early in the course of an attack of yellow fever, the patients complaining of a sense of oppression, or weight, in the epigastrium which increases more or less rapidly until severe epigastric pain is experienced, a symptom so common and so marked in this disease as to be of considerable diagnostic importance. Nausea and vomiting are also common, usually most so after the second day of the attack. The *vomitus* at first consists of the gastric secretion streaked with glairy

40102

mucus, somewhat bile-stained, but after the third or fourth day blood may appear, either in the form of dark brown or black specks (the so-called "fly-wing specks") or as reddish or brownish streaks scattered through the vomitus. The amount of vomited blood may increase gradually until finally the vomitus assumes the "coffee-ground" appearance stressed in the older descriptions of the disease. In cases in which severe hemorrhage has occurred in the stomach the classical "black vomit" is seen, the vomited material consisting almost entirely of degenerated blood which has undergone changes in the stomach and become black in color.

Hemorrhage may occur in the intestine but this is comparatively rare and melena is usually due to the passage of the "black vomit" from the stomach into the intestine.

Respiratory System.—During the active stage of congestion a slight cough may be present but usually the respiratory system is not seriously involved in yellow fever. Bronchopneumonia or lobar pneumonia may occur rarely as a complication.

Genito-urinary System.—The yellow fever virus affects the kidneys early in the disease and the great congestion of these organs accounts for the appearance of albumin in the urine usually by the third day but sometimes within forty-eight hours after the onset of the infection. Albuminuria is probably present in most clinically recognizable cases of yellow fever, and Agramonte stated that he was prone to discredit the diagnosis of nonalbuminuric yellow fever. However, this opinion has been proved false by Berry and Kitchen (1931), who found that albumin may never appear in the urine in mild clinical cases of yellow fever. The amount of albumin usually increases and is greatest during the stage of stasis and casts may occur in the urine during this stage. The casts are usually of the granular or hyaline type but epithelial casts may be present. The occurrence of casts has no prognostic significance and they disappear rapidly during convalescence from the infection. In fatal cases death is frequently due to the renal involvement, granular and epithelial casts being numerous in the urine, while the amount of albumin is greatly increased. In such cases the urine is decreased in amount and the patient dies from anuria, accompanied by the symptoms of uremia.

Ehrlich's diazo reaction is not present in the urine in yellow fever except very rarely and is then atypical and of very short duration. Hemorrhage from the urinary tract is rare and hemoglobinuria, if present, is always a complication, usually caused by a malarial infection.

Nervous System.—Yellow fever has a marked effect upon the nervous system, evidenced very early in the disease, the symptoms increasing in severity with the progress of the infection. During the onset, *headache* is a pronounced symptom, usually frontal in location, but sometimes it is present over the occiput or the temples. At the height of the fever the headache may be most pronounced over the vertex of the skull or in the occipital region. It disappears with the initial decline in the temperature but recurs with the secondary rise in the fever. In rare instances the headache may be so severe as to require large doses of morphine in order to control it.

Pain in the back is usually present during the febrile stages of yellow fever, being most pronounced in the lumbar region but often extending to the base of the neck.

Early in the disease the patient may appear to be drowsy but is easily aroused and then appears extremely nervous and apprehensive. In severe cases, as the disease advances, marked cerebral symptoms develop. Delirium may occur and the patient may become very restless, may leave his bed and even wander away if given the opportunity. Tremors, subsultus tendinum, and paralyses of the voluntary muscles may occur, and incontinence of urine and feces is usually present before a fatal ending.

PHYSICAL FINDINGS.—The *facies* in yellow fever is that of other febrile infections during the first few hours after the onset, the skin being congested and red, the conjunctivae much congested and the eyes brilliant. The startled or frightened expression of the patient, described by most students of yellow fever, is not characteristic of this disease but is seen in any febrile condition in which the patient fears a fatal outcome. The reputation of yellow fever among the laity is such that those attacked are often stampeded by fear and this accounts for the facial expression so frequently noted.

The conjunctivae may show slight jaundice as early as the second day of the disease and this may gradually increase until finally the conjunctivae are markedly jaundiced, and the skin of the arms, legs, chest, abdomen and back may be of a lemon-yellow color. In most cases the jaundice in yellow fever is not so pronounced as in Weil's disease, acute yellow atrophy of the liver or in malignant jaundice, but in fatal cases it may be very pronounced, the entire body having an almost mahogany brown color. The jaundice may not be visible in dark-skinned races and is difficult to distinguish in the negro, except in the conjunctivae. The urine is not bile-stained until the latter days of the disease in those cases in which jaundice is pronounced.

In mild infections jaundice, supposed to be so diagnostic of yellow fever, is usually absent, so that the absence of this symptom is not proof that yellow fever is not present.

There are no physical findings of importance in the *lungs* unless a complication is present. It has already been mentioned that findings indicating the existence of *myocarditis* may sometimes occur, and brady-cardia, abnormalities in rhythm of the heart, lessened heart sounds and a feeble apex beat are noted in most cases of average severity and are very pronounced in severe and fatal infections.

Early in the disease there is *abdominal tenderness* upon pressure and this increases as the disease progresses until the *epigastric region* becomes so tender that the least pressure may cause intense pain and may bring about an attack of nausea and vomiting.

The peculiar character of *the pulse* in yellow fever has already been described. The continued fall in the pulse rate after the primary remission in the temperature is so invariably present that it must be considered as a very valuable diagnostic feature, as this lack of corelation between the pulse and temperature is not so pronounced in any other infection. During convalescence the pulse rate may fall as low as 40 to 50 beats per minute and at this time cardiac failure may occur. In fatal cases the pulse often increases in rapidity before death while the temperature may fall, thus reversing the usual picture in these respects. The slow pulse may continue for several weeks after the acute symptoms of the disease have disappeared but eventually it becomes normal

40102

in the vast majority of those patients who recover. In rare instances the damage to the heart is so great that a chronic myocarditis develops and causes the death of the patient.

MILD YELLOW FEVER.—Owing to the occurrence of many cases of yellow fever in which the symptoms are atypical or so mild as scarcely to be recognized, one should be on the lookout for such infections, as their recognition is of the utmost importance from the standpoint of the prevention of the disease. Reference has already been made to the studies of Berry and Kitchen upon the symptomatology of mild infections contracted accidentally in the laboratory by those engaged in the study of this disease. At the time of writing their paper, in 1931, there had occurred thirty-two accidental infections with yellow fever in laboratories, varying in severity between extreme mildness and a fatal termination. The authors studied very thoroughly seven of the infections of mild type, the diagnosis being established by the transfer of the virus to monkeys and to mice by inoculation of the blood of the patients, and by the demonstration of protective antibodies in the blood of the patients after their recovery. Had it not been for these laboratory methods of diagnosis it would have been impossible to have diagnosed most of these cases, so far as the symptomatology of the infections was concerned.

In their report upon the clinical features of these mild infections they say:

"In the mode of onset the light attacks corresponded with classical descriptions. Yet of the signs of the disease commonly recognized as cardinal, i.e., paradoxical pulse-temperature relationship, jaundice, albuminuria and 'black vomit,' only the first was regularly observed, while the others were absent or present in minimal form." From this quotation it is evident that the diagnosis of such mild infections from the clinical symptoms alone would be impossible and thus the diagnosis must depend upon the laboratory methods that have been mentioned.

Diagnosis.—The diagnosis of yellow fever during the early stage of the disease is very difficult and even impossible, in many instances, especially in the milder types of the infection. Yet it is at this time that the diagnosis is most important, not only from the standpoint of the welfare of the patient, but because it is during the first three or four days of the symptomatic infection that it is transmissible to mosquitoes and hence capable of initiating an epidemic. If an epidemic is already present, any febrile condition having a sudden onset, accompanied by marked prostration, nausea or vomiting, epigastric tenderness and pain, a rapid pulse, congestion of the mucous membranes and albuminuria, appearing after the first twenty-four to thirty-six hours, should be regarded as yellow fever and precautions taken accordingly. Later in the disease the occurrence of Faget's sign, marked albuminuria, hemorrhages, the vomiting of blood, and jaundice, make the clinical diagnosis comparatively easy. Of special significance is the daily increase in the amount of albumin in the urine and the slowing of the pulse after the secondary rise in temperature, symptoms practically peculiar to this disease after the first three or four days from the onset.

In the mildest attacks of yellow fever it is impossible to make a diagnosis from the symptoms and signs alone, and one must depend upon laboratory tests for this purpose.

The daily testing of the urine for albumin is most important in diagnosis. If tested upon the first day after the onset no albumin will be found, but thereafter each day will show an increase in the amount until by the seventh day, in severe cases, it will fill half of the test tube or even more. This daily increase in the amount of albumin in the urine is almost diagnostic of yellow fever when accompanied by other suspicious symptoms or during an epidemic of the disease.

The *leukocyte count* in yellow fever is of some importance in the diagnosis, as there is a considerable decrease in the number of leukocytes, instead of an increase, as in most febrile infections. This decrease, along with albuminuria, is very suggestive in the presence of an epidemic and is practically diagnostic.

LABORATORY METHODS OF DIAGNOSIS.—The *intracerebral inoculation* of mice with the patient's blood during the first three days of the disease will enable one to make a diagnosis of yellow fever. For this purpose the blood should be collected from a vein in the arm *during the first three days* after the onset of symptoms, and 0.03 cc. of the separated serum should be injected intracerebrally into each of six mice and these animals observed for a period of two weeks. If any of them develop symptoms of encephalitis, subinoculations should be made into normal mice and these sent to a yellow fever laboratory for further study and experiment. The development of an encephalitis in any of the inoculated mice should be considered as positive evidence of yellow fever; but as this test cannot usually be completed until after the patient has either recovered or died, it is of value as a corroborative test rather than as a primary diagnostic one.

The employment of the *mouse protection test* is of the utmost value in determining whether a given case was one of yellow fever or of some other infection or disease. About 25 to 30 cc. of blood should be taken from a vein in the patient's arm during the first three days after the onset of the disease and again in three or four weeks after the onset, and sent to a yellow fever laboratory for study. If the blood is from a patient suffering from yellow fever the injection of it into mice previously inoculated with the virus will give the following results: The blood taken during the first three days will not protect the animals who will develop yellow fever, as no antibodies are present during this early period of the disease, but the blood taken three or four weeks after the onset will protect the mice, as antibodies will be present if the patient suffered from the disease.

In handling blood from yellow fever patients it must be remembered that the virus is present in the blood during the first three or four days and the blood is very infective. The utmost care must be exercised that none of it comes in contact with the skin as infection may result and many laboratory infections have been contracted in this manner, in all probability.

In addition to the mouse protection test the *microscopic examination of liver tissue* removed by means of the viscerotome is a most useful method of diagnosing the disease in fatal cases. The viscerotome is an instrument devised to remove a small section of liver by plunging it into that organ, thus avoiding the necessity of an autopsy. By means of this instrument it was shown that fatal cases of yellow fever were occurring in many localities in Brazil where the disease was unsuspected. The

40102

tissue removed by the viscerotome is sent to a yellow fever laboratory and examined for the characteristic pathology of yellow fever as shown in the liver. In Brazil all patients dying of a febrile infection are thus examined.

By means of the viscerotome examination, which demonstrates, if positive, the presence of the disease at the time of the examination, and of the mouse protection test, which demonstrates past infection with yellow fever, it is possible to survey accurately any locality and ascertain whether yellow fever is, or has been, present.

DIFFERENTIAL DIAGNOSIS.—Almost any acute febrile disease may simulate yellow fever during the first day or two after onset and at this time an accurate differential diagnosis is usually impossible without the aid of laboratory procedures. Of the diseases that are most apt to be mistaken for yellow fever later in the course of this infection may be mentioned dengue fever, influenza, the eruptive fevers, the malarial fevers, typhoid fever, and infectious jaundice, or Weil's disease.

Dengue Fever.—Perhaps no disease has been so frequently confused with yellow fever as has dengue fever and, in fact, the first cases of yellow fever occurring in a community have almost invariably been diagnosed as dengue fever. The acute onset, the congested appearance of the face, the severe neuralgic pains in the back and legs, and the general prostration of dengue fever all simulate the early symptoms of yellow fever, but after the first three days the absence of albuminuria, hemorrhages, jaundice and Faget's sign in dengue distinguishes it from yellow fever. The absence of fatal cases during an epidemic of dengue fever is also of the greatest importance in the differential diagnosis, for death is seldom, if ever, caused by dengue, whereas there are always fatal cases of yellow fever during any epidemic of the latter infection. As a matter of fact the diagnosis of yellow fever cases as dengue during the early part of an epidemic is usually made as a protective gesture by the health authorities, rather than because there is any real confusion between the two infections. The local health authorities are always loath to admit the presence of yellow fever in a locality because of the quarantine measures that must be adopted if this disease is known to be present in a community.

Influenza.—One would hardly believe that influenza and yellow fever could be confused but it is true that mild cases of yellow fever have been repeatedly diagnosed as cases of influenza, especially in the presence of an epidemic of the latter disease. It is noted by Berry and Kitchen (*loc cit.*) that the mild cases of yellow fever contracted in the laboratory and studied by them were diagnosed by local physicians as influenza. As catarrhal symptoms are very rarely encountered in yellow fever it is probable that this mistake in diagnosis was not made upon the character of the symptoms present but because influenza was present at the time in epidemic form, and at such times physicians are very apt to diagnose any febrile condition as influenza. The absence of catarrhal symptoms, of albuminuria and jaundice, as well as of Faget's sign and hemorrhages in influenza, should suffice to make such a mistake in diagnosis impossible in all but the mildest cases of yellow fever and even in such cases the absence of catarrhal symptoms should obviate such an error.

It should be remembered, however, that influenza is not invariably accompanied by catarrhal symptoms, especially in the tropics and subtropics, and this may lead to confusion in the differential diagnosis. The same statement is true of the so-called "intestinal flu," but diarrhea, which is a prominent symptom of this type of influenza, is not usually present in the early stage of yellow fever.

The Eruptive Fevers.—Of the eruptive fevers, scarlet fever, measles and smallpox are most apt to cause confusion in the diagnosis of yellow fever during the first days of that infection. In *scarlet fever* the sore throat serves to differentiate the two conditions as an angina does not occur in yellow fever. The catarrhal symptoms of *measles,* together with the presence of Koplik's spots, should serve to differentiate it, while in *smallpox* there is no remission of the fever before the occurrence of the eruption and jaundice is absent. In all of these infections the appearance of the characteristic eruption serves to differentiate them from yellow fever, and mistakes in diagnosis could occur only before the eruptions appear and then are almost inexcusable.

Malaria.—In most regions where yellow fever is endemic and in regions where epidemics may occur, the malarial fevers are endemic and may cause confusion in diagnosis. The onset of tertian and quartan malaria may simulate that of yellow fever, but the absence of albuminuria and jaundice during the first few days is characteristic of these types of malaria. If albuminuria should occur it is slight in amount and later in developing than in yellow fever. In some attacks of malaria, caused by the estivo-autumnal plasmodium, *Plasmodium falciparum,* albuminuria may develop early and slight jaundice may be present, and in such cases it may be difficult to make a differential diagnosis. The absence of Faget's sign, of hemorrhages and the vomiting of blood, and of jaundice usually serves to distinguish such cases of malaria from yellow fever. The quick response of malaria to quinine, and if this drug has not been administered, the demonstration of the malaria plasmodia in the blood, should enable one to make a differential diagnosis with little difficulty. Combined infections with yellow fever and malaria may rarely occur and render the diagnosis most difficult.

In some malarial infections jaundice may be present but in such cases the enlargement of the liver and spleen should assist in clarifying the diagnosis. In hemoglobinuric, or blackwater, fever, albuminuria may be intense and hemoglobinuria is present, but if the urine is bloody in yellow fever the condition is one of hematuria and this is rare. The blood count in malaria does not exhibit the leukopenia present in yellow fever and pigment is absent from the blood in the latter disease.

Typhoid Fever.—It would be impossible to confuse yellow fever and typhoid fever except during the first week of the latter disease, during which time the symptomatology may sometimes be similar; but in typhoid during this time albuminuria is absent, hemorrhage, if it occurs, is from the nose and the gums do not bleed, a leukocytosis is present and Faget's sign is absent. In addition, the rose spots of typhoid, the absence of jaundice and the enlargement of the spleen should serve as additional evidences of the typhoidal nature of the infection. The onset of typhoid is much more gradual than that of yellow fever and if blood cultures are made early, the typhoid bacillus can usually be demonstrated. Later, after the first week or ten days, a positive Widal reaction will be present in typhoid while the diazo reaction will also be positive if typhoid is present.

40102

Weil's Disease.—The disease which most closely resembles yellow fever in its symptomatology is infectious jaundice, or Weil's disease, and the differential diagnosis is often very difficult. The experience of Noguchi, in Guayaquil, where he discovered the spirochete which he believed to be the cause of yellow fever, is an excellent illustration of the truth of this statement. The patients he studied were diagnosed by physicians expert in the recognition of yellow fever, but, despite this fact, several cases of Weil's disease were certified by them as cases of yellow fever and it was in the blood of these patients that Noguchi found the spirochete which in reality was *Leptospira icterohaemorrhagiae,* the cause of the latter disease.

In Weil's disease the sudden onset, intense congestion of the face and mucous membranes, and the severe muscular pain and prostration are almost identical with the onset and early symptomatology of yellow fever; but, while albuminuria and jaundice are present, they do not appear as early as in yellow fever, and the jaundice of Weil's disease, in well-marked cases, is more severe and of a darker color than in the average case of yellow fever. Hemorrhages may occur into the skin and conjunctivae in both infections but hemorrhages from other sites are rarely observed in Weil's disease although in very severe cases of the latter disease the vomitus may be bloodstained and resemble the "black vomit" of yellow fever. Jaundice occurs in from 50 to 60 per cent of cases of Weil's disease but is absent in the mild cases. The fever in Weil's disease does not remit upon the third or fourth day as in yellow fever, but usually persists for two to three weeks. Faget's sign is not present in Weil's disease and there is a leukocytosis instead of a leukopenia with an increase in the neutrophilic leukocytes and a shift to the left in the Arneth index. The spleen and lymphatic glands are enlarged in Weil's disease but not in yellow fever.

Very mild cases of Weil's disease, terminating in from three to five days, cannot be distinguished from yellow fever save by the use of laboratory methods of diagnosis. The method found most useful is the intraperitoneal injection of 5 to 6 cc. of the patient's blood into guinea pigs. If the disease present is yellow fever the guinea pigs will show no symptoms, but if it is Weil's disease a fatal infection will result accompanied by jaundice, albuminuria, hemorrhages in the viscera, and *Leptospira icterohaemorrhagiae* may be demonstrated in the infected animal. After the twelfth day of the disease catheterized urine may be employed for the injections instead of the blood. The direct examination of the blood for the spirochete is usually unsuccessful, but centrifugalization of the blood and the examination of properly prepared specimens of the plasma often results in the demonstration of the spirochete.

The microscopic examination of centrifugalized specimens of urine for *Leptospira icterohaemorrhagiae* is an excellent method of diagnosis but does not usually give positive results until after the tenth or twelfth day of the disease. It is also possible to obtain cultures of the spirochete upon blood agar. Martin, Pettit and Vaudremer have developed an agglutination test, using cultures, and agglutination occurs in titers of from 1 : 500 to as high as 1 : 30,000, the agglutinins appearing in the patient's blood about the tenth or twelfth day after the occurrence of symptoms, and persisting for months or years. Other serologic methods of diagnosis are the use of formalized cultures, as suggested by Schüffner, and the adhesion test of Brown and Davis, which consists in bringing the blood serum of the patient into contact with the spirochetes in the presence of an indicator, as blood platelets, to which the spirochetes adhere, if the patient's blood serum is positive.

An immunity test has been developed for the diagnosis of Weil's disease which is applicable after the second week of the disease. It consists in mixing about 1 cc. of the patient's blood serum with several lethal doses of *Leptospira icterohaemorrhagiae* and injecting the mixture into guinea pigs after it has been allowed to stand for fifteen minutes. If the patient's blood serum contains immune bodies the injected guinea pigs will remain well whereas controls will die. This is an excellent test and is specific for this spirochete.

Other conditions that may possibly be confused with yellow fever are *acute yellow atrophy of the liver, catarrhal jaundice,* and various forms of *endemic jaundice* observed in different localities. Attention to the symptomatology of these conditions and the utilization of the various laboratory methods which are available should serve to distinguish them from yellow fever.

Complications.—Because of its short duration, yellow fever is not apt to be complicated by other infections or diseases, although in endemic regions *malaria* is frequently a complication. In alcoholics, kidney complications may arise and either *parenchymatous* or *interstitial nephritis* may occur, and in such cases a fatal result sometimes occurs from uremia. *Pulmonary complications* are rarely observed. *Cardiac complications,* usually due to secondary infection, are not common; but in patient's suffering from *cardiac disease,* yellow fever is very frequently fatal, and even in patients free from such disease there is always danger of sudden failure of the heart during the course of the infection and during convalescence.

Sequelae.—Considering the severity of yellow fever in many patients, the sequelae which have been recorded are remarkably few in number. Perhaps the most frequently observed is *parotitis,* confined to one parotid gland, and evidenced by fever, swelling of the gland, and usually subsiding without suppuration. This sequela generally occurs during convalescence and in rare instances an *abscess* of the gland may develop. *Abscesses of the skin, small boils,* and a more or less *chronic diarrhea* may also occur as sequelae. The entire intestinal tract is usually very sensitive after an attack of yellow fever and great care is necessary to prevent sequelae connected with this tract.

Because of the profound effect of the yellow fever virus upon the heart, one would expect that sequelae connected with this organ would be frequently observed but, as a matter of fact, such sequelae are exceedingly rare. A *chronic form of myocarditis* has been reported as following yellow fever, and the writer has personal knowledge of a fatal case of chronic myocarditis following an unusually severe attack of yellow fever.

Treatment.—At the present time we do not possess any specific for the treatment of yellow fever and the most that one can do is to treat the symptoms as they arise. Immune serum is of no value in treatment after the occurrence of symptoms but it would undoubtedly modify their severity if it were possible to administer it during the incubation stage of the disease. The earlier the infection is diagnosed, the better the prognosis under proper symptomatic treatment.

40102

Complete rest in bed and **careful nursing** are the most essential parts of the treatment of this disease. A yellow fever patient should never be moved after the first twenty-four hours following the appearance of the symptoms and many patients have been killed by unnecessary trips in ambulances. While treatment in a hospital is preferable to home treatment, removal to the hospital after the second day of the disease is not to be recommended, if home care can be provided. The excitement attendant upon such a move is always detrimental to the patient and may prove fatal in severe infections. In moving yellow fever patients from the home to the hospital the utmost care should be taken to prevent possible infection of mosquitoes and this may be accomplished by the use of a mosquito bar placed over the patient during removal. After removal from the home, the house should be promptly fumigated to destroy any mosquitoes that may have bitten the patient and become infected.

Whether the patient be treated at home or in a hospital, the room in which he is being treated should be well ventilated and thoroughly screened, the windows and doors being protected by wire mosquito netting containing 18 meshes to the linear inch. If, for any reason, it is impossible thus to screen the room, a mosquito bed net should be used.

Yellow fever is a disease that demands the most careful nursing and a trained nurse should always be employed, if possible. The regular and careful taking of the temperature, the pulse, and the careful recording of the symptoms as they appear are of the greatest value to the physician in the treatment of this infection, and the nursing of yellow fever patients should never be left to ignorant or careless individuals. As the prompt and intelligent treatment of symptoms means so much in the favorable prognosis of this infection, it follows that the care which can only be afforded by a trained nurse is essential in the management of this disease.

If constipation is present at the beginning of the disease it should be relieved by a mild purgative. The choice of such a purgative may be left to the physician but, in view of the irritated condition of the intestinal tract, especially of the stomach, which is usually present, as evidenced by nausea and epigastric discomfort or pain, one should be selected that is as little irritating as is possible. Many authorities recommend calomel in minute doses, followed by a mild mineral water, but if there are marked symptoms of gastric irritation it is preferable to give an enema to clean out the lower bowel. It is undoubtedly best to abstain from all internal medication during the first three days of the disease, if possible, for the more quiet the patient is kept during this time, the better is the prognosis.

During the first three days of the disease **no food** should be allowed; if the symptoms are very severe, no food should be allowed during the first four days. The patient's blood sugar should be carefully watched and carbohydrates should be supplied by the intravenous injection of glucose. Rectal feeding may have to be employed in rare instances. If vomiting is severe and precludes the administration of fluids by mouth, the intravenous injection of glucose and normal saline by hypodermoclysis may be employed and water may be given per rectum. Acidosis, which is always present to some degree in yellow fever, should be combated by small, frequent draughts of an alkaline water, as Vichy, or bicarbonate of soda may be added to tap water. The administration of lemonade or diluted orange or grapefruit juices is often beneficial, helps to control the thirst and to reduce the acidosis. The chances of hemorrhage from the stomach (black vomit) occurring are very markedly reduced by depriving the patient of all food during the first three days of the disease. After this period, if the stomach is not too irritable and the fever is not above 39° C. (102.2° F.), food may be cautiously given, beginning with rice water, chicken soup, gelatin, ice cream and soft gruels. Milk is not usually well borne by the yellow fever patient and it must be administered in small amounts mixed with limewater or an alkaline mineral water. Later, when the stomach is less irritable, milk may be given in larger amounts, as it is a most valuable food, and a return to a more liberal diet is usually possible after the tenth day from the commencement of the symptoms. One should always remember that most serious results and even death have followed too liberal feeding during the convalescence from yellow fever.

Nausea and vomiting are most distressing symptoms in many patients suffering from yellow fever. Usually the abstention from food will control these symptoms, but, if not, sinapisms, the sucking of ice, the sipping of champagne or ginger ale, and the application of an ice bag over the epigastrium may be sufficient. If necessary, small doses of cocaine may be administered but **morphine should never be employed. Atropine** or **tincture of belladonna** is useful in controlling the gastrointestinal symptoms. Care must be taken that the amount of fluid ingested is not sufficient to further irritate the stomach.

If the vomitus is bloodstained or "black vomit" occurs, the administration of **tincture of chloride of iron,** as recommended by Agramonte, is useful, 5 drops of the tincture being given every two or three hours in a small amount of lime juice and glycerin. Hypodermic injections of adrenalin may be administered if the hemorrhage is severe but are seldom needed and are really of doubtful value. Bleeding from the gums may be controlled by local astringents and the mouth should be frequently rinsed out with a mild antiseptic solution, such as **Dobell's solution.**

In the presence of "black vomit" all attempts to supply nourishment by mouth should be suspended and **rectal feeding** at once instituted, together with the administration of **glucose intravenously.** A useful formula for rectal feeding is that recommended by Agramonte, as follows:

Milk .... 90 cc. (3 ounces)
Whisky .... 15 cc. (½ ounce)
Normal salt solution .... 90 cc. (3 ounces)

A cleansing enema should be given and then this mixture injected into the rectum very slowly and retained.

Guanidine intoxication may occur in yellow fever, due to the destruction of the liver tissue, and this is best treated by the administration of calcium. If the drug is given by mouth, **calcium lactate** in doses of 5 Gm. (75 grains) daily is preferable, but if oral administration is impossible **calcium gluconate** in a saturated solution (7.5 per cent) should be injected intramuscularly, in 10 cc. amounts. Calcium should not be administered intravenously in any form.

It may be necessary to administer morphine to control very severe vomiting, but this drug should never be used unless absolutely necessary, and if the kidneys are seriously involved it should not be employed at all.

40102

Fever seldom requires special treatment as it is rarely excessive in yellow fever and does not last for long periods of time, as in typhoid infection. Hyperpyrexia does rarely occur and should be controlled by cold sponging. If the temperature rises above 39.5° C. (103.1° F.) it should be lowered by sponging with water of a temperature not lower than 21° C. (69.8° F.). If the temperature remains elevated, water at temperatures of 16 to 10° C. (60.8 to 50° F.) should be employed in sponging. Under no circumstances should the patient be subjected to a tub bath for lowering the temperature, and sponging should not be repeated oftener than every four hours. Antipyretic drugs are dangerous in yellow fever owing to the weakened heart muscle caused by the yellow fever toxin, but in case sponging is contraindicated a mixture of acetyl-salicylic acid and caffeine is the least dangerous of the antipyretics.

The condition of the *kidneys* is most important in yellow fever and most authorities agree that failure of these organs and the occurrence of *anuria* is almost invariably followed by death. The possible occurrence of anuria, as evidenced by a diminished excretion of urine, should be carefully guarded against by the use of **warm mustard baths** and, according to Carroll, by the administration of **urea** hypodermically, doses as large as 1 Gm. (15 grains) being allowable.

It should be remembered that the amount of albumin present in the urine is not a true guide as to the real condition of the kidneys, for many patients showing a large amount of albumin and many casts in their urine recover, while others showing a small amount of albumin and few casts may die from anuria. Rectal enemas of cold normal saline solution are useful if the quantity of the urine lessens and fluids cannot be administered by mouth, as such enemas increase the secretion of urine and may also lower the temperature. One to two pints of normal saline should be given rectally and retained, the injection being made very slowly.

For *cardiac weakness* stimulation should be secured by the hypodermic injection of **strychnine** or **digitalin,** and Agramonte regarded the latter drug as especially useful as it also increases the amount of urine secreted, although he warned against the use of digitalin for the latter purpose alone. Alcohol is a useful stimulant but, owing to the irritability of the stomach, it can seldom be employed unless by rectal injection. The condition of the patient, as regards the irritability of the digestive tract, should always govern the administration of alcoholics and of these, iced champagne will be found least irritating and most useful. Sudden heart failure should be treated by injections of **adrenalin** or **camphor.** If renal complications are present alcohol, in any form, is contraindicated.

During the early stage of yellow fever the use of **external applications** of various kinds will alleviate some of the unpleasant symptoms. An ice bag to the head or ice compresses upon the forehead will often help the headache and are preferable to the use of any drug for this purpose. Warm applications to the lumbar region will relieve the lumbar pain which is often severe, while gentle rubbing of the muscles with an oily lotion helps to alleviate muscle ache, provided the patient is not too much disturbed by the massage.

TREATMENT OF CONVALESCENCE.—Convalescence after an attack of yellow fever is usually rapid and uneventful, but in those having very severe attacks or who are suffering from other disease conditions, convalescence may be prolonged and, according to some observers, relapse may occur. **Good nursing** is almost as important during convalescence as in the acute stage of the disease. **Absolute rest in bed** should be insisted upon for several days and the patient should not be allowed to wait upon himself or to leave his bed under any circumstances until convalescence is well advanced. A bed pan should be used and the patient should not be allowed to assume an upright position in bed or to use a commode during the early period of convalescence.

Diet during convalescence is very important, for too liberal a diet or the feeding of indigestible foods may result in a relapse or the appearance of serious symptoms, and many deaths have occurred from overfeeding during the convalescence of the patient. If the stomach has been very irritable during the acute attack, a liquid diet should be persisted in for the first week, at least, of convalescence, and extreme caution should be exercised in the institution of a semifluid or solid diet in such cases. In convalescence from severe attacks no meats or solids should be fed until toward the end of the second week and then with care. If the patient has suffered from a light attack, a semifluid or solid diet may be given during the latter portion of the first week of convalescence, but even in such cases it will frequently be found that the stomach does not digest well and the appearance of the slightest distress after eating should be a signal to return to a fluid or semifluid diet, consisting of milk, junket, gelatin, soft puddings, meat broth, eggs and cream.

The *condition of the kidneys* should be watched closely and, if albumin continues to appear in the urine in considerable quantities, milk and gruels should constitute the diet; but if the albumin steadily diminishes in amount, a more liberal diet may be allowed, the urine being tested daily in order to estimate the condition of the kidneys.

Jaundice sometimes becomes more marked during convalescence than during the acute stage of yellow fever and sometimes persists for several weeks after the patient has entirely recovered. This simply indicates that the damage to the liver tissue by the yellow fever toxin has been considerable and is being slowly repaired. The occurrence of this symptom does not call for treatment of any kind.

If *complicating conditions* are present during convalescence they should be properly treated. The use of tonics is beneficial together with the administration of the vitamins.

RELAPSES IN YELLOW FEVER.—A rise in temperature followed by two or three days of fever, after what has appeared to be the terminal fall in the temperature, sometimes occurs, and some authorities have improperly called such exacerbations of the fever a relapse. True relapses, occurring from a week or two or more weeks after convalescence has been established, are reported by some observers, but are undoubtedly very rare in yellow fever. They have been observed following excesses in food or drink or after improper physical exertion. The symptomatology of these relapses is atypical and most recent students of this disease appear to doubt that relapse really occurs in yellow fever, regarding the cases described as relapses as disturbances in digestion and irritability of the intestinal tract. The entire subject of relapse in yellow fever requires more careful study before one can make a definite statement as regards their occurrence or their number. The fact that so strong an immunity follows an attack of this disease and is so rapidly acquired, negatives the idea that relapses are very frequent and casts great doubt upon their occurrence, unless in very mild infections in which immunity may be weaker and more slowly acquired.

Prophylaxis.—The prevention of yellow fever depends upon the elimination of the insects, especially *Aedes aegypti*, transmitting the virus causing the disease, and upon protective vaccination of exposed individuals. For convenience of description the subject may be divided into *personal* and *general* prophylaxis.

PERSONAL PROPHYLAXIS.—The most important personal prophylactic measure against yellow fever is **vaccination** with a living yellow fever virus, and all individuals who are liable to exposure should be vaccinated. At the present time the most valuable vaccine employed in prevention is that prepared from the virus known as 17 D, a modified strain of the yellow fever virus cultivated upon the chicken embryo media for several generations until the viscerotropic and neurotropic properties are markedly reduced. This vaccine is prepared in the laboratories of the Rockefeller Foundation, New York City, and cannot be obtained commercially but only through government and research institutions, i.e., the Rockefeller Institute or the Hygienic Laboratory of the Public Health Service of the United States. During 1939, 581,-513 persons in Brazil were vaccinated with this vaccine, while to date (1940) over two million persons have been vaccinated without any serious complications and with most excellent results.

Sawyer (1939) states that the strain of the yellow fever virus used in the vaccine can be maintained indefinitely in tissue cultures but that before use it is passed through a single passage in living chick embryo within the egg, which increases the virus content of the vaccine. According to Sawyer, the method of preparing the vaccine is as follows: The ground-up embryo is suspended in normal human serum, centrifuged to remove particles, passed through a Seitz filter and dried in the frozen state in ampules which afterward are sealed with a blast lamp. Each lot is tested for sterility, virulence, quantity of virus and also for neurotropic properties by intracerebral inoculation of a Rhesus monkey.

The *dose of the vaccine* is from 0.5 to 1 cc. of the rehydrated vaccine, administered subcutaneously at the insertion of the deltoid muscle of either arm. No reaction follows at the site of inoculation, but a rise in temperature, accompanied by headache and aching in the muscles, is frequently observed from the sixth to the seventh day following vaccination. Protective bodies appear in the vaccinated individual's blood between the seventh and the twenty-first day following vaccination. At the present time we do not know how long protection afforded by this vaccine may last but we do have evidence that it may last for several years.

The possibility of introducing yellow fever into countries free from this disease by means of vaccinated individuals has been feared by some, as the virus employed in vaccination is a living one, and theoretically might be presumed to multiply to such an extent in the vaccinated individual's blood as to enable him to infect susceptible mosquitoes or other insects, should they bite such individuals shortly after they were vaccinated. The experience of the French, who have employed a living virus vaccine for some years, negatives such a fear, and the Rockefeller Foundation believes that such a risk can be ignored so far as the vaccine developed by the Rockefeller Institute is concerned.

Experimentally, it has been found that it is impossible to tranfer the virus from vaccinated individuals to monkeys through the bite of *Aedes aegypti* which has fed upon a vaccinated person; however, the Rockefeller Foundation recommends that the living virus should not be employed as a vaccine in yellow fever-free localities without the consent of the national or local health authorities.

If it is impossible for an individual to be vaccinated certain precautions may be taken which will lessen the chances of infection. Localities that are known to be endemic or epidemic foci of yellow fever should be avoided, if possible, but if one is forced to live in, or visit, such localities, the use of gloves, head nets and boots, during the day, and sleeping in a screened room or beneath a bed net at night, are efficient methods for the prevention of possible infection by the bites of transmitting mosquitoes. If one is nursing or coming in contact with yellow fever patients it should be remembered that the blood during the first three or four days of the disease contains the virus and that infection is possible if such blood comes in contact with the skin of an uninfected person. In some patients hemorrhages from the nose or gums may occur during this period and such blood is infectious; precautions should be taken that it does not come in contact with either the broken or unbroken skin of non-immune individuals. As already stated, most of the laboratory infections with this disease have apparently been contracted in this way and its possible importance is not fully realized by many authorities in discussing the prevention of this disease.

GENERAL PROPHYLAXIS.—The general prophylaxis of yellow fever consists in the protection of communities from the mosquitoes transmitting the infection, from individuals already infected and in either the incubation or acute stages of the disease, and the institution of general vaccination against the infection.

Before considering the general prophylaxis of yellow fever from the standpoint of protection from the transmitting mosquitoes, it is essential that one have a good general knowledge of the biology of *Aedes aegypti*, the mosquito most often concerned in transmission. This mosquito may be easily recognized by the presence upon the thorax, just in front of the insertion of the wings, of white lines formed by scales, arranged in the form of a lyre, the foot of the instrument being toward the head of the insect. In addition, the short palpi of the female have a white termination and the legs present white bands, marking the bases of the tarsi.

Aedes aegypti is a domestic mosquito breeding in water contained in cisterns, clogged gutters, rain barrels, fountains, unused toilet basins, water closet tanks, tin cans and, in fact, in any collection of water available around the habitations of man. The eggs are laid in such water and the period necessary for the entire development of this mosquito from the egg to the adult insect is approximately from ten to twelve days under the most favorable circumstances. Only the females bite man and infected mosquitoes remain so during their lifetime, the length of which in nature is unknown, but in captivity infected mosquitoes have lived for as long as 200 days.

40102

Aedes aegypti is a house mosquito and it seldom flies far from human habitations. It may be carried by winds for long distances, but its natural flight is limited and it prefers to remain close to its birthplace if blood meals are obtainable.

In the general prophylaxis of yellow fever two measures relating to the mosquitoes transmitting the infections must be considered, i.e., the *destruction of the mosquito,* either in the larval or adult stage of development, and the *protection of man from the bites* of the infective mosquitoes. Theoretically, either of these measures should prevent infection, but it is usually necessary to combine the two in practice.

Destruction of the Transmitting Mosquito.—The destruction of the usual transmitting insect, *Aedes aegypti,* is comparatively easy and is most effectively accomplished by the prevention of the breeding of this insect. It has been already noted that this mosquito breeds in any collection of water near human habitations and breeding may be prevented by getting rid of such collections of water. All receptacles that harbor water and which are not needed for domestic or other purposes should be destroyed. Those that must be retained should be screened with wire copper netting containing 18 meshes to the linear inch. If screening is not possible, such water receptacles should be emptied at least once a week, thus preventing the development of the adult mosquito. Unused hoppers of toilets and water traps should be thoroughly flushed once a week and all gutters and drains should be carefully inspected at weekly intervals to see that they are not clogged. Suitable collections of water that cannot be otherwise dealt with should be oiled at intervals of eight to ten days.

In many localities water buckets are kept outside barracks, houses and other buildings for use in case of fire and, unless these are properly cared for, they will serve as prolific breeding places for mosquitoes. All that is necessary to prevent the development of mosquito larvae in such buckets is to empty them once a week, being careful to see that they are not emptied into a sewer or stream but upon the ground in bright sunlight, where the water will quickly evaporate and the sun will kill the larvae or pupae, if present. Care should be taken to see that no larvae or pupae are present in the buckets before they are refilled. If desired, wire cover screens may be used to cover these buckets, but such covers are expensive and unnecessary. One frequently observes that the water in fire buckets is kept oiled, but this practice is a foolish one and is simply an evidence of unfamiliarity with the life cycle of *Aedes aegypti* by the one ordering such a procedure.

Water troughs for domestic animals should be frequently flushed and in no case should water be allowed to remain within such troughs if not in use. The tanks in water closets, sewer traps and open cesspools should be frequently inspected and properly treated, the tanks and sewer traps by either weekly flushing or oiling and the cesspools by oiling at intervals of two weeks.

Fountains and other artificial collections of water made for beautifying the grounds surrounding habitations or other buildings should be drained and kept dry if yellow fever is present in a locality. At other times such collections of water should be stocked with some species of fish known to feed upon mosquito larvae. The fish that are most useful in this respect are the roach, carp, top minnows, and goldfish, the roach and top minnows being especially active in this respect.

The most effective method of accomplishing the abolition of the breeding places of *Aedes aegypti* in any locality is to place the work under the charge of a trained sanitary or health officer, who should be assisted by the requisite number of trained inspectors. The locality to be inspected should be divided into districts, varying in number with the size of the village, town or city in which yellow fever is occurring. Daily inspections should be made of all premises in each district by the inspector assigned to that particular district and all possible breeding places of the mosquito discovered and eliminated. It is not safe, during a yellow fever epidemic, to leave the inspection of premises to the owners, as they are usually ignorant of the biology of mosquitoes and cannot recognize their breeding places.

The *destruction of adult mosquitoes* may be accomplished by the use of various chemicals, employed in fumigation, and by catching the insects by hand in houses or in properly constructed traps.

A large number of *chemicals* have been recommended for the destruction of mosquitoes but the most generally useful are pyrethrum powder and sulfur dioxide. The burning of **pyrethrum powder,** commonly known as Persian or Dalmatian insect powder, is useful when it is impossible to screen habitations or when one is exposed to mosquitoes while occupying unscreened rooms. This powder is made from the dried flower heads of plants belonging to the genus *Chrysanthemum* and should be as freshly prepared as is possible.

For the purpose of destroying mosquitoes the powder is burned in the unoccupied or occupied room, being placed upon a tin or dish and a lighted match touched to it. The powder burns slowly and gives off a large volume of smoke having a peculiar, but not disagreeable, odor, or it may be obtained in the form of solid cones or pastilles and these may be burned. The smoke is not harmful to persons or the contents of rooms, and if the rooms be closed the smoke will stupefy all mosquitoes within them and they may then be swept up from the floor and destroyed. While the burning of pyrethrum powder is of service in protecting one from mosquitoes under the conditions mentioned, it is really of limited value and should not be relied upon for protection if better methods are available.

Sulfur dioxide is employed for the fumigation of rooms or buildings and will kill all adult mosquitoes that may be present. This gas was employed for this purpose in Havana, Panama and Rio de Janeiro with marked success during yellow fever epidemics, and entire blocks of buildings may be fumigated at one operation, as was done in Havana by United States Army authorities.

In employing sulfur dioxide it must be remembered that it injures most metallic substances and some fabrics and these should be removed from the rooms to be fumigated. All windows and doors should be closed and porches should be enclosed by canvas or sailcloth; paper should be pasted over all cracks which will admit air and around the exterior and interior doors and windows. The building should be divided into parts for fumigation and the necessary amount of sulfur burned in each part. Closets, clothes presses, bureau drawers and trunks should be opened before fumigation is begun in order that any mosquitoes within them may be exposed to the gas. In poorly constructed buildings which it is

40102

impossible to make airtight, the entire building should be covered with canvas or sailcloth in order to fumigate it properly.

The powdered sulfur is placed in iron pans which, in turn, should be placed in large receptacles containing water, in order to avoid the danger of fire, as the sulfur sputters in burning and the water is intended to catch the burning particles and extinguish them. The amount of sulfur to be employed in fumigation can be ascertained by dividing the number of cubic feet in the rooms to be fumigated by 500, and reading the result in pounds or fractions of pounds of sulfur.

Hydrocyanic acid gas is largely used for the fumigation of ships coming from ports where yellow fever may be present and for large-scale fumigation of buildings in localities where the disease may be occurring. This gas is more efficient than is sulfur dioxide when properly employed but its extremely toxic nature renders it unsuitable for use except by skilled operatives. As is well known, hydrocyanic acid gas is almost instantly fatal to man when inhaled and fatal accidents have repeatedly occurred during its use as a fumigant. Consequently, the greatest precautions should be taken while using it and a gas mask should be worn in the fumigation of ships or buildings with this agent. The same methods are used to render the premises airtight as in fumigation with sulfur dioxide and a generating apparatus may be employed carrying the gas through a rubber hose to the room to be fumigated; or if entire buildings or compartments of ships are to be fumigated the gas is generated by placing the requisite amount of sulfuric acid in a wooden, earthenware or lead-lined receptacle and adding to it the proper quantity of potassium cyanide which should be wrapped in paper, in order to give the operator time to leave the compartment or building before any gas is generated. Ten to 15 Gm. of potassium cyanide are required for each 1,000 cubic feet of space to be fumigated. The gas should be allowed to act for three to four hours, after which the building, rooms or compartments are opened from the outside and not entered until sufficient time has elapsed for thorough ventilation and the removal of the gas by such ventilation. This method of fumigation must be performed by experts in handling this dangerous gas.

The *adequacy of fumigation* may be tested by placing cages containing mosquitoes in the rooms to be fumigated, and this should be done, if possible, if an epidemic of yellow fever is prevailing.

In the fumigation of ships, either by sulfur dioxide or hydrocyanic acid gas, the gas is usually generated in a boat placed alongside the vessel to be fumigated and led into the holds or compartments of the ship through canvas hose.

Catching adult mosquitoes in rooms is a useful method for the prevention of yellow fever and is especially important in houses in which a case of this disease has originated and where fumigation cannot be efficiently accomplished. In catching mosquitoes the chloroform tube is most generally useful, consisting of a large test tube at the bottom of which rubber parings or a small amount of cotton is placed and saturated with chloroform. When not in use the open end of the tube should be tightly plugged with cotton. When in use the cotton plug is removed, the open end of the tube gently placed over the mosquito as it rests upon a surface, then slightly moved across the surface, when the insect will fly toward the closed end, whereupon the open end is quickly removed from the resting surface and plugged with the cotton. The chloroform quickly stupefies the mosquitoes and they can then be destroyed. In addition to the chloroform tube the mosquito hunter should be provided with an ordinary "fly swatter" and instructed to catch or to "swat" every mosquito observed. *Aedes aegypti* and other mosquitoes should be searched for in the dark corners of rooms, upon the walls or baseboards, under beds, in closets, beneath sinks, behind pictures, behind clothing hanging in closets, beneath toilet fixtures and within mosquito bed nets.

Mosquitoes may also be caught in properly constructed mosquito traps and then destroyed. It must be remembered that in times of epidemics of yellow fever every *Aedes aegypti* mosquito is a potential source for the infection of man and should be destroyed if possible.

The *protection of man from the bites of mosquitoes* is a very important method of prophylaxis and is accomplished by the screening of patients and of human habitations. The prompt screening of patients suffering from yellow fever is most important and any febrile patient should be screened during an epidemic of this disease until the true nature of the fever has been ascertained. If possible, the patient should be kept in a screened room and by this is meant a room in which not only the windows are screened but also the doors. This will prevent the mosquitoes not only from leaving the sickroom through the windows but from invading other portions of the house, should they be present. If it is impossible to screen the sickroom the patient should be kept under a mosquito bed net containing at least 18 meshes to the linear inch. All habitations should be thoroughly screened, employing wire netting of the same number of meshes, and if one is obliged to be outdoors the use of gloves and a head net is indicated if *Aedes* mosquitoes are numerous and an epidemic of yellow fever is present. It should be remembered that *Aedes aegypti* bites in the daytime as well as at night.

The proper methods of screening are discussed in Volume III, under the subject "Malaria," to which the reader is referred.

As already stated, in moving yellow fever patients from home to a hospital care should be taken to avoid possible infection of mosquitoes in transit. This is easily accomplished by covering the patient with a mosquito net raised above the body by means of sticks fastened at the corners of the litter.

Maritime Prophylaxis.—In order to prevent the introduction of yellow fever into ports by vessels coming from an infected port it is necessary to apply well-known rules governing quarantine and fumigation adopted by the public health authorities of the country in which the non-infected port is situated. It is not the province of this contribution to discuss maritime prophylaxis, as space forbids, and, in addition, such prophylactic measures are under the control of the officers of the United States Public Health Service, so far as this country is concerned, who are trained and expert in the application of the necessary measures for the prevention of the introduction of this disease into this country.

Airplane Prophylaxis.—The great increase in air transport and the rapidity of journeys thus performed has rendered the subject of the possible importation into localities of contagious and infectious disease by means of the airplane of great importance. It has been shown by numerous observers that mosquitoes transmitting disease, as malaria and yellow fever, can be easily transported by means of airplanes, and it has

been necessary to take this fact into account in the prevention of yellow
fever. It would be possible for individuals in the incubation stage of
this disease to leave endemic areas in South America and reach the
United States by airplane long before the incubation stage is completed,
while infected *Aedes aegypti* or other mosquitoes could also be thus introduced into this and other countries. At the present time the prevention of the introduction into this country by airplanes is under the
control of the U. S. Public Health Service, and upon the arrival of every
airplane from South America all of the passengers are inspected; an
inspector searches the plane for mosquitoes before it is beached, if a clip-
per, or immediately after landing, if a land plane; while afterward it is
thoroughly fumigated with hydrocyanic acid gas. These measures have
so far proved effective. Passengers are also vaccinated against yellow
fever if they so desire, while the personnel of the airplanes are also
vaccinated.

In addition to the measures already described for the protection of
a community there are certain general measures regarding quarantine,
etc., that have to be enforced by the local health authorities. All persons
coming from a known infected region should be kept isolated and their
temperature taken at regular intervals for the period of time necessary to
complete the longest known incubation of yellow fever. If conclusive
evidence can be submitted that an individual has suffered from yellow
fever, thus being an "immune," such isolation is not necessary, and it
is sometimes considered by health authorities that all persons who have
lived for ten years in known endemic areas must have suffered from the
disease or are naturally immune. Children of less than ten years of
age are considered as nonimmune unless there is decisive evidence that
they have had an attack of yellow fever.

The immediate notification of every case of fever during an epidemic
of yellow fever is most essential, and a census of the nonimmune population should be taken in order that such persons may be watched by the
sanitary authorities and immediately isolated if any suspicious symptoms
are noted. A house-to-house inspection should be made during an epidemic by qualified inspectors whose duty it should be to discover any
cases of illness, and all cases of fever should be regarded as yellow fever
and the patients isolated and kept in mosquito-proof rooms or beneath a
mosquito net until the nature of the illness is ascertained.

An educational campaign regarding the etiology and methods of transmission and prevention of yellow fever should be at once instituted in
areas where the disease is present, in order that the general public may
be informed regarding these matters.

Prognosis.—The death rate of yellow fever has varied so greatly
in different epidemics that it is practically impossible to state definitely
the average mortality of this infection. In some epidemics it has been
stated to be as high as 70 per cent while in others it has varied between
5 and 10 per cent. In Havana, between 1886 and 1896, the mortality
from yellow fever was reported as 33.3 per cent, while Carter (1922)
states that in the epidemic of 1897, in the United States, the mortality
was between 6 and 10 per cent, and in 1898 it was probably from 4 to 6
per cent. However, Carter states that in Panama, in 1904 and 1905,
the reported mortality, which he regarded as quite accurate, was about
16.6 per cent. Much higher mortalities have been reported in other
epidemics, as already noted.

With the more recent methods available for the diagnosis of this disease it will probably be found that its mortality is not so great as has been reported in the past when the mild infections went unrecognized and unreported.

The prognosis is better in negroes than in whites, apparently due to a partial immunity of the negroes to the infection. *Age* is very important in prognosis, yellow fever being much less fatal in children than in adults, while the prognosis in old people is very grave. In *alcoholics* and in individuals suffering from *liver, kidney* or *heart disease* the prognosis is bad.

Among the clinical symptoms and signs that render the prognosis more grave are the following: early appearance of *jaundice;* the occurrence of marked *hemorrhages* and of *"black vomit";* the occurrence of a *temperature* above 39° C. (102.2° F.) and a continued high temperature without the usual remission; the *absence of Faget's sign,* i.e., a falling pulse with a stationary or rising fever; and a decrease in the quantity of urine or anuria. The amount of albumin in the urine has little prognostic significance, but a decrease in the quantity excreted is most important. Carter states that the secretion of less than a pint a day is usually followed by death.

The gravity of the prognosis is increased if the patient is moved after the second day of illness and too early feeding of solid food accounts for many deaths in patients who would otherwise have recovered.

While yellow fever must be regarded as a disease which may be attended by a high mortality, and, because of this, the prognosis must always be a guarded one, it should be remembered that in many epidemics the mortality has been comparatively low and that careful nursing and the proper treatment of serious symptoms have a marked effect upon the prognosis, many severe cases recovering under such conditions which would otherwise have proved fatal.

Pathology.—The pathology of yellow fever is so characteristic that a diagnosis of this infection may be made by a study of the lesions produced by the virus, especially those produced in the liver. This fact has made the viscerotome a most useful diagnostic instrument and its use has rendered a complete autopsy unnecessary, although most desirable, if it can be obtained.

MACROSCOPIC PATHOLOGY.—Most patients dying of yellow fever present a markedly jaundiced appearance, the entire body being of a bright yellow color, the jaundice after death being much more marked than during life. In some cases the entire skin is of a light mahogany color and, much more rarely, little jaundice may be noted. The mouth may contain blood or "black vomit" and the gums are frequently hemorrhagic, while marked ecchymoses may be present upon the skin.

On opening the body the organs are usually much congested and small hemorrhagic areas may be observed upon the surface of the liver, spleen, intestines and kidneys. The *stomach* contains degenerated blood, the "black vomit," and petechial hemorrhages are present in the mucous membrane, especially at the cardiac end of the stomach. The intestines contain extravasated blood, and the duodenum, for about one quarter of its length, may contain more or less degenerated blood from the stomach, while the mucous membrane may show areas of superficial necrosis and hemorrhage. The *liver* is markedly yellow in color externally and in
40102

some cases of a peculiar reddish-yellow color, which has given rise to
the name "boxwood liver." Hemorrhagic areas may be noted beneath
the capsule and the organ is friable, the consistence being considerably
decreased. The *spleen* may be slightly enlarged but is usually about
normal in size and in general appearance. The *kidneys* are enlarged
and may show petechial hemorrhages beneath the capsule. The cortex
may be pale or congested and often has a distinctly yellow color. The
lungs may show marked congestion and hemorrhagic areas may be present upon their surfaces, especially of the lower lobes. Hemorrhages
may also be present within the parenchyma of the lungs. The *heart* is
of a pale yellow color, flabby in consistence, and usually normal in size.
The *pericardial cavity* may contain an excess of fluid and minute hemorrhagic areas may be present in the pericardium, while the *endocardium*
is pale yellow in color and may also present small hemorrhagic areas.
Endocarditis does not occur as a result of infection with the yellow fever
virus. The *pancreas* may be enlarged, paler than normal, and of decreased consistence. The *brain* usually appears normal, but there may
be slight congestion, and minute hemorrhagic areas may be present upon
the surface of the cortex.

MICROSCOPIC PATHOLOGY.—It is the microscopic pathology of yellow
fever that is diagnostic. The *liver* presents microscopic changes that are
characteristic and diagnostic, and similar changes do not occur in this
organ in any other infectious disease, although somewhat similar lesions
may rarely be observed in poisoning by phosphorus or carbon tetrachloride, but the symptoms which accompany such poisonings easily
serve to distinguish them from those which accompany a fatal attack of
yellow fever.

The microscopic pathology of the liver in this infection has been
carefully studied and described by Rocha-Lima (1912), N. Paul Hudson
(1928), Torres (1928), Klotz and Belt (1930), Hoffmann (1928–1938)
and others. There is an intense coagulation necrosis and fatty degeneration of the liver tissue, commencing at the mid-zone of the lobules
and extending toward the periphery. In some cases all that remains
of the cellular structure of the lobule are a few parenchymatous cells
situated at the periphery. The liver cells are either necrotic or filled
with fat globules, the cytoplasm being hyaline in appearance and acidophilic in its staining reactions. In the central zone of the lobule around
the central vein the necrosis and fatty degeneration may be pronounced;
in the intermediate zone both necrotic and fatty degenerated cells are
present; and, in addition, cells undergoing a peculiar hyaline or coagulation necrosis, the so-called "Councilman bodies," are noted. In the
peripheral zone of the liver lobules the cells show the same changes as
in the intermediate zone but here apparently normal liver cells may be
present.

The "Councilman bodies" or, as Hoffmann prefers to call them, the
"yellow fever bodies" are large, rounded, granular acidophilic staining
bodies which do not contain a nucleus and which are considered by
Hoffmann and others as very characteristic.

In 1928 Torres described intranuclear acidophilic bodies occurring
in the nuclei of degenerating liver cells in yellow fever, similar to bodies
occurring in the tissue cells in some other virus diseases. They are
found most frequently in the liver cells during the early stages of the

infection, before the advent of marked necrosis, according to Cowdry and Kitchen (1930). The intranuclear inclusion bodies of Torres vary from 1 to 4 microns in diameter, lack any definite internal structure, are acidophilic in their staining reactions, and are sometimes surrounded by an unstained halo. Their number varies but several may be observed within the nucleus of a single cell. These bodies are believed to represent the reaction of the nucleus of the liver cells to the yellow fever virus.

In addition to the lesions described minute hemorrhages are observed within the parenchyma of the liver and the sinuses contain degenerated leukocytes. The Kupffer cells show granular degeneration, the cytoplasm containing iron pigment and bile, while the nuclei are pyknotic.

Of the changes mentioned above, the most characteristic of yellow fever are the mid-zonal necrosis and fatty degeneration, which, as first noted by Rocha-Lima, are found only in yellow fever and are, therefore, diagnostic of this infection.

The *kidneys,* microscopically, show fatty degeneration and acidophilic necrosis of the epithelium of the tubules, while the glomeruli are enlarged and congested, and hyaline and granular casts may occur in the tubules. Hoffmann (1937) has called attention to the presence of renal lime casts in the tubules in the kidney in yellow fever and considers their occurrence of diagnostic value.

The *spleen* in fatal cases of yellow fever has been studied microscopically by Klotz and Belt (1930), who noted absence of hyperplasia of the fixed tissues of the parenchyma but that the malpighian corpuscles contained mononuclear cells, that there was a hyperplasia of the corpuscles, and that a marked eosinophilia occurred in very severe infections. A waxy degeneration of the spleen was commonly noted by these observers.

The *heart* shows fatty degeneration and cloudy swelling, the fatty degeneration being most marked in the region of the nuclei of the muscle fibers. The pathology of the heart in yellow fever has been especially studied by Cannell (1928), who examined this organ in 29 fatal cases of the disease. He considered that the lesions in the heart were not diagnostic and could find no lesions that would explain the bradycardia so characteristic of this infection.

The microscopic pathology of the *brain* has been carefully studied by Nicolau, Mathis and Baffet (1937) in a single fatal case of yellow fever. They found the meninges normal, perivascular infiltration of mononuclear cells around the blood vessels, and intranuclear inclusion bodies in the nerve cells and glia cells of the cerebral cortex. Stevenson (1939) studied the microscopic pathology of the brain in 20 cases of yellow fever and found that the chief lesion consisted in perivascular hemorrhages, occurring most frequently in the subthalamic and periventricular region at the level of the mammillary bodies, with lesser involvement in the temporal pole and the cerebellum. In 9 cases a perivascular lymphocytic infiltration was noted. The changes in the nerve cells were very slight and they could find no inclusion bodies, or definite evidence of neurotropism of the virus in the cases they studied.

The *pancreas, pituitary body, glandular structures* and *lungs* show no characteristic microscopic lesions, but hemorrhagic areas may occur in all of these structures.

40102

REGENERATION OF TISSUES AFTER YELLOW FEVER.—As already stated, the sequelae of yellow fever are usually negligible, despite the fact that the finding at autopsy demonstrates the presence of marked degenerative lesions in the liver and kidneys, so marked in the liver in some cases as to indicate almost total destruction of the organ from a functional standpoint. The same changes, to a lesser degree, must be present in individuals who recover from a severe attack, yet total regeneration of the injured tissue evidently occurs in a remarkably short time as demonstrated by the perfect functioning of the diseased organs during and after convalescence.

The question of the regeneration of the tissues of the liver and kidneys has been studied by Klotz and Belt (1930) and they found that in all instances complete regeneration of the tissues quickly occurred, the regeneration originating from the undamaged areas of the parenchyma of the organs. They conclude that the absence of fibrotic changes in these organs is due to the immunity which the connective tissue possesses to the yellow fever virus and to the fact that the pathologic changes are noninflammatory and nonautolytic in type, which accounts for the absence of thrombi in the smaller blood vessels and the lack of reaction of the connective tissue during the active stages of the infection.

History.—The history of yellow fever has been very completely covered by Carter (1931), in his classical work entitled, *Yellow Fever: An Epidemiological and Historical Study of its Place of Origin.* Carter decided, after a very exhaustive survey of the subject, that yellow fever probably originated in Africa, but the recent discovery of jungle yellow fever in South America tends to negative this conclusion, as it may well be that this infection was present in the jungles of South America prior to its discovery as an urban infection, and thus it is not necessary to predicate that it must have been introduced into the Western Hemisphere through the importation of slaves from Africa or the personnel of sailing vessels from that continent. It is also true that yellow fever was described in America before it was recognized in Africa, for Carter states that the first accurate description of this disease in America dates back to 1648, and it was not until 1778 that Schotte described it as occurring in Senegal.

For a period of two and one-half centuries after the description of yellow fever in man nothing was known as to the exact cause of the infection or the actual method of transmission, although it was generally regarded as a most contagious disease transmitted by fomites. Numerous organisms were described, from time to time, as the causative agents, such as the cryptococcus of Freire, the bacillus of Sanarelli, and the leptospira of Noguchi, and all of these were accepted for a time as the veritable cause of the infection.

To Carlos Finlay, of Havana, belongs the credit for first suggesting, and offering experimental evidence to prove, that yellow fever is transmitted by mosquitoes. However, Finlay's work did not receive the attention that it deserved and his results were not generally accepted by the medical profession. In 1900 the United States Army Board, composed of Reed, Carroll, Lazear and Agramonte, was sent to Cuba to investigate yellow fever, and their work resulted in the demonstration that the disease is transmitted by the mosquito, *Aedes aegypti,* after a period of incubation in the insect; that the blood of patients suffering from the disease is not infectious to the mosquito after the third or fourth day from the appearance of symptoms; that the disease is not contagious and is not transmitted by fomites, and that the cause is a filtrable virus. All of these findings have been confirmed by many subsequent students of the subject and much has been added to our knowledge of the etiology and epidemiology within more recent years.

No account of the etiology of yellow fever would be complete without mentioning the work of Hideyo Noguchi, the eminent Japanese scientist, upon this subject. In 1925 Noguchi was sent by the Rockefeller Foundation to Guayaquil to ascertain, if possible, the cause of this infection, and in a few of the patients certified to him as suffering from the disease by Guayaquil physicians, who were supposedly experts, he demonstrated in the blood a spirochete which he was able to isolate in culture and to which he gave the name *Leptospira icteroides.* The inoculation of pure cultures of this spirochete into guinea pigs resulted in the death of these animals and the pathologic findings were similar to those seen in fatal cases of yellow fever occurring in man. For several years the medical profession generally accepted *Leptospira icteroides* as the cause of yellow fever, although a few investigators, notably Agramonte and Sellards, refused to accept Noguchi's findings. Sellards believed *Leptospira icteroides* to be identical with *Leptospira icterohaemorrhagiae* and was finally able to prove his contention by comparing cultures of *Leptospira icteroides,* sent him by Noguchi, with cultures of *Leptospira icterohaemorrhagiae.* Sellards' conclusions were supported by the failure of the Yellow Fever Board, of the Rockefeller Foundation in Africa, whose members were unable to demonstrate Noguchi's spirochete in yellow fever patients studied by them. Noguchi later went to Africa and was unable, himself, to demonstrate the spirochete, falling a victim to the disease while studying its etiology. It is now accepted that the patients in whom Noguchi found the spirochete were in reality suffering from Weil's disease and not from yellow fever.

Within recent years the researches of members of the International Health Division of the Rockefeller Foundation, working in Africa and South America, have contributed many important data to the history of yellow fever. Thus, in 1928, Stokes, Bauer and Hudson discovered the susceptibility of Indian monkeys, as *Macacus rhesus,* to experimental infection with yellow fever virus; Soper, Rickard and Crawford (1934) demonstrated the diagnostic importance of routine examinations of liver tissue removed by the viscerotome; Sawyer and Lloyd (1931) developed the intraperitoneal mouse protection test; Soper, Penna, Cardosa, Serafim, Frobisher and Pinheiro (1933) discovered jungle yellow fever, and Soper (1936) and others by means of surveys demonstrated the distribution of this type of the disease; Lloyd, Theiler and Ricci (1936), and Theiler and Smith (1937) cultivated the virus in pure culture; Sawyer (1937), Lloyd, Theiler and Ricci (1936), and Theiler and Smith (1937) developed an efficient method of vaccination of man with the living virus, while many other workers, as Hindle, Hindle and Finlay, Hughes, Findlay and MacCallum, Jadin and others have contributed much to our present knowledge of the yellow fever virus. It is probable that the history of this disease, so far as methods of transmission, relation to other animals than man, and its epidemiology are concerned, is still far from complete and that within the next few years discoveries may be made that will still further revolutionize our ideas regarding this most important and interesting infection.

The knowledge that we at present possess in regard to yellow fever has been obtained at the expense of many heroic lives, for many students of this infection have perished from the disease. The names of Lazear, Adrian Stokes, Hideyo Noguchi, William A. Young, Paul Lewis and Theodore Hayne will always be remembered as having given their all that our knowledge of yellow fever might be more complete.

In most discussions of the history of this disease several pages are devoted to an analysis of the numerous epidemics that have occurred throughout the world, from time to time. Space forbids such a discussion here and the reader is referred to the work by Carter, mentioned previously, for a complete summary of such epidemics. No less than 70 epidemics of yellow fever were reported in the period between 1833 and 1936, in the West Indies and in North, Central and South America. Some of these were localized and of small extent, while others were widely distributed and of most serious character. So far as the United States is concerned, yellow fever has appeared many times, during the last one hundred years, in New Orleans, and repeatedly in Memphis, Mobile, Galveston, Charleston and other southern cities, while even in New York and Philadelphia this disease caused serious epidemics during the early part of the present century.

Geographic Distribution.—The geographic distribution of yellow fever at the present time appears to be confined to Africa and South and Central America. But in the past this disease was carried to many parts of the world which are now, and have been for many years, free from the infection.

In Europe, where yellow fever was introduced by sailing vessels between the years 1700 and 1878, according to Hirsch (1883), epidemics occurred in Cadiz, Lisbon, Oporto, Malaga, Madrid, Cartagena, Gibraltar, Granada, Tortosa, Barcelona, Brest, Saint-Nazaire, Swansea and Southampton. The last epidemic in Spain occurred in Barcelona in 1821, while the last cases occurred in England, at Swansea, in 1865, and at Southampton in 1867. Aside from the epidemics mentioned above occurring in Europe and in the United States, yellow fever has been practically confined to Africa and the countries of Central and South America, and the West Indies, especially Cuba, since its first description by Du Tertre, in Guadeloupe, in 1635.

Within recent years it has been possible to ascertain with greater accuracy the distribution of this disease, through the use of the viscerotome and the mouse protection test. Results obtained in surveys, by employing these methods, have shown that the disease is present in many localities where its existence was not suspected. By means of the mouse protection test a world-wide survey of the presence of immunity to yellow fever has been made by the Rockefeller Foundation and it has been found that Europe, the Orient, North, East and South Africa, Australia and Canada were negative so far as any yellow fever immunity in their populations was concerned, and that in the United States, Mexico, the West Indies, Central America, the portion of South America west of the Andes, and the northern portion of South America such immunity was limited to individuals who were old enough to have suffered from the disease during previous known epidemics. On the other hand Soper (1937) states that the surveys have shown that yellow fever is now present in all but a few of the southern states of Brazil, in Bolivia, Paraguay, Peru, Ecuador, Colombia and Venezuela, and that it occurs in many localities where the common transmitting mosquito, *Aedes aegypti,* does not exist. In both South America and Africa there are immense areas in which it exists as an endemic infection in the form of "jungle yellow fever" and such areas are potential sources of widespread infection of man should nonimmunes enter such regions. In these endemic areas the disease is essentially one of some lower animal, in all probability some species of monkeys.

In Africa the surveys have shown the presence of yellow fever in a great area extending from the coast of Senegal to the upper portion of the Nile, in the Anglo-Egyptian Sudan and southward to approximately 5° S. latitude.

BIBLIOGRAPHY

Agramonte, A.: Boston M. & S. J., 158 : 927, 1908.
———— : Yellow Fever, Tice's Practice of Medicine, Hagerstown, Md., W. F. Prior Co., Inc., Vol. IV, 1929.
Aragao, H. de B.: Mem. Inst. Oswaldo Cruz, 34 : 547, 1939.
Bauer, J. H.: Am. J. Trop. Med., 8 : 261, 1928 ; 11 : 337, 451, 1931.
———— and Hughes, T. P.: Am. J. Hyg., 21 : 101, 1935.
———— and Mahaffy, A. F.: Am. J. Hyg., 12 : 155, 175, 1930.
Berry, G. P. and Kitchen, S. F.: Am. J. Trop. Med., 11 : 365, 1931.
Cannell, D. E.: Am. J. Path., 4 : 431, 1928.
Carter, H. R.: Yellow Fever: An Epidemiological and Historical Study of Its Place of Origin, Baltimore, Williams & Wilkins Co.
———— : Yellow Fever. Practice of Medicine in the Tropics, Byam and Archibald, New York and London, Oxford Univ. Press, 2 : 1228, 1921.
Cowdry, E. V. and Kitchen, S. F.: Am. J. Hyg., 11 : 227, 1930.
Craig, C. F.: Yellow Fever, Brennemann's Practice of Pediatrics, Hagerstown, Md., W. F. Prior Co., Inc., Vol. II, 1939.
Davis, N. C.: Am. J. Trop. Med., 11 : 31, 1931.
———— and Shannon, R. C.: Am. J. Hyg., 11 : 335, 1930.
———— and ————: Am. J. Trop. Med., 11 : 21, 1931.
Findlay, G. M.: Tr. Roy. Soc. Trop. Med. & Hyg., 27 : 437, 1934.
———— and Broom, J. C.: Brit. J. Exper. Path., 14 : 391, 1933.
———— and MacCallum, F. O.: Tr. Roy. Soc. Trop. Med. & Hyg., 30 : 507, 1937 ; 31 : 103, 297, 1937.
Finlay, C. J.: Ann. Acad. Habana, 17 : 449, 482, 1881.
———— : Ann. Acad. Ciencias, 18 : 147, 1881.
Frobisher, M., Jr.: Am. J. Trop. Med., 11 : 127, 1931.
———— : Am. J. Hyg., 18 : 354, 1933.
———— : Davis, N. C. and Shannon, R. C.: Am. J. Hyg., 14 : 142, 1931.
Goodpasture, E.: Am. J. Path., 8 : 137, 1932.
Hindle, E. and Findlay, G. M.: Brit. J. Exper. Path., 11 : 134, 1930.
Hirsch, A.: Handbook and Geographical and Historical Pathology, New Sydenham Soc., London, 1 : 316, 1883.
Hoffmann, W. H.: Virchows Arch., 266 : 769, 1928.

Hoffmann, W. H.: J. Trop. Med. & Hyg., 40 : 149, 1937.
Hudson, N. P.: Am. J. Path., 4 : 395, 407, 419, 1928.
————, Philip, C. B. and Davis, G. E.: Am. J. Trop. Med., 9 : 223, 1929.
Klotz, O. and Belt, T. H.: Am. J. Path., 6 : 655, 663, 689, 1930.
———— and ————: Am. J. Trop. Med., 10 : 299, 1930.
Lloyd, W. and Mahaffy, A. F.: J. Immunol., 25 : 471, 1933.
———— and ————: Am. J. Trop. Med., 15 : 51, 1935 ; 16 : 73, 1936.
———— and Penna, H. A.: Am. J. Trop. Med., 13 : 243, 291, 1933.
————, Theiler, M. and Ricci, N. I.: Tr. Roy. Soc. Trop. Med. & Hyg., 29 : 481, 1936.
Nicolau, S., Mathis, M. and Baffet, O.: Compt. rend. Soc. de biol., 122 : 203, 1936.
————, ———— and ————: Bull. Soc. path. exot., 30 : 615, 1937.
Noguchi, H.: J. Trop. Med., 28 : 185, 1925.
Penna, H. A.: Am. J. Trop. Med., 16 : 331, 1936.
Reed, W.: J. Hyg., 2 : 101, 1902.
———— and Carroll, J.: Am. Med., 3 : 301, 1902.
————, ————, Agramonte, A. and Lazear, J. W.: Senate Documents, Washington, D. C. 61. No. 882, 110. Govt. Print. Office.
da Rocha-Lima, H.: Arch. f. Schiffs- u. Tropenhyg., 16 : 192, 1912.
Sawyer, W. A.: Medicine, 10 : 509, 1931.
———— : Yellow Fever, Oxford Medicine, New York and London, Oxford Univ. Press, 5 : 731, 1939.
———— : Am. J. Trop. Med., 15 : 409, 1935 ; 17 : 35, 1937.
———— : Am. J. Hyg., 25 : 221, 1937.
————, Bauer, J. H. and Whitman, L.: Am. J. Trop. Med., 17 : 137, 1937.
————, Kitchen, S. F. and Lloyd, W.: J. Exper. Med., 55 : 945, 1932.
———— and Lloyd, W. D.: J. Exper. Med., 54 : 533, 1931.
————, ———— and Kitchen, S. F.: J. Exper. Med., 50 : 1, 1929.
Sellards, A. W.: Am. J. Trop. Med., 12 : 79, 1932.
———— : Ann. Trop. Med., 29 : 49, 55, 1935.
———— : New England J. Med., 216 : 455, 1937.
Shannon, R. C., Whitman, L. and Franca, M.: Science, 88 : 110, 1938.

Smith, H. H., Penna, H. A. and Paoliello, A.: Am. J. Trop. Med., 18 : 437, 1938.
—— and Theiler, M.: J. Exper. Med., 65 : 801, 1937.
Soper, F. L.: Am. J. Trop. Med., 17 : 457, 655, 1937.
—— : Tr. Roy. Soc. Trop. Med. & Hyg., 32 : 297, 1938.
—— and others: Am. J. Hyg., 18 : 555, 1933.
——, Rickard, E. R. and Crawford, P. J.: Am. J. Hyg., 19 : 549, 1934.
Stevenson, L. D.: Arch. Path., 27 : 249, 1939.
Stokes, A., Bauer, J. H. and Hudson, N. P.: Am. J. Trop. Med., 8 : 103, 1928.
——, —— and —— : J. Am. M. Ass., 90 : 253, 1928.

Theiler, M.: Ann. Trop. Med., 24 : 249, 1930 ; 25 : 69, 1931.
—— : Am. J. Trop. Med., 13 : 399, 1933.
—— and Hughes, T.: Tr. Roy. Soc. Trop. Med. & Hyg., 28 : 481, 1935.
—— and Sellards, A. W.: Ann. Trop. Med., 22 : 449, 1928.
—— and Smith, H. H.: J. Exper. Med., 65 : 767, 787, 1937.
—— and Whitman, L.: Am. J. Trop. Med., 15 : 347, 1935.
Torres, C. M.: C. R. Soc. Biol., Paris, 99 : 1344, 1928.
Whitman, L.: J. Immunol., 29 : 99, 1935.
—— : J. Exper. Med., 66 : 133, 1937.
—— : Am. J. Trop. Med., 19 : 19, 1939.

There is an intentional break in the continuity of these page numbers. This space will be utilized by future revisions of the text in this volume.

CHAPTER XXI

ASIATIC CHOLERA

By Eugene R. Whitmore, B.S., M.D.

Synonym.—Cholera.

Definition.—Cholera is an acute specific disease, caused by the *Spirillum choleræ asiaticæ*, discovered by Koch in 1883, and characterized clinically by a profuse painless diarrhea, vomiting, rapid collapse, muscular cramps, and suppression of urine.

Etiology.—Predisposing Causes.—There appears to be no difference in sex or age susceptibility. Overcrowding and bad ventilation are predisposing causes; as are worry, underfeeding, acute infectious diseases, overexertion and alcoholism. One of the most important predisposing causes is gastro-intestinal disturbance; and, in the Philippines we expected an increase in the number of cases of cholera after a flight of locusts, on account of the gastro-intestinal disturbance resulting from the eating of the locusts. Healthy persons, carrying the cholera vibrio in their intestine, may develop an attack of cholera after a cathartic, or after some gastro-intestinal disturbance; and it is not uncommon to see a return of the symptoms in a cholera convalescent after some indiscretion of diet.

Exciting Cause: The Organism.—In 1883 Koch discovered the specific cause of cholera, first in Egypt, and later in India. The *Spirillum choleræ asiaticæ* is a short, slightly curved rod, about 1.5 microns long, with a single flagellum at one end, and actively motile. It grows well on all ordinary culture media, and its ability to grow in alkaline media is taken advantage of in developing various special media for its growth.

The El Tor strains of the cholera vibrio produce hemolysis in fluid blood media, while the genuine strains of the cholera vibrio do not produce hemolysis in such media. Both types produce a clear zone around the colony on blood agar; but this is not due to hemolysis in both cases:

49

the genuine cholera vibrios produce this zone as a result of their digestive action on the blood-cells.

A number of laboratory workers have taken cultures into the stomach, partly by accident and partly by intention. In some cases where old cultures were taken there were no symptoms. In a number of accidental laboratory infections there have been all degrees of severity of the infection, from mild diarrhea to rapidly fatal cholera. One of the most interesting experiments is that of Pettenkoffer and Emmerich, who took cholera cultures with the intention of testing whether the cholera vibrio caused cholera. They took some alkali to neutralize the gastric juice, and then drank water to which they had added small amounts of a fresh culture of the cholera vibrio. Pettenkoffer developed a mild diarrhea, but Emmerich developed a severe attack of cholera which came near to costing him his life.

The cholera vibrio does not form spores or any resistant form. Healthy persons, who have not had cholera or diarrhea, may pass cholera vibrios in their stools for a month or two. Following cholera, the vibrios usually disappear from the stools in eight to ten days; but they may persist for over sixty days. Dunbar found living cholera vibrios in stools after being kept at room temperature and on ice for one hundred and sixty-three days. The vibrios stand temperatures well below freezing, and they will stand alternate freezing and thawing. The cholera vibrios die quickly after the death of the patient, and there is no contamination, of the ground in which the body is buried. The vibrios die in guinea pigs, fifteen to twenty days after burial.

The behavior of the cholera vibrio in water is of special importance, as cholera is commonly a water-borne disease. In some waters, the vibrios die very quickly, while they live and multiply in other waters. In sterile water the vibrios will live for a year; and they have frequently been isolated from water in rivers, wells and tanks. In view of the large number of cholera-like vibrios which are found in waters, fish, and in the stools of healthy persons, it is very important to make a complete determination of all vibrios isolated, before concluding that one is dealing with a cholera vibrio. The cholera vibrio does not live more than five or six days on food, and it does not live long in unsterilized milk, on account of the acidity of the milk as soon as it begins to sour. There is danger of infection from green vegetables that have been fertilized with human feces.

The cholera vibrio does not stand drying, and it dies in a few days on clothing kept under ordinary conditions. There is no danger of infection from dust. It resists sunlight for some time, but is killed by 10 minutes' exposure to a temperature of 50° C. (122° F.). It is readily killed by all of the ordinary disinfectants.

Epidemiology.—(*a*) *Source of Infection.*—The source of infection in cholera is man.

In the *clinical case* of cholera, the vibrios are passed in enormous numbers in the stools, and are at times present in the vomitus. Greig found cholera vibrios in the urine of 8 of 55 cases of cholera. He also cultivated the cholera vibrio from the lung of a case of cholera with pneumonia, and he suggested the possibility of spread through the sputum in such cases.

Mild cases of cholera, amounting to little more than a simple diarrhea, are important sources of infection. Convalescent cases rarely excrete the vibrios in the stools for longer than seven to ten days, though they may continue to excrete the vibrios for as long as sixty-five days.

Vibrio carriers are numerous in epidemic centers, and it is very common to find one or more vibrio carriers in a house where a case of cholera has developed. In Manila, six to seven per cent. of the healthy persons in some of the infected neighborhoods were carriers of the cholera vibrio. Heiser reports that of 876 contacts in connection with 72 cases, 40 showed vibrios in the stools, 29 being the cholera vibrio. Munson reports a systematic examination by the Health Stations in Manila: of 29,448 persons examined, 526 (1.78 per cent.) were carriers of the cholera vibrio, this percentage going as high as 2.4 in one health district. None of these persons were cholera suspects. In Bilibid Prison, 5 per cent. of the inmates were carriers of the cholera vibrio. Some of these persons developed cholera after carrying the vibrio for 17 to 18 days, one such case dying within 8 hours after the onset of the illness.

Pottevin examined the feces of 14,158 Egyptian pilgrims at Tor, in the winter of 1912-1913: 13,612 were healthy persons; 480 were sick in the hospital, and 66 were postmortem examinations. Vibrios were found 106 times (7.4 per 1000), 69 (4.8 per 1000) being cholera vibrios. In the 13,612 healthy persons, vibrios were found 40 times (2.8 per 1000); 1.7 per 1000 being cholera vibrios. He also found that persons sick of some other disease than cholera, especially dysentery, were very commonly carriers of the cholera vibrio—the incidence being as high as 79 to 110 per thousand.

Pottevin finds healthy carriers are especially numerous among children. Of 3,173 examinations in St. Petersburg, in 1909-1910, he found 6.6 per cent. of carriers among healthy adults; 9.8 per cent. among children 1 to 15 years old, and 20 per cent. among children less than 1 year old.

It is to be borne in mind that, in the case of carriers, the vibrios may appear in the stools intermittently. For this reason, the Philippine Board of Health insists on repeated examinations of the stools of negative persons in the search for cholera carriers.

Undoubtedly the carriers and the mild cases are of the greatest importance in the spread of the infection in a community and along routes of travel.

There is no evidence that any lower animal harbors the cholera vibrio, or plays a part in its spread to man. In the Philippines, it was suggested that the pig, on account of its special function as a scavenger, might play a part in the spread of the cholera vibrio. Numerous feeding experiments, even to having a part grown pig drink a liter of rice-water stool from a case of cholera, were carried out; but the cholera vibrio was never found in the rectal contents of the pigs, either before or after feeding material containing cholera vibrios.

(b) *Mode of Transmission.*—Cholera is spread in the same way as other diseases in which the infectious agent is contained in the feces, and is taken through the mouth.

Water is one of the commonest modes of transmission of the cholera vibrio. The organism lives for a long time in water, and the fecal discharges of cholera patients or carriers, passing into water supplies, may cause an explosive epidemic. An example of the water-borne epidemic of cholera is the Hamburg epidemic in 1892. The water of the river Elbe, infected by the discharges of cholera patients among some immigrants, was distributed throughout the city for drinking, without purification. Beginning with an occasional case over some weeks, there was a sudden outbreak of the disease, this outbreak reaching its height in ten days with 1000 cases in a day, and then gradually subsiding during the next two months. Vegetables washed in contaminated water may convey the infection.

Milk is not so frequently contaminated, probably on account of the acid reaction that develops when milk sours. However, Heim demonstrated living cholera vibrios in milk that had been sour for six days. Milk may be contaminated by the use of contaminated water, in washing the cans or as an adulterant. Milk is not used to any great extent in many of the countries in which cholera is prevalent.

Contact infection is a common mode of transmission of cholera. This is especially apt to be the case where a number of people live in close contact, and eat and drink from a common dish or bowl, not infrequently dipping the fingers into the·common food dish. An example of contact infection is an epidemic on a ship that left Naples for Brazil, in 1893, with 1472 deck passengers. Cholera broke out among the passengers on the way, and the ship could not land her passengers in Brazil, but had to return to Italy with them. The round trip from Italy occupied nearly two months, and 141 of the passengers died on the trip. Persons handling the clothing and bedding, soiled with the cholera discharges, are not infrequently infected.

Flies transmit the cholera vibrio, just as they transmit the typhoid bacillus, and in the same way. As the cholera vibrio does not stand drying, it is not so readily transmitted by the feces-soiled legs and body of the fly. The cholera vibrio will live in the intestine of a fly for at least three days; and the feeding habits of flies—feeding on fecal matter and on the carbohydrates of man's food—make them especially adapted to carrying the cholera vibrio from feces to man's food. Moreover, the necessity for the fly to take liquid or semi-liquid food accounts for its habit of regurgitating a drop of fluid from its crop onto the food and then sucking up the drop with the dissolved food. Finally, a fly defecates frequently when feeding. Thus, the fly, after walking on, and feeding on, feces containing cholera vibrios, walks on, regurgitates on, and defecates on, the food of man, in that way carrying the cholera vibrio from the contaminated feces to the food.

As the cholera vibrio does not stand drying, there is little danger of transmission through dust or on articles of furniture. The vibrio will live for some days in clothing and bedding that is rolled up without any special attempt at drying.

Where transmission is by contact or by flies, there is not the explosive outbreak that is seen when the transmission is by water. Instead, the so-called "cholera nests" appear about the point where a case develops; and it may be difficult to trace the connection between the cases or between the nests. In some of the towns in the Philippines, these "cholera nests" were very clearly developed after the cholera had been going in the town for some time; and these nests of a few houses were widely scattered through the town, without any traceable connection with each other.

(c) Susceptibility.—All races, all ages, and both sexes are susceptible to infection with the cholera vibrio. Overwork, worry, gastro-intestinal disturbances, and alcoholic excesses increase the susceptibility to infection.

(d) Mechanism of the Disease Process.—In a cholera epidemic, not all persons who take the cholera vibrio into the stomach develop cholera. Among those who develop the disease there are all grades of severity, from mild diarrhea to the severe and rapidly fatal cases. The main reason for the difference in severity of these cases would seem to be in great part due to the difference in resistance of the intestinal epithelium and the general resistance of the person. It is known that cholera is more severe in persons who are weakened from any cause. The causes of natural immunity, and of difference of susceptibility in different individuals, are not known.

When a person takes cholera vibrios into the stomach with water or food, many of the vibrios are killed by the acid in the gastric juice. But large masses of food and large amounts of water may protect the vibrios or dilute the gastric juice to such an extent that the vibrios are not killed in the short time they remain in the stomach before being passed on into the small intestine. If the person has some gastro-intestinal disturbance, or worry, there may be a lessened acidity of the gastric juice; and at times and in some persons the gastric juice is low in acid. When the vibrios reach the small intestine, they find the alkaline reaction of the contents suitable for their rapid multiplication. At times there are no symptoms, and the patient is simply a temporary carrier of the cholera vibrio. Frequently there is a mild diarrhea, which is over in a short time. Under such conditions, any indiscretion in diet or any stopping of peristalsis may lower the resistance of the intestinal epithelium, and the patient may develop a sharp attack of cholera. As long as the cholera vibrio develops in the intestinal contents only, there will not be any very severe symptoms, as it does not secrete a soluble toxin. But, when the resistance of the intestinal epithelium is lowered—or perhaps some strains of the cholera vibrio are more invasive than others—the vibrios invade the epithelium. The vibrios are broken down in the epithelial cells and in the lymph spaces between the epithelial cells; and the toxin thus liberated causes necrosis and desquamation of the epithelium. The toxin is absorbed and causes the acute intoxication of the typical attack of cholera.

The body reacts to the absorption of the toxin by the pouring out of large amounts of fluid into the gastro-intestinal tract. This pouring out of the body fluid causes the dryness and shrinking of the tissues, the concentration of the blood with the resulting low blood pressure, and the suppression of urine. The abundance of albumin and casts in the urine is probably dependent for the most part on the nephritis which develops early in cholera.

The nephritis leads to a marked acidosis in cholera, and it is probable that part of the symptoms are due to this. Thus, the so-called stage of asphyxia and coma may be due to an extreme acidosis. The ammonia excretion is high; the carbon-dioxid content of the blood is diminished; the excretion of acetone bodies is normal. The muscular cramps are usually ascribed to the loss of water from the nerves; but they may be connected with the loss of calcium salts as a result of the great outpouring of fluid into the intestinal tract. The destruction of the intestinal epithelium, and the lowering of the resistance, pave the way for secondary infections.

The cholera vibrio reaches the gall-bladder in a rather large percentage of cases of cholera. Greig found the vibrio in the bile of 80 out of 271 cases of cholera, and in twelve of the cases there were pathological changes in the gall-bladder. In most of the cases in which the cholera vibrio is found in the bile, it is in pure culture.

There is difference of opinion as to the manner in which the cholera vibrio reaches the gall-bladder; and whether there is general infection. Nichols is of the opinion that the gall-bladder infection results from a portal or general septicemia, with elimination of the organism in the bile. Greig is of the opinion that the organism reaches the bile-ducts through the lymph stream and at times goes up the ducts from the duodenum; but that it does not pass through the blood stream. Greig found the cholera vibrio in a lymph gland near the duodenum; in the liver, especially in the region of the gall-bladder; he found it in the exudate in the pulmonary alveoli in cases of cholera with pneumonia, and in the wall of the urinary bladder. This, with the cultivation of the vibrio from the lung and the finding of it in the urine in cases of cholera, leads Greig to the opinion that a septicemia occurs in many cases. Sanarelli, working with young rabbits, was never able to get the cholera vibrio past the stomach; but, when injected subcutaneously or intravenously, the vibrios reached the intestine, and typical cholera occurred. Adult rabbits lost their immunity when the colon bacillus or its products was injected intravenously or into the wall of the appendix. From this, Sanarelli is of the opinion that the cholera vibrio passes through the mucosa of the mouth and the tonsils and reaches the intestine through the blood and lymph channels, first appearing in the region of the ileocecal valve.

Death takes place in the stage of collapse, or later from uremia and acidosis. In cholera sicca, death is due to the profound toxemia, before diarrhea sets in.

The tendency of the disease is to recovery by the production of antibodies. Immunity following an attack is of short duration, and second attacks of cholera are fairly common.

Symptomatology.—CLINICAL HISTORY.—The period of *incubation* is a few hours to five days—usually about three days—during which time there are no symptoms. The disease *sets in* with a mild diarrhea, which is usually painless, but may be accompanied by colicky pains. At first the stools consist of thin fecal matter of about normal color. The diarrhea rapidly increases, and soon the stools become profuse, colorless and watery, rendered slightly opaque by flocculi of intestinal epithelium, giving the appearance of rice-water or thin gruel. The stools are alkaline in reaction, and have an albuminous odor. The stools are passed without colic or tenesmus, there being rather a feeling of relief as the enormous amount of fluid is passed.

Vomiting sets in at the same time the diarrhea increases. At first the stomach contents are vomited; but very soon the vomitus takes on the character of rice-water. The vomiting is projectile, and the fluid gushes from the mouth and soils everything about.

With this great loss of fluid from the body, the tissues very soon become dry and shriveled: the skin is wrinkled and inelastic, giving rise to the washerwoman's fingers; the eyes are sunken; the nose is pinched; and the cheeks sink, leaving the cheek bones prominent. Painful cramps appear in the muscles of the legs, thighs, arms and abdomen. The voice becomes weak and husky. The secretion of sweat and urine is reduced to a minimum. The respirations are rapid and shallow; the heart sounds are faint, and the pulse is feeble; the blood-pressure falling to 50 to 70 mm., or it may be impossible to measure it. The skin becomes cyanotic, especially about the nails and the lips, and the face assumes a dusky gray hue. There is intense thirst.

The rectal temperature may be 38.9°-40° C. (102°-104° F.); but the surface temperature is subnormal: the skin feels cold and clammy, and may be moist with a sticky perspiration. The reflexes are diminished; the mind is clear, though the patient is apathetic; there is complaint of exhaustion, especially from the profuse stools; there is air-hunger, palpitation of the heart and faintness.

All of these symptoms may increase: the cyanosis increases to a dark gray or violet color; the heart-sounds are weak and irregular; the pulse is lost; respiration is shallow and labored, sometimes giving the name of asphyxial stage to the condition; the vomiting and diarrhea gradually cease; there is total suppression of urine; the patient passes into coma and dies.

Instead of progressing to a fatal termination, the symptoms may become less marked, and the patient enters the stage of reaction. The vomiting ceases; the stools become less numerous and gradually return to normal; the pulse returns; the skin becomes warm and regains its elasticity and fullness; the cyanosis disappears, and the skin and mucous membranes become normal in color; the secretion of urine returns; and the patient has returned to complete health in a few days.

But, in many cases, with the stage of reaction, temperature remains elevated to 38.3° or 38.9° C. (101° or 102° F.), the cheeks flushed, and the mucous membranes bright pink in color; the pulse is full and bounding, with the blood-pressure as high as 160 to 180 mm.; there is constipation, and complete suppression of urine. The tongue and lips are dry and cracked, and are covered with brownish sordes. There is headache; the patient becomes apathetic, passes into delirium, and dies in coma.

In some cases, instead of reaction setting in, the cyanosis continues; the pulse is soft, with normal or subnormal blood-pressure; the diarrhea continues and may be bloody; the urinary secretion is not established; and the patient dies on the fourth or fifth day.

Soucek saw cholera rashes rather commonly in an epidemic on the eastern front. One-fourth of the rashes were urticarial, the others macular like measles. The urticarial rash generally appeared about the fifth or sixth day; and the macular rash appeared about the ninth to twelfth day. The macular form appeared on the face, and spread over the body in one to three days. The rash lasted three to six days. The appearance of the rash coincided with improvement in the condition; and Soucek suggests that it is anaphylaxis.

LABORATORY FINDINGS.—In the stage of collapse, the blood is thick and may not flow when a vein is cut. The thickening of the blood is due to the loss of water from the tissues. While in normal blood the corpuscles are about 45 per cent. of the bulk of the blood, in the stage of collapse in cholera, the corpuscles may be as much as 80 per cent. of the bulk of the blood. The red-cell count, as well as the leukocyte count, is high according to the concentration of the blood, there being no evidence of leukocyte reaction. The carbon-dioxid content of the blood is decreased. As early as nine hours after the onset of symptoms, the urine may contain albumin; and later the scanty urine is loaded with albumin, and hyaline and granular casts. The ammonia in the urine is increased; the urea is diminished; there is no change in the acetone bodies. There is increased tolerance to sodium bicarbonate.

Diagnosis.—DIFFERENTIAL DIAGNOSIS ON THE CLINICAL HISTORY.— During an epidemic, the diagnosis is readily made from the clinical picture of profuse painless diarrhea of rice-water stools, vomiting, cyanosis, rapid shallow respiration and feeble pulse, with suppression of urine and muscular cramps. But various metallic and meat-poisonings may give all the symptoms of cholera, and can be differentiated only by bacteriological examination. Bacillary dysentery may be mistaken for cholera, especially those cases of cholera in which the enteritis continues for some days. Pottevin found that dysentery and cholera were at times combined; and it must be remembered that dysentery patients are very frequently carriers of the cholera vibrio.

Cholera must be differentiated from cases of *Bacillus aertrycke* infection: the abdominal pain, absence of suppression of urine, and absence of rice-water stools will help; but a definite diagnosis can be made only by a bacteriological examination of the stools.

In children the meningeal symptoms may be marked; and in Manila it was not uncommon at the postmortem table to find cases of cholera which had been clinically diagnosed as meningitis. Pottevin also noted marked meningeal symptoms in children with cholera.

LABORATORY DIAGNOSIS.—The blood-serum of a cholera patient does not usually develop agglutinins early enough to be of assistance in diagnosis. Greig studied the agglutinins in cases of cholera, and found that fatal cases occasionally agglutinated as high as 1 : 40; but that they usually gave no agglutination. In non-fatal cases, the agglutination increased to the sixth day, and dropped after the twentieth day: high titers—1 : 400 to 1 : 1000—were occasionally obtained. Carriers show agglutination for some time, and this may help in tracing them. When cholera-like vibrios were isolated from a stool which also contained cholera vibrios, there were agglutinins for the cholera vibrio only, and none for the cholera-like vibrio. Normal human serum does not agglutinate the cholera vibrio above 1 : 20, and very rarely above 1 : 10.

Bacteriological diagnosis is the principal method of laboratory diagnosis of cholera; and, as a bacteriological diagnosis can be made very early in the disease, it is of great importance in the fight against cholera.

It may be possible to make a diagnosis by the direct examination of the stool. A small flake of mucus from the stool is placed on a slide, without spreading; it is allowed to dry, and is stained with a 1 :9 dilution of carbolfuchsin. The cholera vibrios appear as typical comma-shaped bacilli, easily distinguished from the other intestinal bacteria. It is necessary to be familiar with the appearance of the normal stool, in order to avoid confusion with the slender spirilla that are common in normal and diarrheal stools.

Dunbar has suggested a method of agglutinating the cholera vibrios directly in the feces. Several shreds of mucus are taken from the stool, and each shred is rubbed up in a drop of peptone water on a cover glass. To some of the cover-glass preparations is added a drop of a 1 : 50 dilution of normal rabbit serum, and to others is added a drop of a 1 : 500 dilution of a high titer cholera-agglutinating serum. In the preparations to which the cholera-agglutinating serum has been added, the cholera vibrios soon lose their motility, while in the controls, to which the normal serum has been added, the cholera vibrios are actively motile. This method is of value in cases where the cholera vibrios are present in almost pure culture; but a negative result is not to be considered as of diagnostic value.

Cultures.—The most satisfactory method of bacteriological diagnosis is to make cultures from the stool or intestinal contents, and to study the organisms in those cultures: cultures must always be made, even when the other methods are used. A shred of mucus is placed in a tube of peptone water, and is rubbed up on the side of the tube. The peptone water tubes are incubated for six to eight hours, and then a loopful of fluid from the surface of the tube is examined by smearing it on a slide, drying with gentle heat, staining with a 1:9 dilution of carbolfuchsin, and examining under the microscope. From any tubes which show comma-shaped bacilli, agar plates are streaked, and are incubated for twelve hours. Agar plates may also be streaked directly from the feces, at the time the peptone water tubes are inoculated.

For the plates, 3 per cent. agar must be used, and the surface must be well dried by inverting the plates in the incubator, with the lid off, for half an hour before streaking them. A glass rod, a platinum loop, or a pledget of cotton can be used for streaking the material on the plates; the requirement being that there shall be isolated colonies on the plates. The vibrio colony has a very characteristic appearance on the agar plate: it appears as a pale disk, which is slightly opalescent and iridescent by transmitted light. At times the colonies are clear and transparent; at other times they may have a yellowish-white appearance, somewhat like colonies of the colon bacillus.

A microscopic slide agglutination is made from the characteristic colonies on the agar plates. A loopful of a 1:500 dilution of a high titer cholera-agglutinating serum is placed on a slide, and with a platinum needle a small amount of material from one of the characteristic colonies is rubbed up in the loopful of serum. Cholera vibrios will be instantly agglutinated to a curdy appearance, while the cholera-like vibrios and other bacteria will rub up to a milky emulsion. The diagnosis is completed by staining some of the material from the colonies which agglutinate in the cholera serum, and by streaking material from the same colonies on agar tubes and studying them further, especially by testing their agglutinability in a cholera agglutinating serum and by testing them by the Pfeiffer phenomenon. In a large number of cases in Manila, in which a diagnosis of cholera was made from the microscopic slide agglutination, we never found the method in error when the organism was carried through further tests. McLaughlin and Whitmore also studied a number of cholera-like vibrios, isolated from various sources, including the stools of persons in the cholera-infected districts; and they were never able to make any of these cholera-like vibrios take on the characteristics of cholera vibrios, and were never able to show that the microscopic slide agglutination method had failed to differentiate a cholera vibrio from a cholera-like vibrio.

In the Philippines, where it was often necessary to send material some distance to the laboratory, agar slants with a sterile swab were sent out to the various health officers. A swab of fecal material, either from a stool, or from the rectum in case the patient was found dead, was spread over the surface of the agar in the tube, and the tube was sent in to the laboratory. We succeeded in isolating cholera vibrios from such tubes when they had been as long as fifteen days in transit to the laboratory, under the ordinary temperature conditions in the tropics. Panganiban and Schöbl have tested various methods of preserving cholera vibrios in stools. They find that salt solution, in concentration from 0.5 to 5 per cent., will preserve the vibrios for five weeks: stronger solutions of salt were not satisfactory. Bile, as suggested by Ottolenghi, was more satisfactory than salt solution. When mixed with a salt solution suspension of feces, so the final mixture contained 25 to 50 per cent. of bile, the vibrios were preserved for seven weeks. It is advisable to emulsify the stool in bile or physiological saline solution for sending to a distant laboratory.

Culture Media.—While peptone solution is satisfactory as an enriching medium in general, where the cholera vibrios are scarce some of the other enriching media will give better results. One of the best of these enriching media is Goldberger's egg-peptone solution, which is made as follows: an egg is shaken up with an equal volume of water; this mixture is mixed with an equal volume of a 5 per cent. solution of sodium carbonate, and the mixture is steamed in the Arnold for one hour. One part of this egg mixture is added to nine parts of peptone solution, and the mixture is filtered and sterilized. The egg-peptone solution is used in the same way as is the ordinary peptone solution.

Instead of ordinary agar for plating, a number of selective media have been developed for the detection of the cholera vibrio, all of these media depending for their usefulness on the fact that the cholera vibrio grows well on a medium of such alkalinity that the common intestinal bacteria do not grow on it.

Dieudonne's alkaline blood medium is one of the most commonly used of these selective media. Equal volumes of defibrinated blood and normal potassium hydrate solution are mixed, and the mixture is sterilized in the autoclave. Seven parts of ordinary agar, neutral to litmus, are mixed with three parts of this alkaline blood, and plates are poured. Before use the plates are allowed to stand at 37° C. for twenty-four hours, or at 60° C. for five minutes. The plates must stand for twenty-four hours before they can be used. The reason for this is that a large amount of ammonia is formed from the alkaline blood mixture, and this inhibits the growth of the cholera vibrios. On this medium, the cholera vibrios and cholera-like vibrios grow well, while the colon bacillus and other bacteria are inhibited. In twelve to twenty-four hours the vibrios appear as large, round colonies, light gray in transmitted light and hyaline in reflected light. A disadvantage of Dieudonne's medium is that the cholera colonies grown on this medium are sometimes difficult to emulsify, and this interferes with the agglutination.

Goldberger's medium for plating is prepared as follows: Ordinary meat infusion is neutralized to litmus with 5.3 per cent. solution of anhydrous sodium carbonate, and then 2.5 c.c. of the 5.3 per cent. sodium carbonate solution is added to each 100 c.c. of the medium; the medium is heated in the Arnold for half an hour and filtered. One part of this alkaline meat infusion agar is mixed with three parts of ordinary 3 per cent. agar, and plates are poured from the mixture. The plates are dried and used in the regular way.

Aronson's medium has been highly recommended. Aronson combined sugars to favor the growth of the cholera vibrio, and the color reaction of Endo's medium, in an alkaline medium to prevent the growth of the ordinary intestinal bacteria. To 100 c.c. of ordinary 3.5

per cent. agar add 6 c.c. of a 10 per cent. solution of sodium carbonate, and steam for 10 to 15 minutes in the Arnold. While it is still hot, add 5 c.c. of a 20 per cent. solution of cane sugar (saccharose), 5 c.c. of a 20 per cent. solution of dextrin, 0.4 c.c. of a saturated alcoholic solution of basic fuchsin, and 2 c.c. of a 10 per cent. solution of sodium sulphite. The solutions of the sugars are sterilized before adding, and the medium is not sterilized after the sugar solutions are added. When completed, the reaction of the medium should be about —3 per cent. to phenolphthalein. In the preparation of the medium, a precipitate forms. This precipitate settles rapidly, and from the supernatant fluid plates are poured, and dried at 50° C. for half an hour before using. A large amount of suspected fecal material can be inoculated directly onto the plate, as the colon bacillus does not grow. Cholera vibrios develop in 10 to 12 hours, and begin to turn red in 15 to 20 hours. The vibrios emulsify well; and the large colonies furnish sufficient material for agglutination and microscopical examination, and for inoculation of plates.

While the colon bacillus does not grow on Aronson's medium, it remains alive and may appear in transplants from cholera vibrio colonies from the plate. For this reason, in order to get the cholera vibrio in pure culture from the Aronson plate, it is necessary to streak from the colony onto a plain agar plate. After 24 hours the colon bacillus may begin to split the sugars in Aronson's medium, and so obscure the colonies of the cholera vibrio.

Volpino found that the cholera vibrios did not always produce red colonies on Aronson's medium when incubated over night. He then examines all colonies that develop on the plate, by agglutination and microscopically. Volpino considers that ordinary agar, of the alkalinity of Aronson's medium, is almost as good as Aronson's medium for rapid diagnosis. It would seem advisable to add the sugars to the ordinary agar in order to hasten the growth of the cholera vibrios.

These selective media make it possible to detect cholera vibrios, even when they are present in small number in the stool, as it is possible to use a large amount of the fecal material for the inoculation. Cholera-like vibrios grow on these selective media; and it is very important that the organisms which develop are tested by agglutination and further culture, in order to determine the nature of the colonies.

The *cholera-red reaction* may be of value in the bacteriological diagnosis; but this reaction very frequently fails unless the culture of the cholera vibrio is pure. It may be tried on the first or second peptone culture, after about 18 hours' incubation; but it is advisable to make the test on a peptone tube inoculated from one of the characteristic colonies on an agar plate. This reaction depends on the fact that the cholera vibrio produces both indol and nitrites in peptone solution and, when a few drops of sulphuric acid are added to the peptone-solution culture, a cherry red color is produced.

Gelatin cultures of the cholera vibrio do not give any information that cannot be obtained other ways; and, since gelatin is difficult to work with, especially in the tropics, it is not advisable to use gelatin cultures.

Complications and Sequelæ.—Since acute nephritis develops in practically all severe cases that survive to the stage of reaction, this condition can hardly be classed as a complication. But the frequency and danger of this condition must be borne in mind. Most of the complications occur during the stage of reaction, and are due to secondary infection. Lobar pneumonia, and diphtheritic inflammation of the mucous membranes of the gastro-intestinal tract are fairly common. Pregnant women usually abort, due to the action of the cholera toxin on the uterine muscle during the cramps. Suppurative parotitis, local suppurations, and gangrene, especially about the genitalia, may occur. Hematuria rarely occurs. If the patient survives the acute nephritis, there is apparently complete recovery of the kidney. Edema rarely occurs in the acute nephritis.

Clinical Varieties.—The typical case of cholera, *cholera gravis,* with the stages of evacuation, collapse and reaction, has been described above.

Cholerine.—Cholerine is a milder form of the disease, in which there is active diarrhea; but there is no collapse, and the urine is not suppressed.

Cholera Sicca.—Cholera sicca is a severe form of the disease, in which the patient dies of the intoxication before diarrhea and vomiting have set in. This form of the disease is more apt to occur in debilitated persons. In the Philippines we saw cases of cholera sicca in persons who had recently had an attack of dengue fever; and there was a case in a soldier who showed, on postmortem examination, extensive tuberculous lesions in the lungs. On postmortem examination, the intestine may be filled with liquid, from which the cholera vibrio is isolated.

At times the clinical picture of cholera is very irregular, and, especially in children, the meningeal symptoms may dominate the picture.

The cases of *cholera carriers,* persons who are not ill but are passing virulent cholera vibrios in their stools, are of great importance. These persons may pass the vibrios in the stools for as long as sixty. days; and, in addition to the danger of spreading the infection to others, these carriers are in danger of developing cholera themselves if they develop any gastro-intestinal disturbance or are given a cathartic.

Treatment.—PROPHYLAXIS.—In any infectious disease there are at least three links in the chain of circumstances which makes it possible for the disease to spread: (1) a source of infection, (2) a mode of transmission, and (3) a susceptible population. A consideration of the epidemiology of a particular disease will indicate where it is best to attack this chain in order to break it.

Prophylactic methods against cholera may be divided into *public* and *personal.*

The *public measures* are generally pretty definitely laid down in the laws of different countries; and consist in control of the source of infection by the **detection and isolation of cases and carriers,** and the control of the mode of transmission by **prevention of pollution of water** and food, and the furnishing of a suitable water supply. Attempts to control the third link in the chain, a susceptible population, consists in **vaccination** with a cholera vaccine.

When a case of suspected cholera occurs, it must be isolated at once, and a bacteriological diagnosis made as soon as possible. If the case is determined to be cholera, it is important to discover the source of infection, and to prevent the spread of the infection. All contacts must be isolated until their stools are examined for the cholera vibrio. Any contact found carrying cholera vibrios must be isolated, the same as a case of cholera, until the stools are free from vibrios. **All discharges** from cases, carriers, and suspected contacts **must be disinfected,** and all linen and bedding must be disinfected. The stools are mixed with an equal volume of 5 per cent. cresol solution, and allowed to stand for at least an hour: a 5 per cent. mixture of chlorinated lime may be used in the same way as the cresol solution. Bedding and linen can be disinfected by immersion in a 2.5 per cent. solution of **cresol.** All food containers should be boiled. As the cholera vibrio does not stand drying, terminal disinfection consists in washing the floor and walls with a 2.5 per cent. solution of cresol.

All cases and carriers must be kept in isolation until the stools are negative for cholera vibrios on three successive days.

It is not necessary to quarantine ships, or to prevent travel; but all persons traveling, by ship or otherwise, if coming from a cholera infected locality, must be detained long enough to make a bacteriological examination of the stools for cholera vibrios. This examination can be completed usually in twenty-four hours, and always in forty-eight hours. Simple detention for five days is not sufficient, as cholera carriers can be detected only by examination of the stools for cholera vibrios.

In the same way, it is not advisable to undertake any general quarantine on food supplies, as the advantages do not offset the disadvantages. It is necessary to investigate the source of the food supply, and to take proper precautions against any article of food that seems to be carrying infection. Pottevin considers that foodstuffs are not dangerous in the spread of cholera where several days elapse between the time the food leaves a cholera district and the time it arrives in a new district; but, if the time is short, the food may be a real danger. As water is the common medium by which the infection is spread, it is necessary to **guard carefully against any contamination of the water supply.** All vegetables which are eaten uncooked must be guarded against contamination; and it is best to urge the people to avoid as much as possible the use of uncooked food of any kind. An active campaign must be waged against flies.

Personal prophylaxis is very important, and consists in **drinking** only **boiled water;** in **eating no uncooked food,** especially fresh vegetables; in carefully washing the hands after going to the toilet, and before eating; avoiding all foods which lead to gastro-intestinal irritation; prompt treatment of gastro-intestinal disturbances; an active **campaign against**

flies, including the protection of all food from flies; avoiding debilitating influences of any kind; and avoiding bad ventilation and overcrowding.

Vaccination is the principal method of attack on the third link in the chain. While the healthy person has considerable resistance to infection with the cholera vibrio, due partly to the acid condition of the gastric juice and partly to the resistance of the intestinal mucosa to invasion by the cholera vibrio, it is only too evident that this resistance is not enough to protect in a great percentage of persons. Since it appears that there is at least a temporary immunity following an attack of cholera, and it is possible to demonstrate antibodies in the serum of lower animals and men after vaccination with a cholera vaccine, attempts have been made to specifically raise the resistance of persons to the cholera vibrio by **vaccination.**

1. *Living cultures* of the cholera vibrio have been used in a vaccine. Ferran was the first to try vaccination as a prophylactic against cholera, and he used living virulent cultures, recently isolated from cases. Gamaleia used living attenuated cultures. Haffkine carried out vaccination on a large scale in India. His first vaccinations were with a living attenuated culture, followed by a virulent culture: later, he used only the virulent culture. The general results of Haffkine's vaccination are that the incidence of cholera is lowered among the vaccinated; but the mortality is nearly as high in cholera cases among the vaccinated as among the unvaccinated.

2. *Killed cultures* are more convenient than living cultures to use in a vaccine. Gamaleia also used killed cultures in vaccination. Kolle used a vaccine made by growing the cholera vibrios on agar, suspending them in saline solution, heating to 58° C. for one hour, and adding 0.5 per cent. phenol to the suspension. The dose was 2 mg., moist weight, of the bacterial mass as scraped from the agar.

Murata, in Japan, tried a vaccine prepared according to the Kolle method in 1902. Using the dose of 2 mg., moist weight, of the bacterial mass, he reduced the incidence and the mortality of cholera among the vaccinated. When he increased the dose to 4 mg., moist weight, of the bacterial mass, there were no more cases of cholera among the vaccinated.

3. Various vaccines have been prepared from *filtrates* from cholera cultures, and from various *autolysates* and *extracts* of the cholera vibrio. Bartarelli prepared an autolysate by suspending agar cultures of the cholera vibrio in saline solution, heating to 60° C. for one hour, allowing it to autolyse in the incubator at 37° C. for two days, and filtering. The filtrate is the vaccine, and Bartarelli demonstrated antibody production in the serum of rabbits vaccinated with this vaccine. Strong has used such an autolysate in the vaccination of a considerable number of people, and there is considerable evidence that such an autolysate gives protection against cholera.

It appears that a strain of the cholera vibrio of low virulence is as satisfactory for a vaccine as is a strain of high virulence; but it is necessary to choose a strain that gives good antibody production. Some strains of the cholera vibrio do not give good antibody production regardless of whether the virulence is high or low.

Cholera vaccination has been tried out rather extensively in the recent war, and the results have been fairly satisfactory. The indication is that there is good protection for three months; but that the protection has disappeared by the end of six months, and revaccination must be practiced by the end of that time. In general, the vaccine used has been heat-killed cholera vibrios suspended in saline solution. The United States Army has used experimentally heat-killed cholera vibrios suspended in oil in the form of a single dose lipovaccine.

Arnaud reports on cholera vaccination in the Greek army in the second Balkan war: 93,868 men were vaccinated, and 14,332 were not vaccinated. Of the vaccinated, 72,652 received two doses of vaccine; 21,216 received one dose of vaccine. The incidence of cholera in the unvaccinated was 5.75 per cent.; in those who had one dose of vaccine it was 3.12 per cent.; and in those who had two doses of vaccine it was 0.43 per cent. Similar results are reported by von Roemer in Batavia, and by Kersten on the vaccination of German troops in a Turkish town in 1917. In von Roemer's work, the mortality was not reduced among the vaccinated who contracted cholera.

Generally the local and general reaction following cholera vaccination is very slight. Simicek saw a case of pemphigoid eruption in a man, following the second injection of cholera vaccine, and he considered it due to hypersensitiveness.

The use of anticholera serum has not given any satisfaction in prophylaxis.

CURATIVE TREATMENT.—In treating a case of cholera, it is to be borne in mind that the patient may die in the stage of collapse, that he may die of uremia following the stage of reaction, and that there is danger of relapse as a result of errors of diet in the first few days of convalescence.

The patient is to remain strictly in **bed,** and provision is to be made at once to disinfect the stools and vomitus. Vomiting makes it impossible for the patient to take any nourishment, and it usually makes it impossible to give any medicine by mouth. **Cracked ice** will to some extent relieve the vomiting and the great thirst. **Morphin** may be given to relieve the vomiting and the muscular cramps, but it is generally agreed that morphin is to be used sparingly or not at all.

The room is to be airy and well ventilated; but the patient is to be kept warm, and external heat applied when collapse sets in.

Rogers advocates the use of **permanganates,** on account of their property of destroying toxins. The patient is given all he can drink of **calcium permanganate water** (1 to 6 grains [0.065 to 0.4 gram] to the pint); and is given a 2-grain pill (0.13 gram) of **potassium permanganate** every fifteen minutes for two hours, then every half hour until the stools become less copious and are green and more fecal in character: this occurs in twelve to twenty-four hours. Then six to eight pills are administered during twenty-four hours. The pills are made with vaselin or kaolin, and are coated with a mixture of five parts of sandarach varnish and one part of salol; or they may be put in gelatin capsules, the junction of the halves of the capsule sealed with gelatin, and exposed to formaldehyd vapor until the gelatin is keratinized. Rogers uses atropin sulphate, in the dose of 1/100 grain, hypodermically, night and morning; and he finds that it greatly decreases the danger of collapse.

Stumpf recommended the use of **kaolin** in the treatment of cholera; and Arneth and Kuhne report excellent results from its use in the recent war. The kaolin is used as a prophylactic by putting it in the drinking water. In treatment, the patient is given the suspension to drink; and the suspension is injected into the bowel. Kuhne reports that with the kaolin treatment, the mortality from cholera was reduced from 45 per cent. to 2 or 3 per cent., in an extensive experience in Serbia. He finds it useful in prophylaxis and treatment of all forms of diarrhea. Arneth advises the usual methods of treatment, in addition to the use of kaolin.

There is general agreement that the loss of fluid and the acidosis must be combated early, as the two indications are to tide the patient over the collapse stage and to prevent his dying of uremia after the stage of reaction. These indications are met by the intravenous injection of fluid.

In the collapse stage, when the blood-pressure falls below 70 mm. of mercury, it is necessary to give an *intravenous injection*. Rogers uses the specific gravity of the blood as a guide in determining when intravenous injection is necessary. To determine the specific gravity of the blood, he uses mixtures of glycerin and water of specific gravities varying from 1.048 to 1.070. A drop of blood is placed in these glycerin-water mixtures until it is determined which mixture is the same specific gravity as the blood. If the specific gravity of the blood is over 1.062, at least a liter of fluid is injected; if the specific gravity is 1.066, at least two liters of fluid is injected. The temperature of the injected fluid is varied according to the rectal temperature: if the rectal temperature is about normal, the fluid is run in at a temperature of about 37.8° C. (100° F.); if the rectal temperature is below normal, the fluid is warmed to 38.9° to 40° C. (102° to 104° F.); if the rectal temperature is high, the fluid is run in at a temperature below the normal temperature of the body.

Normal saline solution is satisfactory for making up the loss of fluid from the body; but Rogers recommends the use of a hypertonic solution containing 120 grains (7.8 grams) of sodium chlorid, 6 grains (0.4 gram) of potassium chlorid, and 4 grains (0.26 gram) of calcium chlorid to the pint of water.

Sellards has shown that intravenous injection of a solution of **sodium bicarbonate** has great advantage over the injection of physiological or hypertonic saline solution, as it not only makes up the loss of fluid, but also meets the great requirement of overcoming the acidosis and relieving the anuria.

Sellards and Shaklee used the following solution in the stage of collapse:

Sodium chlorid .... 0.4   per cent.
Potassium chlorid .... 0.042   per cent.
Sodium bicarbonate .... 0.5   per cent.

They gave injections of two liters (4.22 pints) of this solution intravenously, with an interval varying from 4 to 29 hours. At times they gave four liters (8.5 pints) for the first injection; and they occupied 15 to 30 minutes in running the solution into the vein. Though they started the injections early, the urine remained acid until the stage of reaction set in—after as many as six injections; and the urinary secretion never started until after the reaction set in. The injections are repeated when the pulse becomes weak and rapid and the blood pressure falls to 50-70 mm. of mercury. The blood-pressure rises to normal or above in one to three hours after the injection.

In the stage of reaction they used a 1.5 per cent. solution of sodium bicarbonate without the addition of any other salt, giving two liters of the solution. In the stage of reaction, it is necessary to watch the reaction of the urine, as it is necessary to reduce the amount of sodium bicarbonate injected, as soon as the urine becomes alkaline.

The use of the alkaline solution may also produce muscular twitchings and cramps; possibly as a result of the precipitation of the calcium salts by the sodium carbonate.

The sodium bicarbonate solution, given early in the disease, prevented death from uremia; while, when given late in the disease, the course was modified, and the anuria was at times relieved, but the final outcome of the disease was not changed.

It is advisable to use sodium bicarbonate solution, as sodium carbonate solution is hemolytic; and Sellards found that it produced convulsions in one case. The sterilization of the sodium bicarbonate is somewhat difficult, as the salt changes to the carbonate during sterilization. In the solution used for collapse, Sellards and Shaklee added the sodium bicarbonate to the sterile solution, just before injection.

To sterilize the sodium bicarbonate solution, fill strong, narrow-mouthed bottles as full as possible with the solution, leaving only spaces for expansion of the fluid when hot; tie tightly-fitting stoppers in place. It is an advantage to sterilize the solutions in an atmosphere of carbon dioxid; this can be done by placing a dish of boiling water in the bottom of the autoclave and, just before closing the autoclave, adding a handful of sodium bicarbonate to the dish of water, then closing the door and leaving the vent open at the top until the carbon dioxid has driven the air out. The autoclave is tightly closed during the sterilization—7 pounds for 45 minutes—and is cooled down to room temperature before opening. Such solutions do not have over three per cent. of sodium bicarbonate changed to carbonate; and they keep well if tightly stoppered. The solution may be sterilized in the ordinary way, and a current of carbon dioxid passed through it to convert the carbonate into the bicarbonate.

While there is possibility that attempt should be made to replace the calcium lost from the body, it is not advisable to include the calcium in the alkaline solution, as the carbonate formed in the sterilization precipitates it out.

Rogers now includes intravenous injections of sodium bicarbonate in his treatment of cholera; and reports the reduction of the mortality due to uremia from 11.1 per cent. without alkalis to 3.25 per cent. with alkalis.

Goff and Denney used continuous proctoclysis in the treatment of cholera; and they report that this method of treatment induced evacuation in the "sicca" cases, and encouraged kidney elimination.

Segale showed that the glycogen disappeared from the blood and there was a mere trace left in the liver in cholera. The carbohydrate metabolism does not appear to be disturbed in cholera; and it is not possible to introduce nourishment through the gastro-intestinal tract during the stage of collapse. This, with the good results from intravenous injections of glucose in other acute infectious diseases, would indicate the advisability of its use in cholera. Kausch uses a 5 per cent. solution of glucose for subcutaneous injection, and a 10 per cent. solution for intravenous injection, giving 1000 c.c. twice a day, for nutritive purposes. Strauss advises a 4.5 per cent. solution intravenously. Gaertner adds glucose to the saline solution given intravenously. All three agree that the results are good; there being increased flow of urine, with possible washing out of toxins.

The use of **anticholera serum** has not given very encouraging results. If serum is to be used at all, it must be given early, and be given intravenously in doses of 50 to 100 c.c., with an interval of eight to twelve hours.

No food can be given during the stage of collapse; but as soon as the vomiting ceases, the patient may take albumin water, broths, milk diluted with soda water and thin gruels. It is necessary to be very careful in increasing the diet, as there is danger of bringing on a relapse with all the dangers of the original attack.

Prognosis.—The average mortality is about 50 per cent., varying from 30 to 80 per cent.; about 35 per cent. of the cases dying in collapse, and about 15 per cent. of the cases dying of uremia. The mortality is usually higher at the beginning of an epidemic. Recent acute illness, or debility of any kind, kidney disease, intemperance, and youth or old age, make for a bad prognosis. If the collapse sets in early, the prognosis is bad.

Pathology.—MACROSCOPIC.—When the patient dies in collapse, the skin is dry and wrinkled, and the fingernails are cyanotic. Rigor mortis is early and marked; so a limb may be moved, or the head may be turned from one side to the other. All of the tissues are dry, and the muscles are dark red in color. The appearance in the peritoneal cavity is striking. The omentum is shrunken and dry, and the peritoneum is dull, dry and sticky. The ileum is purplish-pink or rose-red in color, while the colon is normal in color; this appearance of the intestine is almost characteristic of cholera. The liver, spleen and lungs are shrunken and dry; and the heart contains dark, thick blood. The intestines are filled with rice-water material; the lymphoid follicles in the ileum are prominent; the blood-vessels about the follicles are injected, and there may be hemorrhages about the follicles. The liver is congested; the kidneys are swollen, congested, and may be ecchymotic.

The gall-bladder frequently shows a catarrhal inflammation; but the inflammation may be hemorrhagic or necrotic. It is probable that the more severe inflammation of the gall-bladder is due to mixed infection with other bacteria.

There is surprisingly small evidence of gross pathological change in cases that have died as a result of a pure infection with the cholera vibrio.

MICROSCOPIC.—The epithelium of the intestinal mucosa is necrotic, and the cholera vibrios have penetrated deeply into the mucosa or even into the submucosa. There is generally little parenchymatous change in the organs; but the liver, and especially the kidneys, show early cloudy swelling. The kidneys show necrosis of the epithelial cells, and the tubules are blocked with granular debris.

When the process continues longer, the parenchymatous changes in the kidneys are especially marked, the epithelium showing necrosis and fatty degeneration. The lungs may show lobar pneumonia as a complication.

When the patient dies in the condition of cholera typhoid, the change in the intestinal mucosa may be marked, amounting to a necrosis of the mucosa: this change is especially marked just above the ileocecal valve. This change is due to secondary invasion by other bacteria, and the cholera vibrio is not generally found in such lesions.

Greig has studied the lesions in the gall-bladder, and in different organs. In the gall-bladder, the epithelium is gone, and the wall is thickened and infiltrated with round cells, with evidence of hemorrhagic infiltration. The cholera vibrios are found in areas in the liver, near the gall-bladder; and the liver cells are necrotic in these areas. In a congested and edematous lower lobe of the lung the alveoli were filled with cellular exudate, and congestion in the alveolar walls. He found cholera vibrios in the spaces of a lymph gland near the small intestine, deep in the wall of the gall-bladder, in the liver near the gall-bladder, in the exudate in the pulmonary alveoli, and in the submucosa of the urinary bladder. Schöbl found cholera vibrios in infiltrated and necrotic areas in the liver of his experimental animals, after inoculation of a virulent culture of the vibrio into the gall-bladder.

History.—Cholera has been known in India from ancient times, and Susruta described an epidemic in the seventh century, A. D. It appears to have been endemic in the Delta of the Ganges, from where it spread as repeated epidemics over India; and there were numerous epidemics from the fifteenth to the seventeenth century. But it does not appear that cholera was known outside India until the Indian epidemic of 1817, which spread through Eastern Asia, reached Africa in 1819 and 1820, and reached Russia in 1823.

The next epidemic started in India in 1826, and spread through Asia to Africa and all of Europe. The disease reached the United States and Canada in 1832, and extended to Mexico, Cuba and the northern part of South America in 1833 and 1834.

The next epidemic started in India in 1846, and spread through Asia, Africa and all of Europe. It reached the United States in 1848, and extended to Canada, Mexico, Central and South America and the West Indies in the following years, up to 1862.

The fourth epidemic, starting in India in 1863, spread through Asia, Africa, and Europe; and reached the West Indies and Ward's Island in 1865, spreading over North, Central and South America during the next years, up to 1873.

The fifth epidemic, starting in India in 1883, extended through Asia, Africa and Europe, and reached South America in 1885 to 1888. In 1893 it was again introduced into the United States and Brazil, extending to Argentine and Uruguay in 1894 and 1895. This epidemic continues throughout Asia and parts of Europe. The disease has been repeatedly brought to the port of New York, notably in 1911; but it has not been able to enter the United States since 1893, and it has not been able to gain a foothold since 1873.

Some parts of the world have remained free from cholera. These are usually cold regions, or islands to which the disease is less likely to be brought. The disease has not yet spread to tropical and southern Africa.

Geographical Distribution.—While the Delta of the Ganges seems to have been the home of cholera, and earlier epidemics are traceable to that origin, it appears that now the disease has become endemic in a number of other regions. The pilgrims, returning from Mecca, rather commonly carry the infection with them to their home country. The disease seems to be endemic in Persia, through India, Indo-China, Java and the Philippine Islands. It is endemic in the Balkans, and has been quite prevalent there during the recent war.

BIBLIOGRAPHY

ARNAUD, F. Le cholera dans l'armée hellenique. Bull. Acad. de méd., Paris, 1914, 3d Ser., lxxi, 384.

ARNETH, J. Zur Behandlung der Cholera. Deutsch. med. Wchnschr., 1916, xlii, 935.

ARONSON, H. Eine neue Methode der bakteriologischen Cholera-diagnose. Deutsch. med. Wchnschr., 1915, xli, 1027 and 1088.

CASTELLANI, A., AND CHALMERS, A. J. Manual of tropical medicine. 1913, 2d Ed., p. 1343. Wm. Wood & Co., New York.

CASTELLANI, A., AND MENDELSON, R. W. Note on the tetravaccine: Typhoid + Paratyphoid A + Paratyphoid B + Cholera. Brit. Med. Jour., 1915, ii, 711.

DUNBAR, W. P. Asiatic cholera. Osler and McCrae, Modern medicine, 1913, 2d Ed., Vol. I, p. 672. Lea & Febiger, Philadelphia.

GAERTNER, G. Bemerkungen zur Pathologie und Therapie der Cholera Asiatica. Wien. med. Wchnschr., 1915, lxv, 182.

GOFF, A. P., AND DENNEY, O. E. Clinical observations on Asiatic cholera in Manila in 1914. Jour. Am. Med. Assn., 1915, lxiv, 1148.

GOLDBERGER, J. Some new cholera selective media. Treasury Dept., U. S. Public Health Service, Hygienic Laboratory Bull., No. 91, 1913.

GREIG, E. D. W. An investigation of the occurrence of the cholera vibrio in the biliary passages. Indian Jour. Med. Research, 1913-14, i, 44.

—————— Preliminary note on the occurrence of the comma bacillus in the urine of cases of cholera. Indian Jour. Med. Research, 1913-14, i, 90.

—————— The invasion of the tissues by the cholera vibrio and further observations on pneumonia in cases of cholera. Indian Jour. Med. Research, 1914-15, ii, 1.

—————— Lesions of the gall-bladder and biliary passages in cholera: a bacteriological, histological and experimental study. Indian Jour. Med. Research, 1914-15, ii, 28.

—————— The agglutinins in the blood of cholera cases. Indian Jour. Med. Research, 1914-15, ii, 733.

—————— Further observations on lesions of the biliary passages of rabbits dying after repeated intravenous injection of living vibrios: a contribution to the study of experimental cholera infection. Indian Jour. Med. Research, 1916, iii, 397.

HEISER, V. G. Cholera in the Philippines during 1913. Med. Rec., New York, 1914, lxxxvi, 827.

HETSCH, H. Choleraimmunität. Handbuch der pathogenen Mikroörganismen. Kolle u. Wassermann, iv, Zweite Auflage, 1913, 110. Gustav Fischer, Jena.

JEX-BLAKE, A. J., AND WILSON, W. J. Notes on three fatal cases of B. aertrycke infection. Brit. Med. Jour., 1918, ii, 310.

KAUSCH, W. Traubenzuckerinfusion bei Cholera. München. med. Wchnschr., 1916, lxiii, 544.

KERSTEN, H. E. Ueber eine Choleraëpidemie, ihre Bekämpfung und die Einfluss der Schutzimpfung auf ihren Verlauf. München. med. Wchnschr., 1918, lxv, 563.

KOLLE, W., AND SCHÜRMANN, W. Cholera Asiatica. Handbuch der pathogenen Mikroörganismen. Kolle u. Wassermann, iv, Zweite Auflage, 1913, 1. Gustav Fischer, Jena.

KUHNE, V. Kaolin in the treatment of cholera. Revue médicale de la Suisse Romande, Geneva, 1918, xxxviii, 555.

MCLAUGHLIN, A. J., AND WHITMORE, E. R. Cholera and cholera-like vibrios encountered in the Philippines. Philippine Jour. Sc., Sect. B., Medical Sciences, 1910, v, 403.

MUNSON, E. L. Cholera carriers in relation to cholera control. Philippine Jour. Sc., Sect. B, Tropical Medicine, 1915, x, 1.

NICHOLS, H. J. Experimental observations on the pathogenesis of gall-bladder infections in typhoid, cholera, and dysentery. Jour. Exper. Med., 1916, xxiv, 497.

PANGANIBAN, C. S., AND SCHÖBL, O. Preservation of cholera stools for delayed bacteriological examination. Philippine Jour. Sc., Sect. B, Tropical Medicine, 1918, xiii, 275.

PAPAMARKU, P. Beiträge zur Frage der Choleraimmunität bei Schutzgeimpften. München. med. Wchnschr., 1917, lxiv, 425.

POTTEVIN, H. Les bases scientifiques de la lutte contre le cholera. (Conference faite a la Société imperiale de médicine de Constantinople.) Bull. de l'Office internat. d'hyg. publique, 1913, v, 953.

—————— Contribution a l'étiologie du cholera. Bull. de l'Office internat. d'hyg. publique, 1913, v, 1158.

VON ROEMER, L. S. A. M. Over de Cholera te Batavia in 1915 en 1916. Geneesk. Tijdschr. v. Nederl.-Indië, 1917, lvii, 295.

ROGERS, L. The results of the hypertonic and permanganate treatment in 1000 cases of cholera; with remarks on the value of alkalis in the prevention of uremia and the rôle of atropin. Lancet, 1915, ii, 219.

—— Further work on the reduction of the alkalinity of the blood in cholera; and sodium bicarbonate injections in the prevention of uremia. Ann. Trop. Med. and Parasitol., 1916, x, 139.

—— The mortality from postcholeraic uremia: a 70 per cent. reduction through intravenous injections of sodium bicarbonate. Lancet, 1917, ii, 745.

ROGERS, L., AND SHORTEN, A. J. The alkalinity of the blood in kala-azar and cholera and the technic of its estimation. Indian Jour. Med. Research, 1915, ii, 867.

SANARELLI, G. Pathogenie du cholera. Reproduction expérimentale de la mâladie. Compt. rend. Acad. de sc., 1916, clxv, 538.

SANTOLIQUIDO. Note de l'administration sanitaire italienne sur les revaccinations antityphoidiques et anticholeriques. Bull. de l'Office internat. d'hyg. pub., 1917, ix, 433.

SCHÖBL, O. Further studies on experimental cholera carriers. Jour. Infect. Dis., 1916, xix, 145.

SEGALE, M. Sul contenuto in glicogeno nel fegato e nel sangue dei colerosi. Policlinico, sez. med., 1912, xix, 441.

SELLARDS, A. W. The principles of acidosis and clinical method for its study. Harvard Univ. Press, Cambridge, Mass., 1917.

SELLARDS, A. W., AND SHAKLEE, A. O. Indications of acid intoxication in Asiatic cholera. Philippine Jour. of Sc., Sect. B., Med. Sci., 1911, vi, 53.

SOUCEK, A. Ueber das Exanthem bei der Cholera asiatica. Wien. med. Wchnschr., 1916, lxvi, 428.

STRAUSS, H. Zuckerinfusionen bei Cholera. Therap. d. Gegenwart., 1915, lvi, 370.

VAN LOGHEM, J. J. Ueber den Unterschied zwichen Cholera- und El Tor-Vibrionen. Centralbl. f. Bakteriol., I Abt., Orig., 1913, lxvii, 410.

VOLPINO, G. L'uso del terreno di Aronson nella diagnosi rapida del vibrione colerigeno. Policlinico, sez. prat., 1916, xxiii, 549.

CHAPTER TWENTY-TWO

LEPROSY

By George W. McCoy, M.D.

Etiology.—PREDISPOSING CAUSES.—While leprosy is, or has been in the past, a disease of all lands and of all climates, it is today confined chiefly to the tropics and subtropics, and to this extent *climate* may be considered a predisposing cause.

Age.—The disease by preference attacks those in youth or in early adult life; one third of the cases occur in the second decade, and over one half between the ages of ten and twenty-five years. It is exceptional to have a case develop in a person beyond fifty or under six.

Sex.—A remarkable and unexplained fact is the preponderance of cases among males. It holds true almost the world over that there are nearly two male lepers for each female leper. Various theories have been advanced to explain this remarkable fact, but none is convincing. Perhaps the simplest one, and one as plausible as any, is the greater opportunity among men for exposure to infection.

Race.—Various races, particularly South Sea Islanders and Orientals, have been regarded as particularly susceptible, but the author is inclined to believe that race per se is not a factor of much importance, and that given equal opportunities for infection, under identical conditions, there is little or no difference in susceptibility among the various races.

Heredity.—The belief in heredity as a predisposing or, indeed, determining factor in the development of leprosy goes back to Biblical times, but it has no substantial foundation. Undoubtedly, leprosy often does occur among children of lepers, but it also occurs among others who come in contact with it. In the Hawaiian experience, the disease is *apparently* acquired about as often from a brother or sister as from the father or the mother. Careful studies in the Hawaiian focus show that when children of lepers are removed from the leprous environment at once after birth, the chances of the development of the disease are small.

EXCITING CAUSE: THE ORGANISM.—We accept the acid-fast organism first described by Hansen as the cause of leprosy, but we are without

39102

73

absolute proof of this. The bacillus is constantly associated with the lesions of leprosy, but as there is some doubt as to whether it has been cultivated, and as the evidence that the disease has been reproduced in animals by the cultures that have been isolated is of the flimsiest sort, clear proof of the etiologic relation is lacking.

Hansen's bacillus is an acid-fast organism which bears considerable resemblance to the tubercle bacillus in size, shape and staining reactions. It is usually found in greater numbers than the latter organism and, as it appears in smear preparations from tissues, is often arranged in bundles.

Numerous observers have, by means of special procedures, cultivated acid-fast organisms, and branching organisms having an acid-fast stage, from leprous lesions. The only organisms that need to be mentioned are those grown by Clegg, and by McKinley and his associates. Both of these workers cultivated acid-fast organisms by special technics but were unable to reproduce the disease in laboratory animals. It has been impossible for these investigators, or indeed any workers, to establish by serologic methods any relation of cultivated organisms to leprosy.

Experimental Inoculation.—Many investigators have attempted to reproduce leprosy in laboratory animals by the inoculation of leprous tissue and, while there are to be found in the literature numerous reports of success in this direction, a careful scrutiny of the experimental data leaves one with the clear impression that the evidence is insufficient to justify the conclusion that leprosy ever has been transmitted to laboratory animals, and a very considerable experience on the part of the author confirms this. This is true, not only for the animals ordinarily used in experimental work, guinea pigs, rabbits, rats and mice, but for monkeys and the higher apes as well. Not only has it proved impossible to infect laboratory animals, but of a large number of experiments on man, but one can be considered as possibly successful, and there is some doubt as to that one. The possible exception is the case of the convict Keanu, a Hawaiian, who was inoculated with leprous tissue by Arning. Two years after this inoculation the subject of the experiment developed leprosy and from it he eventually died. While doubt is thrown on the validity of the experiment by the fact that Keanu lived in a country in which the chances for acquiring leprosy in the natural manner, whatever that may be, were notoriously good, a careful study of the record of the case leaves one with the impression that Arning's experiment probably was successful. There is no satisfactory explanation for the unsuccessful human inoculations, of which there are a considerable number of reports scattered through the literature. There are reports of a few, very few, accidental infections through wounds.

Modes of Conveyance.—We do not know precisely how the causative organism enters the body, but we do know that in some manner the bacilli pass from the sick to the well and in a small proportion of cases cause the disease in a new victim.

Various theories have been advanced to account for transmission, such as infected food, respiratory infection, sexual contact or insect transmission, but proof is lacking that any of these is the usual method of conveyance of the disease. We may consider it a contact disease, and beyond that, in the present state of our knowledge, it is impossible to go.

Symptomatology.—PERIOD OF INCUBATION.—This varies greatly but it is customary to say that the average period is about five years. There are well-authenticated cases in which the time that elapsed between exposure to the infection and the development of symptoms has been as short as two years; and there are others in which twenty years or more have elapsed. During this period usually there are no noteworthy symptoms but there may occur one or more febrile attacks, which, usually, are not regarded as of any significance until cutaneous or nerve lesions draw attention to the underlying condition. Perhaps the most striking thing about the onset and progress of leprosy is the extreme slowness that ordinarily characterizes the development and evolution of the disease. The case is distinctly exceptional in which noteworthy changes occur in periods of weeks, while usually months are required to show any distinct alterations, and often during a period of many years the patient will remain apparently stationary.

CLINICAL TYPES.—For convenience it is desirable to consider the clinical manifestations of leprosy as falling under two types, depending on the prominence of, or the presence, exclusively, of cutaneous or nerve symptoms. The former is often called "tubercular leprosy," though "nodular" is a term to be preferred; and the latter is designated, usually, as the "anesthetic" type, though "nerve leprosy" is a more accurate and descriptive term. While there are many cases that may with certainty be grouped under these headings, there are many others, perhaps a majority, showing manifestations of both types and these are usually indicated by the term "mixed."

(a) *Nodular Leprosy.—The Skin Lesions.*—In this form of the disease the patient's or the physician's attention is usually attracted to red, reddish-brown or fawn-colored patches at one or more points. The skin is found to be slightly thickened, and it may or may not be the site of itching or of burning sensations. These spots are most often found on the exposed parts of the body, though they may also occur on any covered portion. The bronzed or fawn-colored patches are of the greatest diagnostic importance, as they are simulated by few conditions. The author has seen a case in which the body was free from lesions beyond a fawn-colored, very slightly thickened area on the cheek, not more than 1 cm. in diameter, and a similar patch on the forearm, yet a clinical diagnosis of leprosy was made with considerable confidence, and this was verified by microscopic examination. These spots resemble closely the chamois-colored patches of tinea versicolor, but the microscopic examination at once shows the nature of the lesion.

The early lesions may remain a few weeks, disappear, to be replaced by others, or they may be permanent. Sometimes they assume a ringworm appearance with a clear center; indeed they are sometimes mistaken for ringworm. These early lesions are often associated with some general systemic disturbance, but just as frequently the general health remains unaffected. These early spots are not likely to be anesthetic.

After a period that may vary from weeks to years, but one that usually is limited by months, the patches become distinctly nodular and nodules may appear at points that have not been the site of the earlier, more superficial lesions. The nodules vary from the size of a pea to masses that can scarcely be covered by a man's hand, but usually they

39102

range from 1 to 5 cm. in diameter. Rarely the body may be covered with small nodules, each one about the size of a pea, giving an appearance suggestive of a rather scanty eruption of smallpox.

The nodules may be scattered generally over the body, but the face and the backs of the hands and feet are the commonest sites. They are very commonly present on the lobes of the ears, which the experienced examiner never fails to scrutinize most carefully. The cheeks are also favorite sites, and early lesions are often found on the nose, forehead and chin. It is worth noting here that the scalp rarely is involved.

The lesions, as they progress, throw the skin into creases and ridges, giving the face the "leonine" appearance which, while undeniably characteristic, is a relatively late manifestation of the disease; i.e., late in the evolution of the lesions though not necessarily late so far as the life of the patient is concerned. These extensive skin lesions may be accompanied by loss of flesh and strength, but often they have no apparent effect upon the general health of the patient. The author has seen many lepers with typical leonine facies who were able to do a full day's work. The nodular areas are often the seat of ulcerative processes which may start spontaneously or from a slight traumatism.

Subjective Symptoms.—Febrile attacks occasionally occur during the course of nodular leprosy. These may or may not be associated with the development of new nodules. They are usually accompanied by sweating, loss of flesh and weakness.

The Lymphatic Glands.—These, in nodular leprosy, often are swollen but painless. The enlarged gland feels elastic and usually does not exceed the last joint of the little finger in size, but occasionally may be 2 or more centimeters in diameter.

Mucous Membranes.—In any marked case of nodular leprosy there is very likely to be involvement of the mucous membranes. Rhinitis is a usual and annoying symptom that may be associated with epistaxis. Occasionally, nodular infiltration of the nasal mucosa occurs. There is a marked tendency to ulceration of the mucous membranes. This is especially true of lesions of the mouth, throat and larynx. When it occurs in the last situation, it gives rise to the well-known leprous voice, and in severe cases articulation becomes difficult or impossible.

Eye Symptoms.—Among the most common and distressing manifestations of leprosy are those of the eye. There is often a pronounced conjunctivitis, and this may be associated with infiltration at the sclero-corneal junction which finally is likely to involve the whole cornea, leading to more or less complete blindness. At a later date the deeper structures of the eye are involved and, in many cases, softening of sclera and cornea leads to pronounced staphyloma.

(b) *Nerve Leprosy.*—Pure nerve leprosy presents few features which, at first sight, would lead us to consider it as closely related to the form that has just been described. It is in every respect a milder disease. As the name indicates, the symptoms are chiefly referable to the nervous system and often it is called anesthetic leprosy on account of an outstanding symptom. Many cases are so mild as not to pass beyond a paralysis of a part of a hand or of a few facial muscles. On the other hand, in many cases there is most extensive mutilation, such as the loss of a hand or foot, manifestations which justify the term "mutilating leprosy" sometimes applied to these cases. Other cases present few or numerous spots of varying size and appearance, which accounts for the term "macular leprosy."

The *skin manifestations* of nerve leprosy may begin by the appearance of reddish patches or of patches showing a deepening of the natural skin color. In other cases there is a loss of pigment, leading to the formation of vitiligo-like spots, frequently called leukodermic areas. In this form of the disease the early skin lesions are more likely to be permanent than in the nodular forms. Sensory changes usually may be demonstrated as soon as the lesions are observed.

Numbness and tingling often are the earliest subjective manifestations associated with, or followed by, impairment of pain perception and of thermic sense.

The eruption, like the early manifestations in nodular leprosy, often appears on the face first, though it may be confined to the covered parts of the body. The patches vary in size from those 1 cm. in diameter to large plaques which can scarcely be covered by the two hands; these latter usually are found over the buttocks and on the back. In many cases the eruption clears in the center, leaving an appearance strikingly like certain forms of ringworm, with which it may be readily confused.

There may be severe *neuralgic pains,* especially in the hands, forearm and the face. Aside from these neuralgic conditions, nerve leprosy is not ordinarily accompanied by painful manifestations.

Nerve Conditions.—In a considerable number of cases a definite *thickening of certain nerve trunks,* particularly the ulnar, may be detected by palpation. The author feels that he should here emphasize a warning against considering any nerve enlarged, unless the swelling can be distinctly felt as a spindle-shaped or cylindric enlargement, or as a definite beading. Hansen called attention to the importance of this, and, if noted, many mistakes will be avoided. Such expressions as "slight thickening" or "moderate enlargement" of a nerve trunk mean little or nothing. Patients often complain of a sense of numbness, or describe a member as dead, when there is involvement of important nerve trunks.

Affection of the Muscles.—Atrophy of certain groups of muscles, with contracture of others, leads to the characteristic deformities of the hands and of the feet. The "leper claw," so commonly seen, is a hand showing atrophy of all muscles of the member, extension of the first joint, and flexion of the last two joints of the fingers. The shrinking of the muscles is most readily observed in the thenar and hypothenar prominences. It is sometimes surprising to observe the good functional utility of a hand that is markedly deformed. Paralysis of the muscles of the lower extremities is less common than that of the upper, but, when it does occur, it leads to abnormalities of the gait, deformity of the foot and sometimes to the inability to walk. Various degrees of facial paralysis may occur, ranging from inability to close an eye, to loss of function of all of the muscles of half or even of the whole face.

Ulceration and Mutilation.—Loss of parts of the hands or of the feet are common. This results from atrophy and from ulceration, which may bring about a melting away of the extremities and sloughing, or spontaneous amputation may occur. The latter may involve a single joint of a finger or may destroy successively parts of the hand or of the foot and may finally result in the loss of the entire member. Carious processes play a conspicuous part in these mutilations, which may be painful and accompanied by swelling and suppuration, requiring surgical measures for relief. The description of nerve leprosy would be incomplete without mention of the trophic ulcers, usually called "perforating" on account of the tendency to deep tissue destruction. They occur chiefly on the sole of the foot, giving rise to the plantar necrosis so common among lepers, though similar ulcers on the palm are not rare. Occasionally these ulcers are painful, but usually they are insensitive and it is no uncommon thing to find a patient walking about in relative comfort on a plantar ulcer as large as a silver dollar and leading to extensively disorganized bone. The absorption of phalanges leading to the shortening of one or more fingers is diagnostically a very important, but not a very common, manifestation of the disease.

Seat of Bacilli.—In this form of leprosy the bacilli are usually difficult to detect microscopically, and in many cases are not to be found in skin or mucous membrane lesions but are confined to the nerve tissues.

Course and Termination.—While a fatal termination is almost always the result in nodular leprosy, in the nerve type the disease may be arrested at any stage; in fact, as the disease usually lasts many years, it is very likely that the victim may die of an intercurrent affection.

(c) *Mixed Leprosy.*—Many cases of leprosy exhibit manifestations of both of the types that have been described. Lesions or symptoms of each type may be present from the outset, or the case may begin as a clean-cut nodular or as a simple nerve case and gradually take on manifestations of the other type.

Generally *the hair* over a lesion falls out. This is especially noticeable when the supra-orbital regions are involved and the eyebrows disappear. As is true of nodular leprosy, the scalp escapes and the hair on it remains unaffected.

LEPROUS FEVER.—The febrile manifestations of leprosy are by no means constant; indeed many cases run for long periods without any fever. Fever may occur as a part of the general disturbance that marks the beginning of the disease, but its nature is not usually recognized. The later manifestations of fever fall into two groups which were differentiated to the writer by Dr. W. J. Goodhue, Medical Superintendent at the Molokai Settlement. First, there is the febrile attack, occurring coincident with and due to a generalization of the infection through the blood stream and followed by the appearance of new tubercles. This may last a few days or a few weeks, but usually the temperature falls to normal, leaving the patient with some new lesions but otherwise not much changed. Second, there is the fever which marks the final decline of the patient. It may run steadily in the neighborhood of 39 to 40° C. (102.2 to 104° F.) for several months and is often associated with profuse sweating, and always with loss of flesh and strength. The temperature often falls to normal or to subnormal during the last days of the life of the victim.

SPECIAL TESTS.—*Microscopic Examination.*—In addition to the clinical features which have been discussed under the symptoms of the disease, we obtain much aid from *microscopic examination* of material from the skin lesions and from the nasal cavities. The specimens for microscopic examination from skin manifestations are prepared in the following manner: An area of thickening, a nodule, or even an area of discoloration, is taken between the thumb and the forefinger and compression made so as to render the area as nearly bloodless as is possible. An incision is next made to a depth of perhaps a sixteenth of an inch and about a quarter of an inch in length. With the blade held at an angle to the sides of the tiny wound, a gentle scraping motion is made. For this purpose a safety razor blade is very convenient, as it can be discarded after each patient. The tissue fluid and tissue elements, secured in the manner described, are smeared on a glass slide, subjected to staining for acid-fast organisms in exactly the same manner as are preparations for the tubercle bacillus, and then examined microscopically.

The acid-fast organisms usually are abundant and are readily recognized. They are found in bundles or groups, as well as scattered through the field, and are often intracellular; occasionally very few organisms are to be seen, perhaps but one or two in a preparation. In this case it is better to make additional preparations from another part of the lesion or from other lesions.

Sections made from excised pieces of cutaneous tissue are sometimes resorted to as an aid in making a diagnosis. The prudent pathologist usually will do no more than express an opinion that a given lesion is consistent with leprosy unless he finds characteristic organisms, when, of course, a positive diagnosis is readily made.

The *examination of smears* from the nasal mucosa is frequently resorted to and often gives valuable information. There are fallacies here, however, that need to be guarded against. A few acid-fast organisms are not rare in the nasal secretions of persons other than those suffering from leprosy. In the nonleprous the bacilli found are usually much plumper than those in leprosy. It was once thought that acid-fast organisms were to be found in the nasal mucus early in the disease. This, however, is usually not the case and as an aid to diagnosis in early cases this examination is not of much importance. The author has seen unfortunate errors made by placing too much dependence on the results of the examination, of nasal smears, and would warn against drawing conclusions from these alone.

Serologic Tests.—There have been a number of serologic tests proposed for the diagnosis of leprosy, but none has been found trustworthy or of practical value. In this connection mention should be made of the fact that a goodly proportion of lepers will give a positive serologic test for syphilis, even in the absence of coexistent syphilis. The reason for this is not clear but the fact seems well established.

A large percentage of lepers react to *tuberculin* given by injection or by inunction. By some, this is regarded as evidence of the nearness, from a biologic point of view, of the leprosy bacillus and the tubercle bacillus.

Diagnosis.—In considering the diagnosis of leprosy we must remember that, generally, a correct diagnosis is of infinitely more importance than in most other diseases, since it may involve the whole future of the patient. With other infectious diseases an error may not do any serious harm, as at most it will merely mean a short period of detention for the patient; but in leprosy, if we err by failing to diagnose a case, we may permit the exposure of many persons, while if a case is diagnosed leprosy erroneously, the greatest injury and injustice is done the patient. He often becomes an outcast and, indeed, in many places loses his civil rights. The importance of these facts is recognized by those who are charged with the administrative control of leprosy and sometimes boards of experts are provided to pass upon cases. That there are very real difficulties of diagnosis encountered, is shown by the fact that boards of examiners are often compelled to defer a final decision until certain obscure lesions have had an opportunity to develop or to disappear.

In countries where leprosy is rarely seen, the chief obstacle to arriving at a correct diagnosis is simply that the disease does not occur to the mind of the examiner, since in marked cases there is no difficulty in reaching a correct decision once suspicion is aroused. Very early cases may defy even the most skillful, while late ones have the diagnosis stamped so plainly upon the features as to require but a glance to reveal the nature of the trouble. Collateral circumstances often are suggestive in aiding to make a diagnosis in a given case. Thus, if a patient never has been in an endemic focus of leprosy there is good reason to believe that some other diagnosis is the correct one; on the other hand, residence in an endemic focus, especially if there are other cases of leprosy among members of the family or other close associates, is to be taken into consideration. Such circumstances never offer conclusive evidence one way or the other, but they may be very helpful.

In cases of leprosy with infiltrated cutaneous lesions it is nearly always possible to confirm the diagnosis by the direct and conclusive evidence furnished by finding *Mycobacterium leprae* (Hansen's bacillus) in properly prepared smears or sections. Histopathologic evidence not supported by the finding of characteristic acid-fast rods is not ordinarily sufficient to justify a positive diagnosis. Probably no great harm would result if a diagnosis were made only when the characteristic organisms are found.

Early neural cases without infiltrated skin lesions may give rise to great difficulty since there is small probability of securing direct microscopic confirmation of one's suspicions. In such cases patchy anesthesia, localized hyperpigmentation or depigmentation, evidence of paralysis of the motor nerves and enlargement of nerve trunks are important signs pointing to leprosy, but it must be admitted that years may elapse before the signs become clear enough to warrant a definite diagnosis.

DIFFERENTIAL DIAGNOSIS.—Leprosy must be differentiated from two groups of diseases:

Cutaneous Diseases.—The skilled leprologist will usually be able to distinguish on clinical grounds the lesions of leprosy from those of diseases that simulate it, but often a microscopic examination is required to settle the point. Syphilis, ringworm, acne indurata, sarcoid, lupus erythematosus, vitiligo and a number of other conditions may lead to an erroneous diagnosis of leprosy. More often the diagnosis of leprosy is not considered and the condition mistakenly diagnosed as being one of those mentioned above, or some other cutaneous disease.

Organic Nerve Disease.—Syringomyelia is sometimes mistaken for leprosy but more often leprosy is mistakenly called syringomyelia. While cases in which there is a clearly defined preservation of tactile sense and loss of pain and thermic perception with lateral curvature of the spine may be labeled syringomyelia, it must be freely admitted that in some cases a definite diagnosis is not possible. Limitation of sensory and trophic changes to the upper extremities speaks for a diagnosis of syringomyelia, while patchy areas of anesthesia and trophic changes favor a diagnosis of leprosy. I have seen a case in which, during life, the diagnosis lay between syringomyelia and leprosy, and, at autopsy, proved to be neither.

Complications.—The leper may, and often does, suffer from the same diseases that affect other persons, but there are several maladies that some writers believe to have a special association with leprosy. These will be discussed briefly.

TUBERCULOSIS.—Pulmonary tuberculosis is a common complication of leprosy and accounts for many of the deaths among lepers. There are no special features of importance in tuberculosis when it develops in victims of leprosy.

SYPHILIS.—It is thought by some that syphilis bears a special relation to leprosy, but the author is convinced that the coincidence of the two infections is without special significance. There is some difficulty in making a diagnosis between the two diseases occasionally, but careful observation usually will serve to make the clinical diagnosis clear. Serologic tests for syphilis are of little value in making a decision as many cases of uncomplicated leprosy show a positive test, as has been stated before.

Treatment.—GENERAL MEASURES.—One of the surprising features in dealing with leprosy is the improvement which cases often show when first brought under isolation at a well-managed institution for the care of these people. Various observers have noted that many cases, perhaps the majority, will begin to improve in general nutrition, as evidenced by a gain in weight and in spirits, and even by a marked change in dermic lesions soon after isolation. Good food, kindly care, and a life now free from the harassing fear of detection must be credited with the amelioration of symptoms that is observed. Certain it is, that the most gratifying changes often occur and that **good surroundings** and **good food** must be considered potent auxiliaries in any plan for the treatment of leprosy.

Certain natural baths, especially several found in Japan, have been held in high esteem in the treatment of leprosy but probably have no definite value.

Artificial baths have also been used. Indeed, a large grove of eucalyptus trees at the Hawaiian leper settlement, Molokai, bear mute testimony to the faith certain physicians had in the use of a bath, which was made of a weak decoction of the aromatic leaves of these trees. Alkalis, notably sodium bicarbonate, are frequently added to the baths. While it is desirable that the patient be encouraged to take frequent warm baths, it seems improbable that any medicament applied in this manner is of any special value.

MEDICINAL TREATMENT.—It is becoming the rather general opinion of many, perhaps of the majority of those experienced in the treatment of leprosy, that medication is of minor importance. Disappointment generally has followed the use of the various alleged specifics. This is true even as regards **chaulmoogra oil** and its derivatives, the **ethyl esters,** preparations that have been used more extensively than any other. While many clinicians continue to claim benefit from the use of chaulmoogra oil (and similar agents) and while it is almost universally used, the physician and the patient must not expect too much from it. When administered by mouth the oil is conveniently given in gelatin capsules, beginning with five drops as a dose two or three times a day after meals, increasing up to as high as the patient will tolerate, sometimes as much as 100 drops thrice daily. The drug, especially in the larger doses, is very likely to nauseate the patient and if this causes distress the dose must be reduced, or the drug discontinued, an occurrence that need not too greatly disturb either the physician or the patient. If the drug is to be given by the hypodermic route the following combination in use at the National Leprosarium at Carville, Louisiana, is as satisfactory as any:

Chaulmoogra oil	90	parts
Olive oil	10	"
Benzocaine	3	"

This is given intramuscularly in doses of 3 to 5 cc. once or twice weekly. Painful indurations occasionally may develop at the site of injections and rarely a cold abscess may form.

Another formula much used is that devised by Dr. Mercado in the Philippines:

Chaulmoogra oil	60 cc.	(fl.oz. ii)
Camphorated oil	60 cc.	(fl.oz. ii)
Resorcin	4 Gm.	(1.03 dr.)

The dose of this is 1 cc. intramuscularly twice weekly, increasing gradually to 5 cc. in each dose.

The ethyl esters of chaulmoogra oil are very popular. They may be given by mouth or by the intramuscular route in doses of 1 to 5 cc. Mercury, the iodides, strychnine, salvarsan, antimony and certain aniline dyes may be mentioned among the many agents that have been employed and lauded for a brief period, but finally have proved to be without specific curative value.

Biologic Agents.—Bacterial vaccines made from acid-fast organisms, grown from leprous tissue, have been employed, but without permanently good results. It would seem likely, considering the experience with other bacterial vaccines, that any agent of this sort should be made from the organism cultivated from the patient to be treated. The dose should be small to begin with—perhaps 50,000,000 organisms at an injection, and the number increased until a reaction is observed. A serum prepared by the immunization of the horse or the sheep with cultures of acid-fast organisms has been used, but it is not considered of any value.

The venom of certain poisonous serpents has been used in the treatment of leprosy, but there is no reason to believe that it is of any benefit.

Under this head it should be mentioned that there are examples reported of the recovery from leprosy after an attack of an infectious disease, as smallpox, and also after vaccination against smallpox.

The treatment of malaria, of hookworm infestation, and of other conditions from which the victim of leprosy may suffer, to be carried on simultaneously with the treatment of leprosy, is strongly stressed by some authorities.

In recent years great stress has been laid on diet in the treatment of leprosy but there is no agreement as to what elements of the **diet** are important beyond those essential to the maintenance of a good general condition of nutrition.

SURGICAL MEASURES.—It is the general experience that wounds in lepers will heal as they do in other persons. Surgical treatment may be undertaken, if necessary, to relieve some threatening complication or for purely cosmetic purposes. Under the former, may be mentioned the amputation of hopelessly necrotic feet, the removal of sequestra from bones of the hand or of the foot, and finally, and perhaps most important, the performance of tracheotomy for the relief of laryngeal stenosis. The latter is an operation demanded rather frequently and the results are so satisfactory that it should be done whenever it is indicated. The author doubts if anywhere in the range of surgery are more gratifying results obtained than in these cases. Under the influence of the rest afforded by the tracheal tube, infiltrated and ulcerated vocal cords may return to a relatively normal condition, and the tube often may be dispensed with after a few weeks or months. Other cases wear the tube for years without serious inconvenience. The author has seen this operation performed many times by Dr. W. J. Goodhue, and always with satisfactory results. Indeed, surgery of leprosy, as practiced by him at the Molokai Settlement, constitutes one of the most beneficial applications of the art.

Nodules may be removed for purely cosmetic purposes and, when the patient wishes such an operation performed, there is no reason why it should not be undertaken. Remarkable improvement in the appearance of the countenance may be brought about by the excision of disfiguring masses of leprous tissue.

LOCAL AGENTS.—Nodular and infiltrated areas have been treated with such **caustic agents** as trichloracetic acid, carbon dioxide snow and chromic acid, and the results appear to justify the use of these drugs though they cannot be regarded as curative.

The *dressing of ulcers* constitutes the largest part of the work at the dispensary of a leper colony. Ordinary surgical principles should be followed. **Balsam of Peru** is much used for lesions that require a mild stimulant; **silver nitrate** when there are extensive granulations, and **phenolated zinc oxide ointment** where a soothing application is required.

Sometimes intractable ulcerations of extremities are much benefited by the application of **Unna's paste** in the shape of a boot. Unna's paste is made by melting together:

Zinc oxide powder	6	parts
Gelatin (Knox)	6	"
Glycerin	12	"
Water	14	"

When it is to be used the mixture is melted in a water bath and painted on the ulcerated area, then a layer of gauze bandage is applied and covered with the melted paste; this is followed by a second and a third layer of bandage, each covered with the paste. The boot may be allowed to remain for ten days or two weeks. Dr. F. A. Johansen of the National Leprosarium at Carville, Louisiana, regards the method as being very valuable for indolent ulcerations.

RESULTS.—We may sum up the results of the treatment of leprosy by saying that, while we cannot expect to see many patients recover, a judicious, persistent application of general medicinal and surgical measures will go far toward ameliorating the distressing manifestations of many cases, and this is a goal well worth the best effort of the physician. Experience and observation have taught the author that lepers almost invariably do everything within their power to help the physician carry out any plan of treatment he may propose. The patience of these unfortunates and their confidence in the ability of the physician to aid them, are outstanding features at all properly conducted institutions for the care of lepers.

Prognosis.—The prognosis of leprosy, as regards life, is of course unfavorable, though the course of the disease is often so slow that there are ample opportunities for intercurrent diseases to cut short the life of the victim. A few die within three or four years of the onset, many survive ten or twelve years, and a not inconsiderable number live much longer than this.

In a fair proportion of cases, perhaps several per cent, active lesions disappear under treatment, or indeed without treatment, and for practical purposes the individual may be regarded as having recovered. Occasionally, all signs of the disease may disappear, or there may remain a slight deformity of the hand or other evidence of nerve involvement. These cases also may be regarded as recovered. Such cases may be discharged on condition that they report to the health authorities every three or four months in order that a recurrence may be detected promptly. In recent years it has become increasingly clear that leprosy may be arrested spontaneously at almost any stage.

Pathology.—Leprosy stands in an almost unique position among bacterial diseases on account of the large number of the specific micro-organisms usually found in the infiltrated lesions. When a section of a leprous nodule, or of an infiltration, is appropriately stained, the whole of the lesion may take the tint of the dye which has special affinities for the micro-organisms, and examination with higher powers of the microscope will show that the tissue spaces and even the cells are literally full of bacilli. Certain lesions of a secondary nature ordinarily do not contain bacilli. The large trophic necroses, such as involve the bones and soft tissues of the extremities, are usually free from acid-fast organisms, a point that must be kept in mind in the microscopic diagnosis of the disease. In many cases that come to autopsy, bacilli are found widely distributed even where the tissues show no gross evidence of disease. Thus, smears from the spleen may show many acid-fast bacilli without the organ showing any change, possibly beyond slight enlargement. Other organs usually show smaller numbers of the bacteria.

There has been much written on the presence of the leprosy bacillus in the circulating blood and rather conflicting observations are on record. The fact seems to be that there may be present, occasionally, a small number of organisms, except during the febrile attacks commonly called leprous fever, when the circulating blood may contain large numbers.

The essential lesion, the leproma, as it is often called, is a soft, elastic, slightly grayish or slightly yellowish mass which may vary in size from a pea to a mass several centimeters in diameter. The structure is made up of round and fusiform cells, sometimes with giant cells. The leprous infiltration is similar in its general characteristics but, as the name indicates, is less clearly circumscribed. All of the structures of the skin and the subcutaneous tissues are involved in the process.

The leprous lesion is often compared with that of tuberculosis, but as is the case with other features of the two diseases, the resemblance is rather superficial. The leprous lesion lacks the tendency to necrosis which is so early and so characteristic of the lesions caused by the tubercle bacillus; indeed, in many respects, the leprous lesions bear a closer resemblance to a neoplasm. In nerve leprosy, bacilli are likely to be scarce and difficult to find. The lymphatic glands, in nodular leprosy, always show infiltration and enlargement with numerous bacilli.

History.—There seems to be no good ground for doubting that Biblical and other ancient writings referring to leprosy do, at least in large part, deal with the same disease we call leprosy today, though there is equally good ground for believing that the leprosy of that day covered many diseases which we now recognize under other designations.

From the twelfth to the seventeenth centuries of the Christian era, leprosy prevailed most extensively over the whole of the civilized world. Indeed, even if we make a liberal discount for errors in diagnosis and for exaggeration in the accounts that have come down to us, there still remains no doubt that this disease was one of the most dreadful scourges that ever has afflicted the human race. During this period the contagious nature of the disease was well recognized, as of course it was in Biblical times, and a very extensive system of hospitals or lazarettos was established. The number of these institutions is said to have run far into the thousands, though most of them had but few inmates. It is claimed that traces of this medieval leprosy still remain in southern and western Europe. Of course we cannot be certain that these small European foci do not represent reinfection such as we know brought about the outbreak in the Memel district of East Prussia in the latter half of the nineteenth century. That the traces of this medieval widespread prevalence of leprosy are in the relatively near past is emphasized by the fact that it was only about the middle of the eighteenth century that the disease disappeared from the north of Scotland.

What often has been called the modern recrudescence of leprosy began in Europe in the early part of the nineteenth century, and it was in Norway that the disease first attracted attention. It is a remarkable fact that shortly after the disease had vanished from the United Kingdom and had practically disappeared from the other countries in western Europe, it began to occur or to increase in Scandinavian countries, particularly Norway, and for about one century constituted one of the serious medical problems of those countries. This recrudescence, however, led to the careful studies that have given us much of our extensive, though still incomplete, knowledge of the disease.

Distribution.—In considering the present-day distribution of leprosy one must carefully differentiate between where the disease *exists* and where it *spreads,* a fact which has a most important bearing on the problem of the official handling of cases. There is no civilized country which does not have its quota of imported lepers, but with rare exceptions the disease shows no tendency to spread. In the large cities of western Europe a considerable number of lepers, infected abroad, are domiciled and only very exceptionally is the infection transmitted. That the disease does not spread in these and in many other places is well established, though why it does not do so we do not know. Obviously, if the disease does not spread in a given locality, we need not be especially concerned about measures for its suppression there. This relative or absolute immunity of certain parts of the world is well exemplified in the United States. There long have been two chief foci of the disease in the United States. One is in the Northwest, chiefly in Minnesota; the other is in the Gulf States, chiefly in parts of Louisiana, Florida and Texas. There is one outstanding difference between these foci. In the former the disease shows a tendency to extinguishment. From a total of perhaps one hundred imported cases there has been a very slight tendency to spread; perhaps half a dozen would cover cases of local origin. On the other hand, in the Gulf Coast foci many cases are of local origin. In other words, the disease spreads in certain parts of the South but does not spread in the Northwest. We know also that there are always a number of lepers in New York City, yet there is no well-authenticated case of local origin—all are imported. This striking fact of the failure of the disease to spread in certain localities is usually accounted for by the better sanitary conditions under which people live as compared with the conditions where the disease does show a tendency to spread. It would not be profitable to discuss this point but it does not seem to be a very satisfactory explanation.

The total number of lepers in the continental United States (1939) is variously estimated. About 350 are in the National Leprosarium near Carville, Louisiana, and probably as many cases are at large. The opinion generally held by leprologists is that the total number in this country is at least 500 and there are some who believe that it will run up to 2,000.

The Insular possessions of the United States have large numbers of lepers and special asylums are provided for them, the most important being the Hawaiian colony at Molokai and the Philippine colony at Culion. The countries of Central and South America are all more or less afflicted with leprosy, Colombia perhaps being the country having the largest number in proportion to the population, and Chile the smallest.

In Europe the disease is disappearing from Scandinavian countries but remains prevalent in parts of Russia, and the Baltic countries, formerly part of Russia, and occurs, although in small numbers, in nearly all the countries bordering on the Mediterranean.

In Africa the disease is widespread and in some parts it is extremely prevalent. Repressive measures have been taken in certain parts that are under European domination.

In Asia the disease is very common. India is estimated to have a million lepers, Japan about forty thousand, and the number in China is very large, but no trustworthy estimate has been made. The Pacific Islands are practically all centers of leprosy, some of them comparatively recent. Thus, leprosy in Hawaii began about the middle of the nineteenth century and within a few years had become so prevalent that at one time more than 2 per cent of the native people were afflicted with the disease. The splendid fight made by the Hawaiian people against the scourge is one which might well be emulated by larger and richer communities. The disease is at present (1939) slowly declining in Hawaii.

REFERENCES

For a detailed discussion of the various problems relating to leprosy, the reader is referred to the *International Journal of Leprosy*, to the files of *Lepra*, and to the publications of the U. S. Public Health Service which record the work of the U. S. Leprosy Investigation Station in Hawaii.

DENGUE FEVER

By Charles F. Craig, M.D., M.A. (Hon.), F.A.C.P., F.A.C.S., Colonel,
U. S. Army Medical Corps (Ret.), D.S.M.

Synonyms.—Breakbone fever, seven-day fever, three-day fever, giraffe fever, bouquet fever, ankle fever.

Definition.—Dengue fever is an acute, infectious disease, caused by a filtrable virus which is transmitted from person to person through the bites of certain mosquitoes, the species most frequently acting as transmitting agents being *Aedes aegypti* and *Aedes albopictus*. Clinically, the disease is characterized by a very sudden onset; severe pains in the muscles, bones and joints; marked leukopenia; a rapidly rising temperature, followed by a recession on the third or fourth day, a secondary rise, and a critical fall to normal or below normal on the fifth, sixth or seventh day; a typical skin eruption usually appearing during the secondary rise in temperature or just before the crisis of the fever; and by marked prostration, both mental and physical.

Etiology.—Dengue fever has been known as a disease entity since 1779, when it was first described by Boylon, in Java, but the best description of it was given by Benjamin Rush, in Philadelphia, in 1880, who studied an epidemic of this infection in that city. Until the researches of Ashburn and Craig, in the Philippine Islands, in 1907, the disease was always regarded as of bacterial origin and as one of the most contagious of all acute infections, and several investigators had described bacteria which they regarded as of etiologic significance. None of these bacteria could be confirmed as the cause of the infection although many attempts at confirmation were made by well-qualified observers. In 1903 Graham produced the disease by the bites of mosquitoes which had bitten dengue patients, and described an organism which he claimed occurred in the blood and which he regarded as a protozoon and the probable cause of the infection. While Graham's protozoon has not been confirmed, numerous investigators have confirmed the transmission of dengue by mosquitoes, as will appear later.

Our accurate knowledge of the etiology of dengue fever dates from the observations of Ashburn and Craig in 1907. At that time the writer, together with the late Colonel P. M. Ashburn, was serving on the United States Army Board for the Study of Tropical Diseases in the Philippines, and the occurrence of an extensive epidemic of dengue among the United States troops afforded us an excellent opportunity for the study of the etiology of this disease. As the result of our experiments and studies we reached the following conclusions regarding the etiology and epidemiology of dengue fever:

1. No organism, either bacterium or protozoon, could be demonstrated in either fresh or stained preparations of dengue blood, with the compound microscope.

2. No organism of etiologic significance occurred in bouillon or citrated cultures of the blood.

3. The intravenous inoculation of unfiltered dengue blood into healthy men is followed by a typical attack of the disease.

4. The intravenous inoculation of filtered dengue blood into healthy men is followed by a typical attack of the disease.

5. The cause of the disease is, therefore, ultramicroscopic, being filtrable.

6. The cause of the disease is present in the blood during the first four days of the disease.

7. Dengue can be transmitted by the mosquito, *Culex fatigans.*

8. Certain individuals are immune to dengue as proved by negative results obtained after intravenous injection of dengue blood.

9. The period of incubation in experimental dengue averaged three days and fourteen hours.

10. Dengue is not a contagious disease, but is infectious in the same manner as are yellow fever and malaria, as proved by our failure to transmit the disease by contact with either the person or clothing of infected individuals.

All of the above conclusions have been confirmed by later investigators and much has been added to our knowledge of the virus of the disease by more recent observers. The fundamental work of Ashburn and the writer was made possible by the courageous action of soldiers of the United States Army, who volunteered for experimental inoculations with the blood of dengue patients, and most of the more recent developments in our knowledge of the etiology and epidemiology of dengue fever have been rendered possible by both soldier and civilian volunteers.

While the work of Ashburn and the writer demonstrated that dengue fever is caused by a filtrable virus and that the disease is not contagious, it has remained for others to add greatly to our knowledge of the properties of the virus and the mechanism of transmission by the mosquitoes concerned. Ashburn and Craig (1907) found that the virus passed through a Lilliput diatomaceous filter that retained the smallest known bacteria, and later Cleland, Bradley and McDonald (1919) found that it could pass the Pasteur-Chamberland F filter; Blanc and Caminopétros (1928), the Pasteur-Chamberland L and L_3 filters; Kligler and Ashner (1928), the Berkefeld N filter; and Simmons, St. John and Reynolds (1931), the Berkefeld V filter. All of these observations prove that the virus of dengue is of small size as compared with many other viruses.

The thermal death point of the dengue virus, according to Manoussakis (1928), is 50° C. (122° F.) maintained for half an hour. It retains its virulence if stored in the icebox at 0° C. (32° F.) for two months, according to Blanc, Caminopétros and Manoussakis (1928), while exposure to direct sunlight for thirty minutes failed to kill the virus. If the virus is dried and frozen it will remain virulent for a long time. Thus, Findlay (1932) successfully inoculated human volunteers in London with dengue blood serum which had been desiccated for several weeks, and Hoffmann, Mertens and Snijders (1932) produced dengue in human volunteers in Amsterdam with dried dengue serum transported from Java and 285 days old at the time of inoculation.

The dengue virus is resistant to certain chemicals, as shown by several observers. It will remain virulent after being exposed to 95 per cent alcohol for several minutes and resists a 1 : 500 solution of neutral red for 7 hours and a 1 : 800 dilution of formalin for 5 hours. It is quickly rendered harmless by weak concentrations of lactic acid, Lugol's solution, potassium permanganate, oleic acid, gentian violet and quinine.

Simmons, St. John and Reynolds (1931) demonstrated that the virus cannot pass through the unbroken skin of man and that it is filtrable as it occurs in the transmitting mosquitoes. Siler, Hall and Hitchens (1926) demonstrated that the virus is in the blood of dengue patients in a suitable condition for infecting mosquitoes for several hours before the occurrence of clinical symptoms and remains in the blood in an infective condition for three days after symptoms occur, while more rarely the blood may remain infective for as long as four days, as shown by Ashburn and Craig (1907).

Apparently almost all of the lower animals are immune to natural infection with the dengue virus, but guinea pigs and monkeys can be infected and, although no clinical symptoms follow such infection, their blood may produce the disease in man. Simmons, St. John and Reynolds (1931) produced an infection in monkeys (*Macacus philippinensis*) caught at an elevation of 4,000 ft. in the mountains of Luzon, where dengue does not occur, but found that monkeys caught in dengue localities were apparently immune to infection. These investigators also produced infection in monkeys imported from Japan. In all of these animals infection was produced by *Aedes* mosquitoes which were allowed to bite infected human volunteers and it was found that, while no symptomatic infections resulted, *Aedes* mosquitoes fed upon the infected monkeys were capable of infecting other monkeys and human volunteers. Simmons (1931) suggests that, in regions where dengue is endemic or epidemic, monkeys may act as reservoirs of infection for man, as in yellow fever. The blood of infected monkeys was found infective to human volunteers from the fifth to the eighth day after inoculation and lost its infectivity after twelve days. Blanc, Caminopétros and Manoussakis (1928) found that the blood of guinea pigs inoculated with dengue blood serum became infective to man in five days after inoculation, and Findlay (1932) demonstrated that the blood of a monkey inoculated with dengue produced the disease in a human volunteer seven days after the inoculation of the animal. No experiments have been reported regarding the possible production of an encephalitis in mice by inoculation of the dengue virus, a method so valuable in the diagnosis of yellow fever, but it would appear probable that success might attend such a procedure and thus furnish us with a useful experimental animal in the study of this infection.

Epidemiology.—The transmission of dengue fever from man to man depends upon the inoculation of the virus by certain species of mosquitoes which have bitten infected persons. Graham (1903) was the first to prove this method of transmission, taking mosquitoes which had bitten dengue patients to an uninfested district and there producing the disease in human volunteers by allowing these mosquitoes to bite them. Graham stated that transmission occurred through the bites of *Culex quinquefasciatus* (*Culex fatigans*), although he admitted that some of the mosquitoes were *Aedes aegypti*. In the light of our present knowledge his successful cases must have been caused by *Aedes aegypti* instead of by *Culex quinquefasciatus*, or by mechanical transmission by the latter.

Bancroft, in Brisbane, Australia, in 1906, claimed to have produced dengue in two human volunteers by the bites of *Aedes aegypti*. It is probable that his claim is correct, although some writers have cast doubt upon his results because an epidemic of dengue fever was raging in Brisbane at that time and the volunteers might have become naturally infected. In 1907 Ashburn and the writer obtained one successful infection in a human volunteer by the bites of *Culex quinquefasciatus*, but this result was undoubtedly due to a mechanical transmission of the virus, as it has been shown that mechanical transmission can occur under certain conditions.

The first investigators to demonstrate beyond doubt the species of mosquito concerned in the transmission of dengue fever were Cleland, Bradley and McDonald (1916) in Australia. These workers proved that dengue is transmitted by *Aedes aegypti* (*Stegomyia fasciata*), the same mosquito that usually transmits yellow fever, and their observations were confirmed in 1926 by Siler, Hall and Hitchens, the latter observers demonstrating that *Culex quinquefasciatus* does not transmit this infection after a period of incubation in the mosquito, and that *Aedes aegypti* is the common transmitting agent, the mosquitoes becoming infective after the virus has incubated in the body of the insects for a period of approximately eleven days after the mosquitoes have fed upon an infected individual.

Mechanical transmission of the dengue virus by other mosquitoes is possible, and probably by other Arthropoda if conditions are favorable. Simmons, St. John and Reynolds (1931) produced infection in human volunteers by the bites of *Culex quinquefasciatus,* if the mosquitoes were allowed to bite the volunteers shortly after biting a patient suffering from dengue fever, but the bites of several mosquitoes were necessary in order to produce an infection. The blood of the patient is carried upon and within the proboscis of the mosquito and remains infective for several hours. Their observations explain the one positive result obtained by Ashburn and the writer (1907), in which experiment many *Culex quinquefasciatus* mosquitoes were allowed to bite a human volunteer shortly after they had bitten a dengue patient, with the production of a typical attack of dengue in the volunteer. How important this method of transmission may be when conditions are favorable, as in a severe epidemic when both *Aedes aegypti* and *Culex quinquefasciatus* are numerous, has not been determined, nor whether other biting or sucking arthropods may transmit the disease mechanically.

Aedes aegypti is the most common transmitter of dengue fever but other mosquitoes have been found capable of transmitting the infection. Morishita (1925), Simmons, St. John and Reynolds (1931), and Snijders, Dinger and Schüffner (1931) have all demonstrated that *Aedes albopictus* is an efficient transmitter of dengue. The latter investigators brought mosquitoes of this species that had bitten dengue patients in Sumatra to Amsterdam, where dengue has never occurred, and produced the disease in human volunteers by the bites of such mosquitoes. In Formosa, Morishita (1925) found that the mosquito, *Armigeres obturbans,* was capable of transmitting dengue, and it is more than probable that further research will demonstrate that still other mosquitoes may act as transmitting agents under favorable conditions.

The fate of the dengue fever virus after being ingested by the transmitting mosquito has been studied by numerous observers. As already stated, mosquitoes may become infected if they bite a dengue fever patient during the last day of the incubation period or for from three to four days after the appearance of clinical symptoms, after which time the virus is in insufficient quantity in the peripheral blood of the patient to be able to infect a mosquito. After biting, a variable period must elapse before the mosquito is able to infect man. This period is usually stated in texts to be from eleven to twelve days but may be shorter or longer, depending upon biologic conditions. Thus, Schule (1928) found that *Aedes aegypti* may become infective as early as eight days after biting a dengue patient and that the length of this period of incubation in the mosquito could be diminished by heat and prolonged by exposure to cold temperatures. Simmons, St. John and Reynolds (1930), in their work with *Aedes albopictus,* found that this species did not become infective to human volunteers until from 13 to 22 days after biting an infected individual, while Blanc and Caminopétros (1929) determined that *Aedes aegypti* is unable to transmit dengue fever if the flies are kept at a temperature below 18° C. (64.4° F.). The virus does not undergo a cycle of development in the mosquito comparable to that of the malaria plasmodia during the stage of incubation, but multiplies until it permeates all of the tissues and reaches the salivary glands and saliva. When this occurs the mosquito becomes infective through the saliva being ejected into the wound made by the proboscis of the fly while feeding. Holt and Kintner (1931) demonstrated the presence of the dengue virus in the salivary glands, the contents of the intestine, the ovaries and the legs of infected *Aedes aegypti,* by inoculating suspensions of these substances into human volunteers. The virus in the mosquito is filtrable.

After becoming infective mosquitoes remain so for life, so far as is known. This fact was first demonstrated by Siler, Hall and Hitchens (1926), and these investigators also showed that the infection is not hereditary in the mosquito, but Simmons, St. John, Holt and Reynolds found that the virus could be transmitted from mosquito to mosquito by copulation, under experimental conditions. Another possible method of transmission of the virus to man from the mosquito, which does not necessitate a period of incubation in these flies, is through the regurgitation of blood from the stomach which sometimes occurs if they are interrupted in feeding. If such flies immediately feed upon another individual, blood is often regurgitated from the stomach and, if it contains the virus, as it would had the flies first fed upon a dengue patient, infection of the second individual bitten might occur.

Immunity to dengue may be natural or acquired by passing through an attack of the disease. Ashburn and the writer (1907) proved that some individuals are naturally immune to dengue by inoculating human volunteers who had never suffered from the disease with dengue blood and with negative results. Our observations were confirmed by the experiments of Siler, Hall and Hitchens (1926) and they also demonstrated that an attack of dengue is followed by an immunity, while Simmons, St. John and Reynolds (1931) found that 100 per cent of individuals who had suffered from an attack of dengue were immune to experimental reinfection one year later. However, in nature, one sometimes sees a second attack of dengue during an epidemic of this disease and some authorities state that third attacks have been observed within a year. Usually an attack does protect for a limited period of time and Sharp and Hollar (1935) state that the immunity resulting from an attack lasts from one to three years. Simmons (1931) found in experimental infections in human volunteers a protective immunity lasting for 13 months, and that natives and monkeys in endemic regions were immune. He suggested that in this disease, as in yellow fever, monkeys may act as a reservoir of infection for man. Immune bodies are in all probability produced in the blood during an attack of dengue, as shown by the work of Shortt (1938), but convalescent serum does not protect against infection.

The great similarity between the viruses of dengue and yellow fever, as well as certain clinical manifestations of these two infections, was stressed by the writer (Craig) in 1911. Both infections are caused by a filtrable virus which is transmitted from man to man by *Aedes aegypti* after a similar period of development in the transmitting mosquitoes; in both, the virus is present in the blood during the latter portion of the period of incubation and for from three to four days after the appearance of symptoms; both may be produced by the injection of the filtered blood of the patient during the period mentioned above; in both the periods of incubation are practically identical; both are accompanied by a leukopenia and slow pulse in relation to the temperature; both present frequently a "saddleback" type of temperature curve; and both may be transmitted by other species of mosquito than *Aedes aegypti* under favorable conditions. In fact, one must admit that the viruses causing dengue and yellow fever are very closely related, the chief difference between them being the much greater virulence of the yellow fever virus, which is frequently fatal to infected individuals, while the virus of dengue very rarely causes death.

The similarity of the viruses has led some authorities to institute experiments to ascertain whether an attack of either disease produced immunity to the other. Thus, Dinger and Snijders (1931) stated that, experimentally, monkeys recovered from dengue fever were immune to yellow fever; but in the later experiments of Snijders, Postmus and Schüffner, in which the mouse protection test was employed in order to demonstrate the possible presence of immunity, it was found that the dengue virus did not possess any protective value against yellow fever. It will be interesting to observe whether the widespread vaccination of man against yellow fever within recent years will have any effect upon the occurrence of epidemics of dengue fever in endemic regions of the disease, as both infections frequently occur in the same localities.

With the exception of influenza, there is no acute infection of man that spreads as rapidly as does dengue fever in a nonimmune population, and no disease exhibits a greater morbidity. In an epidemic observed by Ashburn and the writer, at Fort McKinley, Philippine Islands, over 60 per cent of the entire military command suffered from the disease. Armstrong (1923), in an epidemic in Austin, Texas, states there were 16,000 cases in a population of 22,000 people. As in yellow fever, there is a pause of several days between the first case of dengue and the development of secondary cases, caused by the time required for development within the transmitting mosquito, and this fact leads us to the conclusion that great epidemics of dengue must be due to unusual prevalence of suitable mosquitoes for its transmission, in the presence of a large nonimmune population. In fact, it has often been noted that *Aedes aegypti* mosquitoes were unusually numerous just before and during epidemics of dengue fever. The great rapidity of the spread of this disease renders it one of military importance, for its occurrence in an army in the field might so deplete the number of soldiers as to cause serious military reverses.

The epidemiology of dengue fever depends upon factors having to do with the breeding and development of the transmitting mosquito, which is usually *Aedes aegypti*, and the presence of nonimmune individuals in a community. If the latter are present and an infected individual is introduced, the future history of the disease will depend entirely upon the number of *Aedes aegypti* present. The habits of this mosquito peculiarly fit it for the transmission of the disease, as it is a house mosquito, breeding in close proximity to human habitations and in small domestic collections of water. For a discussion of the breeding places and habits of this mosquito the reader is referred to the chapter on Yellow Fever.

While dengue is one of the most rapidly spreading of all infections it is not contagious, as first proved by Ashburn and the writer in 1907. We allowed human volunteers to sleep in the same garments as had been worn by dengue patients, eat from their table utensils, and live in mosquito-proof tents with dengue patients, and in no instance was the disease contracted from such contact. We also treated 120 patients in our mosquito-proof dengue hospital and none of the hospital attendants contracted the disease although in close contact with the patients for a period of over four months. At the hospital at Fort McKinley, P. I., also screened, where over 600 cases of dengue were treated in the general wards, not a single case of this disease originated among other patients with whom the dengue patients were in contact, thus confirming the results of our experimental observations.

Dengue is usually a disease of subtropical and tropical climates where conditions are most favorable to the development of the transmitting mosquitoes, but it may occur in temperate regions when temperatures favor the breeding of *Aedes aegypti*, as in the late spring, summer and early fall months. Frost quickly terminates dengue epidemics by killing the transmitting mosquitoes, as is the case with yellow fever, so that the disease is essentially one of the warm months in temperate regions. In the tropics epidemics are most apt to occur after the rainy season and the disease is most prevalent along the coast and in the deltas of rivers. The geographic distribution, climatic conditions being favorable, corresponds with the geographic distribution of *Aedes aegypti*, the principal transmitting mosquito, but great epidemics of this disease are only possible if a large nonimmune population is present in the locality.

Symptomatology.—The *period of incubation* in dengue varies considerably, apparently depending upon the dosage of the virus injected by the mosquito and upon the resistance of the individual. Ashburn and the writer (1907) found that it varies from three to eight days in naturally acquired infections and from two and a half to seven days in human volunteers inoculated with blood from dengue patients, the average period being three and three-quarter days. Cleland, Bradley and McDonald (1916) found the period of incubation in indi-

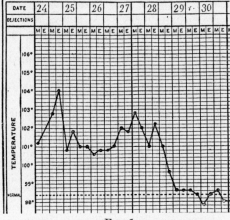

FIG. 1

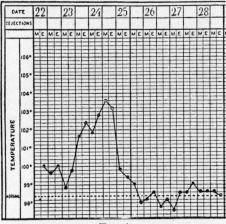

FIG. 4

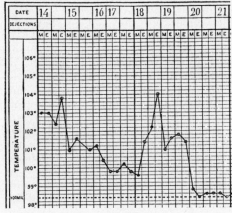

FIG. 2

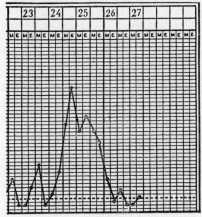

FIG. 5

FIGS. 4 AND 5.—Temperature curves of dengue fever of shorter duration and without "saddleback" type of curve. (After Ashburn and Craig.)

FIG. 3

FIGS. 1, 2 AND 3.—Temperature charts of dengue fever showing typical "saddleback" type of curve. (After Ashburn and Craig.)

42102

FIG. 6.—Temperature curve of dengue fever. A common type of curve. (After Ashburn and Craig.)

viduals experimentally inoculated by infected mosquitoes to vary from six to
ten days; Siler, Hall and Hitchens (1926), from four to six days; and Simmons,
St. John and Reynolds (1931) from three to eleven days, the average being five
and a quarter days. Shorter periods of incubation have been observed after
intravenous inoculation of dengue blood than after infection by the mosquito,
as might be expected, larger amounts of the virus being thus introduced. In nature, periods of incubation varying from four to fifteen days have been observed
but the usual period is from five to eight days.

The *onset* of dengue symptoms is exceedingly sudden in the vast majority
of cases. The patient often is able to date the exact moment of the onset and
almost always can tell the exact hour in which his symptoms appeared. Prodromal symptoms, consisting of loss of appetite, headache, malaise and slight
aching in the muscles, may rarely be present; but usually the muscle ache, headache, prostration and other symptoms of the onset occur very suddenly and
there is no prodromal stage, as in so many other acute infections.

The patient, who is apparently in perfect health, is suddenly overcome by a
sense of extreme lassitude accompanied by severe headache, aching in the muscles, especially of the lumbar region, and weakness of the arms and legs. The
temperature rises rapidly, reaching 39 to 41° C. (102.2 to 105.8° F.) within
twenty-four hours, the average maximum lying between 39.5 and 40° C. (103.1
and 104° F.). In very mild infections the temperature may not go above 38°
C. (100.4° F.) and in the mildest cases may not even reach that point. Along
with the rise in temperature there is, in the average case, severe lumbar aching
which extends into the legs and arms, together with soreness of the muscles of
the eyes and postorbital soreness and sometimes distinct pain in the eyeballs.
The postorbital soreness is considered as peculiar to this disease by some authorities but may be present in other acute infections although not to the same
extent as in dengue. Headache increases in severity and the face is greatly
flushed, the eyes are brilliant and the conjunctivae much congested. The appetite is lost and slight nausea may be present and vomiting may occur. In the
mildest recognizable cases the only symptoms may be slight headache and backache, with general malaise, and there undoubtedly occur cases in which even
these symptoms may not be noted. Such infections are of great importance
from the standpoint of transmission of the disease as they are capable of infecting the mosquito.

Upon the second day of the disease, in a case of moderate severity, the symptoms are well marked. The face is flushed and often appears to be mottled,
the so-called "primary eruption" of the disease. The eyes are sparkling and
the conjunctivae much congested. Movement of the eyeballs is sometimes exceedingly painful and there is pronounced soreness postorbitally upon pressure.
The headache and pains in the back and limbs are often very intense and the
patient complains of pains in the joints and bones. However, these pains are
really in the insertion of the muscles rather than in the bony structures, which
are unaffected in dengue fever. Some patients complain of pain in the joints
upon movement, but in the experience of Ashburn and the writer, the pain was
in the muscle tendons in all cases we observed. Anorexia is usually pronounced
and nausea and vomiting may be present. The mental condition is usually
one of depression and irritability, and in some cases slight delirium may be
present if the temperature is high, or somnolence or stupor may occur. In children, convulsions may occur and mild delirium of a quiescent, muttering type is
frequently present. Constipation is the rule, although some cases are troubled
with a slight diarrhea. Prostration is pronounced, greatly out of proportion to
the seriousness of the infection, and the patient frequently complains of the excessive sense of muscular weakness in the arms and legs. Troubled sleep is a
frequent symptom, the patients falling asleep frequently only to be suddenly
awakened by distressing dreams, and mental depression may be extreme in such
cases.

The typical attack of dengue fever consists in a primary stage, in which the temperature rises and remains above normal for a variable period; a stage of remission during which the fever may fall to normal or slightly above normal; and a terminal stage, in which the fever again rises and finally terminates by crisis.

The primary stage, which has just been described, lasts for three to four days, in the average case, at the end of which time the temperature falls rapidly, often accompanied by profuse perspiration, diarrhea, and polyuria. Usually this remission in the temperature does not reach normal but a degree or two above normal, and lasts for a few hours to one or two days, during which time most of the symptoms disappear and the patient believes himself on the road to recovery. However, in most cases, a secondary rise in the temperature occurs, the fever reaching a point about as high as in the primary rise, and persisting for one or more days, terminating by crisis. During this time the symptoms noted in the primary stage recur but usually less severely, although in some cases the mental depression is much more pronounced and muscular aching may be more severe. The characteristic temperature curve produced by the primary rise, the remission, and the secondary rise gives the so-called "saddleback" appearance to the temperature curve which by some authorities is thought to be typical of dengue fever. The occurrence of many cases in which only one rise in the temperature is noted, and of various modifications of the "typical" curve, renders it of less value as a diagnostic criterion, although, when present, it is certainly very suggestive. Similar curves may occur in other diseases, as yellow fever.

During the second febrile attack the characteristic eruption of dengue appears, usually first upon the dorsum of the hands and feet, then upon the arms and legs, and finally involves the face and the trunk. With the appearance of the eruption, which is of a measly or scarlatiniform character, the crisis in the temperature occurs and the symptoms rapidly disappear, convalescence usually being prompt although it may be prolonged and accompanied by symptoms of marked mental depression. The entire attack, in a case of average severity, covers from five to seven days, but marked variations occur in the clinical types of dengue; some patients show so few symptoms as to make the diagnosis impossible, while others present very severe symptoms and the attack may cover as much as nine to ten days.

ANALYSIS OF SYMPTOMS AND PHYSICAL FINDINGS.—*Skin Eruptions.*—The skin eruptions that occur in this infection are of great diagnostic importance, especially in differentiating dengue from yellow fever, with which it is most often confused. It is probable that in every case of dengue of sufficient severity to cause definite symptoms a skin eruption occurs, while in yellow fever such an eruption is absent. The eruptions that have been reported as occurring in dengue fever have varied considerably in morphology and most of the older writers described a "primary" and a "secondary" eruption. From our observations, Ashburn and the writer concluded that this so-called primary eruption, which occurs at the onset of the infection, is not a true eruption but is simply a general flushing of the skin caused by the dilatation of the capillaries. It is often very evanescent and occurs upon the face, neck, arms, thighs, chest and back, and markedly resembles the rash of scarlatina. Most authorities agree that it should not be regarded as an eruption and it should not be confused with the true eruption, which usually occurs just before the crisis, after the secondary rise in temperature, although it may occur at the time of the secondary rise and even as late as in convalescence. In most cases the eruption occurs between the third and sixth days of the disease, depending upon the time that the secondary rise in temperature occurs.

The true eruption of dengue is often very evanescent and unless carefully watched for is apt to be overlooked. In many patients it does not last for more than two or three hours but it may persist for several days. It is believed that practically all cases of dengue of severity sufficient to cause definite symptoms present this eruption at some time, but, as stated, owing to the fact that it may appear and fade away within a short time, it may be missed. In the writer's experience it occurred in nearly 80 per cent of the cases he has observed and it is probable that many eruptions were missed because of their evanescent character.

The eruption frequently is noted first around the wrists or on the hand near the base of the thumbs and within a short time extends to the trunk, arms, thighs, legs and feet, or covers the entire body. Its morphologic character appears to have varied considerably in different epidemics, if one can believe the descriptions given by different observers. Macular, papular, maculopapular, petechial, measly and scarlatiniform eruptions have all been described as occurring in this disease, but in the writer's experience the most common form observed has been a measles-like eruption but with much finer macules, arranged in smaller groups, and of a brighter red color. The same blotchy appearance may be observed as in measles but there is not the bluish-red color generally present in the eruption of measles. An eruption resembling that of scarlet fever is frequently observed, consisting of minute reddish points so closely arranged as to give the appearance of an almost solid erythema. A petechial eruption is more rarely noted in which minute red or purple dots are superimposed upon the usual eruption, these dots being caused by minute hemorrhages in the skin. The palms of the hands and the soles of the feet frequently present a bright red flushing and all types of the eruption are usually accompanied by some itching or the itching may precede the eruption. Urticarial eruptions have been described by some writers, but the writer has never observed such an eruption.

As already stated, the dengue eruption may last only a few hours but usually it persists for two or three days and, in very severe cases, it may last for as long as a week, but this is exceedingly rare. As the eruption disappears a very fine furfuraceous desquamation occurs in most cases, especially marked in the patients who have had severe infections. The desquamation is usually accompanied by considerable itching and persists for several days. In some blond patients the skin presents a slight brownish discoloration for some time after the eruption has disappeared. Jaundice never occurs in an uncomplicated case of dengue fever.

The Pulse.—In most cases of dengue fever the pulse corresponds with the elevation in temperature during the primary rise of the latter but tends to become slower than would be expected with a corresponding temperature, as the disease advances. The writer has not observed the abnormally slow pulse described by some writers and Faget's sign, i.e., a slowing pulse with a rising temperature, is not observed in dengue as it is in yellow fever. It is during convalescence that a marked slowing of the pulse sometimes occurs, at which time it is usually decreased in tension and may be more or less irregular, following severe infections.

The Alimentary System.—Anorexia is an invariable symptom throughout the entire attack and may persist into convalescence. Nausea is a frequent symptom but vomiting is rather unusual except in very severe cases, and both nausea and vomiting usually disappear after the intermission in the temperature. Constipation is usually present but diarrhea may occur, and pain in the abdomen and abdominal colic are not infrequently observed. The abdomen may be somewhat tender upon pressure and the patient may complain of soreness and tenderness in this region upon movement in bed. The *tongue* presents a somewhat characteristic appearance in many cases, being coated with a cream-colored fur during the first day or two of the disease. This fur becomes thickened and darker in color toward the middle as the disease progresses, at the same time tending to disappear from the edges of the tongue. By the end of the third day the tip and edges of the tongue are clean, while the middle is coated with a yellowish-brown or brown furry coating, which appears moist and free from fissures.

Hemorrhages from any portion of the body are rarely observed in dengue fever and in the experience of Ashburn and the writer, and of Siler, Hall and Hitchens, epistaxis was never observed although this symptom has been described as common by some authorities. Neither has the writer ever observed hemorrhages from the mucous membranes of the mouth or pharynx, or the stomach or intestine, all of which have been described as occurring in some cases of dengue fever. It is the belief of the writer that such cases may have been infections with yellow fever, in which disease hemorrhages are almost always present even in the milder types of the disease. Menstrual hemorrhages may occur in dengue fever and petechiae may be present upon the skin, as already noted.

The Circulatory System.—The heart is not markedly affected in dengue, even in severe infections, but patients sometimes complain of pain or discomfort in the precordium or a sense of suffocation, and syncope may rarely occur. The cardiac rhythm was not altered in any of the patients we observed nor was there any evidence of the production of any lesion of the heart or pericardium.

The Blood.—Certain changes occur in the cellular constitution of the blood that are of much importance in the diagnosis of the disease. The erythrocyte count is not altered and the color index is normal. The most marked and characteristic change in the blood is the occurrence of a very marked leukopenia accompanied by changes in the relative number of the various types of leukocytes. Stitt (1906) called attention to the frequent occurrence of a leukopenia in dengue and noted a reduction in the number of the neutrophilic leukocytes and an increase in the small mononuclears or lymphocytes. Vedder and Ashburn and Craig (1907) confirmed these findings and in our cases we observed that the average leukocyte counts varied between 3,500 and 3,800 leukocytes per c.mm., but we observed patients in whom the count was as low as 1,200 and as high as 5,000 leukocytes per c.mm. of blood. The leukopenia begins as early as the second day after the onset and persists for several days after the temperature returns to normal, usually being most marked upon the sixth or seventh day of the febrile period.

Besides the occurrence of a marked leukopenia there is a decided decrease in the neutrophilic leukocytes and an increase in the mononuclear leukocytes, as demonstrated by Stitt (1906), Ashburn and Craig (1907), Vedder (1907), Simmons, St. John and Reynolds (1931) and others. Simmons, St. John and Reynolds (1931), in their study of many human volunteers in whom the disease was produced by inoculation, or by the bites of infected mosquitoes, found a marked leukopenia in all cases with a marked reduction in mature neutrophilic leukocytes, a great increase in immature neutrophilic polymorphonuclear leukocytes, and an increase in mononuclear leukocytes. The increase in the number of immature neutrophilic leukocytes, i.e., a "shift to the left" in the Schilling index, they regarded as of great diagnostic importance, which, taken in conjunction with the marked leukopenia, renders the diagnosis of dengue practically conclusive. The shift to the left in the Schilling count often began on the day before the onset of the fever and persisted during the entire attack. Simmons and his coworkers found that the leukopenia usually began on the second day of the fever and progressed until the fourth or fifth day, the total count at that time averaging about 2,000 leukocytes per c.mm. of blood. Although the mononuclear leukocytes are relatively increased they are actually decreased in total number, as well as the neutrophilic leukocytes.

The Nervous System.—Dengue markedly affects the nervous system and most of the unpleasant symptoms encountered during the acute attack and convalescence are of nervous origin. Anatomically, Le Gac and Servant (1939) have found that the cerebrospinal fluid shows definite pathologic changes in patients suffering from the disease. The fluid was found to be under increased tension, while there is an increase in albumin and sugar, but it is clear in appearance and there is no increase in the cellular contents. These investigators found that spinal puncture, with the removal of excess fluid, relieved all of the headache and muscular pain, as well as most of the other symptoms of the infection.

Pain is a prominent symptom in all cases of dengue fever except the very mildest, and most prominent in the severe cases of this infection. Pain in the muscles, accompanied by soreness upon pressure, and aggravated by movement, is almost invariably present, and many patients complain of shooting pains or aching in the bones, but the pain is really in the insertions of the muscles to the bones and referred by the patient to the bones. Backache, especially pronounced in the lumbar region, is often very severe and sometimes almost agonizing in cases in which the temperature is markedly elevated. Leg ache and arm ache are prominent symptoms and the muscles of the extremities are often very tender upon pressure. Headache, usually frontal or occipital in type, is a very common and prominent symptom and is sometimes exceedingly severe.

During the febrile period insomnia may be present and, if not, sleep is usually fitful and accompanied by unpleasant dreams. In rare instances delirium may be present, usually of a quiet type but sometimes noisy and violent. Mental depression, both during the attack and during convalescence, is very frequently noted and is sometimes so severe as to lead to attempts at suicide. Ashburn and Craig (1907) observed one patient who attempted suicide while convalescing from an induced attack of dengue fever. Meningeal symptoms have been noted rarely, especially in children, but the writer has never observed such symptoms.

The Genitourinary System.—Unlike yellow fever, which dengue resembles in many respects, there is no indication of involvement of the kidneys, as albumin and casts are not observed in the urine and the progressive albuminuria, so characteristic of yellow fever, is never observed in dengue fever. A slight trace of albumin has been found in the urine by a few observers but has not been observed by the writer.

The Temperature.—The peculiar characteristics of the temperature curve in typical dengue have already been sufficiently described and will not be repeated. Suffice it to say that, if present, the primary rise, the intermission, and the secondary rise and crisis are of great diagnostic importance; but it should be remembered that great variations occur in the temperature curve, the milder infections presenting simply a primary rise and continued fever for a day or two, when the crisis occurs, with no secondary rise in the temperature, while in other cases there may be several days of continued fever without a marked remission and the "saddleback" type of curve does not occur.

The Glandular System.—The spleen is not markedly enlarged in dengue nor are the lymphatic glands enlarged, in the experience of the writer, but some authorities have observed enlargement of the lymphatic glands in some of their cases. It is evident that in some epidemics of this disease enlargement of the lymphatic glands appears to be common while in others it is so rare as to be unnoticed.

The Respiratory System.—Symptoms connected with the respiratory system are very rarely observed in dengue patients. A slight bronchitis has been noted in a very few patients, while a sore throat was complained of in one of the writer's induced infections. The absence of respiratory symptoms is of great diagnostic importance in differentiating dengue from influenza, with which it may be confused.

Complications.—Dengue is a disease of short duration and complications are seldom observed. Rarely an acute bronchitis may occur as a complication and in the very old bronchopneumonia or lobar pneumonia may occur. In patients suffering from cardiac disease collapse may complicate the clinical picture, but in the vast majority of such patients dengue fever appears to have no injurious effect upon the heart, even though cardiac disease is present.

Sequelae.—During convalescence mental depression may be observed, persisting for several weeks in some individuals, and this may be considered a sequela of the disease. Other sequelae are absent in this infection.

Convalescence.—In the writer's experience convalescence from dengue has, in the vast majority of cases, been rapid and most patients were able to resume their occupations within a week after the disappearance of the fever. In rare instances convalescence may be prolonged, the patients being weak and nervous, or mentally depressed for several weeks following the attack. Some authorities state that convalescence is slow and accompanied by great muscular weakness, but this has not been true in our experience.

Diagnosis.—The diagnosis of dengue fever during an epidemic is usually easy but it should be remembered that very mild and atypical cases occur which are easily mistaken for other conditions or remain unrecognized. In the typical case the diagnosis, *clinically*, is based upon the very sudden onset, the extreme prostration with severe aching and pains in the muscles, the saddleback type of temperature, and the characteristic eruption.

LABORATORY DIAGNOSIS.—The laboratory diagnosis is based upon the occurrence of a marked leukopenia, the average number of leukocytes being about 3,500 to 4,000 per c.mm., with a distinct and often great "shift to the left" in the Schilling count, a relative increase in the mononuclear leukocytes and a decrease in the neutrophilic polymorphonuclear leukocytes. These changes in the blood are believed to be practically diagnostic of the disease and a blood examination should be made in every case of fever and the clinical diagnosis confirmed by blood findings, if possible.

DIFFERENTIAL DIAGNOSIS.—Several acute infections may be mistaken for dengue fever and it is most important that this disease be differentiated from such conditions, especially in regions where yellow fever is endemic or epidemic, as the latter infection is probably more often confused with dengue fever than any other infection. The diseases which may be confused with dengue are yellow fever, phlebotomus or pappataci fever, influenza, trench fever, malaria, scarlet fever, measles and smallpox.

Yellow Fever.—The differentiation of dengue and yellow fevers is of the greatest importance, as the two infections are frequently mistaken, the one for the other, and because the early recognition of yellow fever is of fundamental importance in the prevention of this disease and in the control of epidemics. If one inquires into the history of epidemics of yellow fever it will be found that, almost invariably, the first cases of this disease have been called "dengue fever" and not until deaths occurred has the presence of yellow fever in the community been recognized and admitted. The confusion of the two infections in children occurs most frequently because yellow fever in children is a comparatively mild disease and the symptoms closely resemble those observed in an attack of dengue fever. In mild cases of yellow fever in adults the symptoms may resemble those of a moderately severe attack of dengue fever, but the absence of a marked leukopenia and a shift to the left in the Schilling count and the presence of the terminal eruption should serve to distinguish dengue from yellow fever. Likewise, in more severe cases of yellow fever, the presence of albumin in the urine, the slowing pulse with a rising temperature (Faget's sign), the presence of jaundice and hemorrhages from the mouth, nose and stomach, the absence of an eruption and the absence of the characteristic leukopenia with a shift to the left in the Schilling count of dengue, are sufficient to differentiate yellow fever from dengue fever. A slow pulse may be present in dengue but is constant, while in yellow fever we have the phenomenon of a progressively slowing pulse with a rising temperature. Perhaps the most striking difference in the two infections is the early appearance of albumin and casts in the urine in yellow fever and their absence in even the most severe cases of dengue fever. In the presence of an epidemic which is believed to be one of dengue fever, the occurrence of fatal cases at once negatives such a diagnosis, and is decisive as regards the differentiation of this disease from yellow fever. Dengue seldom, if ever, causes death, while yellow fever is accompanied by a high mortality.

Phlebotomus or Pappataci Fever.—This infection, also caused by a filtrable virus, is very apt to be mistaken for dengue as the symptoms are very similar and it occurs in widespread epidemics. This fever persists for only three days and hence is often called "three-day fever." The short duration of the disease should serve to distinguish it from dengue, while the marked leukopenia and the shift to the left in the Schilling count, so characteristic of dengue, are absent in phlebotomus fever, although a slight leukopenia may be present. However, it is true that mild cases of dengue, in which the fever lasts for only two or three days, and which are by no means uncommon, could not be distinguished from phlebotomus fever unless leukopenia were present. There can be no doubt that many epidemics of phlebotomus fever have been thought to be dengue and this has caused some confusion in the clinical descriptions of the two infections.

Influenza.—Strange as it may seem, influenza has been frequently mistaken for dengue, especially in the tropics, where the usual respiratory symptoms of influenza are frequently missing or so slight as to attract little attention. In influenza the aching and tenderness of the muscles, the postorbital pain and tenderness, the prostration and headache may be as marked as in many cases of dengue; but the "saddleback" temperature curve, the terminal eruption, and the marked leukopenia and shift to the left in the Schilling count, all characteristic of dengue, do not occur in influenza and their presence clinches the diagnosis. In the mildest cases of dengue, in which all of these phenomena may be absent, the differentiation of this infection from influenza would be most difficult from a clinical standpoint.

Trench Fever.—The sudden onset of this infection, together with the rapid rise in temperature, the muscular pains, prostration and severe headache cause it to resemble dengue but it may be differentiated by the presence of a leukocytosis, enlargement of the spleen, and tendency to relapse. An erythematous eruption is often present in trench fever but it occurs upon the chest, abdomen and back and does not extend to the arms and legs as in dengue, in which disease the eruption usually occurs first upon the hands, feet, arms and legs, extending later to the trunk.

Malarial Fevers.—The malarial fevers should be easily differentiated from dengue fever by the demonstration of the causative plasmodium in the blood of the patient, by the reduction in the number of red blood corpuscles, which does not occur in dengue, and by the response of the fever to the administration of quinine. In malaria quinine causes a prompt reduction in the temperature, while in dengue it has no effect upon the temperature. Other important differential points are the absence of an eruption in malaria and the leukopenia and marked shift to the left in the Schilling count. Anemia is not a symptom of dengue but is always present in the malarial infections.

Scarlet Fever.—In children scarlet fever may be confused with dengue largely because the so-called "primary eruption" of the latter infection may resemble that of scarlet fever and also because the true dengue eruption may sometimes assume a scarlatinal character. The presence of a desquamation may further confuse the picture. There should be no difficulty in differentiating the two infections if one remembers that in scarlet fever a sore throat is present, there is a leukocytosis, instead of a leukopenia, and the temperature curve is never "saddleback" in type.

Measles.—The fact that the true eruption of dengue frequently resembles that of measles may lead to confusion, but in measles the presence of Koplik's spots, respiratory symptoms and the absence of a leukopenia should enable one easily to differentiate the two infections. Also, the extremely sudden onset in dengue, the "saddleback" temperature curve, and the sudden and extreme prostration would all favor the diagnosis of this disease.

Smallpox.—The severity of the headache, backache and muscular pains at the onset of smallpox renders its differentiation at this time from dengue difficult, but the appearance of the characteristic eruption in smallpox would quickly differentiate the two infections. During an epidemic of dengue smallpox has been mistaken for the latter with very unpleasant results.

Treatment.—The mildest cases of dengue do not require any treatment beyond **rest in bed** and the administration of **acetylsalicylic acid** in sufficient dosage to ease the muscular pains and headache. In all well-marked cases of dengue the prostration is so severe that the patient immediately takes to his bed, and he should be kept in bed during the entire course of the disease and for a week afterward, as weakness may be extreme following the terminal fall in the temperature and rest is essential. At the beginning of the attack a **saline cathartic** should be given and the bowels should be kept open throughout the attack, as constipation is usually present. The headache and muscular pains should be controlled by acetylsalicylic acid and in the rare instances in which this drug does not have the desired effect the use of morphine sulfate is advocated but it is very rarely necessary to resort to this drug. **Cold applications** to the head are often useful if the headache is very severe and cannot be controlled by acetylsalicylic acid. Anorexia is almost invariably present and the **diet** should be fluid or semifluid and the patient should not be urged to eat if nausea and vomiting are present. These symptoms are not of long duration and the failure to take food will not harm the patient. Throughout the attack the fluid intake should be encouraged and iced drinks, as lemonade and fruit juices, may be allowed in unlimited quantities. If the fever rises above 40° C. (104° F.) cold sponging may be employed, but if this causes the patient too much discomfort it should not be insisted upon as the temperature will soon fall below this point without any treatment.

Convalescence from dengue requires careful supervision and the use of **tonics** is indicated, as prostration, loss of appetite, and mental depression are present in many cases. The administration of **vitamins** and the use of a good **wine,** in moderate amounts, will improve the mental condition and hasten complete recovery. Confinement to bed for a week after the temperature has returned to normal is indicated in all except the mildest infections and the patient should not be allowed to resume his usual occupations until the prostration and weakness following the attack have disappeared. The diet during convalescence should be nutritious and full diet should be resumed gradually.

PROPHYLAXIS.—While dengue is not a fatal infection the rapidity with which it spreads in a community, and the large percentage of the population that become infected, render it a disease of much economic importance. Its occurrence in epidemic form among troops during maneuvers or war may so cripple the military forces as to lead to very disastrous results. Thus, the prevention of the disease is important and depends upon the destruction of the mosquitoes transmitting it and protection from their bites. Usually *Aedes aegypti* is the mosquito concerned in transmission, but *Aedes albopictus* has also been incriminated and must be guarded against. The methods of prevention depending upon the destruction of the transmitting mosquitoes and protection from their bites have been discussed in considering the prophylaxis of yellow fever (*q.v.*) and will not be repeated, as the methods available in these respects, in the prevention of yellow fever, are just as efficient in the prevention of dengue, the two infections being transmitted usually by the same mosquito, *Aedes aegypti.*

Patients suffering from dengue should be placed in mosquito-proof rooms or wards in a hospital in order to prevent the transmission of the virus to the mosquito, but isolation is not necessary, as dengue patients may be placed in wards with other patients with no danger of transmitting their infection, provided such wards are thoroughly screened.

At the present time we possess no vaccine or serum which is of proven benefit in the prevention of dengue, although attempts have been made to prepare such agents which would be capable of producing immunity to the infection.

Prognosis.—Except in the very young or old the prognosis in dengue is always excellent as this infection is never fatal in otherwise healthy individuals. While deaths have been reported as occurring from dengue in some epidemics, the data upon which the reports were based were very inaccurate and there is no reason to believe that they were correct. In the great epidemic of dengue that occurred in Greece in 1928, Cardamatis reported the death rate as 1 in 61,000, and Potano stated that the death rate in this epidemic was about 1 per cent. On the other hand, Griffitts and Hanson reported that 32.6 per cent of the deaths occurring in Athens, in August, 1928, during the height of the dengue epidemic, were certified as being caused by dengue, while in Piraeus, where the infection affected approximately 90 per cent of the population, 39.7 per cent of the deaths were attributed to dengue. Such a high mortality rate for this disease is so unheard of in the experience of other observers during epidemics that it is evident that many mistakes must have been made in the diagnosis of the infection and that it is probable, as stated by Strong (1942), that some other virus infection was present at the same time as the dengue epidemic. In the hundreds of cases observed by Ashburn and the writer (1907) in the epidemic in Manila, not a single fatal infection was observed and the writer has never observed a death from dengue in several epidemics of this disease that he has studied. It is certainly true that dengue is never fatal in even very young or old individuals unless some complicating disease is present, as cardiac disease, kidney disease, or pulmonary infections, and even in these conditions it is doubtful whether dengue contributes greatly to the fatal result.

Pathology.—Very little is known of the pathology of dengue for the reason that deaths so rarely occur and necropsy records of such cases are very few in number. Heiser (1937) reported a fatal case in which no pathology was noted beyond some enlargement of the internal lymph nodes, while Photakis (1929) described myocardial degeneration and enlargement of the liver in fatal cases. Meekins (1936) observed hemorrhages in the intestine and cloudy swelling of the liver, spleen and kidneys, while Manson-Bahr (1940) states that pulmonary and intracranial inflammation were the pathologic features which have been most frequently reported. Strong (1942) states that encephalitis and nephritic lesions have been reported and well says: "It seems obvious that we have no definite knowledge of any characteristic pathologic changes in the disease." The very marked leukopenia and the shift to the left in the Schilling count do constitute a feature of the pathology that must be regarded as characteristic, according to Simmons and others.

History.—The history of dengue, as regards its etiology and epidemiology, has been considered already in discussing these phases of the subject. The fundamental historical data are the description of the disease by Boylon (1779) and Rush (1880); the demonstration by Graham (1903) that mosquitoes transmitted the infection; the demonstration by Bancroft (1906) and by Cleland, Bradley and McDonald (1916) that *Aedes aegypti* is the mosquito usually concerned in its transmission; and the demonstration by Ashburn and Craig (1907) that dengue is caused by a filtrable virus. Perhaps the greatest epidemic of this disease of record is that occurring in 1927–1928, in Athens, Greece, where it was estimated that 239,000 cases occurred, and it was in this epidemic that numerous deaths were reported as being caused by this infection.

Geographic Distribution.—Dengue usually occurs in subtropical and tropical regions but epidemics have occurred in temperate regions, as in Philadelphia. The geographic distribution depends upon the distribution of the transmitting mosquito, *Aedes aegypti*, and epidemics of the disease have occurred in the West Indies, Georgia, Florida, Alabama, Mississippi, Louisiana and Texas, in the United States; in Rio de Janeiro, Callao, Lima, Bermuda, Trinidad, Jamaica, Cuba, Vera Cruz, Guadeloupe, Martinique, Barbados, Antigua, the Guianas, and the Central American countries; in Tahiti, and other islands of the Pacific. In the Philippine Islands numerous extensive epidemics have occurred. The disease has also been seen in epidemic form in Port Said, Cairo, Gorée, Tripoli, Mecca, Aden, Jidda, Medina, Zanzibar, the Dutch East Indies, Mauritius and Amoy. In addition, dengue has occurred in Portugal, Spain, Greece, Italy, and it has repeatedly occurred in Australia.

Undifferentiated Fevers Resembling Dengue

From time to time febrile conditions have been described which resemble in their symptomatology dengue fever and to which specific names have been given by the authorities who have described them. The most important of these fevers are the following:

Seven-Day Fever of India.—This fever was first described by Rogers in 1918, who studied it in Calcutta, where he found it to be the most common fever met with in that city. The symptoms are almost identical with those of dengue and Rogers states that the "saddleback" type of temperature curve is characteristic. According to Rogers' description, this fever is accompanied by a slow pulse, pains in the muscles, bones and joints, and a rash appearing first on the extensor surfaces of the forearms upon the fourth to sixth day of the disease, the entire febrile period lasting seven days. There is also a leukopenia with a relative increase in the lymphocytes.

In discussing this fever in 1923, the writer stated:

" It is the opinion of most authorities that Rogers' seven-day fever is really identical with dengue fever, and this opinion is shared by the writer. Certainly there is nothing in Rogers' description of the disease that would differentiate it clinically from many cases of dengue, and some of the clinical features that he regards as most characteristic from a differential standpoint, are very frequently observed in dengue. Thus, the reduction in the leukocyte count and the relative increase of lymphocytes and large mononuclear cells, the slow pulse in comparison with the height of the temperature, and the so-called " saddleback " type of the latter, are all clinical features generally present in cases of dengue. . . . In view of these facts, it may be stated that, at the present time, there is no basis for the belief that seven-day fever is a distinct disease, for the available evidence is all in favor of its being identical with dengue fever."

The conclusion reached above has been concurred in by all experienced observers and today seven-day fever is considered only as a synonym of dengue fever.

Five-Day Fever of van der Sheer.—This fever was described by van der Sheer, in Batavia, Dutch East Indies, as characterized by a febrile course of approximately five days and a macular eruption occurring upon the trunk. The general symptomatology was similar to that of dengue, and DeLangen (1936) considers that it is identical with the latter disease, as it has been determined that it is caused by a filtrable virus and is transmitted by *Aedes* mosquitoes. The observations of Snijders, Dinger and Schüffner (1931) have shown conclusively that the five-day fever of van der Sheer and dengue are identical, as they fed *Aedes aegypti* upon patients suffering from this so-called fever in Sumatra, sent the mosquitoes to Amsterdam where they were allowed to bite human volunteers, and these volunteers developed typical dengue. The virus sometimes caused a "saddleback" type of temperature curve and sometimes a continuous curve, the attacks lasting for from five to seven days. It is thus evident that in different localities dengue may present different aspects and this accounts for the description of the conditions under different specific names. The fever of van der Sheer is undoubtedly identical with dengue fever.

Bwamba Fever.—In 1941 Smithburn, Mahaffy and Paul described a disease occurring in Uganda, Africa, which they regarded as a distinct disease. Clinically, it was characterized by a fever lasting from 5 to 7 days; a slow pulse, averaging about 84 beats per minute, even when the temperature was as high as

102.8° F.; anorexia; headache; backache and muscular pains.   No death occurred and convalescence was rapid and complete.   These investigators were able to isolate a filtrable virus from nine patients suffering from the disease, and the blood of convalescent patients neutralized the virus.   The virus is pathogenic to monkeys when inoculated intracerebrally but does not produce death, although fever is present, while it causes death in mice by intracerebral or intranasal inoculation, the lesions in these animals being practically limited to the brain and consisting of degeneration of the cortical cells and the appearance of intra-nuclear acidophilic bodies which resemble inclusions.

The observations of these investigators have not been confirmed but it is probable that they are correct in stating that Bwamba fever is a distinct dis-ease, although it bears certain resemblances to both dengue and mild yellow fever infections.   Further observations are essential before the identity of the infection is established.

Other fevers, of short duration, have been described which may be identical with dengue fever, as it should be remembered that the latter disease differs greatly in its symptomatology during different epidemics and in different degrees of severity.   Whether these differences are due to different strains of the dengue virus or to differing degrees of resistance of certain races or in-dividuals still remains a question, but that such differences do exist cannot be doubted.

BIBLIOGRAPHY

Ashburn, P. M. and Craig, C. F.: Philippine J. Sc. (B), 2 : 93, 1907.
———— and ————: J. Infect. Dis., 4 : 440, 1907.
Bancroft, T. L.: Austral. M. J., 25 : 17, 1906.
Blanc, G. and Caminopétros, J.: Compt. rend. Acad. d. sc., 187 : 1081, 1928.
———— and ————: Compt. rend Acad. d. sc., 188 : 1273, 1929.
———— and ————: Compt. rend. Soc. de biol., 100 : 31, 1929.
———— and ————: Arch. Inst. Pasteur hellén., 2 : 199; 277, 1930.
————, ———— and Manoussakis, E.: Bull. Soc. path. exot., 21 : 525, 1928.
Cleland, J. B.: M. J. Australia, 2 : 179; 200, 1916.
————, Bradley, B. and McDonald, W.: J. Hyg., 16 : 317, 1917.
Craig, C. F.: N. York M. J., 103 : 360, 1911.
————: Oxford Medicine, New York; London, Oxford University Press, Vol. V, p. 485, 1934.
————: Brennemann's Practice of Pediatrics, Hagerstown, Md., W. F. Prior Company, Inc., Vol. 2, Chap. 36, 1937.
DeLangen, C. D.: Geneesk. tijdschr. v. Nederl.-Indië, 65 : 529, 1925.
Dinger, J. E. and Snijders, E. P.: Arch. f. Schiffs- u. Tropen-Hyg., 35 : 497, 1931.
Findlay, G. M.: Tr. Roy. Soc. Trop. Med. & Hyg., 26 : 157, 1932.
Graham, H.: J. Trop. Med., 6 : 209, 1903.
Griffitts, T. H. D. and Hanson, H.: J. A. M. A., 107 : 1107, 1936.
Hoffmann, J. M., Mertens, W. K. and Snijders, E. P.: Geneesk. tijdschr. v. Nederl.-Indië, 72 : 1195, 1932.
Holt, R. L. and Kintner, J. H.: Am. J. Trop. Med., 11 : 103, 1931.

Kligler, I. J. and Ashner, M.: Ann. Trop. Med., 22 : 151, 1928.
Koizumi, T., Yamaguchi, K. and Tonomura, K.: J. Med. A. Formosa, Nos. 176, 177, 1917; Rev. Trop. Dis. Bull., 12 : 77, 1918.
Le Gac, P. and Servant, J.: Bull. Soc. path. exot., 32 : 888, 1939.
Manoussakis, E.: Bull. Soc. path. exot., 21 : 200, 1928.
————: Rev. d'hyg., 53 : 18, 1931.
Morishita, K.: J. Med. A. Formosa, No. 247, 1925; Rev. Trop. Dis. Bull., 23 : 361, 1926.
Photakis, B. A.: Arch. f. Schiffs- u. Tropen-Hyg., 33 : 333, 1929.
Rogers, L.: Indian M. Gaz., 44 : 36, 1909.
————: Fevers in the Tropics, Ed. 3, London, 1918.
St. John, J. H., Simmons, J. S. and Reynolds, F. H. K.: Am. J. Trop. Med., 10 : 23, 1930.
Schule, P. A.: Am. J. Trop. Med., 8 : 203, 1928.
Siler, J. F., Hall, M. W. and Hitchens, A. P.: Philippine J. Sc., 29 : 1, 1926.
Simmons, J. S., St. John, J. H., Holt, R. L. and Reynolds, F. H. K.: Am. J. Trop. Med., 11 : 199, 1931.
————, ———— and Reynolds, F. H. K.: Philip-pine J. Sc., 44 : 1, 1931.
Smithburn, K. C., Mahaffy, A. F. and Paul, J. H.: Am. J. Trop. Med., 21 : 75, 1941.
Snijders, E. P., Dinger, J. E. and Schüffner, W. A. P.: Am. J. Trop. Med., 11 : 171, 1931.
Stitt, E. R.: Philippine J. Sc. (B), 1 : 513, 1906.
Strong, R. P.: Diagnosis, Prevention and Treat-ment of Tropical Diseases, Philadelphia, The Blakiston Company, Vol. II, p. 905, 1942.
Vedder, E. B.: N. York M. J., 86 : 203, 1907.

CHAPTER TWENTY–FOUR

BRUCELLOSIS

Undulant Fever

By WALTER M. SIMPSON, M.S., M.D., F.A.C.P.

Definition.—Brucellosis (undulant fever, Malta fever, Mediterranean fever, goat fever, contagious or infectious abortion of cattle, Bang's disease, Texas fever, Rio Grande fever, et cetera) is an infectious disease of man, transmitted by cattle, hogs, goats and other domesticated animals. Once regarded as a relatively rare disease, restricted largely to the Mediterranean area, brucellosis is now known to be widely prevalent throughout most parts of the world. The early recognition of the disease along the Mediterranean Coast produced such synonymous designations as Malta fever, Mediterranean fever, Neapolitan fever, Gibraltar fever, Cyprus fever and rock fever.

Etiology.—In 1886 David Bruce [1] isolated the causative organism, a coccobacillus which he later named *Micrococcus melitensis*. Eleven years after Bruce's discovery, Bang,[2] a Danish veterinarian, isolated the organism of infectious abortion of cattle, which he called *Bacillus abortus*. A British Commission, headed by Bruce, investigated the disease on the island of Malta from 1904 to 1907. They demonstrated that the ingestion of raw goat's milk was the common source of infection for man. The prohibition of the use of raw goat's milk by members of the military and naval forces produced an immediate and rapid decline in the incidence of the disease.

For twenty-one years the *Micrococcus melitensis* of Bruce and the *Bacillus abortus* of Bang were regarded as separate, unrelated species. It remained for Alice Evans [3] to make the fundamental discovery in 1918 that the two organisms were indistinguishable morphologically, culturally and by ordinary agglutination tests. In the announcement of her discovery Evans made this prophetic suggestion: "Considering the close relationship between the two organisms, and the reported frequency of *Bacillus abortus* in cows' milk, it would seem remarkable that we do not have a disease resembling Malta fever prevalent in this country."

In 1927 Carpenter [4] recovered an organism indistinguishable from *Bacillus abortus* from the blood of ten human beings with undulant fever; five pregnant heifers inoculated with these cultures promptly aborted. These observations by Evans and Carpenter were soon confirmed by investigators in many countries. Evans' prediction was abundantly fulfilled as it became generally known that the organism which produces infectious abortion in cattle, hogs and other domesticated animals was capable of producing in human beings a disease clinically and bacteriologically similar to Malta fever transmitted by goats.

Since Bruce had described the organism as a coccus and Bang had termed it a bacillus, it became apparent that the *melitensis-abortus* group of organisms should be reclassified. The proposal by Meyer and Shaw [5] that the organisms should be designated by the generic name *Brucella* has met with universal approval. Consistent with this proposal, the name *Brucellosis* has been generally adopted as the single designation for the disease produced in animals and man by the Brucella. The organism usually associated with goat infection is termed *Brucella melitensis,* while the organism of infectious abortion of cattle is called *Brucella abortus.* Traum [6] described a third related organism associated with the infection in swine, which has been designated *Brucella suis.* A fourth and relatively uncommon heterogeneous group of organisms which differs in serologic characteristics from the three chief varieties has been called *Brucella paramelitensis.* The chief significance of these infrequently encountered strains is that the serum of a patient infected with *paramelitensis* organisms may not agglutinate antigens produced from the other more common varieties.

Organisms which have been designated as caprine (*melitensis*) or porcine (*suis*) have been recovered from cow's milk. The antigenic differences are probably best explained on the basis of host adaptation. It seems probable that *Brucella abortus* is the primitive strain from which other strains have developed as the result of passage through various animal hosts.

Epidemiology.—The three common varieties of Brucella produce a group of three closely related, frequently inseparable, diseases. It is generally believed that the *melitensis* variety possesses the highest infectivity, the *abortus* variety the lowest, while the *suis* variety occupies an intermediate position. Such an arbitrary distinction is not entirely valid, however, since any of the varieties may produce either a severe or a mild infection. The goat source of infection is relatively uncommon in this country, except in the goat-raising areas of the southwestern states. *Suis* infections, most common in the hog-raising states of the Middle West, are most often characterized by an abrupt onset and a severe course.

The most common and uniformly widespread cause of brucellosis in the United States is *Brucella abortus.* In a recent survey [7] of the incidence of Bang's disease in this country, involving 11,858,859 cattle, 38 per cent of herds and 8 per cent of cattle were found to be infected. The disease is prevalent in every state; in 12 states over 50 per cent of herds are known to be infected. Although severe, abrupt infections may result from infection with the *abortus* strain, this variety of the organism is more apt to produce symptoms and signs which are more insidious and less severe than those produced by either the *melitensis* or *suis* varieties. There is also convincing evidence that invasion by *abortus* organisms often causes subclinical or asymptomatic infections; anti-Brucella serum agglutinins and positive skin tests with Brucella antigens have been demonstrated in such persons in the absence of clinical evidences of disease.

The two important modes of conveyance of the infection from animals to man are, first, and most commonly, the ingestion of raw cow's or goat's milk or unpasteurized dairy products, and, second, direct contact with infected fresh animal tissues. Among urban populations the chief mode of transmission has been through the raw milk of cattle infected with the *abortus* variety of the organism; most of the city dwellers who have acquired the disease have had no contact with infected cattle, hogs or goats. Farmers, veterinarians, slaughterhouse workers, butchers and laboratory investigators may become infected through the skin as the result of direct contact with the discharges of living animals or with the tissues of animals recently slaughtered. The rate of infectivity is particularly high among veterinarians who have handled the products of conception of infected cows. Hardy [8] demonstrated by animal experiments that the skin may act as a portal of entry of the organism. Morales-Otero [9] has reproduced the disease in human volunteers by inoculations with *abortus* and *suis* strains through abraded skin. There is no definite evidence of man-to-man transmission of the disease.

Horses, dogs and sheep may harbor the infection. There is little evidence, however, that these animals have played any important role in the transmission of the disease to human beings.

Epidemiologically, brucellosis is widely disseminated throughout the United States. The growth of interest in the disease is perhaps best shown by the steady increase in the number of officially reported cases. In 1926 only forty-six cases were reported. By 1930 the number had increased to 1,453. In 1937, 2,497 cases were officially reported to the U. S. Public Health Service by State Health Departments.[10] It is undoubtedly true that the number of cases actually occurring is much larger than that reported. Hardy and coworkers [11] reported the occurrence of 1,669 cases in Iowa from 1925 to 1935.

Brucellosis occurs more commonly in men than in women, in a proportion of about three to one. The disease is uncommon in infants, but about 10 per cent of recorded cases occurred in children between the ages of five and fifteen.

Symptomatology.—As knowledge of the clinical manifestations of brucellosis has advanced, particularly during the past decade, it has become more and more apparent that the older textbook descriptions of the symptomatology of the disease were based largely on experiences with brucellosis of goat origin. The classical clinical picture of a disease characterized by an undulatory, remittent or intermittent fever, drenching sweats, chills, headache, backache, muscular and joint pains, weakness, loss of weight, possibly a palpable spleen, an infrequent skin eruption, leukopenia with lymphocytosis, and secondary anemia, pertains chiefly to the severe acute forms of the disease. In a high proportion of cases the disease pursues a relatively mild, prolonged course, extending over many months or years. The early descriptions by Hughes [12] and Craig [13] included many such cases. Alice Evans and others have more recently directed particular attention to the common chronic ambulatory form of brucellosis, in which the patient, whose spirits are already depressed by continued ill-health, is often given further discouragement when a diagnosis of neurasthenia is made. Many "neurasthenics," whose chief complaints were exhaustion, insomnia, irritability, and a variety of aches and pains, have been found to be victims of chronic brucellosis.

Since the symptomatology of the acute and chronic forms of brucellosis varies so greatly, these two manifestations will be considered separately.

A. ACUTE BRUCELLOSIS.—The incubation period has been found to vary from five days to longer than one month. In accidental laboratory infections the incubation period has varied from ten to twenty days. The prodrome is not unlike that of any general infection, with a gradual onset, although in occasional cases the disease is initiated with a sharp chill and rapid elevation of temperature to 103–105° F. (39.4–40.6° C.). A sense of tiredness and weakness, loss of appetite, constipation, headache and backache are common early symptoms. Usually the patient becomes gradually aware of an afternoon or evening rise in temperature, associated with chills or chilly sensations, nocturnal perspiration and weakness. The patient often feels quite well during the morning hours, particularly in the early stages of the infection. As the temperature rises, during the afternoon or evening, the symptoms gradually return and increase in severity. The nocturnal exacerbations of fever occasionally reach great heights (106–107° F.; 41.1–41.7° C.). There is often a remarkable disparity between the subjective sense of fever and the height of the fever as registered by the clinical thermometer; in many instances the patient does not complain of fever, nor does he present a febrile appearance, but the physician finds, to his surprise, a fever of 101–103° F. (38.3–39.4° C.). As the fever abates, chills and sweating occur. If defervescence is rapid, the perspiration is more apt to be of drenching character. In such cases the sweats, which literally saturate the night clothing and bedding, are one of the most impressive features of the disease. The perspiration often has a peculiar sweetish, fetid odor. The chills may be severe enough to be regarded as true rigors in about one third of the acute cases.[14-17] Many patients experience only mild chilly sensations, while in about one fourth of cases chilliness is absent.

Arthralgia and muscular pains are prominent features of the acute form of the disease in approximately one half of the cases. The joint pains may be more pronounced during the onset or they may persist throughout the course of illness. The myalgia may be accompanied by a feeling of "stiffness" not unlike the muscular soreness which follows vigorous exercise. Hydrarthrosis and transient periarticular swelling have been observed occasionally. Permanent impairment

of the joints usually does not occur. Suppurative osteomyelitis as a complication of brucellosis has been described with increasing frequency during the past
few years.[18] In most of the reported cases the vertebrae, particularly in the
lumbar region, were attacked. In some instances other bones, such as the
humerus, femur, skull and ribs, were affected. While the osteomyelitis sometimes occurred relatively early in the course of the disease, in most cases it was
a late complication, occasionally occurring after apparent recovery from acute
brucellosis. Feldman and Olson [19, 20] found similar examples of Brucella spondylitis in twenty-four hogs, an average occurrence of one in every 6,000 swine
slaughtered.

Marked restlessness and insomnia usually accompany the nocturnal febrile
exacerbations. Delirium occurs in some cases in which the fever reaches great
heights. Regional Brucella localizations in the brain, spinal cord or meninges
may occur during the acute phase of the disease and produce symptoms and signs
of encephalitis, myelitis or meningitis; such complications are, however, more
commonly observed as delayed manifestations of brucellosis. According to Roger
and Poursines,[21] whose recent classical monograph has aroused great interest in
the frequency of central nervous system invasion by Brucella, the meningeal
involvement predominates, and the development of encephalitis or myelitis, or
both, is usually secondary to the meningitis. Because of this predilection for
meningeal localization, Roger and Poursines have termed this form of the disease
"meningo-neurobrucellosis." The involvement of the central nervous system
may produce the first and only symptoms of the disease. The symptomatology
will vary greatly, depending upon the extent of meningeal invasion and the
presence of additional complications involving the brain, spinal cord or peripheral
nerves. In a patient with brucellosis, the development of such symptoms and
signs as severe headache, vertigo, diplopia, nuchal rigidity, aphasia, psychic disturbances, and various forms of paralysis which are often evanescent, calls for
examination of the cerebrospinal fluid. Characteristically, the spinal fluid will
be under increased pressure and will show pleocytosis, increase of albumin, and
a decrease of globulin and sugar. Since the ultimate diagnosis during life depends upon the isolation and identification of Brucella from the spinal fluid, a
particularly diligent effort should be made to recover the organism by culture
and by guinea pig inoculation. De Jong [22] has recorded eleven verified cases of
Brucella meningitis or meningo-encephalitis in which the organism was recovered
from the spinal fluid by culture or by guinea pig inoculation.

The matutinal remissions or intermissions and the nocturnal exacerbations
of fever may last from one week to many months. The name "undulant fever"
refers to recurring relapses of fever following afebrile intermissions. Such
febrile relapses are the exception rather than the rule; most patients experience
but one febrile period, lasting from a few days to several months, and finally
reaching the normal level by lysis.

The essential gastro-intestinal complaints are anorexia and constipation. The
degree of constipation appears often to parallel the severity of the infection.
Diarrhea is of rare occurrence. Nausea and vomiting may occur in the more
severe cases. Abdominal pain is a frequent feature of the disease during its
early manifestations. Among 125 cases studied by Hardy, abdominal pain
occurred in forty; in ten it was the major complaint. Simpson found abdominal
pain to be the chief complaint in sixteen of 142 patients with brucellosis. The
occurrence of abdominal pain has often led to appendicectomy in patients with
unsuspected brucellosis, the correct diagnosis having been made only after the
persistence of febrile symptoms stimulated a further search for the cause. As
in typhoid fever, the gallbladder may become a focus of Brucella infection.
Brucella has been recovered from the excised gallbladder and from the bile
following duodenal drainage in patients with symptoms of cholecystitis.[23-25]

Symptoms referable to the respiratory tract may be an outstanding feature
of the disease in certain instances. Cough, associated with mucoid or mucopuru-
lent sputum production, is frequent during the first few weeks of illness and
may persist for months. Recent reports [26-30] provide convincing evidence that

pulmonary lesions of brucellosis are of frequent occurrence and are often detectable by roentgenographic examination, even in the absence of distinctive physical signs of pneumonia. The lesions most often encountered on x-ray examination are peribronchial infiltrations, hilar infiltrations, and scattered discrete or confluent patchy pneumonic areas. In experimental animals, a patchy, lobular type of pneumonia is a common finding following inoculation with Brucella. Since a bacteremia exists, it is quite likely that the pulmonary lesions are manifestations of blood-borne focal localizations in the lung parenchyma; consequently, the pulmonary manifestations of brucellosis should be regarded as hematogenous lobular pneumonia rather than true bronchopneumonia. Without doubt, pulmonary lesions occur much more commonly than is generally realized. Serial roentgenographic studies often provide an explanation for vague respiratory symptoms.

The most serious cardiovascular complication has been the occasional occurrence of vegetative endocarditis. Smith and Curtis [31] found reports of nine cases of Brucella endocarditis confirmed by postmortem examination, to which they added a similar case. In most instances the vegetations occurred on mitral or aortic valves previously damaged by rheumatic fever.

The name commonly applied to brucellosis of cattle, "infectious abortion," is derived from the well-known predilection of the causative organism for the genital tract. There is strong evidence that the same regional localization sometimes occurs in human beings. Painful swelling of the testes has been described frequently. Acute epididymitis, orchitis, prostatitis and seminal vesiculitis may be early manifestations of the disease. Simpson [15] recovered Brucella abortus from a draining sinus tract which extended from the globus major of the epididymis through the scrotal wall.

There appears to be little doubt that brucellosis is at least an occasional cause of abortion in women who live on farms where they have direct contact with infected animals, or in women who consume raw milk or unpasteurized dairy products. There are reports [32, 33] of human abortion in which the history and serologic findings provide strong circumstantial evidence of the etiologic role of Brucella. In a study of 565 cases of brucellosis, Calder [34] found a history of one or more miscarriages in 32 per cent of the married women; a history of one miscarriage followed by sterility was common; a few women reported as many as five or six abortions. More direct evidence has been provided by Carpenter and Boak,[35] who recovered Brucella abortus from the tissues of a human fetus which was aborted at the end of the fourth month of gestation. Kristensen [36] isolated the abortus variety of the organism from the exudate which covered the uterine site of the placenta of a seven-month fetus. Frei [37] isolated Brucella from the vaginal discharge of a woman who had aborted ten days previously. Cornell and DeYoung [38] tested serologically 1,015 pregnant women in Chicago; none gave definitely positive reactions and in only five instances were there weakly positive reactions. They concluded that brucellosis is not prevalent among pregnant women in Chicago. It should be observed in this connection that practically all of the milk and dairy products consumed in Chicago were pasteurized.

Loss of weight is an almost constant feature of the acute form of the disease. The greatest loss, often from ten to fifty pounds, occurs in those patients who experience high fever, drenching sweats and great prostration.

A transient cutaneous eruption, usually papular, macular or maculopapular, is a relatively infrequent finding. The skin lesions may simulate the roseola of typhoid fever.

B. CHRONIC BRUCELLOSIS.—Many physicians feel that the symptoms and signs of acute brucellosis are often sufficiently characteristic to justify such a provisional diagnosis on the basis of clinical findings. In dealing with chronic brucellosis, however, the physician is often faced with a problem which will tax his diagnostic acumen to the utmost. No disease, not excepting syphilis and tuberculosis, is more protean in its manifestations.

The common employment of the name "undulant fever" has served only to add further difficulties in the recognition of cases of chronic brucellosis. A significant temperature curve, physical signs of disease, and positive agglutination tests and skin tests may be entirely lacking throughout a long period of chronic illness. The recent studies by Evans,[39-41] Poston,[42] Angle,[43] Scoville,[44] Thames,[45] Calder,[34] Hamman and Wainwright,[46] Harris,[47] and Cameron and Wells [48] leave little doubt that a protracted, relatively mild form of brucellosis is widely prevalent and constitutes a major cause of chronic ill-health. Only a small proportion of patients with chronic brucellosis, probably less than 10 per cent, have experienced a previous acute febrile illness, compatible with a diagnosis of acute brucellosis. In many cases the patient is not entirely incapacitated for work, but complains chiefly of weakness and exhaustion, with or without mild fever. Since the commonly employed diagnostic tests are frequently negative in such cases, and since even the most conscientious physician may not find physical abnormalities to account for the patient's complaints, the almost inevitable diagnosis of neurasthenia or psychoneurosis is often made.

Surveys conducted in widely separated parts of the United States during recent years [49, 50] reveal that an ambulatory, partially disabling, chronic form of brucellosis is a widespread cause of prolonged ill-health. Angle, Algie, Baumgartner and Lunsford [51] found that 9 per cent of 7,122 school children gave positive reactions to the intradermal test; 79.3 per cent of the positive reactors consumed raw milk; a high proportion of the children had complaints consistent with the ambulatory type of brucellosis. Gould and Huddleson observed positive reactions in 845 of 8,124 persons (10.3 per cent) tested intradermally with brucellergin. Most of these individuals were residents of an infirmary for homeless indigents and of a mental hospital where unpasteurized milk was consumed and where the supply of dairy products was obtained partly from a herd known to be infected with Brucella. Of the 845 reactors to the skin test only 111 (13.1 per cent) showed a positive agglutination reaction. The unreliability of the agglutination test in detecting chronic brucellosis has been noted by many other workers.

A recitation of all of the symptoms which have been ascribed to chronic brucellosis would serve only to heighten the confusion which as yet surrounds this baffling phase of the disease. In general, it may be stated that the three cardinal features of most cases of chronic brucellosis are weakness, low-grade fever and a lack of objective physical findings. McGinty and Gambrell [52] have listed over 150 different manifestations of chronic brucellosis. The most common complaints and findings have been profound weakness, marked fatigue, exhaustion, prostration, loss of weight, headache, backache, transient or constant myalgia and arthralgia, sweating, chilliness, insomnia, vertigo, cough, pain in the chest, hypotension, bronchitis, palpitation and tachycardia on exertion, anorexia, abdominal pain, constipation, enlargement of the spleen or liver, lymphadenopathy, dysuria, pyuria, cystitis, pyelitis, orchitis, epididymitis, prostatitis, oophoritis, impotence, menstrual disorders, abortion, nervousness, apprehension, depression, paresthesia, encephalitis, meningitis, myelitis, and a macular, papular or morbilliform cutaneous eruption. Mild degrees of fever may be present for many weeks or months; there may be several months of complete freedom from fever; sudden febrile exacerbations may occur, accompanied by an accentuation of the prevailing symptoms, or by the development of evidence of new regional symptoms affecting the respiratory, cardiovascular, genito-urinary, gastro-intestinal, skeletal or nervous systems. Pneumonia, endocarditis, orchitis, epididymitis, prostatitis, oophoritis, cholecystitis, hydrarthrosis, arthritis, spondylitis, osteomyelitis, ocular complications or meningo-encephalitis may be associated with the acute form of the disease, but much more commonly appear several months, or even years, after the often indefinite onset of the chronic type of brucellosis. In some instances such delayed evidences of regional Brucella localization may appear long after apparent recovery from the acute manifestations of the disease. All students of chronic brucellosis have emphasized the almost universal prominence of symptoms which relate to the central nervous system. In addition to the occasional acute invasion of the meninges, brain and spinal cord by Brucella, there is evidence [53] that the endo-antigen of Brucella organisms circulating in the blood has a toxic action upon the central nervous system. These observations led Evans [39] to state: "These facts challenge the right of a physician to make a diagnosis of neurasthenia —a diagnosis regarded as dishonorable by the patient, and also by his family, his employer and his friends—without considering, among other possibilities, the possibility of chronic brucellosis."

Chronic brucellosis should be suspected in all cases of so-called "fever of unknown origin." There are many reports of the isolation of Brucella from the blood, urine, bile or from extirpated tissues in patients who have experienced unexplained long-continued, low-grade fever for years. Hamman and Wainwright [46] re-examined thirty-six such patients; an accurate diagnosis was finally made on ten of them; three were found to have brucellosis.

In contrast to acute brucellosis, it is of particular significance that chronic brucellosis has been recognized in relatively few areas in the United States. The discovery of a large number of cases in these centers has been largely the result of a determined effort on the part of a few investigators to learn of the incidence of the disease in their localities. It seems quite apparent that the vast majority of cases remain unrecognized, since the evidence at hand indicates that chronic brucellosis is widely prevalent in rural communities and in cities and towns in which raw milk is consumed.

A survey conducted by workers of the U. S. Public Health Service [40-42, 54-56] particularly to disclose the prevalence of chronic brucellosis was carried out in three widely separated cities, selected because they represented sections in which the sources of infection differed according to the proportions of cattle, hog and goat populations and in the percentage of raw milk sold (Charlotte, North Carolina, 81 per cent; Kansas City, Kansas, 45 per cent; San Antonio, Texas, 36 per cent). The results of the survey in Charlotte may be cited as an example. The search was made chiefly among patients suffering from unexplained chronic ill-health, particularly among those with long-continued low-grade fever. In contrast to the usual procedure of considering the patient's complaints as due to brucellosis only after positive laboratory tests prompted such an investigation, the patients chosen for this study were selected because they presented clinical pictures suggesting brucellosis. Among 325 patients studied, a definite or probable diagnosis of brucellosis was made in twenty-two; in five cases Brucella was obtained from the blood; in nine cases the tentative clinical diagnosis was supported by a positive agglutination reaction; in eight cases a diagnosis of probable brucellosis was made despite the fact that specific tests failed to confirm the clinical evidence of brucellosis. The inadequacy of specific tests in cases of chronic brucellosis was demonstrated by the fact that of the five patients from whose blood the organism was recovered, none had agglutinin titers as high as 1 : 80 (two had a titer of 1 : 40) ; only one gave a definitely positive intradermal reaction; one gave repeatedly negative opsonocytophagic reactions, while the reactions in the other four varied from weak to strong, and differed in given patients on repeated testing.

LABORATORY FINDINGS.—Since it is exceedingly hazardous to base a diagnosis of brucellosis solely on clinical grounds, recourse must be had to laboratory diagnostic tests. These procedures include (a) primary isolation of the causal organism by cultural methods from blood, spinal fluid, secretions, excretions or excised tissues; (b) indirect recovery of Brucella by culture after animal inoculation; (c) the agglutination test; (d) the intradermal test; and (e) the opsonocytophagic reaction.

The only method by which the diagnosis of brucellosis may be completely established is by the *cultivation and identification of the organism*. While cultural technics have improved greatly during the past few years, with a corresponding increase in the number of reported instances of recovery of the organism, the undertaking is often beset with difficulties and requires skill and, above all, patience. The *melitensis* and *suis* varieties of Brucella ordinarily grow readily under aerobic conditions, while the much more commonly encountered *abortus* variety requires an atmosphere containing 10 per cent carbon dioxide. The procedure used by Poston [42] with notable success is as follows: 15 cc. of blood are obtained from each patient by venipuncture and placed in a small flask containing 4 cc. of sterile 2.5 per cent sodium citrate solution. Four flasks containing 100 cc. of liver infusion broth of pH 6.8 are each inoculated with 2 cc. of the citrated blood. The flasks are incubated at 37° C., two in the room atmosphere and two in an atmosphere containing 10 per cent carbon dioxide. After four days' incubation, daily smears of the broth cultures are made and stained by Gram's method. If no organisms are seen in the smears after ten days' incubation, 5 cc. of the original culture are transplanted to 100 cc. of liver infusion broth every three days for two weeks. Original cultures and transplants are incubated for three weeks before they are reported as negative.

A dehydrated nitrogenous nutrient, bacto-tryptose (Difco), has been used with considerable success [52, 57] as a substitute for liver infusion broth and agar.

In culturing the spinal fluid in suspected cases of Brucella meningo-encephalitis, it is well to use at least 10 cc. of inoculum since relatively few organisms are ordinarily present per cubic centimeter. Urinary specimens for culture should be collected through a sterile catheter. Amoss and Poston [23, 58] have described a successful method for the isolation of Brucella from stools and bile.

The guinea pig is the most suitable laboratory animal for inoculation. Poston inoculates three guinea pigs with blood from each patient; two are injected intraperitoneally with 2 cc. each of citrated blood; one is inoculated in the groin with 1 cc. of citrated blood. The animals are observed daily. Beginning two months after inoculation, tests for specific agglutinins and for cutaneous reaction to Huddleson's brucellergin are made at intervals of a few days. When both tests become positive the animals are killed. Animals which remain negative to the agglutination test and to the skin test are killed four and one-half months after inoculation. Liver infusion broth is planted with the guinea pig's blood and with pieces of organs and is subjected to the cultural procedures previously described. The cultures may then be differentiated into *abortus*, *suis* or *melitensis* varieties by the agglutinin-absorption technic, the bacteriostatic action of dyes, glucose utilization and hydrogen sulfide metabolism.[59-61]

The most commonly used and the most reliable indicator of Brucella infection, in the absence of positive cultures, is the *agglutination test*. This is particularly true in cases of acute brucellosis, in which a high serum agglutinin titer will be found in a great majority of cases. Agglutinins may appear as early as the fifth day of illness, but ordinarily are not found until the second week after the onset. In some instances specific agglutinins may not appear for several weeks. One important source of difficulty in interpreting the results of agglutination tests is the fact that agglutinins may be persistently absent or may be present in low titer in persons from whom Brucella has been cultivated.[41, 62-65] Another source of error in interpreting the agglutination reaction is the fact that the titer may remain at a high level for months or years after recovery. Then, too, some individuals exposed to the infection may develop agglutinins without notable illness. Furthermore, the level of the agglutinin titer may fluctuate widely on repeated testing. These considerations call for the exercise of keen judgment in interpreting the results of the agglutination test. A person suffering from some disease other than brucellosis may have a positive agglutination test merely as the result of a previous symptomatic or asymptomatic Brucella infection.

In the past, diagnostic significance has usually been attributed to titers of 1:80 or above. The choice of such an arbitrary diagnostic titer is not justified in the light of recent studies. In those cases in which the clinical manifestations suggest brucellosis, the absence of agglutinins or their presence in titers of 1:10 to 1:40 should stimulate further bacteriologic and serologic studies.

The difficulties which attend the interpretation of agglutination tests in cases of acute brucellosis are greatly multiplied in cases of chronic brucellosis. While the great majority of patients with the acute form of the disease reveal a positive agglutination test in high titer, a high proportion of patients with chronic brucellosis give repeatedly negative agglutination reactions or positive tests in low titer.   In a group of twenty-eight cases of chronic brucellosis studied by Evans,[54] 46 per cent gave a negative agglutination reaction.

The occasional cross agglutination of *Brucella* and *Bacterium tularense* should be borne in mind.   In cases of tularemia the relatively higher titer with the *B. tularense* antigen and the usually typical history leave little doubt as to the interpretation of the serologic findings.   If the *Brucella* and *B. tularense* titers are the same, or nearly so, agglutinin absorption tests will distinguish between them.

While the agglutination test is undoubtedly of great value, its limitations must be recognized.   Otherwise, errors will be made in two directions: first, the correct diagnosis of brucellosis may not be made because too much reliance is placed in a negative test; or, second, an incorrect diagnosis of brucellosis may be made in a person who has a residual agglutinin titer from a previous invasion by Brucella, but who is suffering from some other disease when the test is made.

The *intradermal test* is used to determine cutaneous hypersensitiveness to specific Brucella antigen.   A positive allergic skin reaction is generally accepted as evidence of past or present Brucella infection.   While the great majority of patients from whose blood Brucella has been recovered show a positive skin test, the test has yielded negative results in a few patients whose infection was proved by culture.

The chief sources of error in interpreting the significance of a positive skin test lie in the fact that the test is frequently positive in exposed individuals with no history of an illness compatible with brucellosis.   Furthermore, the hypersensitiveness, once acquired after symptomatic or subclinical infection, usually persists for may years.   Therefore, it must be emphasized that a positive skin test does not mean that the symptoms from which the patient is suffering at the time of the test are necessarily due to brucellosis.   Students of this disease are only too familiar with instances in which a diagnosis of brucellosis was made only on the basis of a positive skin test and in which further developments revealed the presence of some such disease as active tuberculosis, Hodgkin's disease, leukemia, typhoid fever, malaria, or subacute streptococcic endocarditis.   The intradermal test is regarded by Evans as a less accurate indicator of present infection than the agglutination test because the allergic state usually develops later than agglutinins and because it is generally retained for longer periods after recovery.   Gould and Huddleson,[49] on the other hand, regard the skin test as the most sensitive diagnostic test for brucellosis; these investigators express the belief that if the skin test is negative, brucellosis may usually be ruled out.

A variety of antigens has been used for skin testing.   The two agents most commonly employed are (1) a heat-killed suspension of Brucella in physiologic saline solution (vaccine) and (2) a suspensoid of nucleoprotein isolated from Brucella by chemical separation, known as "brucellergin" (Huddleson).   If commercially available vaccines are used for skin testing, the usual procedure is to dilute the vaccine in a proportion of one part vaccine to nine parts sterile physiologic solution of sodium chloride and to inject 0.1 cc. of the diluted suspension intracutaneously in the ventral surface of the forearm.   It is important to select properly standardized vaccines from a reliable source.   Variations in the manner of preparation, potency and dosage have led to a lack of uniformity in the production and interpretation of cutaneous reactions.   Brucellergin has the advantage of being a standardized preparation, especially designed for skin testing. The brucellergin test is also performed by injecting 0.1 cc. into the skin of the forearm.   A positive reaction by either method is characterized by the development of a circumscribed erythematous, edematous, indurated area at the site of injection.   In a positive test, the area of local reaction averages about three fourths of an inch in diameter, but may vary from one-half inch to three or more inches.   The reaction usually reaches its greatest intensity in twenty-four to forty-eight hours; ordinarily it is best to observe the results of the test forty-eight hours after injection.   The presence of mild, transient erythema, without edema and induration, is of no significance.   In frankly positive cases the induration usually persists for several days.   In hypersensitive persons a positive test may be accompanied by a mild, or in some instances a severe, systemic reaction.   In such cases the lymphatic channels above the site of inoculation may become red, thickened and painful, and the regional axillary lymph nodes may become enlarged and tender. An exacerbation of symptoms may follow the development of a positive skin test. Focal necrosis at the site of inoculation occurs in a small number of cases.

There is evidence [66, 67] that the injection of heat-killed Brucella for the intradermal test stimulates the production of agglutinins. Evans [41] found that the intracutaneous injection of brucellergin in twelve volunteers caused the development of opsonins in seven and agglutinins in five; in one instance the agglutinins rose from zero to a titer of 1 : 320. Hence it is advisable to collect blood specimens for serologic tests before the intradermal test is performed.

The inadequacies of the agglutination test and the intradermal test, particularly in distinguishing between present and past Brucella infection, led Huddleson, Johnson and Hamann [68] to reintroduce the *opsonocytophagic reaction*, a modification of the Leishman-Veitch technic for determining the phagocytic activity of the blood in the presence of serum opsonins and homologous leukocytes. The opsonocytophagic test is employed in conjunction with the intradermal test or the agglutination test, or both, to determine the immunity status of an individual giving positive tests by either or both methods. The test is performed by mixing 0.1 cc. of the patient's citrated blood with 0.1 cc. of a saline suspension of living Brucella which have been grown for forty-eight hours on liver infusion agar. The suspension should contain at least six billion organisms per cubic centimeter of physiologic saline solution (pH 7.0). The mixture is then incubated at 37° C. (98.6° F.) for thirty minutes, after which a small amount of the sedimented cells is removed with a capillary pipette. A smear is then made from a large drop of the cell suspension, dried rapidly and stained with Hastings' stain or Bordet-Gengou's carbol-toluidine blue. The number of bacteria in twenty-five polymorphonuclear neutrophilic leukocytes is determined and classified according to the number of bacteria per polymorphonuclear leukocyte: 0 indicates a negative result; 1 to 20 indicates slight, 21 to 40 moderate, and 41 or more, marked phagocytosis.

According to Huddleson's interpretation, the opsonocytophagic power of the blood is low during the active infective phase of the disease and becomes marked after recovery. On this basis, it is considered that individuals have developed immunity to Brucella if 60 per cent or more of the polymorphonuclear leukocytes show marked phagocytosis. If as many as 40 per cent of the leukocytes show moderate to marked phagocytosis, the patient may be infected and has not yet developed any immunity, or he may be uninfected.

Huddleson has proposed the following system for the diagnosis of brucellosis according to the results of the agglutination test, allergic skin test and opsonocytophagic reaction:

Agglutination Test	Allergic Skin Test	Opsonocytophagic Power of Blood	Status Toward Brucella
Negative	Negative	Cells negative to 20 per cent slight phagocytosis	Susceptible
Negative	Positive	Cells negative to 40 per cent marked phagocytosis	Infected
Positive	Positive	Cells negative to 40 per cent marked phagocytosis	Infected
Negative	Positive	Cells 60 to 100 per cent marked phagocytosis	Immune
Positive	Positive	Cells 60 to 100 per cent marked phagocytosis	Immune

A simplified method for reading the slides and interpreting the results of the opsonocytophagic reaction has been devised by Evans.[41] Foshay and Le Blanc [69] have proposed a simple and ingenious nomogram for the conversion of the four classes of phagocytized bacteria (0, 1–20, 21–40, 40 plus) into a single phagocytic index number.

While theoretical considerations lend support to the contentions of Huddleson and his associates as to the value of the opsonocytophagic test, it still lacks confirmation.   The studies by Calder,[34] and Keller, Pharris and Gaub,[70, 71] provide some support to Huddleson's thesis.   On the other hand, Evans [54] regards the opsonocytophagic test as the least reliable of the diagnostic tests in cases of chronic brucellosis; she found strongly positive (immune) reactions in four cases from which Brucella were cultivated and weak or moderate reactions in recovered cases.   Morales-Otero and Gonzalez [72] tested over 200 individuals (cattle handlers, milkers and laboratory workers exposed to Brucella infection) with a purified Brucella skin-test antigen, agglutination tests, complement fixation tests and opsonocytophagic tests.   They found no correlation between cutaneous allergy to Brucella and the opsonocytophagic reaction.   Fifteen cases that were positive to the opsonocytophagic reaction gave a negative cutaneous reaction, while eighteen showing a positive cutaneous reaction were completely negative to the opsonocytophagic reaction.   Until more extensive studies have been made on culturally proved cases of brucellosis, the results of the opsonocytophagic test should be interpreted with caution.

Hematocytologic studies indicate that leukopenia, with an increase in lymphocytes at the expense of polymorphonuclear leukocytes, occurs in about two thirds of cases; in the remaining third, moderate leukocytosis or normal leukocyte counts occur.   Mild to moderate degrees of secondary anemia are usually present.   The erythrocyte sedimentation rate frequently exhibits a moderate increase.

A lowered basal metabolic rate, vascular hypotension, gastric hypochlorhydria or achlorhydria are commonly observed in patients with chronic brucellosis.

Diagnosis.—Because brucellosis presents many symptoms and signs common to typhoid fever, malaria, tuberculosis and influenza, it is frequently confused with these diseases.   Not infrequently a tardy diagnosis of brucellosis is made only after repeatedly negative Widal reactions, the failure to demonstrate the malarial plasmodium, and the inability to elicit physical signs or roentgenographic evidence of tuberculosis.   Less often, the disease has been confused with rheumatic fever, subacute bacterial endocarditis, bronchitis and appendicitis.

In the acute form of the disease the manifestations are often sufficiently characteristic to justify a provisional clinical diagnosis of brucellosis.   The disease has been recognized most frequently in those areas in which investigators have stimulated their medical colleagues to search for it.   Many victims of the disease do not appear dangerously ill and there is often a natural tendency to neglect the taking of a detailed history and the performance of a thorough physical examination.

In arriving at a diagnosis of brucellosis, careful inquiry should be made regarding exposure to the infection, as a result of the ingestion of infected raw milk or other unpasteurized dairy products, or by direct contact with the tissues, secretions or excretions of infected animals.   The character of the onset of the disease, the sequence of the development of general and localized symptoms, and the physical findings may provide convincing clues.   When clinical suspicion is aroused recourse should be had to the several confirmatory tests.   Since the diagnosis can be established with absolute certainty only by recovery of Brucella, repeated attempts should be made to culture the organism from the blood, urine, bile, spinal fluid, exudates and excised tissues.   Hospitalization is desirable because such bacteriologic studies can be carried out more efficiently in a well-equipped hospital.   If cultural studies yield negative results, or if it is impracticable to carry out such investigations, the next most reliable aid is the agglutination test.   In cases of acute brucellosis with abrupt onset it is unwise to collect the blood specimens for the agglutination test until one week or ten days after the beginning of the disease.   If the onset is insidious, agglutinins may be found at the time of the first examination.   Since the appearance of agglutinins may be delayed, or may fluctuate in titer, repeated tests should be made if the first tests are negative or show agglutination in low titer.   Because of the possibility of producing specific agglutinins or opsonins in the absence of brucellosis, the intradermal test and the opsonocytophagic test should be performed only after repeated agglutination tests are found to be negative.   The value of the agglutination test and the skin test has been adequately demonstrated, but it must be recognized that all of the so-called specific diagnostic tests may yield repeatedly negative results in culturally proved cases of brucellosis, and that none distinguishes with certainty between present and past infection. Thus, in the absence of bacteriologic proof, the finding of positive agglutination tests, skin tests and opsonocytophagic tests must be weighed carefully in the balance of fine critical judgment along with the clinical observations before a decision is reached.

Just as the diagnosis of brucellosis may be missed by too great reliance on any one or all of the diagnostic tests, so also is there danger that the diagnosis may be made much too freely by unjustified reliance on a positive skin test. This hazard pertains particularly to the diagnosis of chronic brucellosis.

Clinical Types.—Five types of the disease are generally recognized: (1) intermittent, (2) ambulatory, (3) undulatory, (4) malignant, and (5) subclinical.

1. INTERMITTENT TYPE.—The disease pursues a subacute course, with fever of an intermittent character; the morning temperatures vary from normal or slightly subnormal to 100° F. (37.8° C.), while the evening temperatures usually range from 101–105° F. (38.3–40.6° C.). The average duration of this type of the illness is from three to four months.

2. AMBULATORY TYPE.—Many persons in this group will remain at their work although aware of the existence of mild fever and a marked sense of weakness. The symptoms and signs of this form of the disease are sometimes the same as in the intermittent type, except that they are less severe. Such cases are frequently confused with influenza. Most of the cases of chronic brucellosis fall into this group.

3. UNDULATORY TYPE.—This form of the disease is characterized by the occurrence of relapses. This feature of the disease was said to be of frequent occurrence in the Mediterranean cases, but has been present in only about 15 per cent of the cases which have occurred in this country. The successive relapses usually decrease in intensity and duration. Physical and mental deterioration are commonly observed in the undulatory form of the disease.

4. MALIGNANT TYPE.—This form of the disease is rare, having occurred in only about 2 per cent of the cases reported in this country. A sudden onset, an acute course with extreme hyperpyrexia and a fatal termination in the majority of cases are the characteristics of this unusual form of the disease. The duration of this type of the disease is usually from one to three weeks.

5. SUBCLINICAL TYPE.—Subclinical Brucella infections have occurred in persons who have been exposed to the infection; anti-Brucella agglutinins have been demonstrated in the serum of such persons in the absence of clinical symptoms or signs of the disease. Carpenter, Boak and Chapman [62] have submitted convincing evidence that anti-Brucella agglutinins develop only when there has been actual invasion of the tissues by living Brucella organisms. There is no evidence that agglutinins are passively absorbed in the intestine from milk containing killed organisms.

Treatment.—The most important consideration in the control of brucellosis is *prophylaxis*. The widespread distribution of the infection among cattle renders it difficult to control the infection at its source. Many cows have Bang's disease and eliminate the organisms in large numbers in the milk and vaginal discharges without manifesting symptoms of the disease (abortion, mastitis, sterility and lessened milk yield). There is but one logical method for preventing the transmission of milk-borne infection to human beings, and that is by **pasteurization.** Brucellosis is only one of the formidable list of diseases transmitted to man through the use of raw milk and other unpasteurized dairy products. Murray, McNutt and Purwin,[73] Boak and Carpenter,[74] and Zwick and Wedeman [75] have demonstrated that complete pasteurization (143–145° F. [61.7–62.8° C.] for thirty minutes) will destroy Brucella. The need for strict supervision of the pasteurization process is apparent. For the protection of the health of those persons whose occupations bring them in direct contact with infected animal tissues, we must rely upon education and the institution of precautionary measures.

For those persons who live on farms, or in small communities where pasteurization is not yet practiced, home pasteurization may be carried out by placing the milk in an aluminum vessel and heating it to 155° F. (68.3° C.), stirring constantly, then immediately setting the vessel in cold water and continuing the stirring until cool.

The *general management* of the patient with brucellosis will be largely determined by the prevailing symptoms and signs. General therapeutic considerations will vary greatly in individual patients. The therapeutic program for patients with acute brucellosis is quite different from that employed for the chronic form of the disease.

In severe cases of acute brucellosis the general management is essentially that employed for any acute febrile disease, characterized by fever, chills and sweats. If the sweating is of a drenching character, special provisions should be made for the protection of the mattress and for changes of bed linen and gowns. If the fever exceeds 104° F. (40° C.) **tepid sponge baths** are indicated; **antipyretic drugs should be avoided.** The patient should remain constantly in. bed during the febrile phase and for at least one week after the temperature has returned to the normal level. Skilled nursing care is an essential requirement in the severe cases. · The same precautions should be taken as regards the disinfection of urine and feces as in cases of typhoid fever. As the fever abates, a **liberal diet of high caloric value** is required, particularly for patients who lose considerable weight. The patient should be cautioned against resuming even moderate activity until there has been an appreciable gain in strength. Two or three additional weeks of rest will often save the patient from several months of partial disability.

In cases of chronic brucellosis the general management must be strictly individualized. Since most of these patients are ambulatory and are at least attempting to perform some work, often at great effort, the program should be directed toward a maximum amount of rest. This may entail a regulation of the hours of work in order to avoid excessive fatigue. Since most of these patients suffer from the symptoms ordinarily ascribed to neurasthenia, a generous amount of practical **psychotherapy,** largely directed toward reassurance, is a fundamental requirement. The members of the patient's family should be fully informed as to the nature of the illness in order to enlist their sympathetic understanding and to avoid their stigmatizing the patient as neurotic or as a malingerer. The common symptoms of headache, backache, joint and muscle pains, insomnia, anorexia, constipation and anemia usually yield to appropriate symptomatic measures.

SPECIFIC THERAPY.—While there is considerable evidence that the employment of various types of serum therapy and vaccine therapy has greatly improved the outlook for most patients suffering from acute or chronic brucellosis, it is extremely difficult to evaluate the effectiveness of any form of specific therapy in a disease characterized by natural remissions and by an extremely variable symptomatology. The reported results of vaccine therapy or serum therapy run the entire gamut from pessimism to hyperenthusiasm. More extensive controlled and systematic studies on a large number of patients, carried out over a period of many years, are necessary before definite statements. can be made. It would appear, however, that sufficient data have been accumulated to justify the continued use of some of the so-called specific agents.

(a) *Serum Therapy.*—Interest in serum therapy, which had waned following the earlier appearance of several unfavorable reports, has been revived by the development of a more potent anti-Brucella serum by Foshay [76, 77] and his associates at the University of Cincinnati. Detoxified Brucella antigens are employed for the development of the antiserums in goats or horses. Several favorable experiences with the Foshay serum have been recorded by other workers.[78] This type of antiserum therapy should be restricted to patients with acute or subacute brucellosis, preferably to those who have had the disease less than eight months. The dosage recommended by Foshay is as follows: For adults suffering from moderately severe to severe manifestations of the disease, the average total dose is 60 cc., given by three daily intravenous or intramuscular injections of 20 cc. each or by two daily injections of 30 cc. each; in unusually severe infections, 90 to 120 cc. may be given in unit doses of 30 cc. during a period of forty-eight to seventy-two hours; for children, a total of 20 to 30 cc. may be given, either intramuscularly or subcutaneously, in daily doses of 10 cc. each.

Serum therapy is not indicated in cases of chronic brucellosis of more than eight months' duration, unless sudden, severe exacerbations occur. Such abrupt relapses are usually the result of regional localizations involving the meninges, brain, spinal cord, heart valves, lungs, liver, spleen and bone marrow. In such cases the dosage of serum would be that recommended for unusually severe infections.

Scattered reports of the use of convalescent human serum, blood transfusions from recovered donors, or immunotransfusions from donors who have received prior injections of heat-killed Brucella, have appeared.[64, 79-82] Even though the number of cases is too small and the period of observation not sufficiently long for accurate evaluation, the results were sufficiently gratifying to justify further trials, particularly as regards immunotransfusions.

(b) *Vaccine Therapy.*—It seems probable that the earlier discrepant reports of the effectiveness of vaccine therapy had their basis in a lack of standardized methods for the preparation of the vaccines, both as regards the choice of suitable strains and the concentration of the vaccine. These difficulties appear to have been largely overcome in recent years by the development of better standards for the preparation of therapeutic vaccines.

Brucella melitensis (varieties *abortus* and *suis*) vaccine, N.N.R., has been widely employed and is available through the usual trade sources. This vaccine is a saline suspension of heat-killed or formalin-killed *Brucella abortus* and *suis* organisms in equal quantities. Vaccines prepared from the *melitensis* variety of the organism should be utilized only in the treatment of the relatively rare *Brucella melitensis* infections.

Experience has taught that no rigidly standardized scheme of dosage of vaccine is applicable to patients with brucellosis. Experience and good judgment are essential requisites in determining the proper dosage for each individual. The usual procedure with the commercially available vaccine is first to test for hypersensitiveness by injecting 0.05 cc. of a 1:10 dilution of the vaccine intracutaneously. If the patient does not experience an excessive local or systemic reaction within the next forty-eight hours, an initial therapeutic dose of 0.25 cc. is injected into the deep subcutaneous tissues, or preferably into the muscle. Local reactions are minimized by intramuscular injections. If no untoward reaction follows the first injection of 0.25 cc., a second dose of 0.25 cc. is given three days later. The dosage is then increased in increments of 0.25 cc., at intervals of three days, until a dosage of 1 cc. is reached. Ordinarily, two injections of 0.5 cc. and two of 0.75 cc. are given before the 1 cc. dosage is attained. Five to eight injections of 1 cc. each may then be given at three-day intervals.

If the patient is highly sensitized, it is wise to begin with intramuscular doses of 0.1 cc., or, in rare instances of extreme sensitization, with doses of 0.1 cc. of a 1:10 to 1:100 dilution of the vaccine, and gradually increase the dosage by 0.1-cc. increments until a dosage of 1 cc. is reached. If, during the course of vaccine injections, an unusually severe local or systemic reaction should occur, it is desirable to reduce the next dose to one half the amount which produced the severe reaction and then cautiously and gradually increase the succeeding doses.

A series of four to six or more sharp systemic, febrile reactions, usually accompanied by a transient exacerbation of symptoms, is the goal of the treatment. Hence, only extreme local or general reactions should be avoided. Elevations of temperature to 103–105° F. (39.4–40.6° C.) are not uncommon within four to eight hours after the injection of vaccine. Such systemic responses may occur following the first injection of a small quantity of vaccine or may not occur until relatively large doses are given. In chronic brucellosis larger doses of the vaccine may be required; if no reaction is provoked after five or six 1-cc. injections, the dosage may be gradually increased by 0.5-cc. increments to 2 or 3 cc.

While some patients who have obtained an apparently satisfactory response to vaccine therapy have had little or no thermal reaction, the most prompt and lasting results have occurred in those who have experienced several such reactions.

Erythema and tenderness at the site of vaccination occur commonly ·for a day or two following injections. In about 5 per cent of cases a local hard tumefaction may persist for much longer periods. In a small proportion of such cases sterile abscesses or local areas of necrosis have developed.

(c) *Brucellin Therapy.*—Brucellin is a fraction of Brucella cells obtained by growing the organism in liver broth. The bacteria-free active agent is recovered from the liver broth filtrate. This preparation was devised by I. F. Huddleson [63], [83], [84] and may be procured at the Central Brucella Station, Michigan State College, East Lansing, Michigan.

The dosage of brucellin must also be adjusted to suit the requirements of individual patients. After the extent of sensitiveness has been determined by the intradermal injection of 0.1 cc. of brucellin, the usual procedure in non-hypersensitive patients is to give repeated injections of 1 cc. at intervals of three days until the morning and evening temperatures between the intervals of injection tend to become subnormal. Here again, one object of this form of therapy is the production of a series of four or more febrile, systemic reactions. If the duration of illness is less than ten weeks, the likelihood of recovery following four 1-cc. injections is greater than if the duration is longer than ten weeks. Patients with long-continued chronic brucellosis require a larger number of injections and may require gradually increasing amounts up to 5 cc. before satisfactory reactions are produced. In highly sensitized persons, it is advisable to start with intramuscular doses of 0.1 cc. If there is no severe systemic reaction following this injection, each succeeding dose may ordinarily be doubled, until the larger dosage is attained.

In children, the initial dose of Brucella vaccine or brucellin should not exceed 0.1 cc. and succeeding doses should be increased by not over 0.1-cc. increments. Considerable dilution of the vaccine is required for hypersensitive children.

A partially oxidized detoxified vaccine, devised by Foshay and O'Neil,[85] has been used with apparent success.[34] Much smaller doses are given subcutaneously at more frequent intervals. The few reports of results indicate the recovery rate equals that of other vaccines or brucellin. Local or constitutional reactions do not occur with the oxidized vaccine. It has been recommended chiefly for the treatment of chronic ·brucellosis.

While it is difficult to evaluate the results of vaccine or brucellin therapy, the experiences of many investigators indicate that about 60 per cent of patients with brucellosis obtain apparently complete recovery after a satisfactory course of either agent. An additional 25 per cent appear to obtain some benefit, while the remaining 15 per cent are not improved.

The contraindications to vaccine or brucellin therapy are heart disease, renal disease, arteriosclerosis, meningeal or cerebral localizations of Brucella or the acute fulminating (malignant) form of the disease.

NONSPECIFIC PROTEIN THERAPY.—Injections of foreign protein substances, such as sterile skimmed milk, typhoid vaccine or typhoid-paratyphoid vaccine have been utilized for the production of nonspecific shock reactions in the treatment of brucellosis.[86-88] Ervin and Hunt [89], [90] reported good results in twenty patients with acute and subacute brucellosis following the intravenous injection of killed typhoid-paratyphoid organisms. The usual initial dose was 30 to 50 million killed organisms, with two to six additional injections, increasing the dosage by increments of 25 million organisms.

CHEMOTHERAPY.—Neoarsphenamine, mercurochrome, acriflavine, metaphen, thionin, methylene blue, methyl violet, gentian violet and other chemical substances have been used in the treatment of brucellosis. In most instances the reports of the apparently successful use of these substances were based upon observations limited to small numbers of patients. The very length of the list argues against the specificity of any of them.

Sulfanilamide and related compounds have been- heralded as effective agents in the treatment of brucellosis since 1936.[91] After the first wave of enthusiasm, usually based on short observations on relatively few patients, other reports of less favorable or entirely negative results have appeared. Blumgart and Gilligan[92] analyzed the results reported in the thirty-one papers which appeared between 1936 and 1939. Twenty-four of the reports were concerned with only one or two patients. Of the seventy-four cases treated with sulfanilamide or allied compounds, there were sixty-eight apparent recoveries and six failures; fourteen of the sixty-eight patients (20 per cent) exhibited relapse after apparent recovery. The daily dosage of sulfanilamide employed in most cases was 4 to 6 Gm. (60 to 90 grains) during the period of fever, with gradually diminishing dosages for three or four days after the fever abated. The administration of the drug was rarely continued for more than twelve days. Bynum[93] reported six cases of brucellosis unsuccessfully treated with large doses of sulfanilamide. Long and Bliss[94] report recurrence of infection in four of five patients whose immediate response to sulfanilamide therapy was apparently quite satisfactory; in two instances Brucella was recovered from the blood after sulfanilamide therapy was discontinued. The writer has had similarly disappointing experiences in several cases treated with large doses of sulfanilamide, controlled by determinations of the sulfanilamide concentration of the blood. Until more extensive and extended studies are made on culturally proved cases, the value of sulfanilamide therapy in cases of brucellosis must be regarded as undetermined. In this connection it might be well to recall the fact that a temporary remission is not synonymous with cure.

ARTIFICIAL FEVER THERAPY.—The observation that recovery from brucellosis often followed the induction of fever by chemical or biologic agents led Prickman and Popp[95] to investigate the possible usefulness of artificial fever induced by physical means in the management of brucellosis. Each of three patients was given three artificial fever treatments, each of five hours' duration, at a rectal temperature of 105–106° F. (40.6–41.1° C.); all were benefited by the treatment. Zeiter[96] described a similarly favorable experience. More recently, Prickman, Bennett and Krusen[97] analyzed the results of treatment with physically induced hyperpyrexia in twenty-one cases of brucellosis; apparent cure resulted in 80.9 per cent of the patients. The duration of the disease prior to artificial fever therapy varied from ten days to two and one-half years. The authors expressed the belief that fever therapy was most efficacious in the acute and subacute febrile stage of the disease. Simpson[98] reserves artificial fever therapy for those refractory patients who do not respond to vaccine therapy. Artificial fever therapy should be carried out only in properly equipped institutions by thoroughly qualified physicians and nurse-technicians.

MISCELLANEOUS THERAPY.—Since some degree of anemia is a common finding in brucellosis, it should be combated with appropriate dietary, iron or liver therapy. Repeated small transfusions (200 cc.) are of value in the management of the more severe grades of anemia. In the more chronic forms of the disease, in which severe anorexia is a prominent feature, vitamin deficiency is common. Large doses of vitamin B, with reinforcement of vitamin A, C and D intake, have been effective in relieving this distressing symptom.

Prognosis.—Fatal outcome is rare, having occurred in about 2 per cent of reported cases. During 1936, 107 deaths from brucellosis were officially recorded in the United States. The importance of the disease is not to be judged by the low mortality rate. The prolonged course and the resulting chronic ill-health in a high proportion of cases make the outlook much more serious than the death rate would indicate. Death is usually the result of overwhelming acute infection, terminating fatally during the first few weeks of illness, or it follows a relapse at any stage of the disease owing to regional localizations of Brucella in such structures as the meninges, brain, heart valves or lungs.

Pathology.—Compared with the wealth of available data on the bacteriology and serology of Brucella infection, relatively little is known concerning any distinctive morbid anatomic changes in man.[99, 100] In guinea pigs inoculated with Brucella, focal nodular reactions in the spleen, liver, lymph nodes, bone marrow and testes may be observed; the focal lesions in the spleen and liver may vary from 0.5 to 2.0 mm. in diameter. Both grossly and microscopically, the splenic and hepatic lesions may show striking resemblance to those of tuberculosis or tularemia, except that caseation necrosis rarely occurs. In other instances, the lesions may grossly resemble tubercles, but the microscopic structure reveals only collections of lymphocytes and fibroblasts, without epithelioid cells or Langhans' giant cells.

In man, similar focal lesions may be found in the spleen, liver, lymph nodes and bone marrow. The essential feature of the morbid anatomy is a proliferation of cells belonging to the reticulo-endothelial system. The spleen is often considerably enlarged, deeply congested and soft, with an increase in the size and number of malpighian corpuscles. The liver rarely shows the same degree of enlargement as the spleen. The distinctive cellular aggregations that are sometimes found in the spleen and lymph nodes may be entirely absent in the liver. Extensive phagocytosis of hemosiderin by reticulo-endothelial phagocytes of the spleen, liver and lymph nodes has been observed in some cases. In many of the cases of Brucella endocarditis or meningitis, no distinctive lesions were found on either gross or microscopic examination of the spleen, liver or lymph nodes. In Brucella meningitis, or meningo-encephalitis, small tubercle-like lesions may be found in the leptomeninges, particularly along the blood vessels; microscopically, these focal lesions are composed of connective tissue cells, lymphocytes and plasma cells, with a smaller number of monocytes and polymorphonuclear leukocytes; the meningeal vessels are often surrounded by a collar of lymphocytes; perivascular lymphocytic infiltrations may be found in the cerebrum. In Brucella endocarditis the valve leaflets are usually rigid and thickened and covered with small, gray, friable vegetations.

Suppurative lesions of brucellosis have occurred in bones, particularly in the lumbar spine. Foci of Brucella infection may occur in the lungs, simulating bronchopneumonia. The generative organs of both men and women are often affected; the lesions may take the form of focal inflammatory areas, in which epithelioid cells, lymphocytes and fibroblasts predominate, or actual suppuration may occur. While involvement of the testes and ovaries is relatively common, the endometrium, fallopian tubes, prostate gland, seminal vesicles and epididymis are less often involved. Parsons, Poston and Wise [100, 101] have described seven cases of lymphadenopathy in which Brucella was recovered by culture from the excised enlarged lymph nodes; the histologic picture in all was regarded by the authors as indistinguishable from Hodgkin's disease; this surprising observation demands further critical investigation before a decision can be reached as to any possible etiologic role of Brucella in the causation of Hodgkin's disease.

Historical Summary.—Hippocrates (400 B.C.) described certain cases of protracted fever, with relapses and remissions and some of the features of tuberculosis, but without a fatal termination. It seems probable that he was describing what we now know as brucellosis. During and following the Crimean War (1854–1856) numerous cases of an obscure irregular fever were reported among the British military forces quartered in the Mediterranean area. Marston, a medical officer stationed in Malta (1863), gave a full and accurate description of the disease, which he termed "Mediterranean remittent fever." The confirmatory reports by Chartres (1865) and Veale (1873) revealed that the disease existed in endemic proportions in the Mediterranean region. Between the years 1860 to 1875, Mediterranean or Malta fever became a distinct clinical entity. In 1886 Bruce cultivated the etiologic agent. In 1897 two great advances were made: Bang discovered *Bacillus abortus* as the cause of contagious abortion of cattle and Wright and Semple first applied the agglutination test to aid in the diagnosis. During this same year the classical monograph by Hughes, on "Mediterranean, Malta or Undulant Fever," appeared. From 1904 to 1907, a commission representing the Army, Navy and Civil Government of Malta conducted monumental studies which provided convincing proof that the drinking of raw goat's milk was the common source of infection. The first cases to be recognized in this country occurred among men recently returned from the tropics (Musser and Sailer, 1899). Craig (1905) not only detected many cases among men in the Army who had served in the Philippine Islands, but also established the diagnosis in a nurse who had never been out of the country and who had had no contact with patients with Malta fever. Craig suggested at this time that many patients with atypical typhoid-like fever might be suffering from Malta fever. A few cases of the disease were reported from goat-raising areas in Texas, New Mexico and Arizona by Gentry and Ferenbaugh (1911) and by Yount and Looney (1913). Then the disease apparently faded from medical consciousness for a decade, when Lake and Watkins (1922) published their startling report of an epidemic of Malta fever in Phoenix, Arizona, which they traced to the infection of raw goat's milk. Up to this time physicians naturally associated undulant fever only with a goat source. It was the monumental observation by Alice Evans (1918), that the organisms of Malta fever and contagious abortion of cattle were for all practical purposes indistinguishable, that led to the discovery of the widespread occurrence of Brucella infection of bovine and porcine origin.

Geographic Distribution.—Following the first report by Keefer (1924) of a case of brucellosis due to the *abortus* variety of the organism, a rapid succession of reports of cases of bovine or porcine origin appeared from South Africa, Canada, Germany, Sweden, Norway, Denmark, Italy, Great Britain, Switzerland, The Netherlands, France, Puerto Rico and New Zealand. Subsequent reports leave little doubt that brucellosis is world-wide in its distribution and is most prevalent in those areas in which Brucella infection of cattle, hogs and goats is widespread.

REFERENCES

1. Bruce, D.: Note on discovery of a micro-coccus in Malta fever, Practitioner, 39: 161, 1887.
2. Bang, B. F.: Etiology of infectious abortion, J. Comp. Path. & Therap., 10: 125, 1897.
3. Evans, A. C.: Bacterium abortus and related bacteria, J. Infect. Dis., 22: 580, 1918.
4. Carpenter, C. M.: Results of injecting pregnant heifers with Brucella abortus isolated from man, J. Am. Vet. M. A., 70: 459, 1927.
5. Meyer, K. F. and Shaw, E. B.: Comparison of morphologic, cultural and biochemical characteristics of B. abortus and B. melitensis, J. Infect. Dis., 27: 173, 1920.
6. Traum, J.: Infectious abortion investigations in pigs, Am. Rep. Dept. Agric., Washington, 86, 1914.
7. Gershenfeld, L. and Butts, D. C. A.: Survey of undulant fever and Bang's disease in United States, Am. J. M. Sc., 194: 678, 1937.
8. Hardy, A. V., Hudson, M. G. and Jordan, C. F.: Skin as portal of entry in Br. melitensis infections, J. Infect. Dis., 45: 271, 1929.
9. Morales-Otero, P.: Experimental infection of Brucella abortus in man, Puerto Rico J. Pub. Health & Trop. Med., 5: 144, 1929. Brucella abortus in Puerto Rico, Puerto Rico J. Pub. Health & Trop. Med., 6: 3, 1930.
10. ——: Prevalence of undulant fever (brucellosis) in United States, Pub. Health Rep., 53: 1195, 1938.
11. Hardy, A. V., Jordan, C. F. and Borts, I. H.: Undulant fever; further epidemiologic and clinical observations in Iowa, J. Am. M. Ass., 107: 559, 1936.
12. Hughes, M. L.: Mediterranean, Malta, or Undulant Fever, London and New York, Macmillan Co., 1897.
13. Craig, C. F.: Symptomatology and diagnosis of Malta fever, with report of additional cases, Internat. Clin., 4: 89, 1906.
14. Hardy, A. V., Jordan, C. F., Borts, I. H. and Hardy, G. C.: Undulant fever, with special reference to study of Brucella infection in Iowa, Pub. Health Rep. 45: 2433; 2525, 1930. Nat. Inst. Health Bull. No. 158, Dec., 1930.
15. Simpson, W. M.: Undulant fever (brucelliasis): clinicopathologic study of 90 cases occurring in and about Dayton, Ohio, Ann. Int. Med., 4: 238, 1930.
16. —— and Fraizer, E.: Undulant fever: report of 63 cases occurring in and about Dayton, Ohio, J. Am. M. Ass., 93: 1958, 1929.
17. ——: Clinical picture of undulant fever, Ohio State M. J., 27: 21, 1931.
18. Kulowski, J. and Vinke, T. H.: Undulant (Malta) fever spondylitis, J. Am. M. Ass., 99: 1656, 1932. Kulowski, J.: Undulant (Malta) fever, osteomyelitis and arthritis, Surg., Gynec. & Obst., 62: 759, 1936. Archer, V. W.: Undulant fever, with report of case simulating Pott's disease, South. M. J., 28: 1, 1935. Snyder, C. H.: Spondylitis in undulant fever: report of 2 cases, J. Michigan M. Soc., 34: 224, 1935. Jensen, J. P.: Spondylitis e Bacillo abortus (Bang), Hospitalstid., 71: 637, 1928. Lassen, H. K.: Et Tilfaelde af Spondylitis pas Basis af Infektion, Med. Bac. Abortus (Bang), Hospitalstid., 73: 64, 1930. Redell, G.: Spondylitis als Komplikation von Febris undulans Bang, Acta chir. Scandinav., 69: 87, 1931. Roger, H.: La spondylite melitococcique, Presse méd., 34: 929, 1926. Vannucci, D. F.: Sulle spondiliti da brucellosi, Gior. di clin. med., 14: 214, 1933.
19. Feldman, W. H. and Olson, C., Jr.: Spondylitis of swine associated with bacteria of Brucella group, Arch. Path., 16: 195, 1933.
20. —— and ——: Isolation of bacteria of the Brucella group in cases of spondylitis of swine; an additional study, J. Am. Vet. M. A., 84: 628, 1934.
21. Roger, H. and Poursines, Y.: Les Méningo-Neurobrucelloses, Paris, Masson & Cie, 1938.
22. De Jong, R. N.: Central nervous system involvement in undulant fever, with report of a case and survey of literature, J. Nerv. & Ment. Dis., 83: 430, 1936.
23. Amoss, H. L. and Poston, M. A.: Cultivation of Brucella from stools and bile, J. Am. M. Ass., 95: 482, 1930.
24. MacQuiddy, E. L. and Martin, J. W.: Cholecystitis due to Brucella melitensis, Nebraska M. J., 19: 227, 1934.

25. Bull, P. and Gram, H. M.: Cholecystitis with pure culture of Micrococcus melitensis, Norsk mag. f. laegevidensk., 72: 1026, 1911.

26. Johnson, R. M.: Pneumonia in undulant fever; report of 3 cases, Am. J. M. Sc., 189: 483, 1935.

27. Bogart, F. B.: Pulmonary changes in undulant fever, South. M. J., 29: 1, 1936.

28. Paretzky, M.: Undulant fever; pulmonary findings simulating tuberculosis, M. Rec., 144: 11, 1936.

29. Lafferty, R. H. and Phillips, C. C.: Pulmonary changes in patients suffering from Malta fever, South. M. J., 30: 595, 1937.

30. Beatty, O. A.: Manifestations of undulant fever in respiratory tract, Am. Rev. Tuberc., 36: 283, 1937.

31. Smith, K. M. and Curtis, A. C.: Brucellosis with endocarditis; report of case with failure of sulfanilamide therapy, Am. J. M. Sc., 198: 342, 1939.

32. De Forest, H. P.: Infectious abortion, Am. J. Obst., 76: 221, 1917. Larson, W. P. and Sedgwick, J. P.: Complement fixation reaction of blood of children and infants, using the Bacillus abortus as antigen, Am. J. Dis. Child., 6: 326, 1913. Sedgwick, J. P. and Larson, W. P.: Further studies on epidemic abortion reactions in children, Am. J. Dis. Child., 10: 197, 1915.

33. Harbinson, J. E.: Undulant fever in California, Ann. Int. Med., 4: 484, 1930.

34. Calder, R. M.: Chronic brucellosis, South. M. J., 32: 451, 1939.

35. Carpenter, C. M. and Boak, R. A.: Isolation of Brucella abortus from human fetus, J. Am. M. Ass., 96: 1212, 1931.

36. Kristensen, M. and Holm, P.: Bakteriologische und statistische Untersuchungen über Febris undulans in Dänemark, Zentralbl. f. Bakteriol. (Abt. 1), 112: 281, 1929.

37. Frei, W.: Uebergang des B. abortus Bang von Haustieren auf Menschen, Schweiz. med. Wchnschr., 59: 334, 1929.

38. Cornell, E. L. and DeYoung, C. R.: Incidence of undulant fever in pregnancy and abortion, Am. J. Obst. & Gynec., 18: 840, 1929.

39. Evans, A. C.: Chronic brucellosis, J. Am. M. Ass., 103: 665, 1934.

40. ———: Studies on chronic brucellosis; introduction, Pub. Health Rep., 52: 1072, 1937.

41. ———: Studies on chronic brucellosis; description of techniques for specific tests, Pub. Health Rep., 52: 1419, 1937.

42. Poston, M. A.: Studies on chronic brucellosis; methods used in obtaining cultures, Pub. Health Rep., 53: 1, 1938.

43. Angle, F. E.: Treatment of acute and chronic brucellosis (undulant fever), J. Am. M. Ass., 105: 939, 1935.

44. Scoville, W. B.: Prevalence of mild Brucella abortus infections, J. Am. M. Ass., 105: 1976, 1935.

45. Thames, E.: Chronic undulant fever. A pathologic debility often resulting in severe nervous disorders, Med. World, 53: 106, 175, 245, 306, 378, 1935.

46. Hamman, L. and Wainwright, C. W.: Diagnosis of obscure fever; diagnosis of unexplained, long-continued low-grade fever, Bull. Johns Hopkins Hosp., 58: 109, 1936.

47. Harris, H. J.: Undulant fever (brucellosis); difficulties in diagnosis and treatment— supplementary report on 51 cases with observations on 120 additional cases, New York State J. Med., 37: 1295, 1937.

48. Cameron, W. R. and Wells, M.: Undulant fever control in Washington County, Maryland, South. M. J., 27: 907, 1934.

49. Gould, S. E. and Huddleson, I. F.: Diagnostic methods in undulant fever (brucellosis) with results of survey of 8,124 persons, J. Am. M. Ass., 109: 1971, 1937.

50. Gersh, I. and Mugrage, E. R.: Incidence of positive immunologic reactions for undulant fever, J. Lab. & Clin. Med., 23: 918, 1938.

51. Angle, F. E., Algie, W. H., Baumgartner, L. and Lunsford, W. F.: Skin testing for brucellosis (undulant fever) in school children, Ann. Int. Med., 12: 495, 1938.

52. McGinty, A. P. and Gambrell, W. E.: Chronic brucellosis, Internat. Clin., 1: 1, 1939.

53. Pinnell, R. B. and Huddleson, I. F.: Chemical Constitution and Biological Properties of the Endo-Antigen of the Brucella group of Microorganisms, Tech. Bull. 156, Mich. State Col., Agric. Exper. Station, Dec., 1937.

54. Evans, A. C., Robinson, F. H. and Baumgartner, L.: Studies on chronic brucellosis; evaluation of diagnostic laboratory tests, Pub. Health Rep., 53: 1507, 1938.

55. ———: Difficulties in diagnosis of chronic brucellosis, Am. J. Trop. Med., 19: 319, 1939.

56. Robinson, F. H. and Evans, A. C.: Chronic brucellosis in Charlotte, N. C., J. Am. M. Ass., 113: 201, 1939.

57. Huddleson, I. F.: Brucellosis in Man and Animals, New York, The Commonwealth Fund, 1939.

58. Amoss, H. L. and Poston, M. A.: Undulant (Malta) fever: isolation of the Brucella organism from stools, J. Am. Ass., 93: 170, 1929.

59. Evans, A. C.: Distribution of Brucella melitensis variety melitensis in United States, Pub. Health Rep., 52: 295, 1937.

60. Huddleson, I. F.: The Differentiation of the Species of the Genus Brucella, Tech. Bull. No. 100, Mich. State College, 1929.

61. ———: Brucella Infections in Animals and Man, Methods of Laboratory Diagnosis, New York, The Commonwealth Fund, 1934.

62. Carpenter, C. M., Boak, R. A. and Chapman, O. D.: Significance of Brucella abortus agglutinins in human serum, J. Immunol., 17: 65, 1929.

63. Huddleson, I. F., Johnson, H. W. and Beattie, C. P.: Studies in Brucella Infection. A Report of 100 Cases Treated with Brucellin, Bull. 149, Agric. Exper. Sta., Mich. State College, May, 1936.

64. Poston, M. A. and Smith, D. T.: Successful treatment of Brucella meningitis with immune human serum: isolation of organism by modified cultural method, New England J. Med., 215: 369, 1936.

65. Huddleson, I. F., Munger, M., Gould, S. E. and Paulson, D.: Study of Brucella infection and immunity in humans, Am. J. Trop. Med., 17: 863, 1937.

66. Goldstein, J. D.: Cutaneous reactions in diagnosis of undulant fever, J. Clin. Investigation, 13: 209, 1934.

67. Heathman, L. S.: Survey of workers in packing plants for evidence of Brucella infection, J. Infect. Dis., 55: 243, 1934.

68. Huddleson, I. F., Johnson, H. W. and Hamann, E. E.: Study of opsono-cytophagic power of blood and allergic skin reaction in Brucella infection and immunity in man, Am. J. Pub. Health, 23: 917, 1933.

69. Foshay, L. and Le Blanc, T. J.: Derivation of index number for opsonocytophagic test, J. Lab. & Clin. Med., 22: 1297, 1937.

70. Keller, A. E., Pharris, C. and Gaub, W. H.: Diagnosis of undulant fever: opsonocytophagic, allergic and agglutination reactions, J. Am. M. Ass., 107: 1369, 1936.

71. ———, ——— and ———: Undulant fever; comparative value of certain diagnostic tests, South. M. J., 31: 1, 1938.

72. Morales-Otero, P. and Gonzalez, L. M.: Allergy in Brucella infections, Proc. Soc. Exper. Biol. & Med., 40: 100, 1939.

73. Murray, C., McNutt, S. H. and Purwin, P.: Effect of pasteurization upon Br. melitensis var. suis, J. Am. Vet. M. A., 33: 336, 1932.

74. Boak, R. and Carpenter, C. M.: Thermal death point of Brucella abortus in milk, J. Infect. Dis., 43: 327, 1928.

75. Zwick and Wedeman: Cited by Boak and Carpenter. J. Infect. Dis., 43: 327, 1928.

76. Wherry, W. B., O'Neil, A. E. and Foshay, L.: Brucellosis in man: treatment with new anti-serum, Am. J. Trop. Med., 15: 415, 1935.

77. Foshay, L.: Serum therapy in human brucellosis. (Abstract.) J. Bact., 33: 42, 1937.

78. Miller, J. L.: Undulant fever, Ann. Int. Med., 8: 570, 1934. Bannick, E. G. and Magath, T. B.: Case of brucellosis treated with antiserum, Proc. Staff Meet., Mayo Clin., 11: 17, 1936. Casey, J. F.: Brucellosis (undulant fever); interesting and important facts about disease with report of severe case occurring in Boston physician, New England J. Med., 215: 1282, 1936. Woodward, L. R.: Brucellosis, J. Iowa M. Soc., 27: 609, 1937. Newman, H. G.: Undulant fever, J. Missouri M. A., 35: 398, 1938.

79. Kennan, T. F.: Convalescent serum in treatment of undulant fever, Virginia M. Monthly, 62: 34, 1935.

80. Creswell, S. M. and Wallace, C. E.: Immunotransfusion in undulant fever; report of 2 cases, J. Am. M. Ass., 106: 1384, 1936.

81. Kretzler, H. H.: Undulant fever; case treated by immune serum, Northwest Med., 34: 261, 1935.

82. Smith, D. T. and Poston, M. A.: Some unusual cases of Brucella infection, Tr. Am. Clin. & Climatol. A., 1937.

83. Huddleson, I. F. and Johnson, H. W.: "Brucellin," possible specific for undulant fever in man, Am. J. Trop. Med., 13: 485, 1933.

84. ———: Brucellosis. Causes, Sources of Infection. Clinical Diagnosis, Laboratory Diagnosis, Treatment, Bull., Central Brucella Station, Mich. State College, 1938.

85. O'Neil, A. E.: Preliminary note on treatment of undulant fever in man with detoxified vaccine and with antiserum, Ohio State M. J., 29: 438, 1933.

86. Budtz-Olsen, J.: Ten cases of undulant fever treated with typhoid vaccine, Ugesk. f. laeger, 92: 596, 1930.

87. Miller, S.: Protein shock therapy in undulant fever, Lancet, 1: 1177, 1933.

88. Manson-Bahr, P.: Undulant fever of abortus type treated by protein shock, Lancet, 1: 1178, 1933.

89. Ervin, C. E. and Hunt, H. F.: Diagnosis and treatment of undulant fever, J. Am. M. Ass., 109: 1966, 1937.

90. ———, ——— and Niles, J. S., Jr.: Foreign protein therapy; treatment of undulant fever by intravenous injection of killed typhoid-paratyphoid "A" and paratyphoid "B" bacilli, Am. J. M. Sc., 192: 234, 1936.

91. Grouès, P.: Sur quelques cas de mélitococcie traités par le rubiazol seul ou associé à des agents thérapeutiques spécifiques de l'affection, Lyon méd., 158: 615, 1936. Thévenet, V.: Un cas de mélitococcie traité par le rubiazol (per os). Terminaison favorable relativement rapide de la maladie, Lyon méd., 158: 668, 1936. Berger, W. and Schnetz, H.: Ein Behandlungserfolg bei Morbus Bang mit Prontosil, Med. Klin., 33: 594, 1937. Suchier, W.: Zur Behandlung der Bangschen Krankheit, Fortschr. d. Therap., 13: 305, 1937. Béthoux, L., Gourdon, E. and Rochedix, J.: Mélitococcie traitée par le chlorhydrate de sulfamino-chrysoïdine, amélioration clinique, persistance des germes dans le sang, Bull. et mém. Soc. méd. d. hôp. de Paris, 53: 678, 1937. Ahringsmann, H.: Heilung der Bangschen Krankheit durch Prontosil, München. med. Wchnschr., 84: 1778, 1937. Bethoux, L., Gourdon, E. and Rochedix, J.: Fièvre ondulante guérie cliniquement et bactériologiquement par l'emploi de dérivés sulfamidés non azoïques, Bull. et mém. Soc. méd. d. hôp. de Paris, 53: 1297, 1937. Bevan, L. E. W.: Abortus fever: some notes from Southern Rhodesia; treatment of human case with prosepticine, J. Comp. Path. & Therap., 50: 338, 1937. Lloyd, J. H.: Sulfonamide-P in Brucella abortus infection, Brit. M. J., 1: 145, 1938. Richardson, L. A.: Infection with Brucella abortus treated with prontosil, Lancet, 1: 495, 1938. Francis, A. E.: Sulfanilamide in treatment of undulant fever. Lancet, 1: 496, 1938. Stern, R. L. and Blake, K. W.: Undulant fever; its treatment with sulfanilamide, J. Am. M. Ass., 110: 1550, 1938. Manson-Bahr, P.: Action of sulphanilamide on Brucella abortus infections, Practitioner, 140: 740, 1938. Hall, L. T. and Dunlap, R. L.: Report of case of Brucella abortus infection treated with sulfanilamide, Nebraska M. J., 23: 252, 1938. Welch, H., Wentworth, J. A. and Mickle, F. L.: Use of sulfanilamide in diagnosis and treatment of brucellosis, J. Am. M. Ass., 111: 226, 1938. Sheppe, W. M.: Sulfanilamide in treatment of undulant fever, J. Chemotherapy, 15: 38, 1938. Blumgart, H. L.: Recovery of patient with undulant fever treated with sulfanilamide, J. Am. M. Ass., 111: 521, 1938. Petzetakis, M.: Abortivbehandlung des Maltafiebers durch Prontosil, Deutsche med. Wchnschr., 64: 1147, 1938. Punch, A. L.: Undulant fever treated with prontosil, Lancet, 2: 429, 1938. Thomson, A. P.: Treatment of Brucella abortus infection with fouadin and prontosil, Brit. M. J., 2: 884, 1938. Fraser, R. H., White, F. D. and Perrin, M. B.: Résumé on undulant fever: use of prontosil and prontylin (report of 2 cases), Canad. M. A. J., 39: 455, 1938. Matthews, N.: Brucella abortus infection treated by sulfanilamide, Brit. M. J., 1: 483, 1938. Page, W. A.: Brucella abortus infection treated by sulfanilamide, Brit. M. J., 1: 594, 1938. Traut, E. F. and Logan, C. E.: Undulant fever treated with sulfanilamide, J. Am. M. Ass., 111: 1092, 1938. Neumann, C. Z.: Treatment of undulant fever with prontosil, Brit. M. J., 2: 342, 1938. Toone, E. C., Jr. and Jenkins, A. M.: Undulant fever (brucellosis) treated with sulfanilamide; report of case with recovery, South. M. J., 31: 478, 1938. Haden, R. L.: Treatment of undulant fever with sulfanilamide; report of case, Cleveland Clin. Quart., 5: 241, 1938. Livingston, A. E.: Undulant fever treated with sulfanilamide, Rocky Mountain M. J., 35: 787, 1938. Bartels, E. C.: Sulfanilamide in undulant fever, New England J. Med., 219: 988, 1938. Gaffney, M.: Report on 5 cases of Brucella abortus infection, Brit. M. J., 2: 885, 1938.

92. Blumgart, H. L. and Gilligan, D. R.: Treatment of undulant fever with sulfanilamide and related compounds, M. Clin. North America, 23: 1193, 1939.

93. Bynum, W. T.: Recurrences of undulant fever (brucellosis) following administration of sulfanilamide, J. Am. M. Ass., 112: 835, 1939.

94. Long, P. H. and Bliss, E. A.: The Clinical and Experimental Use of Sulfanilamide, Sulfapyridine and Allied Compounds, New York, Macmillan Co. 209, 1939.

95. Prickman, L. E. and Popp, W. C.: Treatment of brucellosis by hyperpyrexia induced by Simpson-Kettering hypertherm, Proc. Staff Meet., Mayo Clin., 11: 506, 1936.

96. Zeiter, W. J.: Treatment of undulant fever by artificial fever therapy; report of case, Cleveland Clin. Quart., 4: 309, 1937.

97. Prickman, L. E., Bennett, R. L. and Krusen, F. H.: Treatment of brucellosis by physically induced hyperpyrexia, Proc. Staff Meet., Mayo Clin., 13: 321, 1938.

98. Simpson, W. M.: Discussion of paper by Ervin, C. E. and Hunt, H. F.: Diagnosis and treatment of undulant fever, J. Am. M. Ass., 109: 1970, 1937.

99. Sharp, W. B.: Pathology of undulant fever, Arch. Path., 18: 72, 1934.

100. Parsons, P. B. and Poston, M. A.: Pathology of human brucellosis; report of four cases with one autopsy, South. M. J., 32: 7, 1939.

101. ———, ——— and Wise, B.: Pathology of human brucelliasis, Am. J. Path., 15: 634, 1939.

CHAPTER TWENTY-FIVE

PLAGUE

By Charles F. Craig, M.D. (Hon.), F.A.C.P., F.A.C.S., Colonel, U. S. Army
Medical Corps (Ret.), D.S.M.

Synonyms.—Oriental plague, black death, pestis.

Definition.—Plague is an acute, infectious, specific disease, caused by *Pasteurella pestis* (*Bacillus pestis*), and characterized by enlargement of the lymphatic glands, toxemia, an initial lesion, in the bubonic type, and by a specific form of pneumonia or septicemia, in the pneumonic and septicemic types. Plague is primarily a disease of rats and other rodents and is transmitted from man to man by certain species of fleas.

Etiology.—The cause of plague is a bacillus discovered by Yersin and by Kitasato, working independently, in 1904. It is called *Pasteurella pestis* and is an oval-shaped bacillus, showing polar staining with ordinary bacterial stains. It is gram-negative and can be cultivated without difficulty upon most of the ordinary laboratory media. It grows best at 37° C. and upon nutrient agar it is pleomorphic, the organisms being rod-shaped, filamentous, irregular or coccoid, especially if 3 per cent of sodium chloride has been added to the medium. Upon a mixture of melted butter and bouillon there is a very characteristic stalactite growth, while in plain bouillon there is a heavy sediment. The organism may be isolated from the enlarged glands, the buboes; from the sputum in the pneumonic type, and from the blood in the septicemic type of plague.

The causative relationship of *Pasteurella pestis* to plague has been demonstrated by numerous laboratory infections from pure cultures in man and by the production of the disease in susceptible animals, especially rats, either by inoculation or by rubbing the pure culture into the shaved skin of the abdomen of the experimental animal.

Epidemiology.—In considering the epidemiology of plague it should be remembered that it is primarily a disease of rats or other rodents and is only secondarily a disease of man. The latter is infected by the bite of certain species of flea, especially by the rat fleas, *Xenopsylla cheopis* and *Ceratophyllus fasciatus*. Numerous other rodents besides the rat are naturally infected with plague, the most important in this country being the ground squirrel of California, and the fleas infesting such rodents may convey the infection to man. The disease in rodents is transmitted by fleas as in man, the fleas transmitting the infection from rodent to rodent, from rodent to man, and from man to man. The rats most commonly infected are the brown or sewer rat, *Rattus norvegicus,* and the black or house rat, *Rattus rattus.* The rat fleas will not usually leave a living rat to bite man, but when the animal dies of the plague the fleas will leave the dead body and, in the absence of other rats or rodents, will bite man. The habits of rats explain many of the epidemiologic aspects of plague and before the occurrence of an epidemic of this disease in man there is always a preceding increase in the mortality of the rats of the vicinity, due to a preceding epidemic among these animals.

The bubonic type of plague is not contagious but the pneumonic type is intensely contagious and is transmitted from man to man by droplet infection,

4041

whereas in the bubonic type the method of transmission is by the bite of infective fleas. The mechanism of transmission by the flea is important and most interesting, and was first demonstrated by Bacot and Martin in 1914. When fleas feed upon infected rodents or man, the plague bacilli are taken into the stomach but multiply very rapidly in the proventriculus, forming masses of the bacterium which occlude the proventriculus and distend the esophagus, thus preventing the blood from reaching the stomach when the flea tries to feed again. The efforts made by the flea in endeavoring to pump the blood into the stomach lead to regurgitation of a mixture of blood and plague bacilli into the wound made by biting, and thus the bitten individual receives an enormous dose of plague bacilli. These so-called "blocked fleas" are the principal source of infection although infection may be conveyed mechanically by fleabites. The "blocked fleas" may live and remain infective for as long as 70 days. Some observers believe that the .bedbug may also transmit infection to man. Clothing may act as a transmitting agent, for infected fleas may hide in it, and thus the disease may be transmitted from place to place. Pneumonic plague is very contagious and is transmitted directly from man to man by droplet infection and direct contact with the sputum which contains myriads of the bacilli. Epidemics of pneumonic plague originate from cases of pneumonia occurring in patients suffering from the bubonic type.

The plague occurring in rats, ground squirrels, and other rodents is often referred to as "sylvatic plague." The ground squirrels of California are infected and the infection has spread from this state into Oregon, Montana, and other states of the Union, and man has become infected from these animals wherever the squirrels have been found infected. Rats suffer from a chronic form of plague and apparently "healthy carriers" of this organism are found among these animals and other rodents, and thus the disease is perpetuated and becomes endemic in certain regions.

There is no natural immunity to plague in any race and all ages and both sexes are susceptible. Epidemics are most common when the mean temperature is between 50 and 85° F. (10 and 29.4° C.), but the bacillus resists freezing. It is quickly killed by exposure to direct sunlight or drying. In the tropics epidemics of plague are most frequent during the rainy season.

Symptomatology.—The *incubation period* of plague is believed to be from two to five days. Clinically, the disease is divided into *pestis minor* and *pestis major*, the latter being subdivided into *bubonic, pneumonic* and *septicemic* plague.

Pestis minor includes those cases of mild plague characterized by slight fever, enlarged lymphatic glands in the region of the fleabite, and mild general symptoms, including headache, aching in the back and limbs, anorexia and general malaise. The fleabite in these mild cases may often be observed, being evidenced by a vesicle or pustule surrounded by an area of inflammation. Many of these mild cases of plague are undoubtedly unrecognized and serve as foci of infection during epidemics.

Bubonic plague, the most frequently observed form of the disease, has a sudden onset in most cases, although a definite period of malaise may precede the onset. The patient is rapidly overcome by the toxemia present and often presents the appearance of alcoholic intoxication. The fever rises rapidly to 103 or 104° F. (39.4 to 40° C.) or higher; the face is pale and anxious at first but, as the fever rises, becomes flushed; the conjunctivae are congested, and the skin is hot and dry. Chills or chilly sensations may be present, the pulse and respirations are increased with the fever, and there is usually extreme prostration. After the fever has reached its height the mental condition is one of stupor, the patient appearing stupid when questioned, there being marked difficulty in concentrating, while speech is interfered with and there may be slight delirium. At this time patients clinically resemble intoxicated individuals and instances have occurred in which they have been arrested for intoxication and jailed.

At the height of the attack the face is greatly flushed, vomiting and diarrhea may be present, and symptoms of toxemia are prominent. Albumin may appear in the urine and there may be marked delirium. In cases that recover the temperature is remittent in type and falls by lysis on the fifth or sixth day, while in fatal cases it may remain elevated until death occurs. In such cases prostration is extreme, delirium or stupor is present, the heart action is feeble, and the liver and spleen are enlarged. The tongue is furred, the breath very offensive, and coma occurs before death. Fatal infections usually last from three to six days before death occurs.

In the bubonic type of plague the enlargement of the group of lymphatic glands draining the region of the fleabite, or the bubo, is initiated by a feeling of tension and pain followed by enlargement of the glands upon the second or third day after the appearance of symptoms. In practically two thirds of the cases the bubo is located in the inguinal region, the axillary bubo being next in order of frequency, while the submaxillary and cervical glands are seldom involved. Buboes may be multiple and there may be general enlargement of the lymphatic glands. The bubo may suppurate or may be distended by hemorrhage into the tissues, and such hemorrhages may occur elsewhere in the skin, leading to the formation of "carbuncles" or necrosis. If suppuration occurs the temperature is irregular and persists as long as suppuration continues. The bubo may disappear slowly; but if suppuration takes place, healing is delayed, thus prolonging convalescence.

Pneumonic plague is rare and the onset is very sudden with a rise in temperature to 102 to 104° F. (38.9 to 40° C.) and an exaggeration of the symptoms if this complication occurs during an attack of bubonic plague. There are cough, dyspnea, rapid respirations, pain in the chest, marked toxemia, and the expectoration of large amounts of brownish sputum, the "prune-juice" sputum of this type of plague, containing enormous numbers of plague bacilli. The physical signs are indefinite, resembling those of bronchopneumonia, there being moist râles over the bases of the lungs and limited areas of consolidation scattered throughout the organs. In primary cases of pneumonic plague the superficial lymphatic glands may be tender and enlarged. This form of the disease is invariably fatal, death occurring in from three to four days in most cases.

Septicemic plague resembles in its symptomatology the bubonic type, but buboes do not occur and the course of the disease is very rapid, death occurring in from two to three days. In this form the bacilli occur in large numbers in the peripheral blood and smears of this fluid may show them, but blood cultures should be relied upon in diagnosis. Toxemia is very marked and may kill the infected individual within twenty-four hours. There may be little fever, but prostration is most severe and mental torpidity, delirium or coma is present before death. In children this form is more frequent than in adults and may resemble meningitis in symptomatology. The septicemic form of plague is really a very severe form of bubonic plague in which a fatal toxemia develops before buboes have time to form.

Plague is a disease of very short duration, death or recovery occurring within a few days. Thus, *complications* and *sequelae* are not often observed, although cardiac failure not infrequently causes death or complicates convalescence. In pregnant women abortion invariably occurs and a form of myocarditis sometimes follows a severe infection. Suppurations of the skin may occur as sequelae.

Diagnosis.—The diagnosis of plague should rest upon the results of laboratory examinations. The isolation of the plague bacillus from the blood, sputum, bubo contents, enlarged glands or tissues is essential in order to demonstrate the presence of plague and fortunately such isolation and cultivation are not difficult. Perhaps the most useful method of laboratory diagnosis is the inoculation of susceptible animals. If a shaved area of the abdominal skin of a guinea pig is rubbed with a small amount of material from a bubo or a culture obtained from the blood, sputum or glands, the animal will die within seven days, while if a white mouse is inoculated with similar material at the base of the tail, it will die within forty-eight hours. For various methods of cultivating *Pasteurella pestis* the reader is referred to standard works upon clinical diagnosis.

In times of epidemic occurrence of plague the diagnosis may be made from the clinical symptomatology, the occurrence of many cases showing buboes with the characteristic toxemic symptoms being sufficient upon which to diagnose the disease, but even in such cases the diagnosis should be confirmed by laboratory methods and the organism demonstrated, if possible. Pneumonic plague and septicemic plague are impossible to diagnose clinically and the diagnosis must be made by demonstrating the organism in the sputum and blood respectively, or by animal inoculation. Mild cases of bubonic plague are frequently overlooked or wrongly diagnosed. It is wise to remember that in regions where plague is known to be endemic, or where it is epidemic, all rapidly fatal conditions accompanied by buboes, pneumonia or symptoms of toxemia should be regarded as suspicious and most carefully examined for *Pasteurella pestis.*

Conditions which may be clinically confused with plague are climatic bubo, glandular fever, tularemia, typhus, influenza, the early stage of yellow fever and buboes caused by venereal disease and pyogenic infections. Most of these conditions can be easily differentiated by laboratory methods, but if such are not available it is sometimes very difficult to be sure of a diagnosis. *Typhus fever* very closely resembles plague in its onset, but the presence of the characteristic eruption and of the Weil-Felix reaction should serve to differentiate it *Influenza,* accompanied by pneumonia, has often been confused with pneumonic plague and during the great epidemic of 1918 many cases of influenzal pneumonia were suspected to be plague because of the rapidly fatal result. Only by the use of laboratory methods can a differential diagnosis be made between pneumonic plague and influenzal pneumonia. Significant clinical differences are the more watery character and larger amount of the sputum in plague pneumonia and the fact that the latter occurs as a primary condition, whereas influenzal pneumonia occurs as a complication. However, plague pneumonia may occur as a complication of bubonic plague, but the presence of buboes in such cases should help in the differentiation. The other conditions mentioned may be differentiated through a careful study of the clinical and physical findings and the application of proper laboratory methods.

Treatment.—The treatment of plague is not satisfactory. **Plague serum,** when employed in the earliest stages of the disease, in 100-cc. doses, has been reported upon favorably. **Human convalescent serum,** in 20-cc. doses, upon three successive days, has been found to reduce the mortality about one half. Bacteriophage treatment has not proved of any value, according to most of those who have used it.

The treatment of either *pneumonic* or *septicemic plague* is useless as all patients suffering from these forms of the infection invariably die.

The treatment of the *bubonic type,* aside from the use of specific serums, is purely symptomatic. If the fever is unusually high it may be reduced by sponging with lukewarm water but it should be remembered that in such cases prostration is extreme and cardiac failure is common. If vomiting is present it may be relieved by sucking ice or by a full dose of calomel followed by a saline. The application of a mustard plaster over the epigastrium is often efficient in relieving this symptom. If collapse occurs cardiac stimulants are indicated and morphia should be employed to relieve pain or control severe nervous symptoms, as delirium. The intravenous injection of **mercurochrome** in a 1 per cent solution in water, the dose employed being 2 to 5 mg. per kilo of body weight, has been reported upon favorably by some practitioners. The usual dose for an adult is 20 cc. of a 1 per cent solution. A liquid **diet** is indicated during the active symptoms and a full diet during convalescence.

The treatment of the bubo is important and adds much to the comfort of the patient. If the case is seen early the complete enucleation of the bubo is recommended by some authorities, but it is to be remembered that general infection has occurred before the bubo is noticeable and enucleation is not recommended by the vast majority of physicians who have had an extended experience with the treatment of plague. The injection of a mixture of equal parts of **camphor** and **thymol** in doses of 0.5 to 1 cc. into the bubo, or of **iodine,** employing a 1 per cent solution containing double the quantity of potassium iodide, and injecting 5 to 10 cc. daily for a period of four days, has been recommended. The local treatment of the bubo with applications of glycerin and belladonna is favored and if suppuration occurs the bubo should be at once incised and drained. If the buboes become actively inflamed, poultices should be applied in order to hasten suppuration, when they should be incised, cleansed, and dressed with an iodoform dressing.

During convalescence great care should be taken to **avoid unnecessary exertion,** as cardiac failure may occur.

Prevention.—Bubonic plague and septicemic plague are transmitted almost entirely through the bites of infected fleas, and it is extremely doubtful if fomites ever transmit the infection unless infected fleas are transported in clothing or other materials. The protection of man from fleas is thus the most important prophylactic measure and this is accomplished by the **trapping** or **destruction** in other ways **of rats and other rodents,** and the wearing of **flea-proof clothing** if one is exposed to possible fleabites in attending patients or in frequenting rat-infested buildings. The poisoning of rats is an effective method for their destruction and this may be accomplished with strychnine, barium carbonate, arsenic or phosphorus; while trapping, the employment of the Danysz virus containing an organism of the Salmonella group fatal to these animals, fumigation of ships, warehouses and dwellings with sulfur or other gases which will destroy rats, and the use of flea insecticides, are all valuable preventive measures when properly employed.

While fomites are not generally regarded as responsible for the transmission of plague, there are some observations on record which appear to prove that under certain conditions clothes, fabrics of various kinds, animal skins, and other articles may harbor the plague bacillus in a living condition, and it is the part of wisdom to disinfect such articles if there is reason to believe they have become infested with the organism. The most active **disinfectants** for the purpose are live steam, lysol, chloride of lime, 5 per cent carbolic acid and 2 per cent formalin solution.

In attending plague patients, doctors and nurses should wear **gauze masks** (especially in attending pneumonic plague patients), **gloves** and **boots,** and the legs should be protected by tightly wound puttees. Animals should be prevented from entering the house in which there is a plague patient and all who have no reason to be present should be rigidly excluded. The usual quarantine measures for infectious diseases should be strictly enforced and, if an epidemic of either bubonic or pneumonic plague is present, all public gatherings should be forbidden and schools, churches and theaters should be closed. **Ratproofing** of all **buildings** is an essential part of plague prophylaxis and is most important.

Prophylactic immunization with a plague **vaccine** is a most valuable preventive measure. In the presence of epidemics all of the inhabitants of the affected region should be vaccinated, the vaccine usually employed being Haffkine's, consisting of heat-killed cultures of *Pasteurella pestis.* This vaccine has been very extensively used in India and has reduced the incidence of the disease about three quarters and the mortality about one third, the protection lasting about one year. The reactions following the use of this vaccine, especially in children, are apt to be severe, and the first dose administered should be a small one. The dose varies from 0.5 to 4 cc., according to the age of the patient, and three injections apparently give good results.

The prevention of *pneumonic plague* consists in the administration of the plague vaccine to all exposed individuals and the prevention of droplet infection by the wearing of masks made of cotton covered with muslin, as gauze masks are not so efficient as the muslin cotton mask introduced by Strong. In addition, the usual precautions should be taken regarding clothing, already mentioned, and care should be exercised in handling bedding and all articles that have come into contact with the patient, and all such articles should be disinfected.

Plague patients should be treated in **well-ventilated wards** or **rooms,** and this is especially important in the case of pneumonic plague.

Pathology.—The pathology of plague is that of a severe septicemia, the bacilli reaching the blood through the lymphatics draining the site of the infective fleabite.

The primary lesion in bubonic plague, the *bubo,* consists of a marked enlargement of a group of lymphatic glands, soft in consistence, and filled with a hemorrhagic exudate, surrounded by an area of hemorrhagic edematous tissue. The exudate contains plague bacilli which disappear when suppuration occurs.

Rigor mortis occurs rapidly and the skin of the patient may present hemorrhagic areas of a purple or almost black color, which gave the name "Black Death" to this infection. Such hemorrhagic areas are especially numerous in septicemic plague. Upon opening the body all of the organs are congested and hemorrhagic; the serous cavities, stomach and intestines often contain much blood; the liver and spleen are enlarged and mottled, and the kidneys hemorrhagic; the lungs are greatly congested and edematous and, in cases of pneumonic plague, there are present a fibrinous pleuritis and the usual evidences of severe bronchopneumonia. The bronchial glands, trachea and larynx are greatly congested, and in the vessels of all of these organs bacilli are present in large numbers. In the septicemic form of plague the meninges are greatly congested and the brain is edematous.

Geographic Distribution.—During epidemics plague has spread to almost every country in the world, but the present endemic centers are in Mesopotamia, India, China, Uganda, the Philippine Islands, and a small center upon the island of Hawaii. Sylvatic plague is endemic in Siberia and other countries, and in California and other northwestern states of the United States the ground squirrels are infected. Outbreaks of plague frequently occur in various parts of the world but are quickly controlled by the application of proper preventive measures. Only in India is plague a constant cause of high morbidity and mortality.

History.—The history of plague is fascinating and has been well covered in many works devoted to the subject and in general literature, as in Defoe's "History of the Plague Year" and in Gibbon's "Rise and Fall of the Roman Empire." There is abundant evidence that the Indian physicians recognized this infection hundreds of years before Christ, and the great epidemic occurring in the reign of Justinian (6th century A.D.) is well described by Gibbon. Many great pandemics of this disease have occurred, during which Europe, Asia, Africa and North and South America have been invaded, and the name "Black Death" was given to the great pandemic originating in China during the 14th century.

The cause of plague, *Pasteurella pestis,* was discovered independently by Yersin and by Kitasato, in 1904; the method of transmission by the flea by the Indian Plague Commission, in 1905; and the mechanism of transmission by the flea, by Bacot and Martin, in 1914.

BIBLIOGRAPHY

Bacot, A. W. and Martin, C. J.: J. Hyg. (Plague Supplement III), 13 : 423, 1914 ; 23 : 98, 1924.
Haffkine, W. M.: Brit. M. J., 2 : 1461, 1897.
Kitasato, S.: Lancet, 2 : 428, 1894.
McCoy, G. W.: J. Infect. Dis., 6 : 170, 288, 1909.
Manson-Bahr, P. H.: Manson's Tropical Diseases, Ed. 10, London and New York, 1936.

Petrie, G. F.: System of Bacteriology, London, Med. Res. Council, 3 : 137, 1929.
Strong, R. P.: Philippine J. Sc., 1 : 181, 1906 ; 2 : 155, 1907.
Wu Lien-Teh : A Treatise on Pneumonic Plague, League of Nations, Geneva, 1926.
Yersin, F.: C. R. Acad. Sc., 119 : 356, 1894.

CHAPTER TWENTY–SIX

THE MYCOSES

By Richard L. Sutton, Sr., M.D., and Richard L. Sutton, Jr., M.D.

In the plant kingdom there are many kinds of parasites which affect the human being. The mycoses are the diseases caused by fungi. Bacteria, the Schizomycetes, botanically are members of the fungi, but they are not to be considered here. They seem to be almost wholly unrelated to other groups of fungi, although some of the higher forms are suggestive of Myxophyceae which have lost their chlorophyll. Schizomycetes are typically unicellular plants; the cells are usually small and relatively primitive in organization. Higher fungi form a large, heterogeneous group of plants including all those lacking chlorophyll. In most of them the vegetative body is surrounded by cell walls and usually appears as septate filaments called *hyphae*. The vegetative hyphae are collectively known as *mycelium*. Hyphae grow by the sprouting of small protuberances, which enlarge, round off and are cut off from the mother cells by septums. Daughter cells, or sprout cells, are known as *blastospores*. Among the yeasts this is the only type of vegetative body. When growth conditions are unfavorable, resting cells are formed, called *chlamydospores*. When circumstances become favorable, the chlamydospores develop normal, vegetative mycelium. Hyphae generally are intertwined in silky masses, which generally are capable of absorbing food at any point. Various specialized structures develop from them. Most fungi, at certain ages and under favorable conditions of nutrition, develop reproductive structures on the mycelium. These are usually *spores*. Spores are cells or groups of cells characteristically formed and able to grow independently into new individuals. In many fungi there is a sexual function involving the two processes: (1) *fertilization*, comprising the fusion of two nuclei, thereby doubling the number of chromosomes; and (2) *miosis*, in which there is a return to the single chromosome number. Some fungi live without such reconstruction of their nuclei and propagate themselves by imperfect stages only. Such fungi with incomplete or with incompletely known life cycles are called *fungi imperfecti*.

Historical Review of Fungus Diseases.—Hooke in 1677 made a lens which enabled him to see filaments of the fungus productive of yellow spot disease in the damask rose. Malpighi knew of "plants which grow on other plants." In 1729 Micheli wrote about many fungi and described *Aspergillus*. Linnaeus (1752) collected all the facts then known, and named many species. The first important human pathogen to be seen was observed by Langenbeck (1839), that of thrush; and in the same year Schönlein found that of favus. Charles Robin in 1843 named Langenbeck's organism *Oidium albicans*. Lebert named Schönlein's fungus *Oidium schoenleini*, and Remak changed this to *Achorion*. In 1844 Gruby found fungi of ringworm and differentiated the large spore type from the small spore.

4042

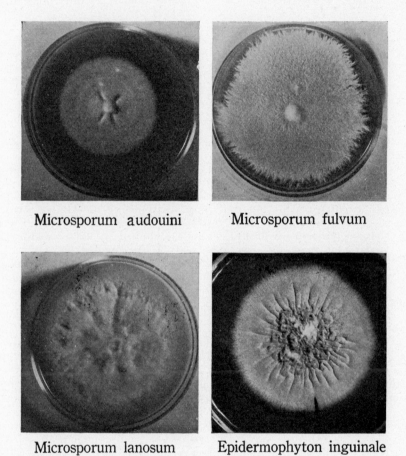

Microsporum audouini   Microsporum fulvum

Microsporum lanosum   Epidermophyton inguinale

Fig. 1.—Giant colonies of common pathogenic fungi. Half natural size. (Courtesy of Dr. George M. Lewis and Dr. Mary Hopper, New York Skin and Cancer Unit.)

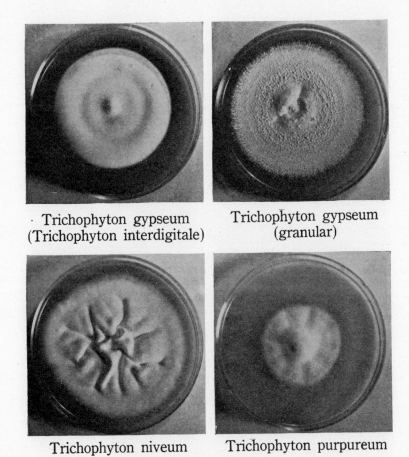

Trichophyton gypseum
(Trichophyton interdigitale)

Trichophyton gypseum
(granular)

Trichophyton niveum

Trichophyton purpureum

FIG. 2.—Giant colonies of common pathogenic fungi. Half natural size. (Courtesy of Dr. George M. Lewis and Dr. Mary Hopper, New York Skin and Cancer Unit.)

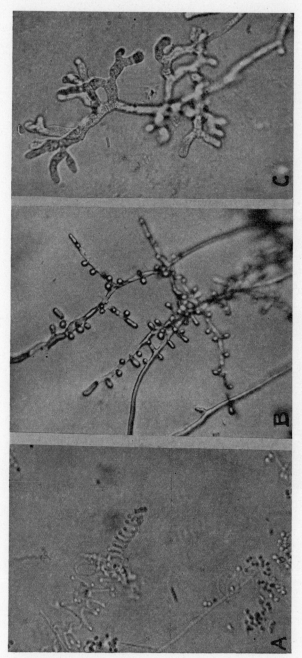

Fig. 3.—Microscopic characters of common pathogenic fungi. (Courtesy of Dr. G. M. Lewis and Dr. Mary Hopper, New York Skin and Cancer Unit.)

A. *Trichophyton gypseum.* The spirals are characteristic of this species.

B. *Trichophyton crateriforme.* Microconidia may be attached or unattached singly or in clusters, and are seen in many species of fungi.

C. *Achorion schoenleini.* Favic chandeliers are characteristic of this species.

Classification.—The list of classes of fungi from Dodge's *Medical Mycology* illustrates the main subdivisions. It must be admitted that the taxonomic distribution of the pathogenic species is by no means at the stage of final agreement.

1. **Schizomycetes**—bacteria in the larger sense.
2. **Myxomycetes**—slime molds having many resemblances to Protozoa in some stages of their life cycle.
3. **Phycomycetes**—fungi in which a number of united protoplasts form a single large cell.
4. **Ascomycetes**—a large, polymorphic group possessing a common method of spore formation in asci.
5. **Basidiomycetes**—a large group with spores borne on specialized organs.
6. **Fungi Imperfecti**—the heterogeneous group with unknown life cycles which may perhaps have degenerated until sexuality has been lost.

Mycotic Diseases are by no means limited to the skin, but their conspicuous manifestations are most often cutaneous. The point of view of this article is that of the dermatologist.

Diseases of the Skin Caused by Fungi might be described on the basis of the specific etiologic agent, for example, *"Epidermophyton inguinale* disease" or *"Trichophyton purpureum* disease." That this can and will be done seems inevitable in our opinion, for favus has long been so separated. It is sometimes possible, by judging from characteristic cutaneous manifestations, to recognize that an infection of the skin is caused by a particular pathogen. Bilateral, superficial, circumscribed, erythematous and scaly eruptions of the upper parts of the inner aspects of the thigh are commonly caused by *Epidermophyton cruris.* One may often correctly suspect that an infection of the scalp is caused by *Microsporum lanosum* from the history of contact with an infected animal, the short duration, the tendency to heal spontaneously and the inflammatory character of the lesion. Infections of the skin due to *Monilia albicans* and the lesions of blastomycosis, actinomycosis and sporotrichosis have clinical expressions characteristic of the infective organism. One can usually recognize the identity of *Trichophyton purpureum* as the infecting organism from clinical inspection alone.

However, the diseases produced by closely related organisms may not be distinguishable clinically; and this fact, in addition to the botanical confusion of families, genera and species, makes the undertaking unprofitable now. As the use of cultural methods for identifying particular agents in particular cases becomes more common, one may look forward to specificity and accuracy in the future. It is probable that efficient methods of treatment will come to be correlated with individual types of infection. It is practical to discuss dermatomycoses according to their sites.

Dermatomycosis is the generic term including all infections due to fungi, both superficial and deep.

Dermatophytosis is applicable to superficial infections, especially of the hands and feet.

Epidermophytosis implies infection with an *Epidermophyton.*

Trichophytosis is similarly limited to parasitism with a *Trichophyton.*

TINEA

Synonyms.—Ringworm; Dermatomycosis.

Tinea is infection of the skin, hair or nails produced by various fungi. Such infections are common and are at times serious. The peculiar ability of the dermatophytes to grow on keratin constitutes the advantage they have over most other fungi, and it forms the basis of their parasitic relationship with the human host. The existence of sensitivity to trichophytin in superficial ringworm infections, as well as in deep ones, has been shown to be almost constantly present. There are analogies between the immunologic biology of dermatomycosis and of

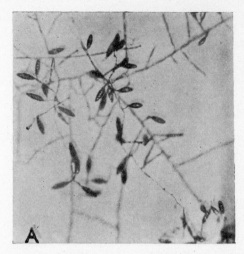 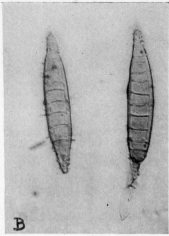

FIG. 4.—Microscopic characters of common pathogenic fungi. (Courtesy of Dr. G. M. Lewis and Dr. Mary Hopper, New York Skin and Cancer Unit.)
A. Microsporum fulvum. Macroconidia, or fuseaux, attached to hyphae, this feature being indicative of *M. fulvum* or *M. lanosum.*
B. Microsporum lanosum. Detached macroconidia showing septations.

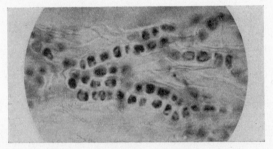

FIG. 5.—Trichophyton; stained preparation highly magnified. (Courtesy of Dr. B. B. Beeson.)

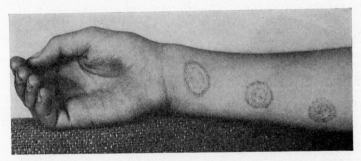

FIG. 6.—Tinea corporis, showing concentric rings of activity, with central healing.

tuberculosis. Infectious diseases in general are characterized by the appearance of a primary lesion at the site of inoculation and by the appearance of lesions of the skin under allergic conditions. Such latter dermatoses comprise the "ids." Allergy is the *sine qua non* of their existence. During the existence of a trichophytid the trichophytin reaction is positive. The existence of disease depends on the presence in the integumentary tissues of the parasite, which may or may not grow actively. The form of the disease which results depends on (1) the growth, activity and virulence of the fungus, and (2) the reaction of the tissues to its presence, reactivity which may be hyperergic, hypo-ergic or anergic. Tinea of the nails, for instance, may be entirely asymptomatic; it may be asymptomatic locally and yet serve as the source of repeated attacks of cutaneous infection; and on occasion it may maintain pruritic dermatomycosis about the anus or crotch, or some other clinical manifestation of fungus disease.

Environmental circumstances influence the equilibrium of the parasitic relationship so that the fungus may thrive or the tissues prevail. Moisture, warmth, darkness, and traumatic or chemical irritation favor the fungus. Ventilation, coolness and dryness favor the tissues, as, of course, do mechanical débridement (washing), avoidance of injury, and the application of nonirritating antiparasitic chemicals.

Classification.—In general, clinical infections with fungi may be considered individually with clinical satisfaction without regard to systematic botany. Pathogenic fungi causative of tinea damage only the skin, even when they have been injected intravenously. As a rule they damage the skin only superficially. Nevertheless, their activity results in humoral alteration, and tinea, like many other dermatoses, is by no means a purely cutaneous phenomenon.

We look upon eczematous tinea as the equivalent of dermatitis venenata due to a self-reproductive chemical substance on the skin. This point of view is of course semidiagrammatic; it simplifies the understanding, however, of the host-parasite relationship.

Clinical Forms.—One sees lesions of the following forms: vesicular, scaling, macular, macerated, fissured, papular, callous, keratotic and lichenified. The nails are often infected.

Fungi which are principally pathogenic to animals cause in animals lesions which are not very deep and inflammatory, disease which is readily transmissible from animal to animal, lesions which contain numerous organisms easy to demonstrate, lesions which are difficult to cure. The same organisms in the human being produce deeper and more inflammatory lesions, strong reactivity to trichophytin, disease which is not readily transmissible, lesions in which organisms are few and demonstrable with difficulty, and lesions which tend toward spontaneous cure or are comparatively easy to cure. Fungi which are principally pathogenic to human beings cause chronic, resistant, noninflammatory disease in human beings, and in animals cause deeply inflammatory lesions. The distinction between "animal" and "human" infections is a rough distinction.

TINEA CORPORIS.—Tinea of the glabrous skin usually begins as flattened, reddish papules. The lesions tend to spread peripherally and to heal in the center. Within a few days an annular patch is formed. The central portion is pinkish or reddish in color and has a smooth or faintly scaling surface. The margin of the plaque is sharply defined, slightly elevated, actively inflamed, more or less scaly, and often vesicular in places, Circinate lesions gradually enlarge until a diameter of 5 to 10 cm. or more is attained, then they remain stationary for several days. Occasionally two or more patches coalesce, giving rise to arcuate figures. They may disappear spontaneously, leaving no trace. The tendency to undergo central involution is less marked or even lacking in some cases. The eruption may consist partially or entirely of several solid, pinkish, reddish, or brownish, scurfy, ill-defined, rounded or oval patches. Concentric rings of activity are common. The lesions range in number from a few to a dozen or more. Itching or burning of slight degree may be present, but

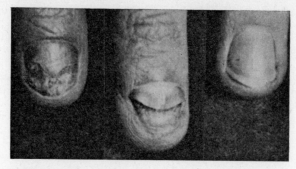

FIG. 7.—*T. purpureum* infection. The typical onychomycosis produced by this species. (Courtesy of Drs. Lewis, Hopper, and Montgomery.)

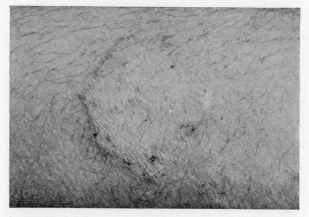

FIG. 8.—*T. purpureum* infection. The typical lichenoid involvement of glabrous skin produced by this organism. (Courtesy of Drs. Lewis, Hopper, and Montgomery.)

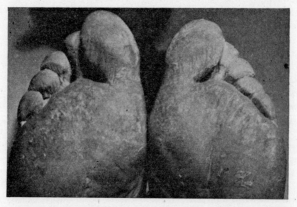

FIG. 9.—*T. purpureum* infection. The typical involvement of the soles produced by this species. (Courtesy of Drs. Lewis, Hopper, and Montgomery.)

symptoms are seldom prominent. The sites of predilection are the uncovered surfaces of the body, the face, neck and hands. The palms are sometimes attacked and the disease may be limited to this location. Tinea often affects the soles and interdigital spaces, the fingers and hands being involved secondarily. Mucous membranes usually escape, and we have never seen buccal tinea, although instances have been noted. The perianal skin is often involved, and this constitutes one variety of pruritus ani. Mycotic vaginitis is usually monilial (see Moniliasis).

In trichophytosis, a state of resistance to inoculation with more of the same organism exists in the healed zone, although areas outside the margins of these patches are vulnerable.

Diagnosis.—The distribution, history and course of the lesions are usually distinctive. In scales removed from the margin of a lesion, mounted in a 10 per cent aqueous solution of potassium hydroxide and then examined microscopically, one finds the pathognomonic mycelium and spores. In pityriasis rosea the eruption is usually confined to the trunk and commonly begins with the appearance of a "mother spot"; the lesions are numerous, develop quickly, and pursue a relatively rapid course. In seborrheic dermatitis the sternal and interscapular regions generally are affected after the scalp, and the lesions, while often circinate, are usually irregular. The scales are unctuous, and vesicles are not present excepting when secondary infection exists. The lesions in psoriasis at times are annular, but they are usually dry and never acutely inflammatory; on scraping off the superficial scales the typical bleeding points are exposed; and the extensor distribution of the eruption is more or less characteristic. Local deep tineal infection may be mistaken for carbuncle, from which it differs in being less acute and far less painful. Diagnosis should be positive by demonstration of fungi rather than being made by exclusion.

TINEA CRURIS (ECZEMA MARGINATUM; DHOBIE ITCH).—This clinical variety of dermatomycosis may occur also in the axillae or beneath pendulous breasts. It is usually due to *Epidermophyton inguinale*. The infection at first may resemble intertrigo, that is, monilial or streptococcic dermatitis; but usually the primary eruption consists of a few, superficial, circinate patches which sooner or later coalesce to form confluent, symmetric, bat-wing-shape inflammatory areas which have sharply defined, elevated borders. The margins may be straight, but usually they present a festooned appearance with more or less infiltration. The patches are generally located on the inner surfaces of the thighs, contiguous with the scrotum or labia and the intergluteal regions. In women the mucosa of the vulva is sometimes involved. In either sex the umbilical region may be affected. Extensions along the sagittal line anteriorly and posteriorly give rise respectively to involvement of the mons veneris and the perianal region and intergluteal fold. About the anus and over the coccyx, fissuring is particularly likely to occur, and distressing and chronic pruritus results. The lesions of tinea cruris are usually moist at first, and they readily become macerated, secondarily infected, and painful as well as merely itchy. As they heal, they become dry, scaly and less edematous. Recurrences are common, for the eradication of all fungi is almost impossible, while friction, sweating, warm weather, tight clothing and obesity combine to favor luxuriation of the organism. Tinea of the pedal interdigital spaces and of the nails commonly serves as the source of reinfection, and the feet, usually requiring treatment, must always be examined in cases of tinea cruris. Crural dermatomycosis due to *Blastomyces* is vegetative and papillomatous in contrast with the macular disease produced by *Epidermophyton*. Any of several species of fungi may infect this region. Clinical distinctions independent of cultural differentiations have not as yet been clarified.

Dhobie itch or washerwoman's itch is tropical epidermophytosis. Warmth and perspiration combine to aggravate the symptoms. Scratching and secondary infection render the parts raw and inflamed.

4042

Tinea of the crotch may be confused with contact dermatitis, seborrheic dermatitis and erythrasma. The location and character of the eruption, its history and the presence of satellite lesions serve for recognition. In monilial vulvovaginitis, mycotic dermatitis of the near-by regions of the skin is likely to be present. Tinea of the crotch in women calls for an examination of the vaginal secretions and for the use of douches, such as **1: 5000 potassium permanganate,** on general principles. In erythrasma the patches are superficial and only slightly inflammatory, and the causative organism, *Actinomyces minutissimus,* is readily differentiated from *Epidermophyton inguinale.* Positive diagnosis depends on discovery of the fungus.

TINEA OF THE HANDS AND FEET.—*Epidermophyton, Trichophyton* and *Monilia albicans* and other yeastlike organisms are often active here. Tinea of the hands often depends on the existence of tinea of the feet, where the infection may involve the skin or the nails, or both. Dermatophytids of the hands are more common than actually demonstrable tineal infection, and many a case of tinea-like pompholyx can be cured by applying treatment to the feet or to some other focus without particular regard to the hands. Streptococcic and staphylococcic dermatitis of the hands, recalcitrant perhaps because of focal infection, is likely to be the correct diagnosis when the hands alone are inflamed in the absence of lesions of the feet. The differentiation between mycotic and coccic infections of the extremities is important, for the treatment of the one is not effective for the other.

Three main groups of cases are seen:

(1) Vesicular, in which the lesions are grouped and are accompanied by marked itching, being characterized by sago-grain vesicles and occurring mostly in hot weather;
(2) Squamous, resembling scaling dyshidrosis, usually with a central primary lesion which results from the drying of confluent vesicles, and
(3) Pyodermic, resulting from secondary infection.

The essential lesions are probably vesicles, and these may be solitary or multiple, grouped or widely scattered. The vesicle is deeply seated, only slightly elevated, and has the appearance of a boiled sago grain embedded in the epidermis. Its content is usually clear, and as a rule there is no erythema surrounding new vesicles. Within a few days the fluid is absorbed, leaving a brownish macule. Eventually the roof of the dried vesicle becomes torn, exposing a red, smooth, shiny surface with a collarette of upturned scales. In acute cases the vesicles may be grouped and may become confluent, even forming bullae. In extensive, acute bullous infections the patient is incapacitated. When vesicles are grouped in a dry area such as the palm or sole, desquamation occurs, leaving a circular, well-defined, shiny, reddish area denuded of its corneum. This may heal spontaneously, or new vesicles may continue to develop about the periphery, and extension may occur in all directions. Groups of vesicles may appear in a dry or moist, well-defined, eczematous area. The areas affected, in their order of frequency, are: (1) the fourth interdigital space of the foot, (2) the plantar surface of the arch, and (3) over the tuberosity of the fifth metatarsal. At the base of the fifth toe a fissure, partly interdigital and partly plantar, is commonly present. Similar fissures may occur beneath all the flexural folds of the toes. Maceration of the exfoliated epidermis in the fourth interspace produces a white, sodden, thickened, adherent mass of epithelium. Hyperhidrosis is usually an associated symptom. The patient's complaint is of itching, which may be moderate or severe. Sensitiveness, pain and incapacitation occur in acute, bullous cases.

Inguinal lymphadenitis occurs in many severe and acute cases involving the feet. *Trichophyton interdigitale* has been secured by culture from a swollen inguinal node, the same organism being recovered from the focus.

Diagnosis.—Tinea of the palms and soles is to be distinguished from contact dermatitis, which is ordinarily not interdigital, is manifest as severely pruritic

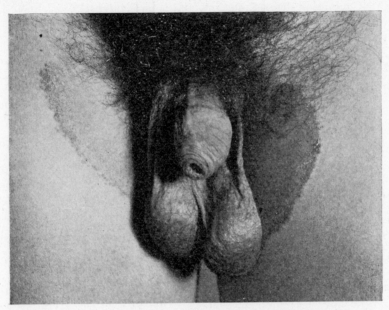

Fig. 10.—Tinea of the crotch; inguinal epidermophytosis. Always examine, and usually treat, the feet as well as the crotch in these cases.

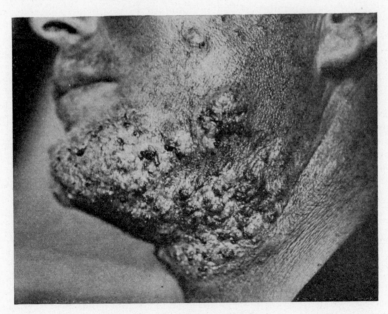

Fig. 11.—Tinea barbae, with kerion.

patches with fading, ill-defined margins, and is most intensely vesicular, if vesicular at all, in the central part of the inflamed areas rather than at the periphery. Impetigo and infectious eczematoid dermatitis are acutely inflammatory, are interdigitally located when they complicate scabies but rarely otherwise, spread rapidly with vesicles which are not multilocular, and produce separation of the epithelium from the dermis rather than multiple intra-epithelial vesiculation. Streptococcic or staphylococcic dermatitis often begins from a specific and remembered minor injury, upon which salves have been applied to the therapeutic detriment rather than betterment of the lesion. Coccic dermatitis is more painful and more speedy in its progress than mycotic dermatitis. Oozing, undermining, rapidly spreading, tinea-like dermatitis involving the dorsum of the feet or involving the hands and not the feet is usually coccic and cannot be treated with success by ointments, but responds well to **gentian violet** and **1: 10,000 bichloride of mercury** soaks. Fungus infection of asymptomatic character often spreads swiftly and increases in virulence when eczematous dermatitis occurs. Microscopic study is necessary for positive diagnosis.

TINEA BARBAE.—Two clinical types of tinea of the hairy regions are recognized, superficial and deep. In the superficial form the process may involve several hair shafts to a greater or less extent, but seldom to the degree seen in tinea capitis. Infected hairs become dry and brittle and can usually be extracted readily, the diseased root-sheath being often adherent to the shaft. The skin is somewhat reddened and thickened, and there are more or less scaling and slight itching. Vesiculation and pustulation are commonly absent. The disease frequently remains superficial throughout its course, involvement of the hairs being slight or even lacking.

Deep inflammation occurs in many cases, however, either from the beginning of the attack or after the disease has been present for several days or weeks in superficial form. The lesions may be few or many. Numerous, disseminated lesions constitute **sycosis** in contradistinction with **kerion,** in which the lesions are large and few in number. The inflammatory tumors are flat or oval and reddish, and are studded with dead or broken hairs or with gaping follicular orifices. The nodules may ulcerate in the center, but ordinarily pus and seropurulent material are discharged through inflamed, dilated, follicular openings. The common sité for the lesions is the skin beneath the jaw and in the cervicomaxillary fold. The entire bearded region may be involved, but as a rule the upper lip escapes. The severe form of tinea barbae usually develops slowly and is sluggish in its course, but it exhibits a tendency to undergo self-healing in time.

Kerion celsi, or tinea kerion, is deeply seated, acutely inflammatory tinea of the scalp, manifest by the formation of a rounded, boggy, oozing tumor. Similar carbuncular lesions on the dorsum of the hand or forearm may be called **agminate folliculitis.** The surface of the lesion is reddish or purplish and is marked by numerous pinhead- to split pea-sized pustules and gaping follicular orifices. The subcutaneous tissue is honeycombed with purulent matter, which often may be squeezed out through the follicular opening. Tumors may be single or multiple. They are extremely sensitive to pressure and may give rise to considerable pain. As a result of long-continued inflammation with its ensuing symptomatic but transient alopecia, this type of tinea may undergo spontaneous cure.

Diagnosis.—In seborrheic dermatitis and contact dermatitis the process is superficial, and the hair shafts are not involved. Syphilis gives rise to more or less tissular destruction followed by atrophic scarring and pigmentation. The characteristic lesions of sycosis are superficial, hair-pierced pustules or papules; the shafts seldom drop out spontaneously, and the upper lip is generally involved early in the course of the attack. In the deep type of tinea the lesions may simulate carbuncle. Actinomycosis must be distinguished.

Suppurative Tinea is a name designed to include kerion, sycosis and agminate folliculitis. *Trichophyton album* and *T. gypseum* are common offenders.

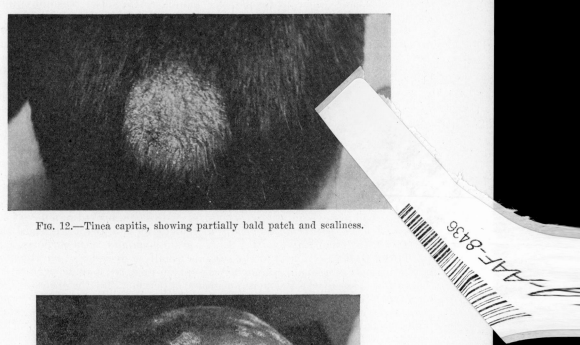

Fig. 12.—Tinea capitis, showing partially bald patch and scaliness.

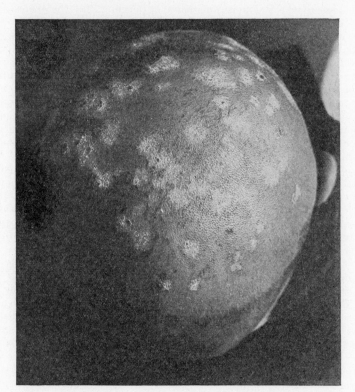

Fig. 13.—Tinea capitis, after roentgen depilation.
(Courtesy of Dr. George Miller MacKee.)

Many such cases occur in people who handle cattle. The trichophytin test is usually positive in suppurative tinea.

Granuloma Trichophyticum, or Majocchian granuloma, is a type of deep ringworm differing from kerion chiefly in its chronicity and its milder degree of inflammatory intensity. It does not suppurate until late or unless it becomes secondarily infected. It occurs on the scalp and beard in connection with pre-existent fungus infection, and on the backs of the hands and forearms. The lesions are sharply defined and have smooth surfaces. They are skin color, not tender, and of the size of a small nut. They may persist for months or years. Sometimes they are hard and keloid-like with deformed hairs at the periphery. The nodules usually occur in groups, but they may be solitary. They may occur on the leg and are readily mistaken for stasis or varicose dermatitis. In all cases of ulcer of the leg the nails should be examined for fungus infection, treatment of which may be prerequisite to success in treatment of the leg ulcer. *Trichophyton violaceum* is the usual organism in Majocchian granuloma.

Lichenoid Form of Deep Ringworm.—This type of nonsuppurative infection, dependent on pre-existing tinea, is manifest with scale-covered papules seen at the orifices of hairs, occurring especially at the elbows and knees. It constitutes an intergradient lesion between Majocchian granuloma and tinea corporis.

TINEA CAPITIS.—Tinea of the scalp is usually a disorder of childhood. The earliest lesion is a small, rounded, scaly patch or a red papule perforated by a hair. The base of the lesion is somewhat hyperemic, but the scales are whitish or grayish in color. As the patch slowly widens, it shows no tendency to undergo central involution such as occurs in lesions involving the glabrous skin. The hair shafts become dry, lusterless, whitish and brittle. They break off, and so occasion symptomatic alopecia, but the loss of hair is incomplete and young shafts are mingled with dead and broken stumps. Occasionally the inflammation may be so acute as to give rise to vesiculation and pustulation. The patches range in size up to several centimeters in diameter, and they may coalesce. Itching is the principal symptom, and scratching may lead to secondary infection.

"Disseminated ringworm" is the title applied to cases presenting small scattered patches of the disease. "Black dot ringworm" is so called because of a tendency of the hair to break off flush with the follicular orifices. "Bald ringworm" is characterized by such baldness as may be almost indistinguishable from alopecia areata. *Microsporum lanosum* produces well-defined patches of alopecia with marked inflammatory reaction, consisting of erythema, scaling, pustulation and crusting, and this may lead to spontaneous cure. *Microsporum audouini* infection is not so inflammatory, produces gray patches ("gray patch ringworm") and is much less readily healed. In fact, *Microsporum audouini* infections are so resistant that roentgen epilation is generally required to cure them, while in other types of infection local applications alone are likely to suffice. *Trichophyton violaceum* tends to produce permanent alopecia when it infects the scalp. *Epidermophyton inguinale* has been known to cause pityriasis capitis.

Tinea Capitis in Adults.—While infection of the adult scalp is uncommon, it is sometimes seen. The organism is usually a trichophyton invading the hair shaft, microsporum infection being quite rare. The eyelids may be involved in tinea, one form being folliculitis, with redness, swelling and perhaps exudation. There may occur edema of the lid margins without scaling, or there may occur scarring followed by the loss of the lashes. The usual organisms are *Trichophyton sulphureum* and *Trichophyton violaceum*.

Diagnosis.—The symptoms of ordinary tinea of the scalp are characteristic. The youth of the patient and the presence of partly bald, well-defined, scaly areas marked by lusterless and brittle or broken hairs, and dilated or debris-stuffed follicular orifices, are typical. One must distinguish seborrheic dermatitis, favus, contact dermatitis and alopecia areata. In seborrheic dermatitis the scales are greasy and are fairly uniformly distributed over the scalp in the familiar form of dandruff. Favus, another kind of dermatomycosis, is discussed in detail elsewhere. Eczematous dermatitis provokes considerable itching and is usually more or less oozing and vesicular. It does not affect the hairs directly. In alopecia areata infected hairs are absent, the bald region is in no way inflamed, and the circular patch of bald scalp is not scaly. For positive diagnosis, microscopic examination is requisite. A broken, whitish stub is chosen and is extracted with an epilating forceps. It is placed in a drop of 10 per cent potassium hydroxide solution on a glass slide, and after a few minutes it is examined under the microscope. Fungi are ordinarily easy to find if they are present, and a fruitless careful search is one criterion of cure.

Wood Light is ultraviolet light comprising wavelengths of about 3650 A° which pass a Wood filter, made of glass containing nickel oxide. Exposed to this light in a dark room, infected tissues fluoresce, and hairs can quickly be differentiated by their brilliant appearance if they are infected with *Microsporum*, but they do not fluoresce when *Trichophyton* is the agent. *Microsporum* infection is revealed by the luminous, short, yellowish-green stubs; *Trichophyton endothrix* makes them dull and bluish. *Achorion schoenleini* is greenish, less luminous than *Microsporum*. Tinea versicolor and patches of erythrasma show individual colors sufficient both to diagnose and to delimit the extent of involvement. Other fungi do not fluoresce characteristically.

TINEA OF THE NAILS.—*Trichophyton gypseum* and *T. purpureum,* as well as *Monilia albicans* and the organism of favus, are the vegetable parasites which commonly attack the nails. They are capable of living in the nail substance, which they invade more or less deeply—*Trichophyton purpureum* attacks especially deeply—and so they cause the nail to become thickened, lusterless, friable, and yellowish or whitish in color. The progress toward the root of the nail exceeds the rate of outward extrusion of the nail in its normal growth, so that eventually the entire nail plate may be supplanted by a scaling and horny, malformed, infected mass. The nails may be primarily involved, or secondarily to cutaneous infection. Chronic interdigital tinea of the feet eventuates in infection of the nails almost invariably. When the nails have become infected, they serve as foci for the dissemination of parasites, and cutaneous infection nearby then becomes unresponsive to lasting cure. Chronic infection of the nails often serves as a focus of infection for repeated attacks of distant dermatophytosis or dermatophytid.

The process of invasion of the nail is gradual. The free extremity of the nail, particularly at the side, first is involved. Several nails may be infected, but the times of onset are separate. Infection of all nails is rare, but it is sometimes seen. Sharply demarcated patches of opacity within the nail substance, asbestos-like and generally angulated in outline, are known as **leukonychia trichophytica.** There may be no inflammatory paronychial disease, for no inflammation is provoked by *Trichophyton* unless the fungi provoke local tissular hyperergy. The organisms are distributed throughout the infected, ungual structures. They can readily be detected in scrapings subjected to the action of 20 per cent potassium hydroxide solution. They may be stained and cultivated.

Onychomycosis is extremely persistent and has no tendency to undergo spontaneous healing. Mechanical riddance of the major portion of fungus-bearing tissue is an important part of successful treatment. The nails should be filed or pared down or drilled once a week. The removal of corneous material can be facilitated by the cautious application of **10 per cent potassium hydroxide** preliminary to scraping. Such mechanical débridement must be pursued energetically. We find **saturated alcoholic solution of silver nitrate** a satisfactory agent to apply to the scraped nails. **Strong, alcoholic solution of iodine** has been recommended. **One per cent bichloride of mercury in aqueous solution** may be used. Ointments are not satisfactory. The best effect the medicinal agent can produce is to serve as a fungistatic while the nail grows forth at the rate of a millimeter a week. If fungistasis is secured, the nail will eventually replace itself. Some six months of persistent treatment may be expected to be necessary in onychomycosis.

TRICHOPHYTON PURPUREUM INFECTION.—Lewis, Montgomery and Hopper (1936) led the way in defining specific dermatoses produced by specific tineal organisms. Disease provoked by *Trichophyton purpureum* is sufficiently distinctive, they demonstrated, to be recognized from its clinical manifestations alone with a fair degree of certainty. The lesions are palm size or larger and commonly affect the groins, back, thighs or umbilical region. The central region of the patch is lichenified and the borders, where spreading occurs, show follicular papules. The infection is highly pruritic and resistant to treatment. The nails are often affected.

On the hands and feet the appearance of the eruption seems to be peculiar to this organism. Lesions of the feet may involve the soles, sides, dorsa, toes and nails. The plantar surface is a common site. When the hands are involved, the palms, dorsa, fingers or nails may be affected. The entire sole is often involved, but the infection may be localized to a small area around the heel or on the ball of the foot. The infected skin is dull red and slightly thickened or indurated. Scaling, a constant feature, is usually fine and branny as compared with the large, flaky scaling of psoriasis and of some types of dermatophytosis. The absence of visible vesiculation is a feature. There is usually a sharply marginated border along the outer side of the foot between the infected skin and the normal skin on the dorsum. Small, irregular, infiltrated, erythematous and scaly patches may be found on the dorsum of the foot and toes. There is no tendency to clear in the center. On the undersurfaces of the toes and in the interdigital webs there is some maceration. When the entire area about the toe is infected, the skin is thickened and dry. Painful fissuring may occur about the joints. The eruption on the hands is similar to that on the feet. All the palmar skin may show the characteristic thickening, scaling and dull red color. Erythema may be slight, so that the condition may be mistaken for callus. Irregular, isolated patches may be present about the dorsum of the hand and fingers. Sometimes the skin of an entire finger is affected. Redness of the skin over the joints of the hands, with or without scaling, may be noted. Fissuring of the affected patches about the joints is a fairly common feature. The absence of vesiculation is notable. Sweating is diminished.

Nails infected with *T. purpureum* commonly have features peculiar to this organism. Unlike ungual infections with *T. gypseum,* there is not frequent concomitant involvement of the interdigital webs. The nail is infected deeply, not superficially. The progress is slow as compared with the more rapid progress of *T. gypseum.* Toenails and even the feet may be found to be infected without the knowledge of the patient. There is little inflammatory reaction in the subungual and paronychial tissues. Yellow or white longitudinal streaks may appear in the nail, and they seem to be the result of the separation of the nail plate from its bed. The streaks gradually widen, the nails separate more and more, and debris accumulates. The nail itself becomes thinned by the gradual invasion of the fungus. It becomes brittle and may be broken off at the distal portion, leaving only the proximal part. Sometimes the entire nail plate is lost, leaving the nail bed covered with scales and accumulated debris. The organisms cannot be isolated from the surface of the nails, but when deep portions of the nail are planted on agar slides *T. purpureum* in pure cultures may be obtained.

On the glabrous skin the lesions may be circinate, somewhat resembling tinea circinata, or they are more likely to be of the solid, flat type. Sometimes the shape is bizarre and configurate. Rarely the lesions resemble tinea imbricata, and they may suggest ichthyosis.

In the groin, involvement of the intergluteal fold, scrotum, pubis, and near-by areas of the skin is common. The lesions have the same characteristics as the solid plaque type seen on the glabrous skin. Pruritus is a distressing symptom.

In treatment, resistance is a notable feature. Trichophytin has been tried without success, and roentgen and ultraviolet therapy are likewise ineffective. In all forms of the infection the persistent use of strong, antiparasitic remedies over a long period of time has given the best results. **Chrysarobin, anthralin, compound tincture of benzoic acid, salicylic acid in alcohol,** and **strong potassium permanganate solution** are all of value. Such irritating remedies must be temporarily abandoned from time to time and smoothing agents substituted. Nails must be mechanically scraped before each application of the medicament.

MYCOTIC PARONYCHIA.—The paronychial tissues are susceptible to fungus infection. The disease may be acute, subacute or chronic. Inflammation, maceration, vesiculation and fissuring between and about the fingers frequently are concomitant. The disease tends to be an occupational one, affecting individuals exposed to pathogenic fungi while their hands are wet at work. *Fruit canners' dermatitis* is of this sort, and soda fountain clerks and washerwomen are susceptible. Manicuring may serve to inoculate the infection. Inconspicuous infection of the nails may provoke repeated attacks of mycotic paronychia. Budding organisms are the usual causes. In treatment, avoidance of long-continued moisture is important. Prevention in industrial circumstances may be obtained by hygienic measures: the prompt discarding and sterilizing of infected containers, the use of rubber gloves, and the prompt segregation and effectual treatment of infected workers. **Gentian violet** is particularly useful in monilial cases. Soaks in **1: 5000 potassium permanganate,** and the local application of a paste of **sodium perborate** about the lesions, are excellent measures.

DERMATOPHYTID.—In mycotic infections there may occur widespread, disseminated eruptions due to allergy to fungi as well as to dissemination of the fungi themselves. Dermatophytid is the general name for such eruptions, which differ widely in their clinical forms. *Epidermophytid, moniliid* and *trichophytid* are specific names, applicable when the specific causative agent is known. The incubation period is usually a few weeks, although the eruption may follow infection within a few days or it may follow treatment of tinea by x-ray or by trichophytin. The eruption may be violent or mild. During it, the specific test is always positive and is generally accompanied with focal flare. **Lichen trichophytica** is the name applied to a dermatophytid occurring in tinea of the scalp, in which the eruption is composed of scant or numerous, small red papules located on the back and shoulders, becoming scaly as they disappear. Dermatophytic erythema multiforme and erythema nodosum have been seen, the nodules in the latter being covered with delicate, follicular papules, while the eruption is accompanied by considerable fever. The commonest dermatophytid is **pompholyx** of the hands in vesicular tinea of the feet. If the focus is not controlled, the eruption may spread to involve the arms in scattered, discrete and confluent patches of erythema, later becoming eczematous and scaly. The sides of the neck and the face may become involved, and the eruption as a whole may become a widespread, oozing one involving the head, the extremities and much of the body. This is the extreme case, however.

Dermatophytids are free from demonstrable fungi. They depend on hyperergy to products of fungi. Injections of trichophytin into the skin regularly reduce sensitivity and increase tolerance, and hyposensitization so produced is sometimes accompanied by clinical improvement, but there is no satisfaction in treating tinea and its allergy by means of trichophytin, in our experience. One does better to attack the focus with appropriate means and, in treating the "ids," to use bland, nonspecific remedies such as **1: 500 aluminum acetate** for wet dressings or **calamine lotion with phenol.** Deep forms of trichophytic infection may be associated with fever, anorexia, headache, lymphadenitis and lymphangitis. Erysipelas-like, recurrent inflammation of the legs sometimes accompanies active dermatophytosis of the feet. These are not cases of true erysipelas or of chronic or recurrent streptococcic infection, but they are cases in which the reaction to fungus vaccine is hyperergic and in which passively transferable reagins exist. Such cases respond to treatment of the mycotic disorder of the feet, which must be cured if attacks are to be prevented. Urticaria and eruptions resembling pityriasis rosea or erythema annulare centrifugum may be due to tineal infection and allergy.

Dermatomycins.—Vaccinal preparations of fungi have been studied with regard to their academic and practical significance. Reactions to trichophytin include the immediate urticarial reaction, the late tuberculoid inflammatory reaction to intradermal tests, and the eczematous reaction to patch tests. Efforts to obtain practical therapeutic results by the use of vaccinal agents may summarily be considered fruitless. While this statement is debatable, it gives our present opinion.

Precipitins, agglutinins, and complement fixation antibodies circulate in human beings who are hypersensitive to dermatomycins. There vaccinal fungus materials can be used in diagnosis, much as tuberculin and luetin are used. Again the practical importance is slight because allergy from past infections, presently unimportant, may persist so that a positive test has no trustworthy significance as to the nature of the dermatosis at hand. Furthermore, in acute, severe, and actively spreading infections with fungi, sensitivity is absent or has not as yet developed, so that the negative test is without diagnostic indication. The reaction probably is actually specific, but the specificity is determined by genus rather than by species of fungus. Different species differ greatly in their ability to sensitize. The reaction is always positive in the presence of a dermatophytid. Repeated injections of trichophytin for testing purposes probably do not lead to the development of sensitivity. Some patients react to weak dilutions, others only to stronger ones. The patch test is less delicate and less reliable than the intracutaneous test. The uncommon immediate wheal reaction is usually associated with the presence of passively transferable antibodies. Positive reaction, while not diagnostic, does confirm other findings, signifies a hopeful prognosis and suggests the advisability of conservative treatment. If the test is negative in the face of proved infection, the immediate prognosis is poor, for immunity has not developed or is inadequate, and treatment must be sustained and vigorous. If the test is negative and fungi are not locally demonstrable, the eruption is not mycotic; this is important in the differentiation of contact dermatitis, particularly when the hands or feet are involved.

ETIOLOGY AND PATHOLOGY OF TINEA.—Mycotic infections of the skin are common disorders. Infection may occur immediately or through contact with contaminated articles such as towels, slippers, bath mats and the like. Mycotic infections of animals are readily transferred to human beings, sources being cats, dogs, horses, cattle and even birds. Epidemics are commonplace, and schools, colleges, armies and other communities where personal contact is close, are disseminating sources. There are individual differences in susceptibility to infection, but lasting immunity apparently develops in no one, and reinfections are common. Moisture, warmth and darkness are predisposing environmental circumstances.

The organisms most commonly met in the United States are listed, with their identifying features, for which we are indebted to Dr. George Lewis and Dr. Mary Hopper, of the New York Skin and Cancer Unit:

Direct examination, in these descriptions, usually refers to the microscopic appearance of the organisms following the mounting of a specimen in 10 per cent aqueous solution of potassium hydroxide. *Cultural characteristics* are as seen after isolation on a solid medium containing 4 per cent crude American dextrose, 1 per cent Fairchild's peptone, and 1.8 per cent agar. *Culture mount* refers to the microscopic appearance of a cultural growth as seen in a hanging-drop preparation, in a Henrici slide culture, or in a direct mount from a culture of material in 10 per cent potassium hydroxide solution. The last type of mount is not advisable for routine use because, so prepared, the arrangement of fungus elements cannot be studied satisfactorily.

Microsporum audouini (commonly causative of tinea capitis).

Direct Examination.—Short, broken-off hairs are chosen for examination. The spores are round, small, and grouped to form a mosaic sheath around the infected hairs. There is usually no tendency to the formation of chains.

Cultural Characteristics.—Beginning as a cottony elevation, the growth after 2 weeks is grayish-white and fluffy, and the aerial growth is sparse. There is usually a central elevation. Radial grooves seldom develop on dextrose peptone medium, though, on maltose agar, radial grooves almost invariably appear. Pleomorphism is uncommon.

Culture Mount.—Fuseaux and microconidia are occasionally seen. Chlamydospores and pectinate bodies are frequent.

Microsporum lanosum (commonly causative of tinea capitis).

Direct Examination.—Hair infected with *M. lanosum* cannot be distinguished from hair infected with *M. audouini*. In scrapings from lesions of tinea circinata, segmented mycelium may be noted.

Cultural Characteristics.—The growth appears first as a downy fluff, and it develops fairly rapidly. After 2 weeks the colony is woolly, and the aerial material is abundant. The color is buff tan. This development of yellow pigment on the undersurface of the colony is characteristic. Grooves may be radial or concentric. Pleomorphism begins after 4 or 5 weeks. The appearance under the filtered ultraviolet rays (Wood light) is distinctively lavender blue or shell pink toward the center of the colony, the colors being bright and clear.

Culture Mount.—The feature of this fungus is the presence of large numbers of fuseaux of the tapering sort Microconidia and some other forms may also be noted.

Microsporum fulvum (Tinea).

Direct Examination.—A hair infected with *M. fulvum* may resemble in appearance a hair infected with any other *Microsporum*. Sometimes spores in linear arrangement may be observed.

Cultural Characteristics.—The growth is flat, felty, and cinnamon brown. A central umbo may be present. Concentric furrows sometimes appear. Pleomorphism is usually manifest after several weeks.

Culture Mount.—Numerous fuseaux are present. Racquet mycelium, nodular organs, and small round spores may also be seen.

Achorion schoenleini (Favus).

Direct Examination.—Large spores in chains are noted in the substance of the hair. The presence of air bubbles is almost of diagnostic significance. Sporulated mycelium will be found in large amounts in scutula but are few in number in infected nails or in superficial lesions of the smooth skin.

Cultural Characteristics.—After 3 or 4 weeks the growth is smooth, compact and waxy. The surface shows numerous folds. Pleomorphism is rare. The submergence of the colony usually results in cracking of the agar.

Culture Mount.—Favic chandeliers may be noted. Chlamydospores in large numbers may also be observed.

Trichophyton violaceum (Tinea).

Direct Examination.—Large spores in linear arrangement may be seen invading the shaft of an infected hair or in scales or nail tissue.

Cultural Characteristics.—The colony is compact, smooth and shiny, and it has a typical deep violet color. The surface shows convolutions. Pleomorphism is rare.

Culture Mount.—The mycelium shows irregular and oddly shaped branches. No free or attached spores are developed. Chlamydospores are seen in older colonies.

Trichophyton crateriforme (Tinea).

Direct Examination.—Large spores in chains are seen in the shaft of the infected hair, usually in large numbers.

Cultural Characteristics.—The growth is compact, creamy white, and velvety. The central portion is broken and depressed, being yellow. Pleomorphism is rare.

Culture Mount.—Conidia in clusters (grapes) or on stalks (thyrses) are to be noted. Chlamydospores are common.

Trichophyton gypseum (Tinea).

Direct Examination.—In a follicular infection, small, round spores in chains may be found external to the hair. In scales, macerated tissue, or in nail scrapings, chains of spores or segmented mycelium with little branching will be noted.

Cultural Characteristics.—There are 4 types of growth which we believe are closely related genetically:

1. The usual type. This begins as a white, fluffy growth. After about 2 weeks, the surface becomes velvety and buff-colored. There is usually a boss at the center and a few irregular folds.

2. The granular variety. The surface is powdery and is light buff or maize yellow in color. Fluffy changes develop with age.

3. The *T. interdigitale* type. This begins as a downy projection, developing into a white, fluffy, diffuse growth covering an agar slant within 2 weeks.

4. The *T. niveum* type. This is white and fluffy at first, later becoming compact. Surface irregularities are present.

Culture Mount.—

1. The usual type. Spirals may be seen. Small numbers of fuseaux, nodular organs, pectinate bodies, racquet mycelium, and chlamydospores may be noted. Microconidia are present.

4042

2. The granular type. Numerous fuseaux are present and dense masses of microconidia are to be seen. Few spirals will be seen. Chlamydospores and racquet mycelium may be found in the subsurface growth.

3. The *T. interdigitale* and *T. niveum* types. A large number of filaments and a few clusters of microconidia are observed. Nodular organs and racquet mycelium may be found. Spirals and fuseaux are usually absent.

Trichophyton purpureum (Tinea).

There is nothing characteristic in the microscopic appearance of the fungus in scrapings. While the amount of fungus material may be sparse, large numbers of organisms have been noted in an occasional specimen. The mycelium is about the same size as that of *T. gypseum*, being 3 or 4 microns in diameter.

The culture on dextrose agar, in primary growth, at first is fluffy, pure white and hemispherical. The edge of the colony becomes less fluffy and at times is granular. The undersurface of the colony shows the typical rose-purple color, which gradually spreads to the edge of the colony and may be noted in varying degrees throughout the colony. Pleomorphism occurs eventually. Under filtered ultraviolet rays (Wood light) the cultures show colors which are bright but hazy. The central half of the colony is mauve; the remainder is a light, soft blue-violet. There are many sterile vegetative hyphae and many microconidia in thyrses and in grapelike clusters in culture mount. Fuseaux are few. Chlamydospores develop in older growths. Inoculation of animals is occasionally successful. The index of sensitization is low.

Monilia albicans (Moniliasis) .

Cultures.—The growth is smooth, pasty and cream-colored, and it grows rapidly on dextrose medium. The central portion later appears honeycombed. On corn meal agar, mycelium, characteristic spore clusters and chlamydospores develop. Ascospores are not formed.

Agglutination Reaction.—The organism agglutinates in a serum prepared against *Monilia albicans* (Benham, 1931).

Animal Inoculation.—Benham (1931) found that the intravenous injection of 1 cc. of a 1:1000 suspension of a live culture, kills a rabbit in 4 or 5 days. Abscesses in which *Monilia albicans* may be recovered develop in the kidneys and other organs.

Differential Diagnosis.—Cryptococci do not develop mycelium, and other species of *Monilia* may be distinguished from *Monilia albicans* by the absence of chlamydospores when grown on corn meal agar. *Mycoderma* may usually be recognized by its gross appearance in culture; a culture mount reveals arthrospores. *Endomyces* and *Saccharomyces* form ascospores; the former also develops mycelium.

Epidermophyton inguinale.

Direct Examination.—The scales contain chains of spores in which the elements tend to be flattened. The amount of fungus material is often plentiful.

Cultural Characteristics.—After 2 or 3 weeks the growth is apparent. It develops a velvety surface with irregular folds and is characteristically grayish olive drab or greenish drab in color. Pleomorphism develops early.

Culture Mount.—Fuseaux of the blunt-end variety are to be seen in groups. Chlamydospores and racquet mycelium may also be observed.

Malassezia furfur (*Microsporum furfur*) (Tinea versicolor).

Direct Examination.—Fungus elements are usually present in profusion and the picture is characteristic. They consist of round or ovoid, refractile spores in clusters. Mycelia, moderate in length but rather fragile, occur in considerable numbers.

Cultures.—Doubtfully successful. See Tinea versicolor.

Actinomyces minutissimus (Erythrasma).

Direct Examination.—On examination with the high power of the microscope, fine threads may be noted. If the oil-immersion lens is used, the threads are visible, being long, tortuous and interlacing. A few spores may be seen.

Cultural Characteristics.—There is not general agreement that this micro-organism has been cultured.

Endodermophyton tropicale (Tinea imbricata).

Direct Examination.—Numerous segmented hyphae are noted.

Cultural Characteristics.—The growth is compact and gray to brown in color, and it shows an uneven surface. There is superficial resemblance to *Achorion schoenleini*.

Culture Mount.—Vegetative forms may be noted. Microconidia are not present.

Hormodendron pedrosoi (Chromomycosis).

Direct Examination.—So-called sclerotic cells (Medlar) are present. These may be septate and are usually in groups. Small septate filaments may also be noted.

Cultural Characteristics.—The growth is compact, limited and felty. Concentric zones, colored brownish olive, olive black, olive gray, and gray, may be noted.

Culture Mount.—Olive brown spores are borne on conidiophores. Disjunctors are also usually present.

Actinomyces bovis (Actinomycosis).

Direct Examination.—This is the most important laboratory investigation of a patient suspected of infection with this micro-organism. The granule is seen to consist of one or more colonies in which in the mid-zone there is a mass of twisted mycelium, and at the periphery a palisaded arrangement of hyphae, forming a fringe. These latter organs are enlarged at one end and are striated. The ray fungus is gram-positive. The central mycelium takes the basic dye and the peripheral zone takes the acidic dye.

Cultural Characteristics.—There is considerable difficulty in obtaining a cultural growth, and it usually dies quickly. The colonies are pasty but of variable consistency and configuration.

Culture Mount.—Sterile mycelium without characteristic spore forms.

Rhinocladium (Sporotrichum) schencki (Sporotrichosis).

Direct Examination.—Cigar-shaped cells may be noted, but fungus material is usually absent.

Cultural Characteristics.—After 2 weeks, a moist growth is noted which is light brown in color, but with age it becomes dark brown. The central portion shows irregular foldings. White excrescences form on the surface.

Cultural Mount.—Pear-shaped conidia are situated irregularly along the mycelium and arranged also as terminal triads and tetrads.

Blastomyces dermatitidis (Blastomycosis of Gilchrist).

Direct Examination.—Budding, thick-walled, round or oval, granular cells, 8 to 20 microns in diameter, are to be found.

Cultural Characteristics.—The central portion of the colony is gray and smooth, becoming white and filamentous. A peripheral moist zone is usually present. Yeastlike growths are obtained on blood agar.

Culture Mount.—Microconidia, chlamydospores, and racquet mycelium may be noted. Budding cells may be obtained from the yeastlike growth.

Coccidioides immitis (Blastomycosis of Rixford and Gilchrist).

Direct Examination.—The micro-organism is a sphere with a doubly contoured capsule, from 5 to 60 microns in diameter, and it contains 6 to 20 endospores.

Cultural Characteristics.—The growth is white and filamentous; a brownish shade develops with age.

Culture Mounts.—Septate mycelium is profuse. Arthrospores and chlamydospores may be distinguished.

Torula histolytica (Torulosis).

Direct Examination.—Various-sized budding cells will be seen. A wet India-ink preparation reveals a wide capsule.

Cultural Characteristics.—The colony is moist and cream-colored, later changing to yellow and then to brown.

Culture Mount.—Round or oval, various-sized budding cells will be seen (India-ink technic). No mycelium and no ascospores will be found.

DEMONSTRATION OF FUNGI.—One tears off the cap of a blister, including the margin of it, and immerses this in 10 per cent aqueous potassium hydroxide. After maceration the bit is crushed under the cover slip and dim light is used in examination. Experience is necessary for distinguishing hyphae and spores from droplets of fat, epithelial cells and detritus. Fungi may be stained (Swartz and Conant, 1936) by the following method: heat the scales on a slide in a drop of:

℞ Lactic acid	1.0
Phenol crystals	1.0
Glycerol	2.0
Cotton blue (C4B Poirrier)	0.5 per cent
Distilled water	1.0

Berberian (1937) used this technic:

Cover scales in small bits with 50 per cent glacial acetic acid in water, and dry in incubator, causing adherence of scales to slide; defat by flooding with ether several times, with acetone several times, with alcohol in diminishing concentrations; stain in Martinotti's toluidine blue; wash in water; differentiate with 0.5 per cent acetic acid; dehydrate in absolute acetone; pass through xylene; mount in euparol or balsam.

4042

Hairs may be examined as follows:

The diseased stump is put on a slide, and washed with ether, to defat. It is then treated with aniline gentian-violet solution for 5 minutes, blotted, treated with potassium iodide solution for from 1 to 5 minutes, blotted, treated with aniline oil, then a mixture of equal parts of aniline oil and dilute hydrochloric acid to decolorize, finally with aniline oil, followed by xylol; then it is mounted in balsam.

Mosaic fungus, so-called, is perhaps not fungus at all, for it dissolves in ether, absolute alcohol and phenol. It seems to be a degeneration product, for it has been observed that mosaic material and *T. gypseum* in transition forms are in contiguity in mycotic scales. During the healing of the lesions, mosaic fungus increases and living fungus diminishes.

PROGNOSIS.—The outlook in mycotic infection varies with the location, extent, duration of the disease, the specific cause, and the reactivity of the particular patient. Tinea corporis usually responds readily and favorably to treatment, although *T. purpureum* infections are exceptions to this rule. In extensive cases of tinea of the scalp the infection is extremely rebellious in some cases, easier to cure in others, depending on the infecting organism. In cases in which kerion occurs, baldness due to scarring may result. Great care must be exercised in examining a case before discharging it as cured. Good treatment, which implies attention to detail and to the following of correct broad principles, is materially advantageous. Patients with manifestations which confused and baffled dermatologists in 1930 are being managed with much greater confidence a decade later. Attention must be paid to all foci of mycotic infection, especially the nails. All infected areas must be treated simultaneously so that dissemination cannot occur. Fungi, like bacteria, breed speedily under suitable conditions. Animal and human sources of reinfection, along with inanimate sources such as clothing and shoes, must be recognized and dealt with. Dermatitis venenata due to medication must be recognized and avoided. In difficult cases the patient must co-operate by devoting himself exclusively to treatment.

TREATMENT OF TINEA.—Success depends on correct interpretation of the case at hand. Correct diagnosis is essential. The distinction of tinea from dermatitis venenata and from coccic disease is important. Tineal dermatitis is due to mold-like fungi which primarily parasitize the dead horny cells of the epidermis and secondarily provoke inflammation, allergy, eczematous dermatitis, and antibody production. The antibodies may be sessile (local) or circulatory and associated with distant allergic manifestations, the dermatophytids. In the places where the living fungi are present, treatment is aimed at (1) their mechanical removal and (2) chemical destruction of them. These aims must be carried out by means which are compatible with the welfare of the host's tissues. Violent chemical measures are not successful. In the lesions due to allergy, the aims are (1) soothing the inflamed skin where pathogenic fungi are not present, and giving symptomatic relief to the patient; (2) attacking foci whence dissemination originates and where fungi are present. As a mushroom grows overnight from an invisible spore when circumstances are favorable, so a focus of inconspicuous fungi can luxuriate overnight and cause clinical disease.

Many chemical substances are serviceable, and no one of them is specific. The physician's job consists not in extermination of parasites but rather in tipping the equilibrium between host and parasite in favor of the host, while one trusts to the natural responses to attend to the healing. The host's immunity is of considerable importance (see discussion of Dermatomycins).

Débridement is important. Vesicles should be opened so that chemicals may get into them. No greasy preparation is ordinarily satisfactory when applied to an acute, vesicular lesion, but astringent soaks and antiseptic powders are. Inflamed skin treated with soaks and without grease readily becomes cracked and fissured if it is flexed, but it regains its normal flexibility when the inflammation disappears. The use of unguents, while comforting, proves to be a disappointment and a waste of time, and immobilization, along with the repeated application of soaks, is to be preferred. The patient may wish to continue to use his sore hands or feet; he must be advised not to do so. Medicinal agents may provoke alterations of the skin. This must be recognized when it occurs, and the medicine must be stopped before it does harm. Wet packs of a suitable dilution become too strong if they dry without being rinsed and refreshed. It is as important to stop the use of a medicine as it is to start it. The plan of treatment must be individualized. Routine treatment fails as often as it succeeds.

Conditions of the Background.—Obesity predisposes to mycotic infections, for the fat person is usually warm and moist, particularly in the folds of the body. In diabetes the sweat is laden with sugar, which serves as pabulum especially for *Monilia.* Summertime is of course the time when mycoses flourish. Tight clothes, especially girdles, underwear, and trousers combine to keep the crural regions continually moist and ill ventilated so that tinea of the crotch may be impossible to cure until these conditions have been altered. Shoes which are tight across the toes, holding them in continuous juxtaposition, make it next to impossible to cure interdigital tinea. In such cases, the shoes should be changed and the feet dried during the middle of the day, and broad-toed shoes ought to be worn.

Constitutional remedies are of little or no value. Arsphenamines are decidedly dangerous as well as useless, for the sensitivity of the skin is precarious during mycotic infection. Alkalis are usually without value, but dilute hydrochloric acid sometimes seems to help, perhaps by altering the pH of the sweat. Vaccinal therapy has been completely disappointing in our hands.

Roentgen therapy in treating tinea must be used with greater wisdom than in most other conditions for which it is useful. X-ray energy does not act by killing the fungus; in fact, it takes some fifty times the dose which will necrotize the skin to influence pathogenic mycotic organisms as they grow in vitro. Roentgen therapy stops hyperhidrosis and so plays a useful part. It provokes the dissolution of the inflammatory reaction and helps to cause vesicles to resorb. It inhibits the ability of the skin to respond to the presence of the fungus, and on this account its use is generally followed by several days of symptomatic remission. When roentgen therapy is used time after time as the disease repeatedly reappears, the result is atrophy or burn, and the disease continues to be superimposed on skin which has been treated beyond tolerance. We find roentgen therapy practically never necessary and only seldom desirable in the treatment of tinea.

Chemical Agents.—The remedies we find most useful are:

1. 1:5000 potassium permanganate:

    ℞ Potassium permanganate .... ℥ii
        Water .... ℥viii

    Sig.: ℥i to 1 qt. water for soaks.

2. 1:10,000 bichloride of mercury:

    ℞ Bichloride of mercury .... gr.xxx
        Water .... ℥ii

    Sig.: POISON. ℥i to 1 qt. water for soaks or wet packs.

3. 1:500 aluminum acetate:

    ℞ Aluminum acetate (basic) .... ℥ii
    Div. in caps. no. viii.

    Sig.: One capsule to one pint of water for moist packs.

4. 5 per cent, 10 per cent and sometimes 20 per cent silver nitrate in water, for occasional topical application, serving as a protein precipitant capable of some penetration between epithelial cells and of rendering the epidermis uninhabitable by fungi.

5. 10 per cent silver nitrate in alcohol for painting infected nails after filing them.

4042

6. Soap and water, along with a scrubbing brush sometimes, and perhaps reinforced with sandpaper for attacking thick collections of scales in chronic, squamous tinea of the feet.

7. 10 per cent salicylic acid in alcohol, a potent provocator of scaling which in itself is a means of débridement.

8. Gentian violet, the 2 per cent aqueous solution being the best, a medicament which is fungicidal for gram-positive organisms, is not toxic, and is astringent, providing a protective dry crust over an oozing surface.

9. A dusting powder with active ingredients such as camphor, precipitated sulfur, boric acid and salicylic acid, the vehicle being zinc oxide, zinc stearate and starch:

> ℞ Camphor .... ℨss
> Salicylic acid .... gr.x
> Zinc oxide
> Cornstarch
> Zinc stearate ....of each to ℨi

Sig.: Dust between toes and into shoes to keep feet dry.

10. Whitfield's ointment, a medicament which provokes scaling and which must commonly be diluted:

> ℞ Phenol .... ♏v
> Salicylic acid .... gr.xxx
> Benzoic acid .... ℨi
> White Vaseline .... to ℨi

Sig.: Full-strength Whitfield's ointment; may be diluted with vaseline.

11. Lassar's paste, simply a soothing medicament:

> ℞ Phenol .... ♏v
> Salicylic acid .... gr.x
> Zinc oxide
> Cornstarch .... of each ℨi to ℨii
> White Vaseline .... to ℨi

Sig.: Soothing ointment to allay itching.

12. Schalek's paste, an excellent antiparasitic agent:

> ℞ Phenol .... ♏v
> Salicylic acid .... gr.xx
> Precipitated sulfur .... gr.xxx
> Zinc oxide
> Cornstarch .... of each ℨi to ℨii
> White Vaseline .... to ℨi

Sig.: Modified sulfur parasiticidal ointment; rub in twice daily, wash off with soap once daily.

There are few cases of tinea which will not respond to one or a combination of these agents correctly used. For débridement soap and water have no rival, but the allowance must be meager, bathing being performed only daily, and hurriedly, and with the use of water that is not hot. All alkali must be rinsed off thoroughly and the parts dried carefully. If the response to soap and water is unfavorable, they must be discontinued.

Medicaments may incorporate the following parasiticidal agents in the percentages indicated:

Ammoniated mercury (5 to 10 per cent), parasiticidal.
Balsam of Peru (5 to 10 per cent), antiparasitic.
Benzoic acid (5 to 15 per cent), antiseptic and scaling.
Betanaphthol (3 to 10 per cent), parasiticidal.
Chrysarobin (1 to 10 per cent)—dangerous about the eyes—exfoliative, reducing agent.
Iodine, the tincture—incompatible with sulfur—antiseptic.
Oil of cinnamon (0.2 per cent)—liable to irritate.
Phenol (1 per cent), antipruritic.

Pyrogallol (1 to 10 per cent), reducing agent comparable with chrysarobin.

Salicylic acid (2 to 10 per cent), provocator of desquamation; not strongly antiseptic itself.

Resorcinol (2 to 10 per cent), similar to salicylic acid.

Sodium thiosulfate, isotonic to saturated solutions, weakly antiparasitic, sometimes irritating, usefulness overestimated.

Sulfur (2 to 15 per cent), excellent fungicidal agent, activity enhanced by combination with salicylic acid.

Crude coal tar (2 to 20 per cent) in lanolin and vaseline, messy but effectively antiparasitic and rarely irritating.

Thymol (0.5 per cent or weaker), fungicidal, liable to irritate.

Treatment of Tinea Corporis.—The disease as a rule responds to any of the strong parasiticides. Daily applications of **iodine** for four or five days may prove curative. **Ammoniated mercury ointment** serves admirably in some cases. An ointment containing **10 per cent tar** or **5 to 10 per cent sulfur** is prescribed. **Five per cent chrysarobin in vaseline** is a useful agent, but it promptly makes the skin red and sore and must be kept from the eyes with care. **Schalek's paste** is useful; it should be rubbed in repeatedly until the skin becomes slightly sore and scaly, then treatment should be stopped for several days while one waits to see whether more is required.

Tinea of the Feet is the commonest form of human mycotic infection, probably because of the favorable environment there offered the fungus by continued moisture, warmth and darkness. Into the feet first, infection is commonly inoculated in swimming pools, locker rooms and shower baths. A few spores reaching the hands would be far less likely, than if they reached the feet, to find favorable circumstances for their growth, or would be washed away.

Circumstances favoring the organisms may be altered by washing the feet with soap each night, using plain, nonmedicated soap and rinsing them well in order to carry away the scaly accumulations which provide pabulum. The toes should be dried carefully after bathing, so that they are actually dry. A dusting powder is then useful.

The shoes should be loose, particularly at the toe. The shoes and hose should be changed during the middle of the day, so as to break the long 16-hour period during which the feet are continually moist and dark and the toes are held in juxtaposition.

In acute cases, characterized by vesiculation, the vesicles should be opened and the bases painted with **5 or 10 per cent aqueous solution of silver nitrate.** The feet should be soaked in some antiseptic foot bath such as **1: 5000 potassium permanganate** or **1: 10,000 bichloride of mercury.** The soaks may last 10 minutes, two to six or eight times a day, using lukewarm water. In severe cases the patient should be off his feet, which between soakings should be dry and exposed to the air. In mild cases the patient will remain ambulatory. In severe, acute, vesicular and spreading cases immediate control can scarcely be obtained, for the parasite is so virulent that, until time for immune response on the part of the host has passed, the disease continues to spread. It is such cases that are particularly often associated with dermatophytid. The vesicles should be opened and the lesions swabbed with **5 per cent silver nitrate** or **2 per cent gentian violet** or **1: 100 potassium permanganate,** all of which act as astringent antiseptics; and wet packs, using **1: 10,000 bichloride of mercury,** may be applied for half an hour, then left off for half an hour or so. The skin will crack if it is flexed, and the patient is temporarily incapacitated.

In chronic infections with interdigital maceration and scaling about the toes and on the soles, daily washing and dusting are advisable. **Silver nitrate** is especially useful swabbed over the involved areas. Ointments which provoke scaling, such as **Schalek's paste** or **Whitfield's ointment** (which may be diluted half and half with vaseline), may be rubbed in twice a day, the feet being washed once a day with soap and water. *Scaling provoked by the medicament must not be mistaken for scaling provoked by infection. The ointment may be used for several days, then omitted for several days,* during which time the

4042

physician takes stock of what his remedies have accomplished. We seldom use ointments, finding ourselves able to manage tinea of the feet more satisfactorily with astringent swabs, soaks and débridement. Chronic ringworm of the toes is commonly maintained by foci in the nails, and the nails must be examined and treated appropriately if infection is present.

Tinea of the Crotch and Axilla.—Infection in these locations commonly depends on the presence of infections elsewhere, particularly of the feet, which must be examined and treated appropriately. The application of **5 per cent silver nitrate,** and the use of **1 : 10,000 bichloride of mercury** as cool wet poultices applied for 10 or 15 minutes two to six times a day, generally serve to control the infection. The underwear and trousers must be loose so that the parts are well ventilated. Sometimes one obtains excellent results by rubbing in an ointment composed of **4 per cent salicylic acid and 6 per cent precipitated sulfur in vaseline,** which is left on overnight and washed off with soap and water the next morning. Sometimes the activity of the disease is too great to allow the use of potent remedies at first, and a day or two is well spent using moist, soothing applications, with intervals of allowing the sore skin to dry in the air or under a heat lamp. After partial healing, stronger remedies may be applied without discommoding the patient. In women mycotic infection of the crotch is likely to be an external manifestation of mycotic vulvovaginitis, and **1 : 5000 potassium permanganate douches** given twice a day should supplement the external therapy. Ointments cannot be used for more than a day or two in the hairy regions of the crotch and axilla without promoting staphylococcic complication and furuncles, which one wishes anxiously to avoid.

Tinea of the Beard.—Localized inflammatory mycotic infection, kerion, is treated by the **removal of loose hairs,** the **application of wet packs of 1 : 10,000 bichloride of mercury,** and **small doses of roentgen therapy.** When the infection is disseminated and chronic rather than deeply inflammatory and localized, the problem is more difficult. Ormsby recommended that the **parts be kept moistened with olive oil for two days,** then **shampooed with soap, freed from crusts,** and **shaved clean.** Following shaving, the face should be bathed in hot **boric acid solution** for 10 minutes. Then, while bathing, the pustules should be opened with an aseptic needle. The face should be sponged with **10 per cent sodium thiosulfate solution** and allowed to dry. It is washed again with warm water, dried gently, and smeared with **10 to 20 per cent sulfur ointment,** which is left on overnight. In the morning the face is washed, the **thiosulfate** is swabbed over it, and it is dusted with a **salicylic acid powder** for the day. The shaving, inunction and bathing may be repeated as the growth of the beard indicates. After healing progresses, the ointment at night is eventually superseded by the dusting powder alone. Diseased hairs are removed by epilation with forceps. Roentgen epilation is seldom necessary. Cleanliness and prevention of contamination are as important as in treating an infected scalp. The disease is readily communicated by razors and other toilet articles.

Tinea of the Scalp.—This readily transmitted infection is often epidemic among children. Prophylactic measures are essential. The hair should be closely clipped or shaved, and a snugly fitting paper cap (conveniently made by cutting off and discarding the top two thirds of a grocer's paper sack) should be worn continually, being refreshed daily and the old one burned. The scalp should be washed with **nonmedicated soap and water** once a day or once in two days, depending on its soreness. Infections with *Microsporum audouini* are highly resistant, and their cure depends on epilation, generally most conveniently accomplished by means of **x-ray.** Epilation with forceps is an important adjunct. *M. lanosum* infection may be treated successfully by showing the mother how to remove all infected hairs with a good forceps (a cheap instrument being worthless), with instructions to shampoo the head daily and to follow drying after the shampoo with a thorough rubbing in of **4 per cent salicylic acid and 6 per cent sulfur in vaseline,** an ointment which in our experience is highly effectual. If the head becomes too sore to continue with this forceful treatment, it should be left alone for a few days, then the treatment should be taken up and carried on. Any of the many parasiticidal drugs may be used; the sulfur-salicylic acid combination is quite satisfactory. Epilation can be carried out at daily sessions, every hair in the patch and those in the margin also being removed carefully and discarded into paper containers which may be burned.

Roentgen epilation of the scalp is safe if it is done by an expert. The epilating dose of unfiltered rays is about 300 r. It is the superficial, noninflammatory "human" type of infection which is likely to require epilation, while the more inflamed, "animal" type can often be cured by local measures alone. Roentgen epilation is fully discussed by George MacKee in his *X-ray and Radium in the Treatment of Diseases of the Skin*, Ed. 3, 1938. Epilation can be accomplished by the use of thallium acetate, a deadly poison in overdosage. Taken internally in a single dose not exceeding 8.5 mg. per kilo of body weight, *never* being given to children *older* than eleven years, the hair loosens and may be extracted easily by the use of an epilating wax within 12 to 24 days. We do not recommend this method, its dangers, excepting under special circumstances, outweighing its advantages.

Pusey's wax, a good one, is made thus: (1) beeswax, 1 part by weight, and (2) powdered rosin, 4 parts; melt "1" and pour in "2" slowly while mixing.

Kerion of the scalp is treated like kerion of the beard (*q.v.*).

FAVUS

Favus is the dermatosis due to infection of the skin with *Achorion schoenleini* or with any of several closely related organisms. It is characterized clinically by the occurrence of pinhead- to pea-sized, saucer-shaped, yellowish crusts or scutula. Infection may involve the hair, nails or glabrous skin, or all of these. The scalp is the commonest site. The lesions commence as small, whitish, scaly patches. Within a few weeks crusts assume definite shape as small, sulfur-colored disks, each of which is usually perforated by a hair. Of saucer shape, these cups, with slightly elevated fringelike edges, are tightly fixed to the skin, and atrophy occurs beneath them. When the crust is detached, the depressed, torn surface is covered with serous or bloodstained fluid. A scutulum tends to enlarge peripherally, and neighboring lesions coalesce to form thick, mortarlike masses. The crusts may slowly enlarge, and the central, oldest portion becomes whitish or pearly in color, while the peripheral, younger portion remains yellow and exhibits furrows in concentric rings: or perhaps a scutulum, having attained a certain size, ceases to spread peripherally and builds up on the surface, forming a crusted mass. The scutula possess a peculiar, characteristic odor like that of a mouse nest. The hairs become dull, dry, lusterless and brittle. In long-standing cases the follicles undergo atrophic obliteration. The disease progresses tediously and it may endure over a period of many years. On the glabrous skin manifestations are more acute, and the patches are reddish, scaly and discoid, while atrophy is a less prominent feature than on the scalp. Favus of the nails is distinguished from tinea only by cultivation of the organism or by the concomitant presence of typical favus elsewhere.

Cutaneous eruptions dependent on allergy occur in favus and are called **favids.** They are the analogues of trichophytids.

Etiology.—*Achorion schoenleini* is the common cause of favus. *A. gallinae, A. quinckeanum, A. gypseum* and *A. violaceum* cause similar disease, and are distinguished by their cultural characteristics.

The disease may be transferred by handling infected animals, such as rats, cats, mice, cattle and horses. Transference from infected human beings to other human beings is of course the usual route.

Diagnosis.—The disease persists for many years but tends to undergo spontaneous cure with cicatricial atrophy. It is responsive to good treatment.

4042

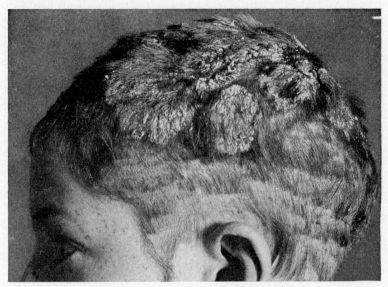

FIG. 14.—Favus of the scalp, showing typical crusting.
(Courtesy of Dr. George Miller MacKee.)

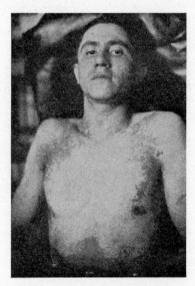

FIG. 15.—Tinea versicolor.

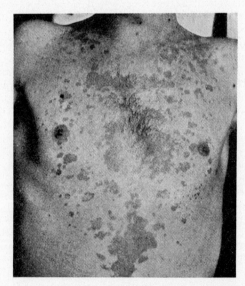

FIG. 16.—Tinea versicolor.

Treatment.—The treatment of favus of the scalp is essentially that of tinea capitis. **Roentgen epilation** is highly desirable. The parasiticides commonly used are those enumerated under the treatment of tinea. Simultaneous treatment is necessary for all infected members of the family and of all infected parts of the body. Vaccinal therapy is not satisfactory.

TINEA IMBRICATA

Tinea imbricata (Tokelau ringworm) is a dermatomycosis of warm, moist climates, due to various fungi of the genus *Endodermophyton* (*Castellani*). The infection is characterized by the widespread occurrence of scaly patches which often assume a circinate or concentric arrangement. It begins with one or several small reddish macules which soon assume a papular aspect and are accompanied by itching of variable degree. The affected areas gradually enlarge until after several weeks they measure a centimeter or more in diameter. Centrally, the epidermal covering becomes cracked and broken, and the outer layers peel off, giving rise to roughly circular lesions, the margins of which are formed by upcurled lamellae. The free edges are directed toward the centers of the exfoliating areas, and the attached portions become underlaid with more or less pigmentation. Repetitions of the centrifugally moving inflammation and exfoliation result in the development of concentric rings, which coalesce so that the skin comes to present a peculiar mottled and imbricated appearance like the rings of light and dark on the surface of watered silk. The eruption may become universal and the clinical picture may be mistaken for mild ichthyosis.

The face, scalp, palms, soles and nails usually escape. In long-standing cases the scales may become thick and horny. The general health is unaffected. The chronicity of the disease is notable.

Etiology.—The fungus does not penetrate the hairs, but it occurs in great abundance in the scales. *Endodermophyton tropicale* is the usual cause and *E. concentricum*, *E. indicum* and *E. mansoni* are also causative agents. Cultural characters are given under Tinea, etiology (*q.v.*).

Diagnosis.—The disease is to be differentiated from other kinds of tinea and from ichthyosis. Examination of the scales will reveal the fungi.

Prognosis and Treatment.—Tinea imbricata responds only stubbornly even to appropriate treatment, and relapses are common. **Castellani's fuchsin paint** is fairly satisfactory:

 ℞ Saturated alcoholic solution of basic fuchsin 10.0
  5 per cent aqueous solution of phenol 100.0
  Filter, and add
  Boric acid 1.0
  Wait 2 hours, add
  Acetone 5.0
  Wait 2 hours, add
  Resorcinol 10.0

Chrysarobin ointment may be useful. **Deek's ointment** has been highly recommended:

 ℞ Salicylic acid 4.0
  Mercurial ointment 4.0
  Bismuth subnitrate 12.0
  Oil of eucalyptus 12.0
  Anhydrous wool fat .... to 100.0

This burns like fire for some minutes, but the results are so striking that the native patients, who are the ones most commonly affected, willingly submit.

TINEA VERSICOLOR

Tinea versicolor (pityriasis versicolor) is a superficial dermatomycosis due to *Malassezia furfur*. It is characterized clinically by yellowish or brownish macules, usually involving the chest and shoulders. The patients are generally adult. The disease begins with one or more small, rounded macules, which enlarge slowly by peripheral expansion and may reach a diameter of 3 cm. or more. Coalescence gives rise to the formation of large, irregular plaques. These are yellowish or brownish, their surfaces being covered with fine, perforated scales. The lesions may be confined entirely to small areas, but often the eruption is widely spread over the shoulders, back, chest, axillae and upper abdomen. The face may be involved, and so may the scalp. The surface of the patches is smooth and unmarked. Itching of moderate degree may be present. Symptoms are almost wanting as a rule.

Etiology and Pathology.—*Malassezia furfur* is a fungus of which the mycelia are comparatively short and branch frequently. It is easily detected in scrapings immersed in 10 per cent potassium hydroxide. Characteristics are given under Tinea, etiology (*q.v.*). Cultivated by Moore, the cultures are flat and dull, moist and shiny, or mucoid and stringy, and creamy to cinnamon in color, the medium becoming darkened with age. Persons with moist skins, such as sufferers from tuberculosis, seem especially liable to infection.

Diagnosis.—The color, distribution and character of the eruption, its tedious course, and the recognition of the organism in scrapings examined microscopically, serve to distinguish the disease from seborrheic dermatitis, the macular syphilid, pinta and other forms of dermatomycosis.

Tropical Tinea Versicolor, Tinea Flava, Tinea Alba and **Tinea Nigra** were described by Castellani. Tinea, or pityriasis, versicolor is characterized by its yellowish color, the comparative lack of desquamation, and chronicity. Cases in which the yellowish color is practically lacking are called tinea (pityriasis) versicolor alba. The nigra form is characterized by plaques which are dull black and lusterless. The neck and upper part of the chest are most often involved. Castellani reported his finding of *Microsporum tropicum* in the yellow variety, *Microsporum macfadyeni* from the colorless, and *Microsporum mansoni* from the black. Only the last was he able to cultivate.

Treatment.—The disorder is harmless and it responds favorably to appropriate medication. The frequent use of **soap and water,** followed each time by sponging with **saturated aqueous solution of sodium thiosulfate,** may prove curative. The skin may be swabbed with sodium thiosulfate solution and allowed to dry, then swabbed with **3 per cent tartaric acid dilution in water.** Reaction of the acid with the salt frees nascent sulfur and sulfurous acid *in situ*. Only a few applications are required to cure. **Three per cent salicylc acid** and **5 per cent precipitated sulfur** in vaseline will serve fairly satisfactorily. **Half-strength Whitfield's ointment** is useful. **Five per cent crude coal tar in lanolin and vaseline** is messy but effective. The underwear must be sterilized in order to guard against reinoculation.

ACHROMIA PARASITARIA

Depigmentation may result from superficial fungus infections of a sort resembling tinea versicolor. There appear dirty, whitish spots, slightly inflammatory at first but soon losing this aspect, becoming scaly and eventually becoming quite devoid of scales. After depigmentation has occurred, the lesions resemble those of vitiligo or syphilitic leukoderma. Familial incidence of such cases seems to indicate that the disease is infectious. Pardo-Castello has believed that this phenomenon is not a specific clinical entity but is a syndrome which may occur in any of several epidermomycoses in which the fungi disturb the normal pigmentary processes of the skin.

Pseudo-achromia Parasitica.—When cases of pityriasis versicolor and other superficial dermatomycoses are exposed to ultraviolet light, the normal skin reacts and becomes pigmented, while the skin underlying the fungus mass, which is opaque to the ultraviolet light, remains white. Later when the pityriasis has disappeared the white islands in the pigmented areas resemble leukoderma.

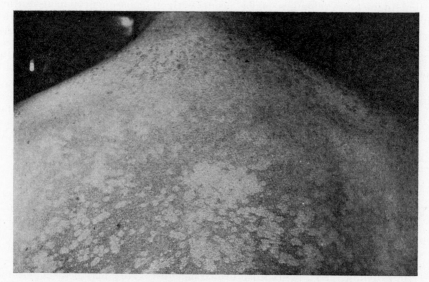

Fig. 17.—Pseudo-achromia parasitica, due to tinea versicolor. Erythema provoked by ultra-violet light therapy is seen between the lesions, in which the fungus acts as an opaque filter.

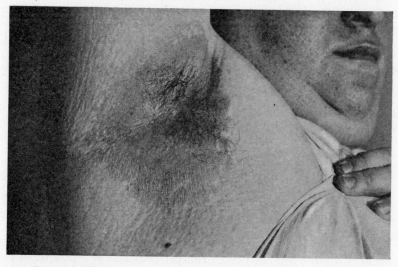

Fig. 18.—Erythrasma. (Courtesy of Dr. George Miller MacKee.)

4042

PINTA

Pinta is a common disorder of Mexico and Central America, characterized by startling pigmentary changes which occur without consequential constitutional symptoms. The cutaneous lesions have been thought to be due to the growth of fungi in the epidermis succeeded by parasitic achromia. The patches show great variability of color. First they are usually erythematous, but later they may become violaceous, yellowish, brownish or quite dark. After several years the affected areas become achromic. They then lack scaliness, are unaltered in texture and are asymptomatic. The etiology of the disorder, commonplace as it is, has been disputed. Recent investigations indicate that a spirochete similar to that of syphilis is to be blamed, for spirochetes may be demonstrated by dark-field examination in scrapings from the lesions in a high proportion of the cases, and patients' serums often give the positive Wassermann reaction. Arsenical medication is said to cure the bluish lesions, which are the lesions that begin the disease and eventuate in depigmentation. Nothing changes the achromia.

ERYTHRASMA

Microsporum (Actinomyces) minutissimum is a delicate fungus with spores and mycelia about 1 micron in diameter. It produces irregular but sharply circumscribed, reddish-brown or reddish-yellow, slowly spreading, finely scaling, dry patches of slightly pruriginous, superficial dermatitis, located usually in the axillary, genitocrural or pubic regions, rarely elsewhere. The earliest lesions are irregularly outlined, dry, reddish-brown macules. They may be orange-colored or of a pale reddish-yellow hue. The scales are fine, dry and flourlike. The patches develop and spread slowly and give rise to few subjective symptoms. In the scales one may find the numerous mycelial filaments. Cultivation is difficult but success has been claimed.

Diagnosis.—The color, size, distribution, number and course of the patches serve to distinguish them from the lesions of tinea versicolor. Pityriasis rosea and tinea cruris follow a different course and present different symptomatology, both being accompanied by well-marked signs of inflammation.

Prognosis and Treatment.—Erythrasma is fairly resistant to medication, and relapses and recurrences are common. Antiparasitic remedies are suitable, such as are used in treating tinea corporis. The axillary hair may profitably be kept shaved, and ointments applied to the hairy regions must be washed off at frequent intervals to prevent furunculosis.

OTOMYCOSIS AND MYRINGOMYCOSIS

Many fungi are capable of provoking integumentary inflammation in the external auditory canal. Itching, stinging, and impairment of hearing if the drum is involved or the canal obstructed, are the results. On the surface of the tympanum the parasites are likely to form a coating which consists of masses of mycelium with blotting paper-like consistency and bad odor. *Aspergillus fumigatus, A. niger, A. glaucus, Penicillium* and *Achorion,* as well as *Monilia, Sporothrix, Blastomyces, Actinomyces, Coccidioides* and other fungi have been found causing dermatitis of the auditory canal. Branny desquamation or moist exfoliation with oozing is seen.

Prognosis and Treatment.—The disease does not undergo spontaneous resolution. It generally responds favorably to mild antiseptics along with careful débridement. Recurrence is likely. **Ten per cent salicylic acid in 70 per cent alcohol** may be dropped into the canal. An ointment of **25 per cent calomel in vaseline** is useful. In the dry, scaly cases **silver nitrate** solution may be swabbed over the affected skin. **Metacresyl acetate** has been highly recommended: one cleans the canal and dries it with a current of warm air, then packs it with cotton moistened with this drug and leaves the pack overnight; the next day after removing the pack, the canal is washed with drops of **1 per cent thymol in 70 per cent alcohol.**

LEPOTHRIX

Lepothrix, also known as **Trichomycosis palmellina, Trichomycosis nodosa,** or **Trichomycosis axillaria** (which may be yellow, black or red), is a dermatomycosis characterized by the occurrence of firm concretions on hairs or by soft sheaths surrounding them. The axillary hair is commonly involved, and adjacent skin is often infected, so that lesions like those of erythrasma or pityriasis versicolor are seen. The disease is by no means confined to the tropics. Concretions on the hairs, yellowish or reddish in color, are composed of masses and chains of micro-organisms, embedded in a homogeneous, chitin-like substance. The hairs become brittle, and fissuring and fracture occur. The nodules in trichomycosis axillaris rubra contain red cocci distributed throughout. In the nigra type there are masses of black cocci scattered in the interstices.

Etiology.—*Actinomyces tenuis* occurs in slender mycelial filaments 0.7 micron in diameter, regular, short, not branching, nonseptate, capable of forming a resistant, hornlike glue. The colonies are small. On hairs it produces nodes which are yellow when the fungus is pure, black when it is associated with *Micrococcus nigrescens,* and red when associated with *Micrococcus castellani* (*rhodococcus*). *Actinomyces sendaiensis,* a polymorphous fungus showing coccic forms, growing in mycelial filaments with ray formation, has been isolated from cases of lepothrix. Pure cultures are black. Inoculations of human hairs have resulted in the appearance of little, isolated or confluent nodules or an adherent, gelatinous sheath, grayish or yellowish in color.

Diagnosis.—The disease is to be differentiated from the following:

Tinea nodosa, which is Beigel's trichosporosis, due to *Trichosporon beigeli.*
Nodular trichosporosis of Behrend, due to *T. ovoides* (Behrend, 1890).
Piedra, or **Trichosporosis tropicalis,** due to *T. giganteum* (Behrend, 1890).
Piedra nostras of Unna, due to *T. ovale* (Unna, 1896).
Trichosporosis of DuBois, due to *T. glycophile* (DuBois, 1910).

Treatment.—The disorder can be cured by removing the sebum by means of benzine and applying **1:1000 alcoholic solution of mercuric chloride.** The hair should be shaved. Recurrences are likely to occur.

Piedra is a disease of the hair seen in some districts of South America. It is characterized by the development of dark, nodular, pin-point to pinhead-sized, gritty masses on the shafts of the hairs of the scalp, eyelashes or beard. The concretions are believed to be due to *Trichosporon giganteum.* Perhaps several kinds of fungi can produce the symptoms. The affected hair should be sponged with benzine to remove the particles, then washed thoroughly with soap and water. **Bichloride of mercury (1: 1000)** may be used daily for several weeks as a parasiticide.

Chignon Disease.—The hairs of wigs and toupees may support the growth of fungi which produce brownish nodules like those of piedra.

Tinea Amiantacea.—This name, signifying asbestos-like tinea, is applied to a disease of the scalp in which heavy scales extend onto the hairs and separate and bind together the proximal portions. It generally appears during childhood and affects the crown of the head. It may be circumscribed or diffuse. It is chronic. It is not followed by atrophy, scarring or alopecia. Preparations examined in potassium hydroxide reveal an abundance of elements resembling fungi, but cultures and inoculations have failed. Ammoniated mercurial ointment is useful in combating the disease.

MONILIASIS

Synonyms.—Thrush; Sprue; Oidiomycosis; Mycotorulosis; Soorpilz; Erosio Interdigitale Blastomycetica (some cases); Intertrigo (some cases); La Perlèche (some cases); Saccharomycetic Dermatitis (some cases); Blastomycosis (a variety).

Monilia albicans (Zopf, 1890), identical with *Oidium albicans* (Ch. Robin, 1853), is the type species of the genus *Mycotorula* (Will, 1916) as given by

Brumpt. Colonies originate by bipolar sprouting of blastospores and the pseudomycelium is composed of ellipsoidal cells. The organism causes the development of a pellicle in liquid medium, liquefies gelatin and ferments sugar. The colonies are creamy, thick and convex. Pseudomycelium is formed by short cells typically crowned by a verticil of blastospores. The terminal cell bears a bouquet of blastospores. Verticils are numerous, simple, regularly spaced, and globular at the end.

Monilia albicans is a "yeastlike" fungus, differing from a true yeast in that a pseudomycelium is formed, whereas true yeasts reproduce by budding, and the daughter cells do not adhere to the mother cell.

This fungus, and others closely related to it, cause many different kinds of clinical manifestations, which may be localized, widespread, or scattered, acute or chronic, inflammatory or indolent, affecting the skin, its appendages, mucous membranes, and gastro-intestinal tract, singly or in combination. They are potent sensitizers, provoking eczematous sensitization as well as passively transferable antibodies.

The clinical forms of moniliasis, as listed by Lewis and Hopper (1938), are:

I. LOCALIZED

Onychia and paronychia

Intertrigo (axillary, submammary, inguinal, interdigital)

Erosio interdigitale blastomycetica (essentially a variety of intertrigo)

Perlèche (essentially a variety of intertrigo)

Intra-oral thrush

Superficial glossitis (beefy tongue)

Stomatitis

Localized patches of "eczema"

Water-bed dermatitis

Dyshidrosis

Vulvovaginitis (with or without symptoms)

Gastro-enteritis (with or without symptoms)

II. GENERALIZED

1. Widespread eruptions usually associated with some of the localized forms. Characteristic flat pustules may usually be observed in some part of the eruption. These pustules become dry, and macerated scales form on the surface. With exfoliation, a bright red, moist surface is left with overhanging edges. Sparse growth of hair may be an additional finding.

2. Moniliids (levurides) in which no fungi can be cultured and which are secondary to a focus of infection with *Monilia albicans*.

III. SYSTEMIC

Not well defined, this group includes cases of pulmonary involvement and instances of massive gastro-intestinal infection associated with cutaneous infection.

Monilial Onychomycosis.—The organisms may inhabit the nail plate, where they produce disease indistinguishable on clinical grounds from other kinds of onychomycosis (*q.v.*).

Monilial Paronychia.—This has been discussed with mycotic paronychia (*q.v.*).

Monilial Intertrigo.—Intertrigo is a clinical name applied to any superficial dermatitis occurring on opposing surfaces, characterized by redness, abrasion and maceration. Hyperhidrosis is followed by fermentation, and the skin becomes abraded and raw. The gluteal and cruro-scrotal folds, the inframammary region and the folds of the neck are common locations. Hot weather, obesity and binding garments are predisposing factors. Monilia are the organisms usually to blame, although streptococci or staphylococci may be the infecting agents. Monilial intertrigo represents biologically the result simply of luxuriation of pathogenic flora of the skin, the flora including pathogens usually because of the existence of foci of infection. Obese women are the commonest sufferers because of their monilial vaginitis, the presence of yeastlike organisms in the vagina being a common circumstance.

In prophylaxis, simple cleanliness and dryness are preventative, achieved by loose clothing, good ventilation and the use of bland dusting powder. Exertion

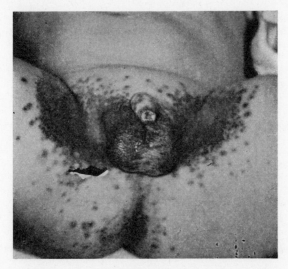

Fig. 19.—Monilial intertrigo provoking "napkin dermatitis" in a boy.

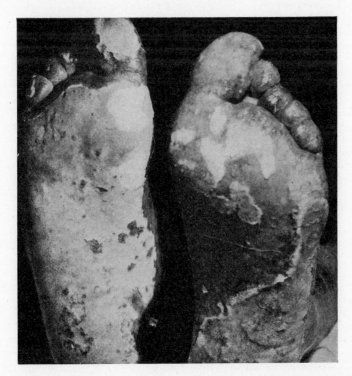

Fig. 20.—Moniliasis, unusually severe. (Courtesy of Dr. Royal Montgomery.)

in hot, moist weather almost inevitably leads to trouble, particularly in fleshy persons and fat babies. Focal infections and sources of reinfection must be controlled. Vaginal douches using **1 : 5000 potassium permanganate** and vaginal swabbings with **1 or 2 per cent aqueous solution of gentian violet** will control mycotic vulvovaginitis. Wet packs are excellent, using cool **1 : 500 aluminum acetate in water,** or **1 : 10,000 bichloride of mercury.** The parts should be dried, perhaps swabbed with **10 per cent aqueous solution of silver nitrate,** and dusted generously with **borated talc.** Often it is desirable to immerse the whole body in medicated baths, and **potassium permanganate,** 100 grains to 15 gallons of cool water, is effective. Ointment preparations meet with little success.

Monilial Stomatitis.—Oral lesions associated with *Monilia* are thrush, glossitis and perlèche.

THRUSH is manifest as superficial, adherent deposits resembling coagulated milk. The lesions bleed if the membrane is forcibly removed. The mucosae of the tongue, cheeks and pharynx are the sites of predilection. The circumoral skin may be involved. *Pityriasis alba* is the name applied to furfuraceous scaling seen about the mouth in children who have oral moniliasis or perhaps perlèche. The disease affects infants and sometimes adults, particularly pellagrins and other debilitated individuals who cannot keep their mouths clean. Epidemics may occur, the organism being transferred by carriers and by unclean utensils. The parasite is readily demonstrated among the epithelial cells scraped from a lesion.

GLOSSITIS associated with *Monilia* occurs in sprue, pellagra and other avitaminoses. Hyperemia of the fungiform papillae and aphthous ulcers occur, along with increased sensitiveness to hot fluids, spices and tobacco smoke. In chronic cases there follows atrophy of the papillae so that the tongue is smooth and red, particularly along the sides. An important relationship certainly exists between dietary deficiency and susceptibility to infection. The stomatitis of pellagra responds promptly and satisfactorily to treatment of the pellagra with nicotinic acid.

PERLÈCHE is an intertriginous inflammation of the labial commissures. It is usually bilateral. The mucosa is thickened and somewhat macerated. The lesions extend a short distance onto the skin and onto the mucous membranes. In severe cases there are deep wrinkles and sore, transverse fissures which cause considerable discomfort when the mouth is open widely. The lesions must be distinguished from the mucous patches and split papules of syphilis. When secondary syphilis affects the mouth, there are always concomitant signs of widespread syphilitic disease. Perlèche seems to be transferable. It has occurred in many individuals in one community, such as an orphanage. Since Sebrell (1938) showed that women on a pellagra-producing diet developed perlèche-like lesions, it is possible that the epidemics have been due rather to food deficiencies affecting a group of individuals than to transference of the disease by contagion. The lack of riboflavine has been known to cause perlèche-like lesions. The disease is treated by the use of **mild astringent mouthwashes,** which may advantageously contain myrrh or sodium perborate. Attention should be given to the **diet,** for it must be **adequate in vitamin B content.** In adults the dentures must be kept meticulously clean with nonirritating chemicals. The lesions themselves may be painted with **10 per cent aqueous solution of silver nitrate,** and a layer of vaseline may be applied at night to protect the fissures from the moisture of drooling while asleep.

Monilial stomatitis in whatever form it appears is responsive to the use of **2 per cent aqueous solution of gentian violet,** a nontoxic but unsightly dye which may be used safely even in the mouths of infants.

Monilial Interdigital Dermatitis.—"Erosio interdigitale blastomycetica" was one name early given this condition when the organisms seen in smears were misinterpreted as nonmycelial and were considered blastomyces. The disorder involves one or both hands and usually appears on the web between the middle and ring fingers. Women, especially laundresses, are particularly susceptible to the disorder. The lesions are superficial, inflammatory and sharply defined, and have slightly undermined, macerated borders, beneath which yeastlike organisms can be found and cultivated. Extension over the dorsum of the hand and up the forearm is not rare. The cases are resistant to treatment, but **dryness, débridement,** and **repeated applications of alcoholic solution of gentian violet** will usually succeed.

Monilial Vulvovaginitis; Pruritus Ani et Vulvae; Vulvovaginitis and Infantile Eczema; Vagina as Focus of Mycotic Infection.—Pruritus ani and pruritus vulvae are often due to *Monilia* (or to other fungi, such as *Epidermophyton*) and the infection is likely to be complicated by medicinal and traumatic irritation. Diabetes promotes pruritus because dextrin encourages the growth of mycotic organisms. Monilial vaginitis is a common cause of pruritus even in women who do not have diabetes. Monilial infestation of the vagina is commonplace and frequently asymptomatic. It occurs in children, virgins, and senile women as well as parous ones. The disease may undergo spontaneous cure, or it may become chronic with exacerbations at times over a period of months or years. Menstruation has the same temporary beneficial effect on the course of the infection as delivery does in cases associated with pregnancy. Infantile oral thrush may result from infection in the birth canal.

The following types of moniliasis are seen:

1. Creamy vaginitis resembling oral thrush, with painful and reddened mucosa.

2. Creamy vulvitis, with considerable discharge, not much redness or inflammation, with or without a small amount of intertrigo, which characteristically consists of small, grouped, shallow vesicopustules.

3. Ulcerative vulvitis, severe, superficially ulcerated, with pain, lymphangitis and inguinal adenitis, possibly with mycotic infection of the bladder.

4. Pseudoleukoplakic vulvitis, in which the mucosa is whitish and opaque and the crusts are hard to remove, but no wrinkling, papillomas or hyperkeratosis exists.

5. Eczematoid vulvitis, with a vesicopustular eruption consisting of small punctiform erosions, spreading and resembling intertrigo.

6. Mycotic pruritus of the vulva, with few erosions, perhaps, and little discharge, diagnosable only by smear and culture.

7. Vesiculopustular cutaneous form, manifesting disseminated involvement principally of external teguments with groups of small vesicopustules, the vesicular stage being brief.

8. Cutaneous intertriginous eczematous form, which is intertrigo-like, with or without demonstrable organisms in the genitocrural plica, the inflammation spreading to the pubis, anal region and medial surfaces of the thighs, with but little visible involvement of the vulva.

9. Inconspicuous vaginitis with disseminated cutaneous involvement in the form of patches of intertriginous dermatitis with small vesicopustules, not amenable to lasting therapeutic effects until the vaginal infestation has been treated properly.

10. Moniliids, often consisting of pompholyx-like patches of tiny, deep-seated vesicles, which may absorb and result in superficial scaling or which may constitute an inflamed and oozing eczematous dermatitis, and which depend solely on vulvovaginitis.

We have seen forms in the male analogous to the types 4, 5, 6, 7 and 8 (excepting the creamy discharge, which is pus plus mucus from the cervical glands) involving the inguinal, pudendal and perianal regions. They respond to similar treatment.

"Infantile eczema," synonymous with infantile dermatitis, is dermatitis resulting from any of several different possible causes. Contact dermatitis in the infant is inconsequentially different from that in the adult. Streptococcic and staphylococcic parasitism of the infant's skin is different mainly because of the comparative flatness of dermal papillae which bind down the epidermis. Infantile dermatomycosis is usually monilial. In the cases of "infantile eczema," so-called, in which there occur deep red, circular and oval, circumscribed but coalescing patches of oozing, itchy dermatitis, the infection is likely to be monilial, and it may have originated in the birth canal. We have treated infantile mycotic dermatitis with great benefit by the widespread application of **2 per cent aqueous solution of gentian violet,** for this drug is efficient, nonirritating and nontoxic. Asymptomatic monilial vaginitis in pregnant women—and it is far more common in pregnancy than at any other time—certainly ought to be treated before parturition. Oral and vaginal monilial organisms are of equal pathogenicity, and they are probably racially but not specifically different from *Monilia albicans.*

Penile infections as well as vaginal are known. They are curable with circumcision and cleanliness unless they are maintained by urethritis or cystitis of mycotic origin, a disease which probably occurs more commonly than it is diagnosed.

DIAGNOSIS OF MONILIAL VULVOVAGINITIS.—The exudate is acidic. Smears show budding yeasts. Mycelia appear in the smears at times of maximum severity of clinical symptoms. After wiping an applicator over the mucosa, one may stir it in 3 cc. of normal saline solution, then examine a drop of this on a slide. Streak Sabouraud's medium to confirm.

Monilial Systemic and Generalized Cutaneous Infection.—Generalized cases are comparatively rare. In these chronic infections, the face, ears, neck, upper chest and mouth are usually involved, and thick, dry, brownish crusts occur on the skin. The majority of such cases, complicated by monilial pneumonitis and gastro-intestinal infection, eventuate fatally. The lesions are dry with a tendency to crust and scale. The patient complains of little itching except when the interdigital spaces are involved. At no time is severe inflammatory reaction present. The condition is afebrile. Massive formation of mycelia and spores can be demonstrated in the lesions. Schultz is aptly quoted as to the "formidable nature of the disorder when it becomes generalized and the remarkable ineffectiveness of any form of treatment."

Moniliids.—These allergic eruptions occurring specifically in moniliasis are the counterparts of trichophytids (*q.v.*). As a rule they consist of tiny, closely aggregated, intra-epidermal vesicles, and they may be set upon a more or less inflamed base, located on the hands, legs or flexures. They may depend on foci in the nails, glabrous skin, tonsils, mouth, vagina, auditory canal or gastro-intestinal tract. It is commonplace to cure pompholyx of the hands by treating tinea of the feet when pompholyx is a trichophytid. We have cured repetitious, pompholyx-like eruptions of the hands by means of douches of **1 : 3000 potassium permanganate** and the application of **gentian violet** to the genitalia, without treating the hands themselves.

Immunology, Skin Tests and Vaccinal Therapy in Moniliasis.—The humoral and tissular reactions to *Monilia* are analogous with those to *Trichophyton*. *Monilia* are potent sensitizers. Treatment by vaccinal hyposensitization has basis in theory, but, in practice, attacks upon the foci of the organisms by means of antiseptics and débridement afford better effect. *Trichophyton* and *Monilia* are immunologically distinct. Skin tests with monilial extracts may be interpreted much as trichophytin tests are. We find them of little practical value.

Etiology.—Infection with monilia, like all infections, depends both upon the soil and the organism. In food deficiencies, particularly avitaminosis B, and in diabetes the individual is more vulnerable. Environmental circumstances may favor or inhibit the growth of the organisms, and moisture, warmth and darkness, as in tinea, enhance the activity of *Monilia*.

Treatment.—To be comprehensive and permanently effective, treatment must be directed at the **eradication of all foci,** both in the skin and elsewhere. Unfortunately, therapy directed at the gastro-intestinal tract is not effective. The accessible parasitized tissues should be kept dry, and ointments have little to commend them, for they allow a film of sweat or ooze to collect, protected from evaporation. **Gentian violet** has been used for many years and it is one of the most effective parasiticides. Baths in **1 : 8000 bichloride of mercury** are useful in altering the flora of the entire body. Douches of **1 : 5000 potassium permanganate** are fairly satisfactory; **bichloride of mercury must not be used** for this purpose. **Cool, moist packs** for 15 to 30 minutes, alternated with drying in a current of air under the influence of **radiant heat,** are effective. Roentgen therapy offers temporary alleviation of inflammation, but it must not be repeated beyond the limit of tolerance, and of itself it is not curative. In paronychia, **5 per cent chrysarobin** in chloroform is a useful paint. In onychomycosis, **débridement, silver nitrate,** and **roentgen therapy** may be used. In stomatitis, cleanliness is an important prophylactic measure. Fingers should not be put into babies' mouths. **Gentian violet** has an important place. **Sodium perborate** may be used both for tooth powder and for mouthwash. The generalized cases tax every resource of the specialist and generally turn out badly after all.

CRYPTOCOCCOSIS

Brownish, dirty-looking patches of dermatitis, unresponsive to soap and water, have been described as being due to yeastlike organisms. Similar organisms have been found in flexural dermatitis and in the scaling and crusting cutaneous lesions of "seborrheic eczema," local or widespread. Cryptococci are simple fungi consisting of globular cells which reproduce by budding. They do not produce mycelium and are thus distinguished from *Monilia.* Clinically the lesions are much like those of moniliasis, from which they are distinguished mainly by botanical studies. They respond to similar treatment.

SEBORRHEIC DERMATITIS

Seborrheic dermatitis is an acute or subacute inflammatory dermatosis which usually begins on the scalp and is characterized by the occurrence of rounded, irregular or circinate lesions covered with yellowish greasy scales. **Pityriasis capitis,** ordinarily called **dandruff,** is the commonest form of the disease. Since this is probably due to *Pityrosporum ovale,* this disease is described with the mycoses.

The lesions may be dry, with a considerable or abundant amount of grayish, branny scales, or they may be oozing and crusted, constituting the "eczema capitis" of older writers. Superinfection accounts for the weeping, however, it is thought; and streptococci and staphylococci commonly complicate seborrheic dermatitis. From the scalp the disease often spreads to the forehead, brows, nose and cheeks, so constituting the "dry skin" of cosmeticians. Psoriasiform patches may occur in the axillae, over the sternum, about the umbilicus and in the crural folds. It is likely that many different but related fungi produce similar clinical syndromes. The margins of the eyelids are involved in many cases and blepharitis may be severe even though the scalp disease is comparatively inconspicuous.

Alopecia probably does not result from dandruff, although in alopecia accompanied by dandruff it is certain that treatment directed against the seborrheic dermatitis will do no harm.

Streptococci may produce scaling, intertrigo and postauricular fissuring, distinguished only with difficulty from seborrheic dermatitis.

Acne vulgaris is usually complicated by pityriasis capitis and pityriasis of the face. This is probably due to the fact that *Pityrosporum ovale* is a lipophile fungus and finds the oily skin of the acne patient a ground where it can luxuriate.

Etiology.—Excessively oily food, particularly milk, cream, butter, chocolate and cod liver oil, is a predisposing factor, and hypothyroidism is also.

Sabouraud reported the following bacteriologic findings:

in pityriasis (simplex) sicca, *P. ovale* is plentiful;

in pityriasis (simplex) oleosa, *P. ovale* is present, and may or may not be accompanied by *Staphylococcus albus;*

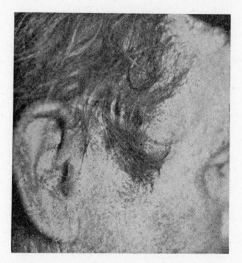

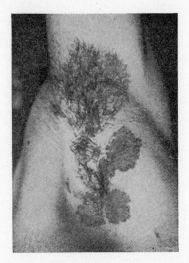

FIG. 21.—Seborrheic dermatitis of scalp and face.

FIG. 22.—Seborrheic dermatitis of axilla.

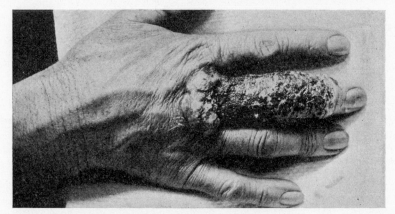

FIG. 23.—Blastomycosis involving the finger. (Courtesy of Dr. Otto L. Castle.)

in seborrhea oleosa, *P. ovale* and staphylococci are present, along with the microbacillus if the hair is falling, but without it if the hair is healthy;

in pityriasis circinate (seborrheic dermatitis), *P. ovale* is usually present, and hair loss is not a feature.

Pityrosporum ovale may be as profuse in scalps of normal appearance as in cases of severe dandruff, according to MacKee and Lewis.

Pityrosporum can be seen in teased potassium hydroxide preparations or stained scales. Most of the cells are ovoid or spherical, with or without budding, being from 2 to 4 microns in long axis, sometimes larger. Moore cultivated the organism from scales on Difco wort agar, the first growth being small, grayish-white colonies which when transplanted to a thicker part of the medium developed into cultures of ocherous salmon to pinkish-buff color.

Whether this agent is or is not the actual causative one, the practitioner can cure seborrheic dermatitis if he treats the scalp as if it were suffering from a form of parasitism to which immunity does not develop and which is almost universally distributed among human beings.

Dermatitis venenata, particularly if it involves the neck or face, and is of long duration, is readily complicated by seborrheic dermatitis. The combination resembles so-called lichenified eczema. It may be cured by first allowing the moiety of the dermatitis which is due to chemical irritation to heal by using bland, soothing applications and avoiding all irritating contacts, then one may use crude coal tar or some other suitable antiparasitic remedy for the remaining parasitic irritation. By interpreting many of our otherwise obscure cases of "eczema" in this manner, we are able to cure patients nowadays who were at one time seemingly insurmountable therapeutic problems.

Treatment.—It may be advisable to put the patient on a **low fat diet,** omitting particularly milk, cream, butter, ice cream, chocolate, cocoa, cod liver oil, pork, shortened foods and canned fish. For the scalp a valuable prescription is:

  ℞   Phenol .... ♏x
    Mercuric chloride .... gr.i
    Euresol (resorcinol monoacetate) .... ℨii
    Spirits of formic acid .... ℨiv
    Alcohol (70%) .... to ℨviii

  Sig.: Rub into scalp several nights a week as directed, particularly after each shampooing. Shampoo every 10 to 14 days. Use no brush because it cannot be sterilized satisfactorily. Use a cheap new comb after each shampoo to avoid reinfection.

An ointment to be rubbed into the scalp is messier than the liquid, but is sometimes more effective:

  ℞   Salicylic acid .... gr.xv
    Ammoniated mercury (or precipitated sulfur).. gr.xxx
    Rose water ointment .... ℥i

  Sig.: Rub in thoroughly one evening a week; shampoo the next morning with ordinary soap.

On the body in widespread cases complicating dermatitis venenata, an ointment rarely irritating, particularly useful in hospitalized patients, is:

  ℞   Crude coal tar .... ℨi
    Lanolin sufficient to mix
    White Vaseline .... to ℨi

  Sig.: 6% crude coal tar. Rub in twice a day for 3 days.

This peels off the seborrheic dermatitis much as chrysarobin peels off the lesions of psoriasis, but it does it more gently. Roentgen therapy has nothing to recommend it.

TORULOSIS

Torulae are yeastlike plants distinguished from higher yeasts in that they form neither endospores nor mycelia, and from *Saccharomyces* in that torulae

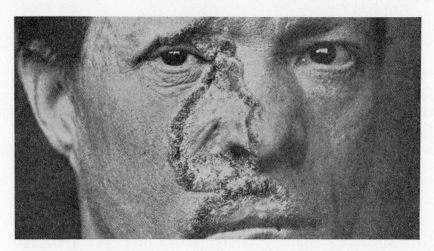

FIG. 24.—Blastomycosis. (Courtesy of Dr. Grover Wende.)

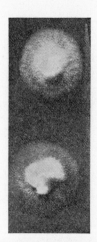

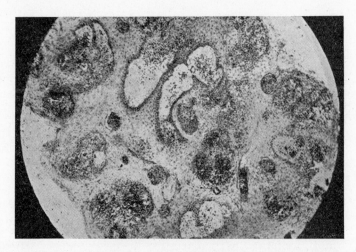

FIG. 25.—Blastomyces, 10-day culture, showing characteristic peripheral zone such as few other fungi produce. (Courtesy of Dr. Fred Weidman.)

FIG. 26.—Blastomycosis. Photomicrograph shows typical abscesses and inflamed papillae surrounded by pseudo-epitheliomatous hyperplasia of the epidermis. (Courtesy of Dr. F. W. Shaw.)

TABLE I

DISEASE	FUNGUS	CLINICAL CHARACTERISTICS	FUNGUS IN TISSUE OR PUS	CULTURE, GROSS	CULTURE, MICROSCOPIC
Coccidioidal granuloma (Posadas' disease, 1892) (Rixford and Gilchrist, 1894)	Coccidioides immitis	Infectious granuloma, acute, subacute or chronic. Protean, with cutaneous, subcutaneous, or systemic lesions, involving generally the respiratory system; lesions may be nodular, ulcerative, verrucoid, gummatous, or cold-abscess-like	Cells isolated or in giant cells; spherical, thick-walled with a reported diameter of approximately 2–80μ; reproduces by endospore formation (ascus); budding absent; wall of ascus often showing radiate formation	Colonies flat, somewhat submerged, grayish, becoming white to light cream, with aerial hyphae; cottony, at times coremioid; color changes to light chamois and to smoky brown with age; growth rapid	Hyphae septate, branching, 0.5–4μ in diameter; hyphal swellings, arthrosporous cells 2.5–7μ in diameter, 5–12μ in long axis; chlamydospores abundant, 5–8μ in diameter; racquet mycelium; terminal hyphospores approximately 5 × 8μ; anaerobic endogenous spore formation
North American blastomycosis (Gilchrist's disease, 1894)	Zymonema dermatitidis, Zymonema capsulatum, Zymonema capsulatum var. isabellinum	Infectious condition often granulomatous, acute to chronic. Protean, with eutaneous or systemic lesions. Cutaneous lesions primary or secondary, papulo-ulcerative, verrucous or papillomatous, gummatous, typically violaceous in color	Simple or budding yeastlike cells, thick-walled, 5–20μ in diameter; usually approximately 7μ	Colonies at first yeastlike, then coremioid, finally profuse and cottony, changing from white to chamois to cinnamon to brown; show radiating ridges and concentric rings of growth; Z. capsulatum remains white, and var. isabellinum is light chamois; growth rapid	Hyphae septate, branching, 2–4μ in diameter; conidia pyriform or round, pedicellate or sessile, 5μ in diameter; racquet mycelium, 5–6 × 3.5μ; chlamydospores terminal or lateral, 5.5–7.5 × 12–15μ or spherical, 7μ in diameter; ascogenous cells spherical, 8–13μ in diameter
European blastomycosis (Busse-Buschke's disease, 1894)	Cryptococcus hominis, Atelosaccharomyces hominis (Torulopsis neoformans)	Similar to Gilchrist's disease but ulcerative type common in cutaneous form, with abscesses, little inflammation; usually found invading cerebrospinal system	Thick-walled, heavily encapsulated, simple or budding cells approximately 5–10μ in diameter, occasionally larger, usually approximately 8μ	Colonies yeasty or pasty, smooth, mucoid to moist, subpulvinate; color light cream, becoming light tan to brown with age; growth fair	Spherical to ovoid budding, encapsulated cells approximately 2–6μ in diameter, rarely larger; no mycelium, pseudomycelium or spores
South American blastomycosis Paracoccidioidal granuloma (Lutz-Splendore-de Almeida disease, 1908) A. Generalized type B. Localized type affecting the buccal mucosa	(a) Paracoccidioides brasiliensis (b) Paracoccidioides tenuis (c) Paracoccidioides cerebriformis	A. Generalized or localized, cutaneous or systemic, granulomatous, papulous, verrucous or ulcerative; acute to chronic; usually lymphangitic in spread B. Lesions localized on buccal mucosa; acute to chronic; verrucous, papillomatous, ulcerative, granulomatous; lymphangitic spread only in terminal stage	(a) and (b) Cells spherical or ovoid, 1–30μ in diameter, rarely larger, with thick walls; simple or multiple budding of minute, spherical, ovoid or bacillary gemmules, of approximately 1μ and larger (c) Cells spherical or ovoid, 3–30μ in diameter, rarely larger, but uniformly larger than those of P. brasiliensis or P. tenuis; thick-walled, with simple or multiple budding of small, spherical, ovoid or elongated gemmules of approximately 3μ or over; cells often found in giant macrophages (pseudococcidioides)	(a) White, adherent to substratum and somewhat hard, well-defined, and somewhat cottony; colonies become light tan with age; growth slow (b) Mycelium mostly submerged; colonies compact, verrucoid or vermiculate at inoculation, showing folds or radiating ridges; white, becoming light tan with age; growth slow (c) On agar, cerebriform to vermiculate, yeastlike, creamy buff, becoming light cinnamon-buff with age; easily separated from substratum, but filamentous, flat and adherent to dry portions of substratum; growth slow	(a) Hyphae septate, branching, 1.5–3.5μ; hyphal swellings 3–9μ; spherical, terminal chlamydospores up to 15μ; intercalary chlamydospores 6–10μ; irregular sclerotic, intercalary cells 7 × 15μ; conidia lateral, sessile or pedicellate, 3–7μ (b) Same as P. brasiliensis, except that corresponding structures are smaller (c) Hyphae irregular, septate, branching, 2–7μ in diameter, with many swellings; cells arthrosporous, oidioid, dumbbell-shaped; chlamydospores spherical, elongate, pyriform or sclerotic, intercalary, lateral or terminal, up to 15μ; conidia lateral, spherical or pyriform, 3–10μ

4042

are pathogenic and do not characteristically ferment sugar. Rarely these organisms produce superficial lesions, but they do not ordinarily invade the skin. Cutaneous cases have not been uniform in their clinical manifestations. There have been described acneform lesions of the forehead, furunculoid lesions of the thighs associated with broad patches of induration of the thigh and popliteal tissues, gummas of the abdomen with hard, purplish nodules of the cheeks, swellings on the forehead, neck, and over the tibia, a granuloma confined to the foot, a mycetoma-like lesion of the foot. Diagnosis depends on identification of the causative fungus. Torulae cause fatal tuberculoid meningitis or encephalitis. They are as often associated with Hodgkin's disease as tuberculosis is. Treatment is unsatisfactory, although roentgen therapy, iodides and gentian violet may be tried, and excision may be performed if feasible.

THE BLASTOMYCOSES

The blastomycoses are chronic infectious diseases due to budding fungi, which commonly attack the skin, giving rise to reddish or purplish, moist, papillomatous lesions, and which frequently invade one or more of the internal organs or subcutaneous tissues, giving rise to granulomatous tumors. Blastomycosis is a general name for infection with any blastomycetic fungus, that is, with any organism which buds. Included are coccidioidal. granuloma due to *Coccidioides immitis*, North American blastomycosis due to *Zymonema dermatitidis* or *Z. capsulatum*, European blastomycosis due to *Cryptococcus hominis*, South American blastomycosis due to *Paracoccidioides brasiliensis*, *Paracoccidioidal* granuloma due to *Paracoccidioides tenuis* and Almeida's disease due to *Paracoccidioides cerebriformis*. Table I, for which we are indebted to Dr. Morris Moore (*Arch. Dermat. & Syph.*, 38: 163, 1938), is informative.

BLASTOMYCOSIS OF GILCHRIST.—Infection with *Zymonema dermatitidis* or with *Z. capsulatum* begins as a rule on some exposed surface, the hands, face and ears being favorite sites. The earliest recognizable lesion is a pinhead- to pea-sized papule or papulopustule which gradually enlarges either by peripheral extension or by the development of new foci until it has attained a diameter of from 1 to 20 cm. Crusting is present almost from the beginning. When the covering is detached, the underlying lesion is found to consist of reddish or purplish, irregular, papillomatous tumors bathed in seropurulent fluid. Usually the subcutaneous cavities are small in size, but sometimes carbunculoid abscesses develop in deep structures. The patches tend to extend peripherally and to heal in the center with the formation of whitish, atrophic scars like those of lupus vulgaris. The disease often involves only the skin, where it may be limited to one or more circumscribed areas. Sometimes it becomes systemic. Both cutaneous and systemic types of blastomycosis are described. The cutaneous forms may be primary when it begins in the epidermis, but it may also be secondary by extension from infection of deeper tissues, the viscera or bony structures. In systemic infections, death usually ensues within a few weeks or months. In localized forms there may be some itching and burning and rarely pain of variable degree. As a rule the symptoms are comparatively trifling.

Etiology.—The infection usually gains entrance at the site of a wound. For diagnosis pus from the micro-abscesses can be transferred to water on a slide (not potassium hydroxide solution), and the fungi may be seen as double-contoured, refractile bodies, many of which are ascogenous and contain granular, shining, sporelike bodies. In sections of tissues, methylene blue and orange tannin are the best dyes for staining the organism. Budding is seen in the tissues, but in cultures where circumstances favor growth the blastomyces luxuriate with a rich mycelium. Beerwort and glycerin, and glucose and agar, are the best mediums. The diasease has been reproduced experimentally in animals, and in monkeys its course has taken the form of development of nodules, involvement of lymph glands, dissemination and eventually death. The organism is pathogenic for mice, rabbits and guinea pigs. Meningitis and dermatitis may be caused by *Zymonema capsulatum*.

Pathology.—Histologically the striking changes occur in the papillary layer of the corium, which is extremely hyperplastic. Freely growing epithelium surrounds the inflamed and enlarged papillae so as to simulate the irregularly sized and shaped epidermal growths of carcinoma. The masses of epithelium in plane sections thus seem to contain miliary abscesses, which are made up of leukocytes, detached epithelial cells, epithelial detritus, red blood corpuscles, blastomyces and giant cells. The basal columnar layer of the epidermis is always preserved, a distinction from carcinoma. Subacute and acute inflammation is present in the corium, and miliary abscesses occur here also. Organisms are found both in the abscesses and in the giant cells.

Diagnosis.—Blastomycosis must be distinguished from tuberculosis of the skin, sporotrichosis, vegetating syphilids, and drug eruptions such as those due to bromides. Similarity to tuberculosis verrucosa cutis may be so close as to require cultural methods for differentiation. A complement fixation test has been devised, using a saline suspension of the organisms as antigen.

Prognosis.—Most of the localized cases do not endanger life, and respond fairly promptly to appropriate treatment. Scarring usually results. The possibility of systemic dissemination is always present and systemic infections are serious. In late stages no therapy avails.

Treatment.—Internally **potassium iodide** in large doses has been recommended. Locally the **x-rays** are particularly useful. The papillomatous lesions may be cleansed by a spray of **hydrogen peroxide** followed by the application of **hexylresorcinol** or **saturated aqueous solution of gentian violet**. **Tincture of iodine** is considered one of the best parasiticides. Destructive agents may be applied to the vegetation, and deep refrigeration with **solid carbon dioxide** or **electrocoagulation** may be used. In systemic cases the state of allergy or immunity importantly influences treatment, for iodides may provoke spreading of the disease rather than cure, particularly if the patient is allergic to his parasites. Sometimes hyposensitization by vaccine followed by iodide therapy may work. Thymol in doses as large as can be tolerated offers a possible recourse.

EUROPEAN BLASTOMYCOSIS.—*Cryptococcus hominis* infected the classic patient of Busse, who was a woman suffering from localized subperiosteal inflammation of the tibia. The abscess opened spontaneously, and the organism was found intracellularly and extracellularly in the pus and in the wall of the abscess. Superficial ulcers developed later on her face, and subperiosteal swellings appeared elsewhere. Death ensued. The same organism has been found in ulcerative cutaneous lesions and abscesses. Diagnosis depends on its identification.

COCCIDIOIDAL GRANULOMA; DERMATITIS COCCIDIOIDES; "VALLEY FEVER."—Infection with *Coccidioides immitis* apparently is commonly acquired through the respiratory tract. Cutaneous lesions may be primary, but often they follow internal infections. The disease may lead to death within a few weeks or after several years, but it is probable that the majority of infected individuals recover.

Clinical types have been described: (1) primary cutaneous infection followed by generalization; (2) primary pulmonary infection, followed by generalization without skin involvement; and (3) primary pulmonary infection and secondary subcutaneous involvement. Additionally, primary nasopharyngeal, pelvic, meningeal and osseous diseases have been described.

Acute infection may be manifested by symptoms of acute respiratory infection, often accompanied by erythema nodosum, from which most patients recover without complications. In miliary coccidioidal granuloma the lesions are found preferentially located on the head, neck, shoulders and upper extremities. They are verrucose and papillomatous. They involve mainly the skin and occasionally the mucosae. Fever is usual and visceral involvement follows. The organisms are easily demonstrated. Prognosis is poor.

In chronic coccidioidal granuloma, typically affected are the sternoclavicular

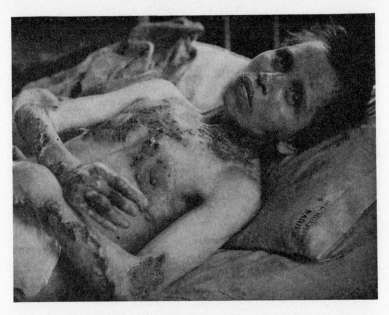

FIG. 27.—Coccidioidal granuloma with widespread cutaneous lesions. (Courtesy of Dr. William Allen Pusey.)

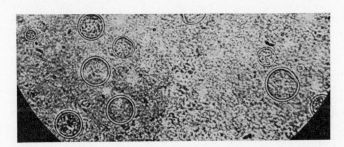

FIG. 28.—*Coccidioides immitis*, in pus. These organisms, much larger than those of *Zymonema*, are readily seen under low magnification. (Courtesy of Dr. Fred Weidman.)

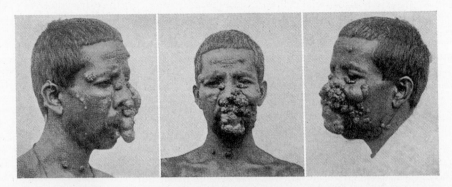

FIG. 29.—Rhinosporidiosis. Mucosal fungations and cutaneous implants in an Indian. (Courtesy of Dr. F. Allen and Dr. M. L. Dave, and the Indian Medical Gazette, 77: 376, 1936.)

joints, the sides of the feet, the neck and the inguinal regions. The lesions are granulomatous abscesses. The connective tissues of deep structures are mainly involved and the mucosae are affected only rarely. The course is slow, with remissions and relapses. Fever is low or absent. The viscera are involved to a lesser extent, the organisms are more difficult to demonstrate, and the outlook is better than in the miliary type of case.

Valley Fever (Desert Fever; California Disease), occurring in the San Joaquin Valley, is acute coccidioidal infection, as Dickson has shown. Some nine days after exposure there appear symptoms of pulmonary involvement, and lesions of erythema nodosum follow. The preliminary illness, resembling a severe cold or bronchopneumonia, is caused by inhalation of the chlamydospores.

Pathology.—The structure of coccidioidal granuloma is that of the infectious granulomas, the causative organisms being found generally within the giant cells of the exudate. They multiply by endogenous formation of spores and do not bud. In the pus they are doubly contoured spheres 5 to 60 microns in diameter with granular protoplasm. They grow on dextrose agar.

Treatment.—Potassium iodide has little effect on the course of the disease. **Antimony** and **potassium tartrate** and **roentgen therapy** have been used with benefit. Coccidioidin, a vaccinal preparation, may perhaps have value. **Gentian violet** has given good effect, both for local injection into the lesion and for topical applications. **Incision and drainage should not be performed.** Thymol, given in doses as great as 6 grams daily, has helped a patient. Sulfanilamide has been recommended.

SOUTH AMERICAN BLASTOMYCOSIS (PARACOCCIDIOIDAL GRANULOMA).— Paracoccidioidal granuloma may be divided into two main groups: (1) the generalized form due to *Paracoccidioides brasiliensis* or to *P. tenuis;* and (2) the localized type affecting the buccal mucosa, due to *P. cerebriformis.* The generalized disease may be acute or chronic. The fungus may enter the buccal tissues by way of the mouth, lodging usually in the gums and forming a hard infiltration which spreads to the lips, nose, and margin of the tongue. The lesions are granulomas. Papillary vegetations may develop on the tonsils and gingivae, giving the appearance of acuminate condyloma. Ulcerative processes may spread to the skin, producing papillary and vegetative lesions on the body. Affecting the skin primarily, a lesion may develop upon an abrasion where the fungi have become lodged. In many cases of chronic paracoccidioidal blastomycosis, the lesions are restricted to the mouth. The germ may penetrate the tonsils and become generalized by way of the lymphatic system. In cases due to *P. cerebriformis* this happens only in the terminal stage. Lymphadenopathy is seen, a difference from Gilchrist's blastomycosis, chromomycosis and verrucose tuberculosis. Diagnosis depends on identification of the causative fungus, but this is difficult to secure in primary culture. *P. brasiliensis* grows slowly, its colonies are dark brown or black, compact, and highly heaped up, and it discolors the underlying medium brown.

CHROMOMYCOSIS is a parasitic dermatosis of polymorphous aspect, with a primarily papular, nodular or verrucose eruption which may progress with ulceration, vegetation and hyperkeratosis. Verrucosities may be isolated or confluent, and may invade the whole foot or leg or other parts of the body. The lymph nodes are not involved. The course is prolonged. Histologically the lesions resemble blastomycosis. There are hyperplasia of the epidermis, papillomatosis of the dermis, and numerous small abscesses. Both free and phagocytized, brownish, ovoid organisms are found in the pus.

Hormodendron pedrosoi, Phialophora verrucosa and *Hormiscium dermatitidis* are among the known causative fungi. Cure is generally obtained by the use of **roentgen or cautery destruction** of the lesions, **débridement** and **antiparasitic topical applications.**

DERMATITIS VEGETANS is an old clinical name for any vegetating, inflammatory dermatosis characterized by the development of exuberantly granulating

plaques, which may range greatly in size and distribution.   Generally they have
developed on oozing, eczematous patches.   The vegetations are deep red in color,
bleed readily, and are crusted and malodorous.   Many such cases have been
blastomycetic dermatitis of various fungus causation, and some have perhaps
been bromide or iodide eruptions.   "Dermatitis vegetans" is a morphologic, not
an etiologic, diagnosis.

RHINOSPORIDIOSIS.—*Rhinosporidium seeberi* is a phycomycetic parasite
occurring in the form of spherules of various dimensions within the polypoid
masses which its presence elicits.   Young cysts some 6 microns in diameter have a
chitinoid envelope, a vacuolar cytoplasm and vesicular nucleus.   Old cysts reach
a diameter of 300 microns and have a cellulose-like envelope enclosing numerous
singly nucleated spores within a mucinous brown ground-substance.   Primarily
affecting the mucous membranes usually of the nose and sometimes of the conjunctivae, the lesions are pedunculated or sessile, strawberry-like or raspberry-
like tumors consisting of tightly packed tendrils suggestive of filiform verrucae.
All seven cases in the United States described through 1938 have been nasal.
Cutaneous lesions, solitary or multiple, are usually the result of inoculation from
foci located elsewhere.   Skin lesions seen in India have been fungating, malodorous tumors which bled readily.   Treatment consists in removal of the tumors
by **excision** and **caustics.**

THE MYCETOMAS

Mycetomas are granulomatous mycotic lesions enclosing fungus grains of
various shapes.   The grains are formed by felted mycelium, and they are discharged through more or less extensive fistulas.   In contrast with the tineas,
which in general produce only superficial disease, the mycetomas are due to other
fungi which produce deeply seated granulomatous inflammation.   They gain
access into the human body through injuries as a rule, and the foot is particularly vulnerable.   **Madura foot** is a clinical entity capable of being caused
by various organisms.   A typical mycetoma, it is characterized by swelling and
gradual disintegration of the subcutaneous structures and the formation of
sinuses which open onto the surface of the skin.

MADUROMYCOSES.—These mycetomas are characterized by grains formed by
voluminous, *septate,* mycelial filaments, possessing definite cross walls and forming chlamydospores.   Maduromycoses may be classed according to the color of
the fungus grains:

MADUROMYCOSIS.   Etiologic Classification According to Brumpt (1936).

Black Grain Type

ALEUROSPORIA
- *Glenospora semoni* (Chalmers and Archibald, 1917), India.
- *G. khartoumensis* (Chalmers and Archibald, 1916), Africa.
- *G. clapieri* (Catanei, 1917), Africa.
- *G. gammeli* (Pollacci and Nannizzi, 1927), North America.
- *Scedosporium sclerotiale* (Pepere, 1914), Europe.

PHIALIDES
- *Aspergillus bouffardi* (Brumpt, 1905), Somaliland.
- *A.* (?) *mycetomi* (Gelonesi, 1927), Somaliland.
- *? Penicillium mycetomagenum* (Mantelli and Negri, 1915), Europe.

TORULAE   *T. jeanselmei* (Langeron, 1928), Antilles.
PHYCOMYCETES   *Mucor* (?) *mycetomi* (Gelonesi, 1927), Somaliland.

HYPHOMYCETES
- *Madurella americana* (Gammel, Miskdjian and Thatcher, 1926), Texas.
- *M. bovoi* (Brumpt, 1910), Italy.
- *M. ikedai* (Gammel, 1927), North America.
- *M. mycetomi* (Laveran, 1902), cosmopolite.
- *M. oswaldoi* (Horta, 1919), Brazil.
- *M. ramiroi* (P. da Silva, 1919), Brazil.
- *M. rifanum* (Gastaminza, 1929), Morocco.
- *M. tabarkae* (Blanc and Brun, 1919), Tunis.
- *M. tozeuri* (Nicolle and Pinoy, 1908), Tunis.

White or Yellowish-White Grain Type

ALEUROSPORIA
{
Scedosporium apiospermum (Saccardo, 1911), cosmopolite.
Indiella mansoni (Brumpt, 1906), Asia.
I. reynieri (Brumpt, 1906), Paris, Greece.
I. brumpti (P. Piraja, 1922), Brazil.
}

SPOROPHORES
{
Cephalosporium recifei (Leão and Lobo, 1924), Brazil.
Acremonium potronii (Vuillemin, 1911), Algeria.
}

PLECTASCALES
{
Sterigmatocystis nidulans (Eidam, 1883), Tunis and Algeria.
Allescheria boydi (Shear, 1921), U. S. A.
}

Greenish-Yellow Grain Type

Aspergillus amstelodami (Mangin, 1900), Brazil.

Red Grain Type

Aspergillus (case of Balfour and Archibald), Africa.
Rubromadurella langeroni (Talice, 1935), Uruguay.

Following the injury, an incised or puncture wound, there develop within a few weeks swelling, edema, and indurated nodules. More nodes develop until the affected patch presents a purplish, knobby appearance as in actinomycosis. Some nodules remain firm and solid, but the majority of them undergo necrosis, so as to become perforated by slender, tortuous channels which extend deeply and let escape variable amounts of seropurulent fluid containing variously colored grains. Spontaneous cure is extremely rare. The course may run for many years. Metastasis ordinarily does not occur, but the progress locally is such as to eventuate almost inevitably in amputation.

The disease is seen in tropical climates, where numerous individuals go barefoot, but an occasional case occurs in North America.

Treatment.—Potassium iodide, copper sulfate and various internal remedies may be tried. Temporary improvement may follow roentgen therapy. **Radical surgical attack** offers the best hope and as a rule offers the only permanent cure.

ACTINOMYCOSIS (ACTINOMYCOTIC MYCETOMA; LUMPY JAW).—Actinomycosis is produced by various closely related fungi which within the tissues form grains of various colors composed of fins, *nonseptate* mycelial filaments, in which the partitions are invisible or difficult to demonstrate and in which chlamydospores are not formed.

ACTINOMYCOSES. Etiologic Classification According to Brumpt (1936).

Black Grain Type

{
Case of Babes (1888), Roumania.
Case of Mironescue (1910), Roumania.
Case of F. de Almeida (1930), hepatic, Brazil.
Case of Beron (1931), Bulgaria.
}

Yellow Grain Type

With clubs

Actinobacillus lignieresi (Brumpt, 1910), cosmopolite.

BREVIORES
{
Actinomyces israeli (Kruse, 1896), cosmopolite.
  [Affects bones; anaerobic.]
A. thibiergei (Ravaut and Pinoy, 1906).
  [Does not affect bones.]
}

MAJORES
{
A. mexicanus (Boyd and Crutchfield, 1921), Mexico and Texas.
A. transvalensis
A. pretorianus
} (Pijper and Pullinger, 1927), South Africa.

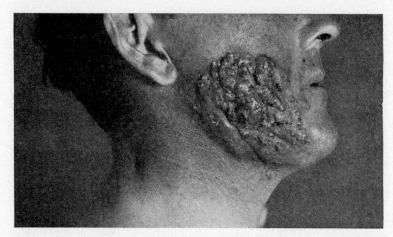

FIG. 30.—Actinomycosis. "Lumpy jaw."

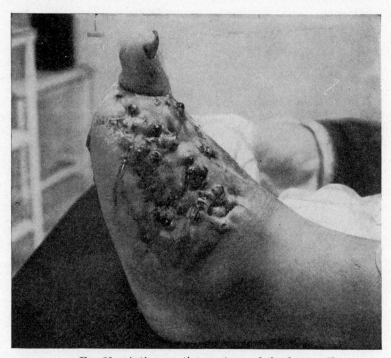

FIG. 31.—Actinomycotic mycetoma of the foot.

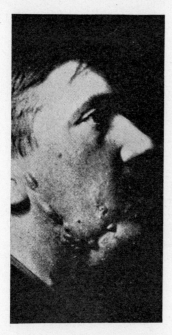

FIG. 32.—Actinomycosis of neck and jaw, showing sinus tracts draining through cutaneous granulomas. (Courtesy of Dr. H. C. Varney.)

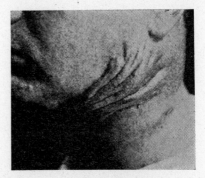

FIG. 33.—Actinomycosis. (Courtesy of Dr. Jabez Jackson.)

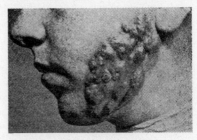

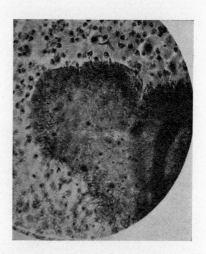

FIG. 34.—Actinomycosis. (Courtesy of Dr. T. W. Allworthy.)

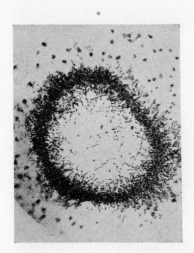

FIG. 35.—Actinomyces. Gram stain showing mycelium within the mass of ray fungus. (Courtesy of Dr. Fred Weidman.)

FIG. 36.—Actinomyces. Ray fungus as seen in a section, showing "clubs." (Courtesy of Dr. Fred Weidman.)

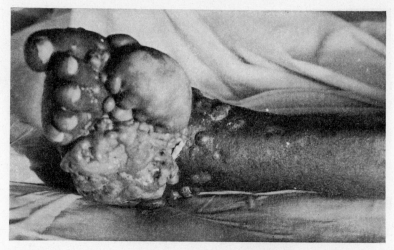

FIG. 37.—Madura foot. Texas case, of Dr. O. Garcia. Advanced state after a duration of more than two years.

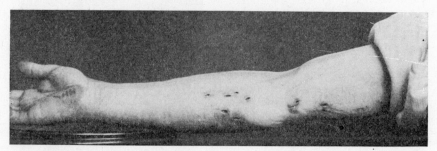

FIG. 38.—Sporotrichosis. The nodules have been incised, and as a result they have ulcerated. Digital primary.

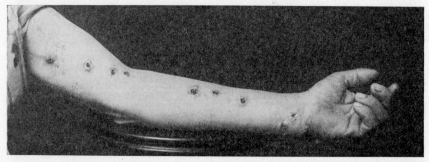

FIG. 39.—Sporotrichosis, showing ulcerative nodules along the channel of lymphatic drainage.

Without clubs

MAJORES
{
A. liquefaciens (Hesse, 1892), Europe.
A. nicollei (Delanoë, 1928), North Africa.
A. garteni (Brumpt, 1910), Europe.
}

MINORES
{
A. asteroides (Eppinger, 1890), cosmopolite.
A. brasiliensis (Lindenberg, 1909), Brazil.
A. brumpti (Bordjoski and Milochevitch, 1915), Jugoslavia.
A. madurae (Vincent, 1894), cosmopolite.
A. convolutus (Chalmers and Christopherson, 1916), Sudan.
}

BREVIORES
{
A. krausei (Chester, 1901), Europe.
A. ponceti (Verdun, 1912), Europe.
}

INCERTAE SEDIS *A. guerrai* (Langeron, 1930), San Salvador [affects bones].

Red or Reddish Grains, Without Clubs

MINORES
{
A. somaliensis (Brumpt, 1906), Africa.
[Affects bones.]
A. bahiensis (P. da Silva, 1919), Brazil.
A. micetomae argentinae (Greco, 1901; Durante, 1911), Argentina.
}

BREVIORES
{
A. pelletieri (Laveran, 1906), Africa.
A. africanus (Pijper and Pullinger, 1927).
[Affects bones.]
A. genesii (Fróes, 1930), Brazil.
}

Actinomyces bovis (cultural characteristics given under Tinea, etiology) is the commonest cause in the United States. It provokes sluggish, nodular, infiltrated lesions which tend to undergo central necrosis and to form chronic subcutaneous abscesses and sinus tracts. The lesions develop slowly. Inoculation through the teeth, gums or tonsils results in the development of infiltration in the jaw and neck. The nodules may require weeks or months to soften and to become fluctuant. Overlying tissues slough, and purulent matter, mixed with small masses of fungi resembling grains of sulfur, discharge from them. The involved region is usually isolated, but generalization may occur.

Cervicofacial cases are the commonest. Pulmonary and deep abdominal cases follow in order of frequency, and any part of the body may be infected. In the tongue, primary actinomycosis has its onset as a painful swelling which is round, tender, and located in the anterior third; it becomes softer, discolored, purplish and painful, and matter discharges through sinuses.

Etiology.—*Actinomyces* may live as saprophytes on some kinds of vegetation and even on human tissues and in tonsillar crypts. Their introduction as parasites is usually due to an injury which of itself may be of seeming inconsequence. According to Brumpt, the Hyphomycetes are fungi which have a white or dusty filamented thallus and which reproduce exclusively by conidia. Hyphomycetes with fine, nonseptate, mycelial filaments, a micron or smaller in diameter, branching laterally, having homogeneous contents and lacking distinct nuclei, often dissociating into bacteroid particles, are Microsiphonales. All of the Microsiphonales parasitic on man may be classed in the genus *Actinomyces*, which is identical with *Nocardia*.

Pathology.—Actinomycotic parasites develop well in all tissues of the body, but clinically they seem to spare the lymph nodes. In sections of the granulomas, macrophages filled with mycelial filaments are numerous near the vessels. Masses of fungi are scattered within the granulation tissue, forming the well-known clubs. The detailed structure of the clubs differs in different kinds of actinomycetic infection and may serve the expert for differentiation, although cultural studies are usually necessary for exact etiologic diagnosis.

Diagnosis.—The yellowish-gray, granular masses of fungi in the discharge should serve to differentiate actinomycosis from syphilis, tuberculosis, sarcoma or carcinoma. The pus may be put into a tube of water and shaken. The sulfur granules sink.

Prognosis.—Most of the localized cases undergo recovery. Most of the systemic cases die. Systemic involvement following upon localized disease is always possible. The disease may heal spontaneously, but this is very exceptional. Its progress causes cachexia, suppuration, reduced resistance, and secondary infection.

Treatment.—The **iodides** constitute the most reliable internal remedy, unless the recently introduced **sulfanilamide** and **sulfapyridine,** reported to be notably successful, prove on further experience to possess dependable merit. Locally, **surgical drainage** and **roentgen therapy** should be employed. **Thymol, 10 to 20 per cent in olive oil,** may be applied locally and injected into the sinuses, and 1 to 2 grams of thymol in capsules may be given by mouth daily on an empty stomach. Myers has found this an effective remedy.

OOSPOROSES.—*Oospora* was the genus name once used, but now obsolete, to apply to the organisms seen in diseases resembling actinomycosis but in which actinomycotic grains were absent.

SPOROTRICHOSIS

Sporothrices are conidiospore fungi (Hyphomycetes) in which the conidia, simple or septate, hyaline or fuliginous, are discrete and are inserted directly into the mycelial filaments. The conidia are mounted on a little pedicle (stipitate) in the genus *Rhinocladium,* a distinction Brumpt made in dividing *Sporothrix* into the two genera, *Rhinocladium* and *Sporotrichum.* Many of these fungi are of common natural occurrence, living as saprophytes; some of the species are able to parasitize man, animals and plants. There is good reason to believe that *Rhinocladium schenki,* isolated in the United States, is the same as *R. beurmanni,* isolated in France. Other pathogenic species include *R. dori, R. gougeroti, R. jeanselmei, R. indicum* and *R. councilmani.* The cultural characteristics are given under Tinea, etiology.

Symptoms.—Sporotrichosis is contracted generally by those who come in contact with the soil and shrubs, and infection follows some trifling injury such as the prick of a barberry thorn or the peck of a chicken. Five clinical types of sporotrichotic manifestation have been enumerated by Lewis and Cudmore (1934):

1. **Localized lymphangitic.**—Most cases in the United States are of this group, in which a primary lesion appears on an exposed part. The chancre is indurated, and softening and abscess formation may take place, or an indolent ulcer or vegetation may develop. Rarely the disease remains localized; but usually, after a week or more, painless inflammation ascends the regional lymphatics, along which secondary nodules form. Regional lymph node enlargement is uncommon, a clinical distinction from tularemia. Systemic symptoms or involvement is uncommon. There is little tendency for spontaneous recovery to occur. After healing has been induced by treatment, scarring of some degree usually remains.

2. **Disseminated subcutaneous.**—Seen more commonly in France than in the United States, this variety is characterized by the appearance of small, hard, painless, subcutaneous nodules of various numbers scattered over the body. Within three to six weeks the overlying skin becomes involved, and the central part of the nodule softens to form an abscess, which may discharge if traumatized, forming a cup-shaped ulcer with an indurated border. A lesion may continue indefinitely in the untreated patient.

3. **Disseminated ulcerative.**—Like the disseminated subcutaneous type, this is distinguished by a tendency to undergo early spontaneous ulceration. The ulcers are varied in size and character. Large crateriform sores may develop, simulating tuberculous ulcers or gummatous syphilids. There is little tendency to heal spontaneously. Untreated, the patient gradually fails.

4. **Epidermic.**—While the primary lesion is practically always subcutaneous, rarely the epidermis at near or remote sites becomes secondarily infected, so that papules, pus-

tules and small ulcers develop. In rare cases the disease has been limited to the skin. Tuberculosis is distinguished with difficulty.

5. **Systemic.**—Invasion of deep tissues and organs may occur. This happens in disseminated cases when treatment is not instituted promptly. The bones or joints may be affected, the tibia being the commonest site. Invasion of muscular and glandular structures may occur, and evidences of pulmonary involvement have been reported. Although the epididymis is the common site of involvement in laboratory animals, it is rarely affected in human beings. Gastro-intestinal and cerebrospinal involvement is extremely uncommon.

Diagnosis.—It is next to impossible to demonstrate the mycelium or conidia in direct smears, but the parasite grows readily on ordinary culture media. Tissular diagnosis is not definitive, for the lesions simulate those of syphilitic, tuberculous, or ecthymiform pyogenic infection. The lymphangitic type, in which the row of nodules follows the lymph channels draining a traumatic lesion that has proved resistant to ordinary treatment, is almost pathognomonic clinically. Complement fixation tests have been devised, and an intradermal skin test using sporotrichin has been investigated, but it is not reliable.

Prognosis and Treatment.—**Iodide,** given internally in the form of sodium or potassium salts, and **iodine** locally as the tincture or diluted as Lugol's solution, are thought to be specific. Surgical intervention generally retards cure rather than hastens it. Roentgen therapy locally has been recommended, but we have not found it successful. Potassium iodide should be given by mouth in doses of 30 to 90 grains a day and should be continued for a month after apparent recovery, which requires something around 10 weeks. When iodide by mouth does not reach a concentration that is efficacious, intravenous medication often succeeds. Sodium iodide is given intravenously in doses of 15 to 30 grains dissolved in 20 cc. of water, daily if necessary.

MISCELLANEOUS UNCOMMON MYCOSES

CEPHALOSPORIOSIS.—*Cephalosporium* is a genus of the sporophore division of the hyphomycetic fungi. The organisms, of which there are several species, have produced nodular, gummatous lesions and dermatomycoses of varied clinical appearance. Diagnosis depends on the demonstration of the fungus and its identification. These infections in general simulate sporotrichosis and are responsive to **potassium iodide** and **roentgen therapy.**

CLADOSPORIOSIS.—*Cladosporium* is a genus of dermatophytes, species of which have produced nodular, gummatous inflammations and dermatomycoses unresponsive to iodide. Diagnosis depends on cultural identification.

HEMISPOROSIS.—*Hemispora* include hyphomycetic fungi which reproduce by accessory spores or hemispores. Species have been found in cases which resembled *Rhinocladium* infections and, like them, were responsive to **iodide therapy.**

ACLADIOSIS.—Conidiospore fungi of the genus *Acladium* have been found in cases characterized by scattered ulcers, sharply defined, round or oval, with red and granulating bases, abundant purulent secretion, and thick yellow crusts, lesions which were gumma-like as well as furuncular, located on the palms and soles or elsewhere. The disease is chronic without tendency to heal spontaneously. It is responsive to **iodide therapy.** It is identified only by cultural study.

ACREMONIOSIS.—*Acremonium potronii* has caused typhoid-like fever and gumma-like swellings which underwent ulceration, but without lymph node involvement. Other cases have resembled mycetoma.

ASPERGILLUS AND PENICILLIUM.—These genera of Ascomycetes bear conidia in chains arising from specialized cells called phialides. They are mold-like fungi. Several species have been known to act as parasites and have produced mycetomas, infections of the lungs, and superficial infections of the ear canals, nasopharynx, skin and cornea. They are found commonly enough as saprophytes on crusted, dirty dermatoses, and one must be critical, though not incredulous, of reports of their pathogenicity.

4042

STERIGMATOCYSTIS.—Superficial, eczematous and epidermal disease has been caused by fungi of this genus. *S. cinnamominus* was found in a Peruvian case resembling tinea versicolor. Species have been found in the ear canals.

SCOPULARIOPSIS is a genus of the Ascomycetes related to *Penicillium*, the conidial apparatus being similar. Species have been isolated from a case resembling sporotrichosis with verrucous chancres and ascending lymphangitis, in onychomycosis, and in the ulcerative mycetomas and gummatous lesions.

The publishers and authors express their appreciation to the C. V. Mosby Company for permission to use a considerable portion of the text and illustrations from the tenth edition of Sutton and Sutton's *Diseases of the Skin*.

BIBLIOGRAPHY

Barrett, C. C.: Arch. Dermat. & Syph., 33 : 126, 1936.
Favus.
Becker, S. W. and Muir, S. K.: Arch. Dermat. & Syph., 20 : 45, 1929.
Tinea amiantacea.
Benham, R. W.: J. Infect. Dis., 57 : 255, 1935.
Cryptococcosis.
Brumpt, E.: Précis de Parasitologie, Ed. 5, Paris, Masson et Cie, 1936.
Exhaustive and excellent treatise on parasitology, both animal and vegetable.
Castellani, A.: J. Cutan. Dis., 26 : 393, 1908.
Tinea versicolor, tropical forms.
—— : J. Trop. Med., 37 : 363, 1934.
Tinea imbricata.
—— and Wilkinson, A. G.: Brit. J. Dermat. & Syph., 34 : 255, 1932.
Trichomycosis axillaris.
Dickson, E. C.: J. Am. M. Ass., 111 : 1362, 1938.
Coccidioidal granuloma.
Dodge, C. W.: Medical Mycology, St. Louis, Mo., C. V. Mosby Company, 1935.
Exhaustive treatise on pathogenic fungi, with bibliography.
Fox, H.: Arch. Dermat. & Syph., 36 : 534, 1937; 39 : 709, 1939.
Pinta.
—— : Arch. Dermat. & Syph., 13 : 398, 1926.
Tinea capitis in adults.
Gammel, J.: Arch. Dermat. & Syph., 15 : 241, 1927.
Mycetoma in United States.
Greenwood, A. M. and Swartz, J. H.: Arch. Dermat. & Syph., 15 : 404, 1927.
Review of literature on tinea, to date.
Gregory, P. H.: Biol. Rev., 10 : 208, 1935.
The dermatophytes, instructive review.
Hopkins, J. G.: Arch. Dermat. & Syph., 25 : 192, 599, 1932.
Moniliasis and moniliids.
Jacobson, H. P.: Fungous Diseases, Springfield, Ill., C. C. Thomas, 1932.
Monograph.
Jordan, J. W. and Weidman, F. D.: Arch. Dermat. & Syph., 33 : 31, 1936.
Blastomycosis.
Lewis, G. M. and Cudmore, J. H.: Ann. Int. Med., 7 : 991, 1934.
Sporotrichosis.
—— and Hopper, M. E.: New York State J. Med., 38 : 859, 1938.
Moniliasis.
—— : Arch. Dermat. & Syph., 35 : 461, 1937.
Correlation of clinical and mycologic features of tinea.
—— : Arch. Dermat. & Syph., 34 : 850, 1936.
Tinea versicolor.

Lewis, G. M. and Hopper, Mary E.: An Introduction to Medical Mycology, Chicago, The Year Book Publishers, Inc., pp. 315, 1939.
Authoritative manual for practical management and laboratory investigation of the mycoses, particularly the dermatomycoses.
Martin and Smith: Am. Rev. Tuberc., 39 : 275, 488, 1939.
Blastomycosis, review and bibliography.
Mitchell, J. H.: Arch. Dermat. & Syph., 5 : 174, 1922.
Tinea of hands and feet.
Mook, W. H. and Moore, M.: Arch. Dermat. & Syph., 33 : 951, 1936.
Torulosis.
Myer, H. B.: J. Am. M. Ass., 108 : 1875, 1937.
Actinomycosis treated with thymol.
Pardo-Castello, V.: Arch. Dermat. & Syph., 25 : 785, 1932.
Achromia parasitaria.
Peck, S. M.: Arch. Dermat. & Syph., 22 : 40, 1930.
Experimental epidermophytosis and immunologic studies.
Report of the Council on Pharmacy: J. Am. M. Ass., 107 : 658, 1936.
Trichophytin and oidiomycin.
Rockwood, E. M.: New England J. Med., 209 : 295, 1933.
Mycotic paronychia.
Shaw, F. W.: J. Lab. & Clin. Med., 20 : 113, 1934; 21 : 343, 1935.
Simplified key to pathogenic fungi.
Shelmire, B.: Arch. Dermat. & Syph., 12 : 789, 1925.
Moniliasis, review to date.
Sulzberger, M. B.: Arch. Dermat. & Syph., 18 : 801, 1939.
Pathogenesis of trichophytids.
—— and others: J. Am. M. Ass., 108 : 2189, 1937.
Erysipelas-like trichophytid.
Sutton, R. L., Jr.: J. Am. M. Ass., 110 : 1733, 1938.
Pompholyx from vulvovaginitis; use of gentian violet; monilial vulvovaginitis.
Sutton, R. L., Sr. and Sutton, R. L., Jr.: Diseases of the Skin, Ed. 10, St. Louis, Mo., C. V. Mosby Company, pp. 1033–1177, 1939.
Whalen, J. E.: J. Am. M. Ass., 111 : 502, 1938.
Otomycosis.
White, C.: J. Am. M. Ass., 103 : 1376, 1934.
Onychomycosis treatment.
White, C. J.: Arch. Dermat. & Syph., 15 : 387, 1927.
Clinical forms of tinea.
Williams, G. M.: Arch. Dermat. & Syph., 4 : 353, 1921.
Trichophytids.

CHAPTER XXVII

SPRUE

BY BAILEY K. ASHFORD, M.D.

Definition.—Sprue is a chronic, wasting disease, generally native to
tropical countries, characterized by an excoriated and sore tongue, excessive intestinal fermentation, and light-colored and frothy stools. It
is usually based on exhaustion processes, especially of the digestive
glandular apparatus, due to nutritional unbalance, low in the complete
protein molecule and high in carbohydrates and fats, and is accompanied
by colonization in the intestinal canal of *Monilia psilosis* Ashford, 1914,
believed by the author and others to be the active causal agent.

Synonyms.—The root-word, "sprouwe," is Teutonic but this was
variously spelled, and employed from ancient times in Holland and Scotland to denote thrush, in which the mouth was covered as if with mealy
chaff, or "spreu." Manson anglicized this to "sprue" in order to distinguish vividly by an unusual folk name a prevalent and fatal disease
of the tropics, then almost universally confused with banal dysenteries
and diarrheas.

There are fully fifty synonyms, including misnomers such as scorbutic diarrhea and chronic dysentery, but a few of the outstanding ones
still employed will be mentioned.

Indische Spruw, by the Dutch; *Psilosis*, by the British; *Aphthae
Tropicae* and *Tropische Moniliasis*, by the Germans; *Diarrhée* or *Entero-
colite des pays chauds*, and *Diarrhée chronique de Cochinchine*, by the
French; *Escorbuto Tropical* (tropical scurvy), *Tisis intestinal* (intestinal phthisis) by the Spanish-speaking population of the West Indies.

Etiology *—CLIMATE.—While sprue is really a disease of warm
climates, it is not climate necessarily that makes it so, as there are many
tropical lands, such as Brazil, and tropical regions surrounded by endemic
zones that seem completely free from it. On the other hand, it exists in
parts of our Southern States and in Korea, in certain sections of which
it appears to be a scourge; indeed, sporadic cases develop from time to
time in frankly temperate and northern climates. Nevertheless, hot
weather seems to favor its development, especially a monotonously warm,
although not strictly high temperature. A sudden change to the chilly
heights of tropical hills in countries where it is endemic often precipitates a bout of sprue. There seems to be no seasonal variation in sprue.

---

* (All numerical statements when not otherwise specified refer to the author's own
series of now over three thousand cases investigated.)

173

RESIDENCE.—One of the most fallacious statements in the literature is to the effect that only persons from northern climates acquire sprue in the tropics and then only after a long residence therein. It is certainly true that such people are much more prone to suffer from the disease and more severely, and that the longer their residence the higher the incidence among them, but an astounding number develop sprue after only a very short stay in endemic zones, even after a short first visit to the tropics. The old belief in immunity of persons native to the soil seems justifiable only when we have a pure race of those who are notoriously immune, such as the negro and the oriental, but for races mixed with the white the conclusion would seem to rest on the unfamiliarity of the observer with the native languages and the lack of opportunity to observe their illnesses.

What is worth while considering is the development of true sprue on return to their northern homes in persons who had previously resided a longer or shorter time in the tropics and who had enjoyed apparent health while there, as well as the sudden appearance of sprue in white or mestizo adults native to the soil who have led an active and often long life in seeming good health in endemic zones.

AGE.—About three-fourths of the writer's patients were between 20 and 60 years of age, and of these two-thirds were between 20 and 40. Children, however, are much more frequently affected than has been previously supposed; one-tenth of the 619 cases of the 1921 series were under ten years of age, 4 being under one year.

SEX.—Of 1452 cases (series 1920 to 1922), 59 per cent were females.

RACE.—Of 211 cases (series 1915 to 1917) there were 174 whites, 21 mulattoes and no negroes. While true sprue has since been seen occasionally in the negro, this ratio has about been sustained in all subsequent series. Sprue is quite rare in the full-blooded negro, and plainly discriminates against the white race in the tropics, particularly in persons whose stock came more recently from the North.

FAMILY AND INDIVIDUAL PREDISPOSITION.—There are families locally known in the community life of Porto Rico as being peculiarly predisposed to sprue, but it is believed to be due to traditionally improper food habits extending over generations. As a complement of this, individual susceptibility is seen among those who are naturally of a weak constitution or who have suffered some serious disease affecting nutrition during childhood, particularly enterocolites of infancy.

ENDEMICITY.—Sprue is a distinctly urban disease, at least in the Antilles. In an expedition of the Institute of Tropical Medicine to the mountains of Porto Rico in which the writer took part in 1913, of 10,140 chiefly rural patients seen in three months and suffering from a great variety of affections, mainly uncinariasis, only 11 cases of true sprue and 19 suspicious ones were found. Our field hospital was then drawing from an area containing approximately 30,000 souls. This should be contrasted with the writer's consulting practice in San Juan where of about 1,500 patients a year, 150 were cases of sprue, the overwhelming majority from towns and mainly from San Juan itself, a city of only 100,000. But sprue has been becoming more and more prevalent in the country districts since good roads, the automobile and employment in the towns have routed the people out of their rural isolation and converted the entire island into a series of suburbs.

SOCIAL CONDITIONS AND HABITS.—Sprue is preëminently a disease of the well-to-do, of the intellectuals, of those who can choose their food. While it does not always pass by the poor man, it is by no means a poor man's disease. It is, above all, frequent among those whose life is a sedentary one, and those who have to work hard to keep up an appearance of affluence; among those whose introspective and imaginative life, with its maze of behavioristic tradition, its prejudices and its self-imposed artificiality, clashes with reality and is continually inhibiting the function of normal digestion. It is also a deadly enemy of those who drift to the Tropics from northern latitudes and who "cannot eat the native food," but gorge themselves on canned goods, cereals and sweets. Of 179 cases in the series 1915–1917, 16 were wealthy, 134 were able to select their food, and 29 were poor.

Besides lack of healthful exercise in sun and air, or its excess which is fully as bad, there is the special factor of insufficient rest. People often work harder in the Tropics than in the North, and certainly for longer hours, and among the reasons therefor is the lack of intelligent initiative on the part of those who are supposed to do the drudgery. The charm of the Tropics also lies in her nights; hence, late hours and lack of rest wear away a bit more of man's resistance to this disease.

INSUFFICIENCY IN VITAL FOOD ELEMENTS.—This is the great underlying factor in most cases of sprue. While the luxuriant vegetation of the Tropics would seem to assure an abundance of vitamin-charged foods, the truth is that most people reside in the Tropics because these countries furnish the highest-priced agricultural crops, tobacco, sugar, citrous fruit, cocoa, coffee, tea, vanilla, spices and other luxuries. The natural tendency, therefore, is to neglect garden products, which if sown or allowed to grow are rarely cultivated or even relished. But in most sprue-ridden countries there is really "protein starvation," i.e., there is an insufficiency of the complete protein molecule with which to replace worn-out body protein, and we therefore have before us the picture of a hot fire under an unattended, unrepaired machine. For example, the average consumption of meat in Porto Rico per individual is 9 pounds a year, as against 180 pounds in the United States; of milk, one ounce a day. The markets are almost empty of succulent vegetables, and such as these are, they are wild, fibrous and uncultivated. This lack of dairy products and fresh leafy and succulent vegetables also brings a certain degree of insufficiency in A-substance and calcium.

Strangely enough, however, although it is no longer so true as it used to be, it has been in times past the poor country dweller of all people in Porto Rico who, though suffering from the nutritional syndrome of this unbalance, rarely contracted sprue. Not only was he so poor as to be unable to buy sweets, bread and all of the grease he wanted, or go into the carbohydrate excesses attained by his more unfortunate urban brother of the sedentary and well-to-do class, but he rarely left his mountain home and remained isolated from urban life. Moreover, he was spared the debilitating heat of the coast and the overcrowding of towns, and, such as they were, he obtained more fresh vegetables and fruits. But he is no longer isolated; his contact with the town is constant. While just as poor or poorer, he spends what he has on more carbohydrates and fats than before, and the intense cultivation of sugar and tobacco has swallowed up the banana patch, the garden patch, the few cattle he used to have, and the shade of the coffee plantation. Moreover, he is now in contact with the carriers of and sufferers from

Monilia psilosis, raised by passage through human beings from the state of a mere saprophyte to that of a pathogen. The excess of sweets, cereals and grease produces acid fermentation, and an ideal medium is thus afforded *Monilia psilosis* which by contact in overcrowded centers of population is passed from one to another until it adapts itself to a parasitic life on man.

GLANDULAR INCOMPETENCE.—There is functional insufficiency not only of digestive glands but of the glands of internal secretion. We need not look to pathologists to demonstrate lesions in these organs for they usually will not be found; it is rather a functional lack. The presumptive evidence of adrenal insufficiency is strong, as seen in the dusky, muddy hue and atrophic condition of the skin, the symmetrical areas of pigmentation, the asthenia, emaciation, low blood pressure, etc. Alteration of ovarian function is often seen in scanty or suppressed menstruation. Parathyroid insufficiency may in part account for tetany, so often noted.

Concerning the participation of the digestive glands there seems to be no reasonable doubt. The liver is notably reduced in size, there is an intermittent reduction in pancreatic output, there is often achylia, and the entire glandular apparatus of the intestine frequently is seen to have suffered an atrophic change. Not only the glandular system but its shadow, the hemopoietic organs, as well as its controlling mechanism, the sympathetic nervous system, to which it is so intimately bound, are also involved, the latter two at times profoundly. Sprue is at bottom an exhaustion process.

The evidence of these conditions is seen in the effect of physiologic strain, such as rage or fear, overwork, intemperance in eating and drinking, too-frequent pregnancies and too-long-continued lactation, even a normal menstrual period, all of which may precipitate a bout of sprue. Not only the strain of life, but also long continued illness from whatsoever cause, even a weakly constitution in nervous, undersized individuals, is often the opening wedge to sprue.

We must keep in mind, however, the fact that sprue does not necessarily require these factors; it often develops very suddenly in persons who are apparently healthy and robust.

The real and practical point in considering glandular insufficiency as a predisposing factor in sprue can be concentrated in what we know scientifically of this condition as it affects digestion and digestive glands prior to the disease, a condition which in turn is exalted when sprue becomes established. Trevor Heaton believes that ''hill diarrhea'' is merely an expression of this glandular insufficiency, and from his description and that of Cunningham of ''famine diarrhea'' the writer is convinced that this is the most frequent preliminary condition to downright sprue. That an illy balanced ration is often the direct cause of this state is apparent merely from McCarrison's experimental work on animals in India.

Such a condition as glandular insufficiency can be recognized the world over but it is not sprue. Undoubtedly many who have not become familiar with tropical sprue where it is endemic have confused this syndrome with the disease in question, as may have happened with distinguished investigators who have gone to the Tropics for the first time to unravel this problem in a period of months in the laboratory. Indeed, probably a reversal to this syndrome, after the causative organism of sprue has been eliminated and only a state of cachexia with permanently atrophied digestive glands remains, has caused others in northern hospitals to deny the relation of *Monilia psilosis* to the disease.

Monilia psilosis Ashford, 1914.—*Monilia albicans* Robin, 1853, represents a plurality of species, one of which, indistinguishable in laboratory

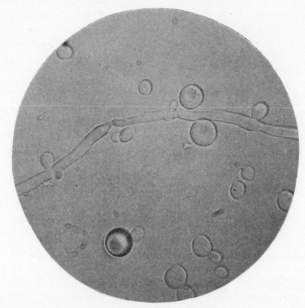

FIG. 1.—Young culture, *Monilia psilosis;* Mycelium, blastospores and budding yeasts.

so far from *Monilia psilosis*, although the latter may prove to be a variant therefrom, is a cause of thrush. It is really not a *Monilia* but *Candida* Berkhout, 1923. Hence the mycologic diagnosis of *Monilia albicans* proposed is: *Candida albicans* (Robin) Berkhout, 1923, *emend.* Ashford, 1930. The species *Monilia albicans* was not clearly delimited when first named and the terminology was altered for the genus with good reason by Berkhout in 1923. Many of Castellani's species of *Monilia,* so often confused with *Monilia psilosis,* were given specific rank practically alone on sugar fermentations, later shown not to be immutable. For a full description of *Monilia psilosis*, reference is made to the bibliography (3d, 4th, 5th, 6th, 11th, 12th and 13th references, Ashford). Awaiting a decision on the change of terminology proposed, the designation *Monilia psilosis* will be used in this text.

In the course of time it is believed that this variety of the thrush fungus will be found to produce clinical pictures of the most varied nature, still considered today separate and distinct diseases, such as sprue, certain bronchomoniliases, tonsillitides, and even some onychomycoses and epidermomycoses. It has been found in the body of man in all of these conditions and considered the causal agent thereof, sometimes by one specific name, again by another. In sprue *Monilia psilosis* has been found by the writer in the circulating blood, and in the bone marrow of a pernicious type of anemia complicating sprue.

Outside the body it is a common saprophyte. To demonstrate how abundant a source of contamination exists, it (or an organism so far indistinguishable therefrom) is found in Nature on fruits (Ashford), in bread for sale in Porto Rico and the yeast used in making the same (Ashford), at times in yeast preparations available to tens of thousands in the United States who seek to increase their vitamins (Ashford in Porto Rico in 1925 and recently again in a well known New York research laboratory). It is constantly found in transit through the intestinal canal of both human beings and animals, *but it is only when it is afforded a propitious medium in the gastro-intestinal tract and has been adapted by passage to parasite man that it colonizes and produces sprue.* As Castellani intimates, but with a different object in view, the common organisms of pus are everywhere; it is only when they effect an invasion of man that they give rise to disease. The same may be said of tuberculosis, as far as that is concerned, but most emphatically for all diseases produced by practically any fungus, notably Actinomyces. Thus is brought out vividly the important distinction between bacteriology and mycology: In the latter, it is the terrain as a rule, not the causal agent, that is of prime importance.

THE COMMUNICABILITY OF SPRUE.—Once adapted for parasiting man, the possibility of communicating sprue must be admitted, but this occurs as a rule only if the intestinal canal of the recipient is in a state favorable to its colonization, *i.e.*, acid and sweet. It seems to have a marked tendency to spread in families. This may be due in part to family habits of eating, but it is notable that many children of parents who have died of sprue have developed the disease many years afterward while living under totally different climatic and food conditions, and infants and young children fed on preserved milk whose mothers were suffering from sprue have contracted severe forms of the disease. French naval surgeons on sick-transports of the slow-going type of 1860, which were repatriating large numbers of soldiers from Indo-China, one-fourth of whom were seriously ill from sprue, reported a large number of instances of contamination of the officers and crew by a disease which from its clear description leaves no reasonable doubt in the reader's mind as to the diagnosis. The communicability of sprue must occur through contact infection; water cannot be considered a vehicle.

Symptomatology.—CLINICAL HISTORY.—As in tuberculosis, the period of latency may be a few days or the best part of a lifetime, and, as in that disease, the symptoms of that period may be merely a long history of failing health and nutrition. Usually there is a period of months or years of "chronic indigestion," the chief manifestation of what has been heretofore termed "nutritional unbalance."

The Syndrome of Nutritional Unbalance Preceding Sprue (Analysis of 286 cases).—The leading features in this condition, in order of their importance, are (1) loss of weight, color and strength; (2) psychic depression and nervous irritability; (3) disordered digestion with gastric dyspepsia, excess of intestinal gas and constipation with occasional loose bowels.

In one-third of the cases the tongue was abnormally sensitive to mild irritants, such as pickles, pepper or smoking tobacco; but there were rarely any lesions to speak of and these, when they occurred, were limited to small aphthae of the buccal cavity or slight excoriation of the tip and edges of the tongue. In 86 per cent of these cases there was a definite complaint of what the patient described as an acid gastric dyspepsia in which a hyperchlorhydria could be frequently verified. In three-fourths of the cases there was an annoying and persistent constipation generally broken by short periods of "loose bowels" or even a yellow diarrhea. In nearly nine-tenths of the cases there was a pronounced excess of intestinal gas, frequently punctuated by fleeting gas pains. Loss of appetite was noted in two-thirds of the cases, and ephemeral nausea in nearly half, occasional vomiting in one-fifth. In the majority of cases there was a steady reduction in the size of the liver.

In nearly all of these patients there was an indefinable "nervousness" or nervous irritability, with psychic depression and a tendency to forget the near-by details of life. Day by day patients are mindful of an increasing asthenia with vague pains in the body, muscle tire, and palpitation and irregularity of the heart. There is a concomitant fall in blood pressure.

In over half the series there was a history of slight numbness of the hands and feet which were cold and tended "to go to sleep." In half of the cases there were cramps in the legs, generally produced on stretching in bed at night or walking on cold cement or tile floors, and in a little over half the series complaint of insomnia was made.

These people are apt to be sallow and listless and to show faint but symmetrical brownish stains on forehead, malar prominences, sides of neck and, at times, around the lips (Fig. 2). These pigmentations were observed in one-half of the series. Reduction in genital vigor in males and menstrual irregularities in females are prominent. The average hemoglobin was 69.1 per cent; the average loss of weight 16.2 pounds. It is notable that in most of these cases there is a decided polycythemia; counts of six million per cubic millimeter and more are by no means unusual. Whether this is due to decreased blood volume or a mild toxic stimulation of bone marrow is not known, but the evident hemoglobinemia is outstanding.

It is upon this condition, so extremely common in these American tropics, and very familiar to temperate and cold climates, that sprue is generally based—not always, however, as will be seen later. In this connection let it be said that a very similar picture is seen to precede and accompany uncinariasis in Porto Rico, not to speak of a number of other slow-going chronic affections. It is not necessary to dilate upon what everyone can see, *i.e.*, that the characteristic picture, not only of mild sprue but of uncinariasis, has heretofore been confused with this great syndrome which the laity from time immemorial has summed up in such expressions as a "run-down condition," "neurasthenia," "effect of tropical climate," etc.

When upon this syndrome *Monilia psilosis* or hookworm is laid, each paints its familiar clinical picture. Without this syndrome a very pathogenic strain of the fungus or a large number of hookworms is apt to be necessary to paint much of anything.

There are two modes of invasion: one, that just recounted, in which little by little the tongue becomes sore, the burning in the stomach and gullet becomes marked, and constipation is replaced by longer and longer periods of a yellowish, fetid, frothy diarrhea with rapid loss of weight; the other, acute in residents of the tropics, especially children and newcomers after a few days' sojourn in endemic zones, which presupposes one or all of three conditions—a high virulence of *Monilia psilosis*, a lack of immunity thereto, or a sudden failure of digestion due to overexertion, excesses in eating and drinking, and overstimulation. In this case, sprue may begin on a definite day as a sudden, acute indigestion which may even simulate dysentery and be accompanied by vomiting, after which the typical picture may develop, generally after a brief interval of apparent betterment.

In the first case, the change that takes place is heralded by symptoms of what the Spanish-speaking people best sum up in the word "irritación," or burning or uncomfortable heat revealed in tongue, bowels, rectum and even vagina. Constipation becomes more and more frequently interrupted by diarrhea, which may follow a strong emotion or dietary indiscretion. Matinal diarrhea with an imperative call to stool in the early hours of the morning, supposed by the French to be due to reflex stimulation of the defecatory muscles by the chilling of the skin of the abdomen at or just before dawn, has been cited in most works as a characteristic phenomenon in sprue. It is said that there is apt to be relative freedom from these outbursts of diarrhea by day, but a careful analysis of the writer's cases has made it evident that this is far from what usually takes place; diarrhea generally occurs throughout the day at very irregular intervals and the movements are not so frequently large as is supposed.

At most irregular intervals, a sudden apparition of small vesicles on the tip and edges of the tongue takes place which may extend over the anterior third of the organ and cause intense discomfort on taking stimulating food. The tongue is red, and its inflamed papillae give it the well known strawberry appearance (Fig. 2). Aphthae may attack the buccal mucous membrane and frenum, even extending to fauces, palate and pharynx.

But the disease may be apparently confined to the tongue or the intestine, as the case may be, and such form instances of what has been termed "incomplete sprue," "tongue sprue," "intestinal sprue."

The Developed Disease.—The patient is now no longer merely out-of-sorts, but clearly sick. The course of the disease is marked by a series of buccal or intestinal exacerbations, each worse than the preceding one, until the extraordinarily obstinate cachexia is reached which is responsible for the gloomy prognosis of early authors. During an intestinal exacerbation the stools become very light in color and foamy, and of a sickening, sour-sweetish, pungent odor. Abdominal pain is slight and fleeting, or absent. These movements are not necessarily very frequent, but apart from the relief which the expulsion of so much gas produces, they leave the patient extremely exhausted. There is usually neither tenesmus, blood nor visible mucus. Distention from gas, mostly colonic, is often quite distressing and may produce tachycardia, cardiac irregularity and even syncope.

The exanthem of the tongue is now no longer limited to tip and edges; it spreads over the visible surface of the organ and gives it the appearance of raw beef. Salivation which has always been noticeable is now often marked, and any food, the swallowing of saliva itself, and even talking cause much suffering. Quite frequently, this saliva is thick and difficult to dislodge and impels constant painful deglutition. When the esophagus is thus affected, the unfortunate patient's cup is full.

All of a sudden, without apparent reason, these lingual symptoms begin to recede and then begins a recrudescence of the diarrhea which from its acrid nature sets up burning of the excoriated rectum and anus.

Indeed, the invasion of the vagina by continuity is not uncommon and a severe vaginitis may be set up from which *Monilia psilosis* usually may be cultivated. During the intervals of relative quiescence of the tongue, the mouth is apt to be hot and dry, and the saliva very thick. There is reason to believe that sudden changes in the *p*H of saliva and intestinal

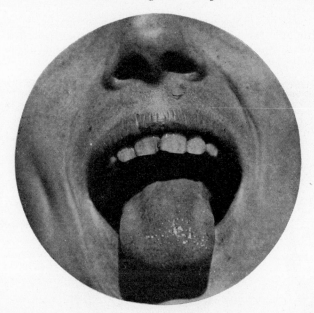

Fig. 2.—Typical strawberry type of tongue seen in early sprue. Use hand lens. Note brownish streak of pigmentation over upper lip. Patient is a female and white.

secretions will explain these very striking exacerbations and their subsequent rapid regression.

During this time, the heaviness and burning in the epigastrium is unremitting. While inconstant, nausea and vomiting are much more common than is usually recognized. Of 193 severe and cachectic grades of the disease, nausea occurred in 60 per cent and vomiting in 45 per cent of the series; in 5.7 per cent this vomiting was frequent.

In 78 per cent of these cases the appetite was said to be diminished; in 24 per cent of the series complete anorexia existed. In many, however, this loss of appetite really does not exist, for at bottom the patient does not eat for fear of consequences and a self-imposed abstention results. Little by little the sick man sacrifices his favorite dishes and his cigarette, and craves bland, pultaceous foods which from the nature of things are precisely what he should not eat: starches, sugars and fats.

As for the rest of the picture, it can be summed up in one phrase: accentuation of that drawn for the preceding syndrome of nutritional unbalance. The symptoms relative to the nervous system are vastly augmented, particularly the mental depression with nervous instability and loss of will power, but at no time is the mind affected. Tetanoid contraction of the muscles of the leg and forearm, felt in fingers and toes, is greatly increased.

Pallor is much more marked, as is a secondary type of anemia with relative lymphocytosis. This pallor is dirty yellow or grayish. Emaciation now becomes very marked; in the series referred to, the average loss of weight was over 27 pounds. The blood pressure falls to around 100 mm. of mercury systolic and 50 diastolic and the asthenia deepens to an extent comprehended only by those who have seen the disease at close range.

The Cachexia of Sprue.—The patient in this stage is usually bed-ridden although the active mind may compel the frail body to drag itself about in spite of its exhausted state. The emaciation of sprue cachexia quite rivals that of any disease, not even excepting cancer, and

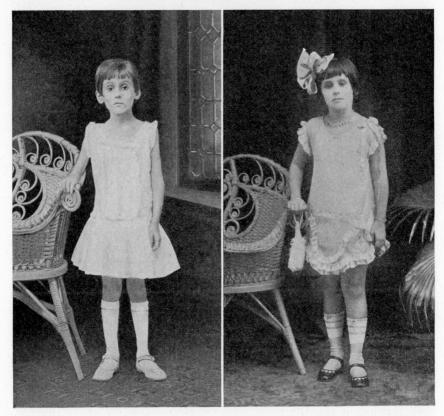

Fig. 3.—A, photograph of patient June 3, 1929. B, same August 13, 1930. This patient, nine years of age, consulted the writer, June 3, 1929, in the cachexia of sprue with a pernicious type of anemia; weight 36 pounds; hemoglobin 45 per cent; erythrocytes 1,620,000. She was photographed, placed on the diet and medicinal treatment recommended in the text, and given three vials of dry liver extract a day. In a week she was free of symptoms (sore tongue, bloating, and diarrhea) and had responded with a reticulocytosis of 16.3 per cent. On June 24th, 1929, she was apparently well; her hemoglobin was 77 per cent, her erythrocytes 3,200,000, and the average diameter of 100 red cells was 8.8 microns.

On the 13th of August, 1930, she returned weighing 87 pounds, with 85 per cent hemoglobin, 5,952,000 erythrocytes, and an average diameter of 7.37 microns in 100 red cells.

As she said that she looked about as she did in the second photograph as far back as December of 1929, this change in her appearance could not have taken over six months.

not only the clothing but the dry, atrophic, irregularly pigmented skin hangs as if upon a skeleton. The writer has frequently received patients whose loss of weight reached 50, 80 and at times 100 pounds. A loss of nearly if not quite half the patient's normal weight is by no means uncommon.

All symptoms heretofore detailed, with few exceptions, are accentuated to their highest expression. The tongue is small, tough like cartilage, and perfectly smooth and glistening, or entirely raw, depending upon the presence or absence of an exacerbation. All filiform papillae are apt to have disappeared. The appetite, however, is often ravenous and unreasonable. George Thin's discovery of the strawberry treatment was due to the sly disobedience of his patient who after months of a monotonous and orthodox milk diet bribed a confederate maid to hide quantities of fresh strawberries under the bed.

Now diarrhea has become constant and is apt to be lienteric, proclaiming the all but total failure of digestion. It is chiefly in the cachectic stage of sprue that a pernicious type of anemia occurs, a fate which awaits over half of these cases.

A terminal pneumonia or a choleriform diarrhea may suddenly carry off the weakened victim, but usually vital functions gradually fade and death occurs from exhaustion, the patient preserving his consciousness practically to the very end.

PHYSICAL FINDINGS.—Aside from descriptions inseparable from the clinical history just given, may be mentioned the frequent presence of slight subcutaneous hemorrhages, even before cachexia occurs, appearing as bruises without any recollection of injury on the part of the mystified patient. Later, during the cachexia, petechiae and extensive purpura, as well as bleeding gums (hence the term "scorbutic diarrhea"), may appear.

On palpation of the abdomen, one is at first struck by the loss of elasticity of the skin, which when grasped between thumb and forefinger and given a half-turn, retains the shape given it by compression quite a few seconds before returning to its normal condition. In a good proportion of cases the liver can be palpated only with difficulty, the spleen not at all, but ptosis of stomach and intestines is very frequent in the advanced grades of the disease and a displaced kidney not unusual. The muscular atrophy of the abdominal wall greatly aids accuracy in palpation.

The skin in general is apt to be dry and rough, although no pellagrous eruption is seen. No enlargement of glands can be noted in uncomplicated cases. The pulse is generally rapid and weak but sometimes very slow. The heart, often unduly small, is feeble, and the lungs yield no abnormal signs. Rectal examination often reveals hemorrhoids or excoriation from the acrid flux. The deep reflexes as a rule are diminished.

LABORATORY FINDINGS.—(a) *The Cytology of the Blood.*—About half the cases which have reached severe grades of the disease show a mild anemia with from 60 to 100 per cent hemoglobin, but as cachexia deepens many of these are apt to follow the other half into either a severe secondary or a true pernicious type of anemia. Of 54 severe and cachectic cases, the average hemoglobin was 52.4 per cent; the extremes were 20 and 95 per cent. The average red cell count was 2,459,044 per mil; the extremes were 5,080,000 and 440,000. Half the cases were clearly those of secondary anemia, the rest primary. With but one exception, normoblasts, and especially megaloblasts, were rare and were seen in only 22 per cent of the cases. There were generally one and never more than six per hundred leukocytes, but in the excepted case there were 144. Poikilocytosis, anisocytosis and polychromatophilia were frequent. There is no typical leukocytosis in sprue, rather a tendency toward leukopenia, but in a number of cases a marked relative lymphocytosis existed.

Excessive reticulocytosis was found a number of times in patients who had just begun a diet high in meat, but this was before Minot's classical work in pernicious anemia and was not understood. The writer began to stain for reticulocytes in sprue anemia in 1924 on the advice of Dr. N. Rosenthal, who insisted upon the importance of a study of these cells. Toward the end of the first experiments on liver extract, the writer received sufficient of this product for a study of 16 cases of anemias in sprue. Fifteen of these cases were pernicious in type (megaloblastic), 8 responding with a reticulocytosis within an average of 5 days, 6 from liver extract, one from a high meat diet, and 1 from Monilia vaccines alone. The other 7 failed to respond to the hormone. This induced the writer to draw the tentative conclusion that in cases which responded there were sufficient megaloblasts in the bone marrow to be stimulated (dysplastic type), and that in those which failed to respond (hypoplastic type) the failure was due to a paucity or lack of megaloblasts in the marrow.

A large number of cases of megaloblastic anemia due to sprue, seen since these investigations were begun, have demonstrated that the hypoplastic or exhausted marrow type is the prevalent one in sprue cachexia and that no amount of liver extract will benefit such cases. The hope of the patient lies in the ingestion of sufficient food of animal origin to restock his marrow with megaloblasts. Then the hormone will probably work; at least it has seemed so from one or two recent cases. This investigation has brought out quite forcibly the necessity for the construction of Price-Jones curves demonstrating the mean and median diameters of red cells and the degree of anisocytosis ("the dispersion"), and this is proving that it is not so much the color index as the information derived from this curve which entitles one to judge the nature of these severe anemias. One of the by-products of this study has been the appearance, shortly after a reticulocytosis due to the megaloblastic hormone, of a decided eosinophilia even to 30 per cent which, by the way, bespeaks a more favorable prognosis.

(b) *Blood Chemistry.*—Most of the chemical changes in the blood seem to be due to nutritional unbalance and are not limited to sprue. In 47 cases, 30 severe, 14 moderate and 3 mild, the averages were about as follows, in milligrams per cent: sugar, 102; creatinine, 2.5; uric acid, 4; urea nitrogen, 15.5; nonprotein nitrogen, 40. It is significant that these values were about the same for 22 cases of the uncomplicated nutritional unbalance syndrome. There is, therefore, retention of nitrogen, which would explain the tendency to neuritis, neuralgia and myalgia, as well as other symptoms. There is a strikingly low figure for cholesterol in many of these cases and a high icteric index.

The calcium content was made the subject of a special study, as Harold Scott had claimed great benefit in sprue from the oral administration of 0.0065 of parathyroid gland extract combined with 0.65

of calcium lactate. The writer gave this treatment three times a day to 45 persons with pure nutritional unbalance for a year, and at the end of that time the total serum calcium averaged 9.09 mg. per cent, the diffusible 4.09. In addition, 22 cases of sprue, many of them severe, were given the same treatment and it was found that after an average of 286 doses the total serum calcium in these cases averaged 8.92 mg. per cent, the diffusible 3.9. An extensive investigation was now planned, comprising 708 persons. The results of an analysis of the calcium content of their serum by Tisdall's modification of Kramer and Tisdall's method can be summarized as follows:

No. cases	Source	Average total Ca.	Average diffusible Ca.	Percentage below norm. min. Total Ca.	Percentage below norm. min. Diffus. Ca.
96	Healthy..........	9.6	4.69	17	38.5
101	Nutritional unbal-				
	ance..........	9.2	4.2	45.6	66.3
55	Sprue............	9.2	4.11	47.2	72.7
456	Inmates insane				
	asylum	8.7	3.69	57.4	79.3

It is therefore a matter of nutrition. The food of the insane was said to be poor and they seemed by all odds the worst nourished of the lot. It is interesting to note here that one-half of the cases of severe and cachectic sprue gave a normal calcium content in the serum.

(c) *Serology of the Blood.*—In the 1920 series, 601 assorted cases suffering from a variety of diseases and conditions were subjected to the complement deviation test, using as antigen killed cultures of *Monilia psilosis* raised in virulence by passage through animals. Of 348 cases of clinical sprue, 90 per cent were positive; of 102 clinically suspicious cases, 61.7 per cent were positive. Only 6 of 151 cases, or 4 per cent, presenting no signs of the disease were positive.

The deviation of the complement, however, proved to be a group reaction, as the same cases positive for *Monilia psilosis* were also positive, although usually in less degree, for antigens of killed cultures of other *Monilia* and even a *Torulopsis*, and the procedure was dropped as fallacious. While for purposes of diagnosis the test is misleading, it is not, however, without considerable value as throwing some light on the true etiology of sprue, shown by Michel's excellent work.

The Chemical Analysis of Gastric and Duodenal Contents.—The Einhorn tube was passed in 41 cases after a test meal of a cup of bouillon or chicken broth skimmed of its fat a half-hour before. Readings were made at intervals of 15 minutes. Achylia was found in 16 cases, or 39 per cent. The estimation of degree of acidity was made by the titration method, using decinormal sodium hydrate solution in all but 8 cases. The average result in these cases on first removal was 26.78 degrees. In 8 cases the *p*H was estimated, the contents of the stomach being received under neutral oil and results were as follows: 2.54, 2.35, 3.23, 3.23.

The duodenal contents showed a high acidity and a reduction in amylase and lipase. However, the results of these experiments are in discord with those of some other investigators. It seems incredible that organs which are reduced to nearly half their size, with the evident insufficiency of gastric and intestinal digestion, should be perfectly normal in function.

Feces.—There is a marked excess of fatty acids over neutral fats (5 to 10:1). In one of the writer's cases, in the enormous output of 1,138.4 gm. of feces for the twenty-four hours on a measured milk diet, the total fat, including fatty acids, soaps and neutral fats, was 53.28 gm. This woman was on a diet of 2,400 c.c. of milk containing 3 per cent of fat, hence she lost 74 per cent of the fat ingested, instead of a normal maximum of 20 per cent for a healthy person. The stools, it is said, contain a normal quantity of bile pigment in the form of leukobilin or urobilinogen, and for this reason are light in color. As a rule they are intensely acid but in the interval between acute exacerbations may be alkaline. This applies quite as forcibly to the saliva.

In the severe and cachectic grades of sprue, *Monilia psilosis* is much more apt to be absent from stool cultures, chiefly for two reasons: (1) In such cases the symptoms are largely due to more or less permanent functional weakness and inactivity of digestive glands and serious anatomical changes in the secretory and absorptive surface of the intestinal canal. It is in this condition that the stools are often alkaline and *Monilia psilosis* does not prosper. (2) Such serious symptoms have compelled the patient to observe a restricted, often an exclusive milk diet before consulting the writer, or other physicians have been sustaining the patient for some time on the writer's sprue diet which is well known to his colleagues in Porto Rico.

Of 280 cases of sprue, 193 were severe or cachectic. In the vast majority of these cases, only one culture of feces was made, 55.3 per cent revealing *Monilia psilosis*. This should be contrasted with 6.6 per cent of positive results in 288 cases of nutritional unbalance, 4.7 per cent in 126 cases of other diseases and 5.6 per cent positive in 178 healthy persons. In a series previous to this one, embracing a smaller proportion of severe cases, 225 cases of clinical sprue gave 75 per cent of positive fecal cultures (series 1914–1917).

Urine: Volume in 24 hours; 37 cases, 1,278 c.c.
    Specific gravity; 148 cases, 1.016.
    Reaction; of 142 cases, 87 per cent were acid.
    Urea; 135 cases, 17.4 gm. per liter.
    Uric acid; 85 cases, 0.45 gm. per liter.
    Chlorides; 131 cases, 8.45 gm. per liter.
    Sulphates; 26 cases, 2 gm. per liter.
    Phosphates; 105 cases, 1.84 gm. per liter.
    Albumin; of 166 cases, 30 per cent yielded albumin, but only 9 per cent more than a trace.
    Sugar; all but 5 of 135 cases were negative; only one had over 1 per cent.
    Indican; in 144 cases, 71 per cent were normal; 19 per cent showed a moderate increase; 10 per cent a great excess.
    Urobilin; not found in 23 cases.
    Bile pigment; of 143 cases, 86 per cent were negative; only 5 per cent had over a trace.
    Sediment; oxalate of calcium crystals were noted in 20 per cent of 55 cases; cells of the renal pelvis in 23 per cent; pyocytes in 63 per cent; hyaline and granular casts in 21 per cent.

Diagnosis.—The diagnosis is made on the clinical history and physical findings and is strengthened by the revelation of an abundant colonization of *Monilia psilosis* in the stool. A history of chronic fermentative diarrhea in warm climates with great loss of weight and without positive evidence of well known bacterial or protozoal causes of intestinal disease, should make one suspicious of sprue and provoke mycological cultures of the feces. When to this the typical tongue and the small liver are added, a reasonable working diagnosis is provided.

Cultures should always be made according to the following standard technic, and always before diet or other treatment has intervened to diminish temporarily the efflorescence of the yeast in the intestinal canal. Sabouraud's glucose agar (peptone 10, glucose 40, agar 20, water 1000, set at pH 6 to 6.5) is the preferred medium. Plates are poured and allowed to solidify. Small particles of the feces are now transferred from a sterile container which are plated in 25 points on the surface of the agar. These are left at from 20° to 30° C. for several days. Generally at the end of the third or fourth day, little, round, glistening, smooth, convex, cream-colored colonies are detected. If only one colony develops out of the 25 points of contact, *Monilia psilosis* may be simply a chance contaminant of fruit or bread, on its way through the bowel like so much waste, but if multiple points of contact show colonies, the higher the number the more the probability of an active colonization in the bowel of the host. This organism is now purified by the usual Koch three-plate method and a pure colony obtained. With this, a U-tube containing a 4 per cent maltose peptone water is inoculated, a stab culture in plain gelatin is made, and a Sabouraud glucose agar slant is sown. If in the course of two days to a week or two, gas is produced in the U-tube, and in two weeks the inverted pine tree in the gelatin and the characteristic macroscopic growth on the slant appear, the chances are that we are dealing with *Monilia psilosis*. This diagnosis will be assured by recognizing the typical organism in a loopful of the sediment from the U-tube under the oil immersion of the microscope. If everything is typical save that maltose is not fermented, either another U-tube is sown or 5 c.c. of the liquid culture are injected into the marginal vein of a rabbit or the belly of a guinea-pig. Retroculture from an animal killed by the organism will usually ferment maltose bouillon. For those who wish to employ the complement deviation test, reference is made to Michel's standard work for the technique (see bibliography).

DIFFERENTIAL DIAGNOSIS.—*The Syndrome of the Pre-sprue Nutritional Unbalance.*—While this syndrome is the shadow of sprue, save for the usual absence of glossitis and diarrhea, there is nothing decisive about the picture and the patient is merely ailing. Cultures of the feces will here be of importance.

Bacillary Dysentery.—The onset is acute and there are fever, tenesmus, abdominal pain, and small, frequent, blood-stained, mucoid stools. Agglutination tests are positive.

Amebic Dysentery.—Recurring bloody and mucoid stools, of a different character from those of sprue, tenderness over the colon, and the presence of *Entameba histolytica* are outstanding.

Chronic Malaria.—There is a history of febrile attacks, splenomegaly and mononucleosis are present, and the plasmodium may be found by thick films or splenic puncture.

Intestinal Tuberculosis.—The character of the diarrhea, fever, abdominal tenderness, foci in the lung or elsewhere, and positive results of inoculation of laboratory animals should clear up the diagnosis. Sprue is an afebrile disease, as a rule; in fact, persistent subnormal temperature is usually observed.

Uncinariasis.—There is a history of ground-itch, absence of the typical excoriation of the tongue and the stools are more apt to be lienteric. There is a tendency to dilated heart and anasarca, generally an eosinophilia, and the ova can easily be found in the stools.

Chronic Pancreatitis.—The neutral fats in the stools are greatly in excess of the fatty acids.

Pellagra.—Pellagra is more apt to attack the poor of rural districts. Seasonal incidence is prominent. The stools are usually pigmented and there is a normal absorption of fats. The tongue is smaller and pointed, the glossitis is more general, and the red color is deeper. Anemia is not a characteristic of pellagra. The skin lesions of pellagra never occur in sprue as the skin is not hypersensitive to the sun's rays. *Monilia psilosis* is usually absent. The mental symptoms of pellagra are missing in sprue and the lesions of brain or cord are constant in the former. Pellagra is not a disease which can be easily confused with sprue, save in pellagra sine pellagra, which is apt to be sprue, not pellagra.

Idiopathic Pernicious Anemia (Addison's Disease).—The subcutaneous fat is preserved; the tongue, while it may be subjectively sensitive, is not characteristically excoriated as in sprue, nor do abrupt appearance and disappearance of the lesions occur. The liver is not usually diminished in size. Diarrhea is not a constant feature and the stools are apt to be pigmented. Distinct cord lesions are manifest.

Gastric Ulcer, Duodenal Ulcer, Cholecystitis, Appendicitis.—All four may be roughly simulated, at times, by gastro-intestinal symptoms in sprue. The sheet anchors here are careful radiographic studies of the digestive tract and laboratory analyses. Erosions and shallow ulceration of stomach and duodenum neither give roentgenologic evidence nor warrant operation.

Tuberculosis of the Tongue.—The lesions are deep and do not appear and disappear rapidly as in sprue. The same may be said of the tongue lesions of tertiary syphilis, different from both.

Geographic Tongue.—This affection is common in the tropics, especially among children. The lesion is very superficial, takes a serpiginous course, and seems neither to cause symptoms nor to be accompanied by constitutional disturbances.

Hereditary Fissured and Rough Tongue.—There are no symptoms and the filiform papillae are hypertrophied.

Complications.—A PERNICIOUS TYPE OF ANEMIA.—The term "pernicious anemia" is believed today to be unscientific and misleading, for what is meant is idiopathic pernicious anemia, or Addison's disease, and in the definition given in medical literature that condition of the blood and hemopoietic organs which is also found in uncinariasis, *Diphyllobothrium latum* anemia, sprue and other diseases is stated or insinuated as fundamental and pathognomonic. Idiopathic pernicious anemia is a disease perfectly distinct from sprue. While the effect on the blood is frequently so nearly like that of Addison's disease as to render differential diagnosis impossible, an additional toxic element, not present in sprue, is apparently responsible for subacute combined degeneration of the cord in the classical idiopathic affection. The megaloblastic anemia of sprue is one of its most dreaded complications and has been described.

GASTRIC AND DUODENAL ULCERS.—These ulcers are apt to be very shallow or, indeed, only a raw condition such as is seen in the tongue may give rise to signs and symptoms of these lesions, with the important exception that radiographic evidence is usually lacking and surgical intervention often harmful.

PROCTITIS AND HEMORRHOIDS.—These may be serious complications. In several instances the writer has seen the constant irritation from a long-standing proctitis result in cancer.

CERTAIN BRONCHOMYCOSES, TONSILLOMYCOSES, EPIDERMOMYCOSES AND ONYCHOMYCOSES are not infrequent complications of sprue, as has been foreshadowed elsewhere.

LEUKOPLAKIA is a not uncommon complication seen by the writer and mentioned here and there in the literature. In a case of sprue treated by the writer it developed without a trace of syphilis in an otherwise healthy young woman.

Sequelae.—ABDOMINAL PTOSES.—Sprue is a disease which diminishes the function of most organs. Now, as the function of supporting connective tissue is mainly to sustain the abdominal organs in their position, when the fibers of this supporting tissue weaken, there is a tendency for these organs to descend toward the pelvis. Thus it is that we find such an abnormal number of ptoses of stomach, intestines, etc., with their consequent operative treatment and often their logical failure to permanently relieve or correct.

INSUFFICIENCY OF DIGESTIVE GLANDS.—This is apt to be permanent in long-standing cases and in the old. It is the chief factor in relapses, sometimes occurring after many years, and the principal obstacle to the return of the patient to the Tropics where the monotonous heat depresses cellular activity. The insufficiency of the liver is particularly apt to be permanent.

Association with Other Diseases.—TUBERCULOSIS.—Undoubtedly this disease claims first rank among those associated with sprue from its tendency to flare up in any long continued condition of malnutrition. About ten per cent of the writer's cases of tuberculosis of the lungs were also far advanced in sprue and, conversely, cure of their sprue frequently brought about such a regression of an incipient tuberculous process as apparently to cure the patient.

SYPHILIS.—This disease acts to greatly enhance the picture of glandular insufficiency, as, naturally, the chronic stages of syphilis are notable for their perturbation of important glandular organs such as the pancreas. It is always well to attack syphilis vigorously by neosalvarsan or its congeners as soon as possible before hoping to secure lasting results from any treatment directed against sprue, but great care should be taken to investigate the state of function of the liver, as the writer suspects that arsenic in this form has precipitated a form of pernicious anemia in several of his cases.

UNCINARIASIS AND MALARIA.—These are formidable adversaries of the sprue patient and specific treatment should be promptly applied. The manifest danger of purging the case of advanced sprue should make one cautious in the administration of vermifuges, and carbon tetrachloride should never be used.

DYSENTERY.—Sprue is so often a sequela of amebic dysentery, in countries where the latter disease is endemic, as to perturb the recognition of the former. This was notable in the history of sprue in Cochin-china where the French were blinded to its true nature in the midst of an acrid dispute over the identity of the two diseases.

Treatment.—Dietetic Treatment.—When one reads that sprue is a singularly intractable disease, tending toward a fatal termination, and then turns to the chapter on treatment and finds that an author counsels a little sugar with this and a ''light cereal'' with that, a rasher of crisp breakfast bacon and plenty of rich milk, it is easy to see why he is pessimistic.   There can be no compromise on the admission of sugar of commerce, cereals and fats in an active case of sprue.   This is fundamental. No matter what particular view the physician may have of the etiology, his success must rest largely on the banishing of these components from the diet of the sprue patient.*

The essentials to recovery in the long run are (1) **prohibition of fatty foods and added fats,** (2) **a sugar- and cereal-free diet,** (3) **a reinforcement to the greatly reduced digestive ferments.**   With an early diagnosis and intervention before too much damage has been wrought, it is by no means necessary, nor is it advisable, to begin with so exacting and monotonous a diet as milk alone.   Patients with a mere dyspepsia and occasional looseness of the bowels, obliged to earn their living, will not tolerate it in practice.   It is the duty of the physician to **return a patient to his normal avocation** as soon as possible, and he should avoid restrictions which diminish the latter's efficiency as a wage-earner in every manner possible, and protect him against the burden of expense entailed by unnecessary idleness.   A milk diet commits both of these faults, as a rule, and should be used only when absolutely necessary. There must be potent reasons for employing a starvation diet in a disease where symptoms are the result of tissue starvation and exhaustion.

The writer has run the gamut of ''cures'' for sprue but has for the last fifteen years finally settled upon a **liberal diet** which not only permits normal activity in the average case, but which starves the fungus that takes a part in causing the disease, not the patient.   In fully 95 per cent of his cases this diet has been quite satisfactory to both patient and physician.   The following is the diet sheet recommended:

Breakfast: Coffee with milk, sweetened with saccharin.
> Two soft-boiled or poached eggs.
> One of the following fruits: oranges, grapefruit, large bananas, apples, pears, peaches, mangoes, ripe pawpaw.

Midday meal: Hot bouillon or chicken broth with small pieces of the vegetables allowed in this diet.
> A half-pound of beefsteak with a little salt, lightly broiled, or lean, rare roast beef or roast chicken. If a tender variety of beef cannot be secured, or for the purpose of varying the diet, a good quality of beef can be chopped up, made into a meat ball and seared over a hot fire. It should be turned out on a previously heated plate and eaten while hot. Fresh fish, broiled or baked, is permitted, as well as are eggs.
> Fresh vegetables from the garden, baked or boiled; okra, cymbelings, squash, carrots, spinach, asparagus, beets, tomatoes, turnips, string beans, lima beans, peas and eggplant. If one is living in the Antillan tropics, the following native vegetables can be used: yautia blanca, boiled or mashed; amarillos, roasted or boiled; casabe (baked); chayote; ñame. A salad on the basis of chopped beet leaves or lettuce with tomatoes, celery, asparagus, beets, cucumbers, pawpaw, chayote, cabbage or fruits. These salads should never be omitted and should be eaten in abundance.

Afternoon repast: Tea or coffee with milk, or skimmed chicken broth.

* Fairley's use of glucose in substitution for sugar of commerce is based on the direct absorption of a monosaccharid without the intervention of any intestinal enzyme. The writer is experimenting in a series of cases with the hope of corroborating the benefit claimed for this addition to the dietary.

Dinner: As for the midday meal.

Supper: A glass of hot milk or some fruit.

Articles prohibited: Sugar and anything that may contain it, such as pastry, preserves and sweetened canned fruits, raisins, dried prunes, ice cream and the product of the soda-water fountain.

Bread and anything containing wheat flour, such as cakes, biscuits, and crackers.

All cereals and flours made from grains such as rice, cornmeal, ''corn flakes'' and other such cereal derivatives with trade names. To this list should be added beans.

Potatoes, sweet potatoes, alligator pears and pineapples.

Remarks: Food should be well prepared and well served. Fried food should not be permitted.

The principal object is to increase the nutrition by providing a diet rich in the elements which are to form muscular tissue, glandular tissue, and nervous tissue, as well as in those containing vitamins. No less than a pound of meat a day is recommended.

(Calorie values should be calculated and should not fall below 1800 C. a day.)

This **diet must be sustained** usually **a long time,** three to six months or a year, and even then the addition of bread, sugar or rice, and, above all, grease, may bring back the earmarks of the old enemy. One must be careful not to become discouraged at a sudden indigestion, often interpreted as a ''relapse,'' in spite of this diet. In reality, if close questioning is resorted to, we will find that some severe physiological strain has brought about a true suspension of digestion. A tablespoonful of **castor oil** and a **day of reduced alimentation in bed** will usually permit the patient to resume his dietetic regimen in twenty-four hours.

This is the diet which should be employed for the benign, the moderate and the moderately severe cases of sprue as well as for its preceding nutritional unbalance. For very **severe and cachectic cases,** one must consider more carefully the digestibility of foods and the tolerance of the patient and for such were created the one-sided diets, known as the ''milk,'' ''fruit'' and ''meat'' cures.

The ''Milk Cure.''—This is adapted to the periods of **violent rawness of tongue and incessant diarrhea** and it should usually be continued until they disappear. A moderate dose of some **aperient** is first given, the patient is **put to bed** in absolute repose of mind and body, if possible a nurse is procured, and **milk** is begun to the exclusion of every other food. The writer has been accustomed to order 1,800 to 2,000 c.c. a day, distributed in two-hourly doses, and taken slowly through a straw. At least eight hours of **sleep** should be provided for, but in case of **great weakness,** one or more feedings should be given between 10 p.m. and 6 a.m. Every four days **increase the quantity** by 250 c.c. until the patient is taking as near 3 to 3½ liters, or more, as he can comfortably tolerate. More than 4 liters is not advised.

In the first week there is apt to be loss of weight, increased amount of intestinal gas, and a longing for solid food combined with a loathing for milk, but the curious unrestful mental state, with inability to concentrate the attention, will give place to a clearness and tranquillity of mind that will outweigh the bodily discomfort.

This diet yields, roughly, from 1,100, at the beginning, to 2,300 calories a day, if the milk is, as it should be, not high in fat. The next week is usually marked by normal bowel movements, healing of the tongue, disappearance or great reduction of intestinal gas and general improvement. After from three to six weeks of a strict milk diet, **fruits** may be added, then **vegetables,** and, last of all, the **full liberal**

sprue diet, the quantity of milk being gradually decreased as these articles are increased.

The **stools** should be **daily seen** by the physician, and if digestion is poor it may be improved by mixing with each feeding a couple of ounces of **banana flour gruel,** one tablespoonful of freshly made banana flour being added to a quart of water and the whole slowly simmered down to a pint.

There is a class of people, relatively small despite the protests of the majority who insist that they cannot tolerate milk, in whom this article of food is not well borne. For such the meat and fruit "cures" were devised.

The "Meat Cure."—This was first recommended by Cantlie, and, for cases not tolerating milk, especially those marked by violent diarrhea, or in whom for any other reason milk cannot be used, it is certainly a boon to the sufferer and to the poor physician, at his wit's end. Here again, **no other food** should be given. Combination of this diet with milk is fraught with disaster.

The patient is **put to bed** and the **diet is sustained** under the same conditions in which the milk was administered. Two pounds of **rump steak or fillet** are minced with a chopping-knife, **not** with the mincing machine, salt is added, and the chopped meat is left on a platter and stored in the ice chest. Every three hours one sixth of this quantity is removed and rapidly and lightly seared in a buttered saucepan, previously well heated over a direct fire. One half hour before each feeding, **hot tea** or **broth, or weak fresh plantain gruel** is served. This diet cannot be endured, as a rule, over a week, as the repugnance for meat has become strong, but this is sufficient time to work a marvelous change in the patient as gas and diarrhea are meanwhile usually dissipated. A gradual induction into the **liberal sprue diet** is now begun.

The "Fruit Cure."—In general, this consists of **gradually increasing small feedings** at very short intervals until several pounds of fruit per day are ingested. **Very acid fruits** should be **avoided.** When the patient begins to improve, the **liberal sprue diet** is in order.

In short, for 95 per cent of all cases of sprue the liberal diet described should be the ideal one. For acute cases, violent bouts of diarrhea and advanced cachexia with raw tongue and diarrhea, the milk diet. For those of the latter class who cannot tolerate milk, either the meat or fruit diet.

MEDICINAL TREATMENT.—The following prescription seems to be of positive benefit in sprue:

```
℞  Pancreatin
   Takadiastase  ........................................  āā 15.
   Magnes. oxid.  ......................................     25.
   Calcii carbonat.  ...................................     50.
          M. et divid. in chart.  No. 50.
          Sig.  One powder after each of the three meals.
```

Strychnine is probably the best general tonic and may be advantageously combined with **dilute hydrochloric acid** and compound tincture of **cardamom.** If a check needs to be placed on too frequent bowel movements, the following has proved useful in the writer's hands:

℞   Tinct. opii deodorat 4
    Bismuth. subnitrat.
    Cret. preparat. .... $\overline{aa}$ 13
    Syr. acaciae 100
    Aquae cinnamon 200
        Sig.   One tablespoonful every two hours until relief.

While certain remedies for special situations may be required, the routine use of other drugs is believed futile if not **harmful;** this is especially applicable to **iron** and **arsenic.** Only in the dysplastic anemia is **liver extract** to be given systematically. The administration of **yeast** is not only a failure; it is a hidden **danger** and it increases intestinal gas. In the hands of the writer, santonin proved to be an utter failure besides being a renal irritant. **Hydrotherapy, massage** and **heliotherapy** are of real value. A change of climate in sprue, from the standpoint of the tropical resident who must earn his living there, is like recommending amputation for a troublesome limb. The vulnerable point in the Tropics is undoubtedly the intestinal canal, but residents of northern climates have a no less vulnerable respiratory apparatus.

In closing this review of the treatment of sprue, let us remember a most important factor in recharging a devitalized body: **rest.** Repose of body and mind, freedom from the strain of work and worry, and a tranquil spirit give the fullest play to whatsoever reparative treatment that may be employed.

PROPHYLAXIS.—The real prophylaxis is the **correction of an unbalanced ration,** and a **defense against unnecessary strain** thrown upon the human organism in the Tropics. In the correction of the ration should be comprehended a radical **curtailing of sweets and cereals** but especially **grease,** an **increase in fresh garden truck,** and a **better and larger supply of dairy products and animal foods.**

Prognosis.—Cases not responding to diet within three months and pernicious types of anemia failing to yield to reticulocytosis after the administration of liver extract are very serious ones and the mortality probably exceeds 50 per cent. This is the sprue of older authors, the cachexia of sprue which has given the disease its bad name. The immense majority of cases which respond to diet within three months tend toward recovery, which is permanent if subsequently the nutritional unbalance originally provoking the disease is avoided. The salvation of the patient lies more in himself than in his physician.

Pathology.—Owing to comparatively few autopsies there is little yet to be said of the morbid anatomy of sprue. The intestinal wall is by no means always thin, as has been reported. There is almost unanimity of findings in the mucosa which usually shows inflammatory changes. Ulceration is not typical of sprue nor are the ulcers deep. They are usually so small and superficial as to be overlooked. The small size of liver, pancreas, spleen, etc., seems due entirely to wasting.

The following is a summary by Dr. E. Koppisch of cases so far studied pathologically in the School of Tropical Medicine of Porto Rico:

"A study of ten cases that came to autopsy failed to reveal pathognomonic lesions. The fat throughout the body was greatly diminished. The tongue showed atrophy of the mucous membrane with desquamation of the superficial layers and more or less complete elimination of the filiform and fungiform papillae. In three cases a fungal growth was present on the surface and mycelium was found penetrating the epithelial layer. Two of these were cultured and *Monilia psilosis* Ashford was obtained. We did not see ulceration of the mucosa of the small intestine. The walls were thin due to atrophy but in the stomach this did not reach the degree seen in idiopathic pernicious anemia. Inflammatory changes were noted in about one-third of the cases; in one, these extended to the submucosa. An acute or chronic colitis, with or without ulceration, was a complicating factor in four cases. In no instance was a mycelial growth found invading the mucosa of the esophagus, stomach or intestine.

"In the liver, fatty changes were frequent and there was much iron-containing pigment in the liver cells and in the Kupffer elements. The amount is much less than in idiopathic pernicious anemia. The peculiar hyaline degeneration of the venous endothelium of the spleen described by Bahr was not observed, and Russell's acid-fuchsin bodies, although present, have not been at all numerous. The pancreas has been invariably normal in its histologic structure, except for slight interacinar fibrosis in two cases. None of the cases studied presented cord changes.

"The bone marrow was completely aplastic in four cases and presented serous atrophy of its fat; in two there was moderate hyperplasia of all elements; in three a marked hyperplasia was in evidence, and the picture was not distinguishable from that found in pernicious anemia. A study of sixteen cases of clinical sprue in which borings of the tibia for the collection of bone marrow during life was performed, in general has given results similar to those above described. There was complete aplasia of the bone marrow in seven; moderate hyperplasia in one; areas of hyperplasia in an aplastic bone marrow in one, and active regeneration in six. One case presented active hyperplasia followed in several months by aplasia.''

History and Distribution.—Sprue was first identified by William Hillary in Barbados in 1766. Throughout a century little or no attention was paid to it as a distinct disease. In 1860, French naval surgeons announced a disease which they claimed to be distinct from dysentery and for twenty years their clinical conviction was pitted against the uncompromising pathologist back in the home country who refused to see in the intestinal flux anything but an evidence of dysentery. As dysentery also existed in those countries, and ulcers were often found in cases with superimposed sprue, the pathologist who was not on the ground apparently won the battle and deprived France of the honor that fell to Sir Patrick Manson, in 1880, of clearly annunciating in a short article of five pages what has ever since been known by the name he gave it.

In 1901, Kohlbrügge described a yeast prevalent in the feces in sprue which he also found invading the mucous membrane and intestine.

In 1905, Castellani began a series of studies on the yeast-budding fungi of the feces of sprue patients, culminating in Bahr's brochure (see bibliography).

In 1914, Ashford described a Monilia very consistently found in the tongue and feces of sprue in Porto Rico which he later named *Monilia psilosis*. The relation of this yeast to sprue is still under discussion.

The best known foci of sprue are found in the Malayan archipelago as a center, extending north to China, south to Australia, east to Korea and the Philippines, and west to India, taking in practically all the intermediate islands, and confining itself largely to tropical regions. In the New World it is a scourge of the West Indies and Central America and is evidently much more prevalent in the south of the United States than has been heretofore realized.

Sociologic Aspects.—The sociologic importance of sprue is that of its chief predisposing factor, the peculiar nutritional unbalance of most tropical countries where the disease exists. Alike a basis also for tuberculosis and uncinariasis, it is this factor that is responsible, more than the organisms which elaborate upon it their well known clinical personality, for most of the high mortality and physical inefficiency of tropical residents is due to ignorance of a balanced diet for the Tropics. This condition, and not so much the diseases it makes possible, should interest the educationalist and statesman, if the Tropics are ever to become again the highest expression of human civilization.

BIBLIOGRAPHY

ANTOINE, F.: Essai sur la diarrhée endémique de Cochinchine, Thèse de Paris, 1873.

ASHFORD, B. K.: Notes on sprue in Porto Rico and the results of treatment by yellowed santonin, Am. J. Trop. Dis. (etc.), 1 : 146–158, 1913.

——: Is sprue a moniliasis of the digestive tract? Am. J. Trop. Dis. (etc.), 3 : 32–46, 1915–16.

——: Further experimentation in animals with a *Monilia* commonly found in sprue, Am. J. M. Sc., 151 : 520–529, 1915.

——: The etiology of sprue, Am. J. M. Sc., 154 : 157–176, 1917.

——: Sprue; Chapter in Oxford Loose-leaf Medicine, Oxford University Press, Amer. Br. edited by Mackenzie and Christian.

——: Observations on the conception that sprue is a mycosis superimposed upon a state of deficiency in certain food elements, Am. J. Trop. Med., 2 : 305, 1922.

——: A clinical investigation of tropical sprue, Am. J. M. Sc., 165 : 157, 1923.

——: Tropical sprue in Porto Rico; a synthesis of fifteen years' work of investigation and two thousand two hundred cases, Proc. Internat. Conference on Health Problems in Trop. Amer., Held at Kingston, Jamaica, B. W. I., pp. 686–708, Med. Depart. United Fruit Comp., 1924.

——: Certain conditions of the gastro-intestinal tract in Porto Rico and their relation to tropical sprue, Am. J. Trop. Med., 8 : 507, 1928.

——: The anemias of sprue; their nature and treatment, Arch. Int. Med., 45 : 647, 1930.

——: The mycology of the intestinal canal in Porto Rico and its relation to tropical sprue, J. Am. M. Ass., 93 : 762, 1929.

——: The significance of mycology in tropical medicine, Arch. Dermat. & Syph., 22 : 7, 1930.

——: The Mycoses, Chapter in Nelson's Loose-leaf Living Medicine, New York, Thomas Nelson & Sons.

—— AND HERNANDEZ, L. G.: Blood-serum calcium in sprue and other pathologic states in the tropics, Am. J. M. Sc., 171 : 575–591, 1926.

BAHR, P. H.: A Report on Researches on Sprue in Ceylon, 1912–14, Brochure of 155 pages, Cambridge University Press, 1915.

——: Sprue, Practice of Medicine in the Tropics, Oxford publications, edited by W. Byam and R. G. Archibald, 3 : 2248.

BAUMGARTENER, E. A. AND SMITH, G. D.: Pernicious anemia and tropical sprue, Arch. Int. Med., 40 : 203–215, 1927.

——: Monilia psilosis as a cause of tropical sprue, Am. J. Trop. Med., 6 : 433, 1926.

BEGGS, C.: Santonin in sprue, Lancet, 1 : 185 (Jan. 15) 1888.

BERTRAND AND FONTAN: De l'entéro-colite chronique endémique des pays chauds, Doin, Paris, 8 : 428, 1887.

BOGGS, T. R. AND PINCOFFS, M. C.: A case of pulmonary moniliasis in the United States, Tr. A. Am. Phys., 30 : 474, 1915; Johns Hopkins Hosp. Bull., 26 : 407–410, 1915.

BOYD, M. F.: Is sprue endemic in the South? South. M. J., 13 : 229–232, 1920.

BROWN, T. R.: The absence of pancreatic secretions in sprue and the employment of pancreatic extract in the treatment of the disease, Am. J. M. Sc., 161 : 501, 1921.

——: The gastro-intestinal findings in a case of sprue, with a note on the treatment based on these findings, Johns Hopkins Hosp. Bull., 26 : 289–291, 1916.

——: Sprue, Johns Hopkins Hosp. Bull., 27 : 289, 1916.

CANTLIE, J.: Sprue and chronic intestinal lesions, J. Trop. Med., 9 : 277–279, 1906.

——: Sprue; its causes, signs and symptoms, pathology and treatment, Internat. Clin., 2 : 113–121, 1898.

CARNEGIE-BROWN, W.: Sprue and Its Treatment, New York, Wm. Wood and Co., 8 : 260.

CASTELLANI, A.: Notes on the hyphomycetes found in sprue, J. Trop. Med., 17: 305–310, 1914.

——: Blastomycosis and some other conditions due to yeast-like fungi, Am. J. Trop. Med., 8: 379–422, 1928.

—— AND LOW, G. C.: The rôle played by fungi in sprue, J. Trop. Med. (etc.), 16: 33–35, 1913.

CUNNINGHAM, J. M.: Fourteenth Annual Report of the Sanitary Commissioner, Calcutta, India, pp. 143–152, 1877.

DALMAU, L. M.: Remarques sur la technique mycologique, Ann. de Parasitologie, 7: 536–545, 1929.

DOLD, H.: The etiology of sprue, China M. J., 31: 387–392, 1917.

—— AND FISCHER, W.: Anatomical findings in experimental sprue, China M. J., 32: 125–131, 1918.

ELDERS, C.: Over Indische spruw, Nederl. Tijdschr. v. Geneesk., 2: 1683–1690, 1919.

——: Over de proeven van McCarrison in verband met de opvatting dat spruw een deficientieziete is., Nederl. Tijdschr. v. Geneesk., 2: 2189, 1920.

——: Over den vorm, het beloop en de prognose van de anaemie bij Indische spruw en over de aetiologie van pernicieuse anaemie, Nederl. Tijdschr. v. Geneesk., 2: 2267–2276, 1922.

ETIENNE, C. J. J.: Un mot sur la diarrhée de Cochinchine et sur son traitement, Thèse de Montpellier, 1877.

FAIRLEY, N. H.: Sprue; its applied pathology, biochemistry and treatment, Tr. Roy. Soc. Trop. Med & Hyg., 24: 131, 1930.

FLEISHER, M. S. AND WACHOWIAK, M.: The presence of yeast-like bodies in the blood of human beings, Am. J. Trop. Med., 3: 59–68, 1923.

——: The relation of Fungi Imperfecti to diarrheal conditions, Am. J. M. Sc., 168: 371–380, 1924.

HEATON, TREVOR: The etiology of sprue, Indian J. M. Research, 7: 810, 1920.

HILLARY, WILLIAM: Observations on the Changes of Air and the Concomitant Epidemical Diseases in the Island of Barbados, Ed. 2, London, printed for L. Hawes, W. Clarke, and R. Collins, 8: 276–297, 1766.

JUSTI, K.: Sprue or Aphthae Tropicae, Arch. f. Schiffs- u. Tropen-Hyg., 17: 517–567, 1913.

KELSCH, L. F. AND KIENER, P. L.: Traité des maladies des pays chauds, Paris, Baillière, 8: 920, 1889.

KOHLBRÜGGE, I. H. F.: Eene Biedrage tot de Aetiologie der Indische Spruw, Nederl. Tijdschr. v. Geneesk., 37: 881–890, 1901.

LANGERON, M.: Blastomycoses, Nouveau Traité de Médecine, part 4, pp. 510–534.

LE DANTEC, A.: Présence d'une levure dans la sprue; sa signification pathogénique, Bull. Soc. path. exot., 1: 342–344, 1908.

LOW, G. C.: Sprue; an analytical study of 150 cases, Quart. J. Med., 21: 523–534, 1928.

MANSON, P.: Notes on sprue, China Imp. Customs Med. Rep., 19–24, 1880–1882.

——: Sprue or Psilosis, System of Medicine, Allbutt and Rolleston, London, Macmillan & Co., 2: 545–566, 1907.

MICHEL, C.: A study of toxins and serological reactions in sprue, Am. J. M. Sc., 154: 177–181, 1917.

——: On the use of a Monilia vaccine in the treatment of sprue, J. Infect. Dis., 22: 53–61, 1918.

PATTERSON, J. B.: Symptoms and treatment of sprue, China M. J., 32: 514–521, 1918.

RABE, HELEN: Diet in tropical sprue, Clifton M. Bull., 14: 55–61, 1928.

ROGERS, J. M.: Isolation of Monilia psilosis in tropical sprue (psilosis), J. Am. M. Ass., 79: 1677–1678, 1922.

SMITH, L. W.: The rôle of Monilia psilosis Ashford in experimental sprue, J. Am. M. Ass., 83: 1549–1554, 1924.

——: Monilia psilosis Ashford in severe anemia associated with the sprue syndrome, Philippine J. Sc., 24: 447–465, 1924.

SOKHEY, S. S. AND MALANDKAR, M. A.: Pancreatic function in sprue, Indian J. M. Research, 15: 921–933, 1928.

——: Liver function in sprue, Indian J. M. Research, 15: 553–563, 1928.

TALAIRACH, P.: Quelques considérations sur l'étiologie et le traitement de la diarrhée endémique de Cochinchine, Thèse de Montpellier, 1874.

THIN, GEORGE: A case of psilosis cured by strawberries and milk, J. Trop. Med., 2: 49, 1899–1900.

THOMSON, J. D.: Some analyses of materials obtained from sprue cases, Tr. Roy. Soc. Trop. Med. & Hyg., 18: 381–382, 1925.

VAN DER BURG, C. L.: Indische Spruw (Aphthae Tropicae), Translation in Chinese Imperial Maritime Customs Medical Reports, (Oct.–March) 1883.

WOOD, E. J.: The existence of sprue in the United States, Am. J. M. Sc., 150: 692–699, 1915.

——: The clinical manifestations of tropical sprue, U. S. Nav. M. Bull., 13: 449, 1919.

——: The existence of sprue in North Carolina, Charlotte M. J., 77: 206–208, 1918.

——: Pernicious anemia in its relationship to sprue, Am. J. M. Sc., 169: 28–38, 1925.

LEISHMANIASIS

By Eugene R. Whitmore, B.S., M.D.

Synonyms.—For the Indian visceral type: Kala-azar, Kala-dukh, Dumdum fever, Tropical splenomegaly. For the Mediterranean visceral type: Splenic anemia of infants, Infantile kala-azar, Ponos. For the Oriental cutaneous type: Sart sore, Oriental sore, Aleppo boil, Biskra button, Bagdad boil, Bouton d'orient, Endemic granuloma. For the American cutaneous type: Forest yaws, Bubas, Uta. Espundia is a term applied to the naso-oral involvement in the American cutaneous type.

Definition.—Under the name leishmaniasis are included the diseases due to protozoa belonging to the genus Leishmania. There are two forms of disease due to Leishmania: one a general or visceral disease which commonly progresses to a fatal termination; and one a cutaneous affection which tends to recovery. Again, each of these two forms of leishmaniasis is divided into two types, mainly according to geographic distribution, in each case the types of the disease tending to differ somewhat clinically.

History of Clinical Varieties.—Kala-azar.—When the British occupied the district of the Garos, in Assam, in 1869, they found an endemic disease which the natives called "kala-azar," meaning black fever, so named from the darkened skin of the affected persons. The disease was considered to be malarial cachexia, and its history is confused with that of malaria up to 1900. With the opening up of human intercommunication, the disease spread to neighboring districts; and, on account of the high death rate, it attracted considerable attention.

In 1900 Leishman found what he considered to be degenerated trypanosomes in the spleen of a soldier who died of dumdum fever at Netley; and he published this finding in May, 1903. In July, 1903, Donovan found the same parasites in blood obtained by splenic puncture during life. Laveran and Mesnil considered the organisms to be piroplasms, and gave the name *Piroplasma donovani.* Ross considered that the organism belonged to a different genus, and he created the genus Leishmania, the organism of kala-azar becoming *Leishmania donovani.* In

1904 Rogers cultivated the organism by adding splenic blood to citrated salt solution; and he observed that the cultural forms had a single flagellum.

INFANTILE KALA-AZAR.—Fede described a febrile splenic anemia in children in Italy. In 1904 Cathoire found peculiar bodies in spleen smears from a child that had died of an ill-defined disease in Tunis, and Laveran considered these bodies to be *Leishmania donovani*. In 1905 Pianese found bodies in the spleen of children dead of Fede's splenic anemia; and he considered these bodies identical with *Leishmania donovani*, at the same time calling attention to the similarity of the symptoms of Fede's disease and kala-azar. In 1907 Nicolle studied the disease in Tunis, and considered the parasite to be related to the parasite of Indian kala-azar but not identical with it; he suggested the name "infantile kala-azar" for the disease, and the name of *Leishmania infantum* for the parasite. Gabbi in 1908 reported that he found the disease among adults, and he considered it to be the same as Indian kala-azar.

ORIENTAL SORE.—In 1756 Russell described Aleppo boil, and stated that the natives considered it was due to the drinking water. The disease was described by various observers from that time on, but it was over one hundred years before anyone seemed to doubt that the drinking water was the cause of the disease. From 1868 to 1902, various workers described ova of worms, bacteria, fungi and protozoa in the tissues of cases of Delhi boil. In 1885 Cunningham described endocellular organisms which he considered as stages of some mycetozoal organism. In 1891 Firth confirmed Cunningham's finding, and gave the name *Sporozoon furunculosum* to the organism. In 1898 Borovsky, a Russian military surgeon at Tashkent, described the clinical picture and pathology of "Sart sore"; accurately described the parasite, and recognized it as a protozoon. Shulgin, a colleague of Borovsky at the Tashkent military hospital, came to the conclusion that Sart sore was transmitted by the bite of some nocturnal insect which served as an intermediate host, just as the mosquito does in malaria. In 1903 Wright found round and oval bodies in endothelial cells in smears from an oriental sore on a boy from Armenia. These bodies were 2 to 4 microns in diameter and Wright gave them the name *Helcosoma tropicum*, which became *Leishmania tropica*.

AMERICAN LEISHMANIASIS.—On his voyage to Brazil in 1648, Pisone saw a disease, known as "bouba," which he considered distinct from syphilis. In Brazil it was thought that the disease was brought in by Negroes from the Calabar coast. Since that time there has been confusion regarding the various ulcerative conditions of the skin in Brazil.

In 1895 Moreira reported that for several years the clinicians in Bahia had noted a peculiar variety of cutaneous lesions, known as "Bahia button," and he expressed the opinion that these lesions were the same as Biskra button. He suggested the name "Bouton endemique des pays chauds," as the condition was not confined to the Orient. Adeodato also considered "Bahia button" to be the same as "oriental sore."

In 1895 Breda studied three cases of skin ulceration with mucous membrane involvement from São Paulo. He concluded that "boubas" was not syphilis, tuberculosis or infectious granuloma, but that it was a special disease. He considered that some endemic skin diseases in the Orient should be called "oriental sore," and that some endemic skin diseases in America and Africa should be called "framboesia." He considered that "boubas" was a variety of "framboesia" that was not limited to the skin, but also involved mucous membranes.

Different workers found different organisms in the ulcerations, and there was difference of opinion as to whether the lesions were syphilis, tuberculosis, yaws or blastomycosis. About 1908, during the building of a railroad in the state of São Paulo, Brazil, it was noted that many of the men were affected on naked parts of the body with chronic ulcers. These ulcers were known as "Bauru ulcers," from the name of the city that was one terminus of the railroad. In 1909 Lindenberg and Carini and Paranhos demonstrated in these ulcers organisms which were identical with *Leishmania tropica.*

In 1909 Nattan-Larrier, Touin and Heckenroth reported cutaneous leishmaniasis from French Guiana; and in 1911 Darling reported it from Panama. Flu reported it from Dutch Guiana in 1911; and Minett and Field reported it from British Guiana in 1913.

In 1911 Carini, studying cases in São Paulo, noted that persons who had Leishmania ulcers on the skin were at times attacked by peculiar lesions of the mucous membrane of the mouth, nose and pharynx, at times by direct continuity from lesions on the neighboring skin, at other times when the ulcer was on a remote part of the body. Carini concluded that the "buba brasilianica," described by Breda, was Leishmania lesions in which the mucous membranes were involved.

Splendore concluded that Breda's "buba brasilianica" was not a good term, as "buba" was a popular term for any form of ulcer, while physicians applied the term exclusively to yaws. Splendore concluded that in Brazil there are two diseases that resemble yaws, but which have a special tendency to involve the mucous membranes. One of these conditions is a form of blastomycosis, and the other is a new form of leishmaniasis.

Escomel in 1911 described a disease that was found in the mountainous regions of Peru and adjacent territory, and gave the name "espundia" to the disease. There was a primary lesion, the "espundial chancre," on the forearm, leg, neck, chest, back or shoulders, more rarely on the face or hands. This primary lesion began as an ulcer or as a button, and healed after a varying length of time, sometimes several years. Some time after the skin ulcer had healed, even several years, the patient developed ulceration of the mucous membrane of the nose, mouth and pharynx. Escomel was not able to find the causative organism; but he pointed out that the disease was not syphilis, tuberculosis, leprosy or glanders. Laveran and Nattan-Larrier found Leishmania in material sent to them by Escomel from cases of espundia.

In Cucuta in 1916 we were told by the physicians that rhinoscleroma was common in that region, and one case was in the hospital at that time. Though there was no history of a chronic skin ulcer, the appearance was that of nasal leishmaniasis. No microscopic examination could be made and leishmaniasis was not known to the physicians there. Mucocutaneous leishmaniasis has been reported from Zulia, Colombia, by Tejera.

In 1913 Migone reported a case of kala-azar in an Italian who had lived in Brazil for thirteen years. The man died after a severe attack of diarrhea. Reports of cases of kala-azar in South America led to a study by the American Kala-Azar Commission, headed by E. Chagas. In

1937, eight cases of kala-azar were discovered in one municipality in the State of Pará, Brazil: seven children, one adult. In the examination for yellow fever, viscerotomy was done postmortem on a large number of bodies, and infection with Leishmania was found in the livers of seventy of these bodies.

Geographic Distribution.—Indian kala-azar is widespread in Assam, in Bengal, in the region of Calcutta, Madras, Ceylon, Turkestan, Indo-China, China, Dutch East Indies, Arabia, Egypt, Sudan and Madagascar.

Infantile kala-azar is found in southern France and Italy, Portugal, Spain, Greece, Crete, Malta, Tunis and Algiers.

Oriental sore is found throughout northern Africa, southern Asia, as far as Greece in Europe, and in New Caledonia.

American leishmaniasis is found in Brazil, Paraguay, Dutch Guiana, English Guiana, French Guiana, Venezuela, Colombia, Panama, Yucatan and Peru. There was an epidemic of dermal leishmaniasis in the Chaco district of Paraguay following the recent war.

Etiology.—THE PARASITES.—The organism found in kala-azar in Sudan can be transmitted to monkeys but not to dogs, and the organism found in kala-azar in Transcaucasia differs somewhat from the organism of Indian kala-azar.

When Wright described the organism from oriental boil, he did not know the name "Leishmania," and he gave the organism the name of *Helcosoma tropicum*. When it was recognized that the organism was a Leishmania, the name became *Leishmania tropica*.

Morphology.—The appearance of all of the Leishmania is very much the same in the body of man. With the Romanowsky stain, the organisms appear as round or oval bodies, 1.5 to 2 microns in diameter and 2 to 4 microns long. The cytoplasm stains blue and two nuclei are seen. The large nucleus is about one quarter the size of the entire organism, lies close to the border of the cell, and stains deep red. The small nucleus lies deep in the substance of the cell, appears as a point or rod and stains more violet than the large nucleus. Leishman suggested that the small nucleus was a blepharoplast and that the organism was related to the trypanosomes. The cytoplasm is quite frequently vacuolated and the large nucleus may appear vacuolated. *Leishmania tropica* is frequently found as long, slender forms, and very large, vacuolated forms are common; otherwise, the different species of Leishmania are morphologically identical.

Leishman suggested that the bodies he found in 1900 were related to the trypanosomes. In Rogers' cultures of the organism of kala-azar, the organisms had a single flagellum taking its origin from the small nucleus; that is, they were the leptomonas form in the order Binucleata which includes the trypanosomes.

All of the Leishmania are cell parasites, being found mainly in the endothelial cells; but they are also found in polymorphonuclear leukocytes, in eosinophils and in myelocytes. At times in smears, especially from cutaneous leishmaniasis, free parasites are found: this probably means that they have escaped from destroyed cells. The parasites have the Leishmania form in the tissue; but Escomel reports the flagellated leptomonas forms in espundia; and Risa and Mustafa saw motile flagellated forms in oriental sore.

Culture.—In 1904 Rogers cultivated the organism of Indian kala-azar by drawing blood from the spleen into sodium citrate solution (1 to 2 cc. of 10 per cent solution in the syringe) and keeping it at 22° C. In 1908 Nicolle cultivated the organism of infantile kala-azar and of oriental sore on Novy-MacNeal medium, and later on a simplified Novy-MacNeal medium. A number of workers failed to cultivate the organism of Indian kala-azar on Novy-MacNeal medium; and this was thought to be a strong indication that the organisms were different. But in 1912 Row cultivated the organism of Indian kala-azar on Nicolle's modification of the Novy-MacNeal medium. The Nicolle modification of the Novy-MacNeal medium is known as the N.N.N.-Agar, which is made as follows:

Distilled water .... 900 cc.
Agar-agar .... 14 grams
Sodium chloride .... 6 grams

This mixture is melted, cooled to 45° C., and one part of defibrinated rabbit blood is added to two parts of the mixture, and slanted. The tubes should be tightly stoppered, so the water of condensation will not dry out. The cultures grow best at 22° C.

In the cultures, from the fourth to the seventh day, the organisms appear as long, slender forms, 15 to 20 microns long, and 2 to 4 microns in diameter. A single flagellum rises from the small nucleus (blepharoplast) and extends as a free flagellum, without any evidence of an undulating membrane; that is, the organism is a leptomonas form. In the culture there are more oval forms, and as the cultures get older, there are oval forms without a flagellum and with vacuolated cytoplasm.

The growth is scant in cultures from Indian kala-azar, more marked in cultures from infantile kala-azar, and there is a heavy growth in cultures from oriental sore. The organism of American leishmaniasis grows even better than does the organism from oriental sore. All of the differences between cultural forms of the organism from oriental sore and those from kala-azar can be accounted for by the better growth of the oriental sore organism in cultures.

Transmission to Animals.—The organism of Indian kala-azar is quite readily transmitted to the hamster, less readily to other animals. Earlier attempts to transmit the infection to monkeys, dogs, rabbits, rats, goats, guinea pigs and pigeons failed. Later, Donovan and Patton both succeeded in infecting dogs with Leishmania by the injection of splenic material from cases of kala-azar; and Row produced subcutaneous nodules in monkeys by rubbing material from the spleen of a case of kala-azar into the skin, and by subcutaneous injection of a culture of *Leishmania donovani.*

The organism of infantile kala-azar is readily transmitted to dogs and monkeys. Other animals, as rabbits, guinea pigs, rats and mice, suffer a light infection. The organism of oriental sore is readily transmitted from man to man; from man to monkeys and dogs; from monkey to monkey; from dog to dog; and from cultures to man, dog and monkey. Gonder obtained general infection of mice by intraperitoneal and intravenous injection of cultures of *Leishmania tropica,* the mice developing in addition ulcerations on the feet and tail. Row obtained general infection of mice by injection of culture of *Leishmania tropica;* but there were no skin ulcerations.

40101

Spontaneous Occurrence of Infection in Animals.—Donovan examined 1,150 dogs in Madras and did not find any of them infected with Leishmania. Castellani has reported a spontaneous infection in a dog in Ceylon.

Nicolle and his associates suggested that domestic animals were connected with the spread of infantile kala-azar; and they found four dogs infected with Leishmania among 253 dogs examined in Tunis. The Leishmania were morphologically and culturally identical with the parasite in man. Other investigators have found dogs infected with Leishmania in a number of places about the Mediterranean. The percentage of infection among dogs varied in different regions, and the regions with the highest percentage of infection among dogs were not the regions with the largest number of cases in the human. In Tunis 1.8 per cent of the dogs were infected; in Athens 13.75 per cent;[*] in Lisbon 5 per cent; in Rome 16 per cent; in Malta 14 per cent; and in Messina 18 per cent. The organisms are found in the spleen, liver and bone marrow. The infection appears in two forms in dogs: an acute and a chronic. In the acute form, usually attacking young dogs, the disease sets in with fever, rapid emaciation, and weakness in the hind quarters, and the dog dies in three to five months. The chronic form usually affects older dogs, and they frequently appear entirely normal. Sergent and his coworkers in Algiers, in a house where there was a child with kala-azar, found a kitten with a few parasites in the bone marrow. Attempts to transmit the infection from dog to dog have failed.

The American Kala-Azar Commission found seven dogs and one cat infected in Brazil.

In French Guiana, Joyeux examined twelve dogs and all were negative.

In some regions where cutaneous leishmaniasis is present, dogs have Leishmania ulcers about the face, as in Teheran and Brazil. Five of the dogs that Brumpt and Pedroso took to the forest with them developed Leishmania ulcers, three of them on the face.

Relation to Insects.—Rogers found that his cultures of the organism from Indian kala-azar grew better when he acidified the sodium citrate solution with citric acid, and he suggested that this might indicate an adaptation to the acid contents of the stomach of insects, and thus indicate insects as the transmitter. He suggested the bedbug as the transmitter; but all of his experiments were negative. Patton followed up experiments with a number of biting insects, but he obtained multiplication of the organisms only in the bedbug (*Cimex rotundatus*): three days after feeding, the stomach of the bug contained flagellate forms that were identical with the flagellates in cultures, and rosette forms were present. Donovan suggested that a cone nose, *Conorhinus rubrofasciatus,* was the transmitter; but there is no experimental evidence that this is so.

Much of recent study has stressed various species of phlebotomus in the transmission of Indian kala-azar. Thus, in North China, Sun and Wu found 7 instances of natural infection with *L. donovani* in *P. chinensis;* and later in 10 of 483 specimens in one village, and in 1 of 54 specimens in another village. They also infected laboratory-bred sandflies (*P. chinensis*) by feeding them on cases of kala-azar or on experimentally infected hamsters.

---

[*] Cardamatis considered Leishmania as a part of the life cycle of Piroplasma; and this percentage may be too high.

Basile carried out a series of experiments to determine whether biting insects transmitted the organism of infantile kala-azar; and he found leptomonas form flagellates in the stomach of fleas that were taken on children with kala-azar and on dogs with Leishmania infection. He also showed that fleas, *Ctenocephalus canis* and *Pulex irritans,* that had fed on cases of infantile kala-azar and on dogs infected with Leishmania, could transmit the infection to dogs. Basile considered that this work not only proved the possibility of transmission of Leishmania by fleas in the Mediterranean regions, but that it also made it very nearly certain that the Leishmania of the dog in those regions is the same as the Leishmania of infantile kala-azar.

Giraud says that the dog is the reservoir of infantile kala-azar in the Marseilles district and that the infection is transmitted to children by the bite of dog ticks.

There is little experimental work on the relation of insects to the organism of cutaneous leishmaniasis. In the regions where oriental sore is found, it is commonly considered that insects are the transmitters of the infection and houseflies are commonly incriminated. Most experiments with houseflies have indicated that the organism of oriental sore dies in a few hours in the stomach of the fly; but Cardamatis and Melissidis found typical Leishmania (not flagellates) in the intestine of flies, six days after feeding, and they suggest that the infection may result from organisms contained in the feces of the fly. Mosquitoes have been incriminated. Wenyon experimented with a number of insects and was able to find development of flagellated forms only in bedbugs and mosquitoes (*Stegomyia fasciata*). But he was of the opinion that this did not indicate that these insects were the transmitters of the infection, but that the large amount of blood they had taken in acted as a culture medium for the organisms. Wenyon thinks that houseflies, and more commonly mosquitoes or phlebotomus, are the transmitters.

In South America, biting flies are commonly incriminated. The history is usually that the person was bitten while in the woods, as indicated by the name "forest yaws"; and it is commonly a tabanid fly that is incriminated. Brumpt and Pedroso think Tabanidae are the most probable transmitters of American leishmaniasis and they suggest the name "American forest leishmaniasis." They consider that the multiplicity of the sores means that the transmitter returns repeatedly to feed; and the Tabanidae do that. In Colombia, mucocutaneous leishmaniasis is so closely associated with the bite of a reduviid bug, that the name for the disease is "picada de pito" (meaning "magpie's bite"), pito being a local name for a reduviid bug.

Various species of sandfly (phlebotomus) are generally considered to be the transmitter in many regions.

It is uncertain whether the organism is mechanically transmitted by different insects, or is transmitted by some insect as intermediate host, with a cycle of development in that insect.

Immunity.—Practically nothing is known regarding immunity after kala-azar under natural conditions, as most of the cases progressed to a fatal termination, until the use of antimony in treatment. In the dog and monkey, some months after recovery from an attack of experimental kala-azar, there is immunity; but for a few weeks after recovery there seems to be increased susceptibility to infection.

An animal that is infected with, or has recovered from, kala-azar is immune to infection with the organism of oriental sore.

After recovery from oriental sore there is increased resistance against kala-azar; but it does not amount to immunity.

During infection with oriental sore there is decreased resistance to infection with the organism of oriental sore, as is indicated by the multiplicity of the ulcers in a large part of the cases.

On the other hand, after recovery from oriental sore, there is immunity to further infection with the organism of oriental sore; and this fact has been taken advantage of by the natives in some localities, who inoculated the children with oriental sore on a covered part of the body, in order to protect them against danger of future infection with the possibility of scar formation on the face.

Relation of the Organisms in Leishmaniasis.—There is a constantly increasing amount of evidence that the organisms causing the different clinical forms of leishmaniasis, in different parts of the world, are merely varieties of one or two species. A clinical difference between American leishmaniasis and oriental sore has been the frequency of involvement of the mucous membranes in the American variety. But Castellani and Chalmers observed two cases of oropharyngeal ulceration in Europeans who had lived for some time in India—in one case they found Leishmania in scrapings from the ulcers; Christopherson observed a case of naso-oral leishmaniasis originating in Sudan, and La Cava noted a similar condition in Italy.

The earlier cultural and animal inoculation differences have been overcome. Wenyon believes that Indian and infantile kala-azar is due to one organism, *Leishmania donovani;* and that probably oriental sore and American dermal leishmaniasis are caused by one organism, *Leishmania tropica.* On this basis the name, *Leishmania infantum,* given by Nicolle to the organism in infantile kala-azar, becomes a synonym of *Leishmania donovani;* and the names *Leishmania brasiliensis,* given by Vianna to the organism in American dermal leishmaniasis, and *Leishmania nilotica,* given by Brumpt to the organism found by Thomson and Balfour in keloid-like skin nodules in Egypt, become synonyms of *Leishmania tropica.* The organism cultivated from the spleen of a case of kala-azar in Brazil, by da Cunha and Chagas, resembles *Leishmania donovani;* but on the basis of some serologic differences they consider it a distinct species, *Leishmania chagasi.*

The conditions caused by Leishmania are most conveniently discussed under two headings: (1) Visceral Leishmaniasis, and (2) Cutaneous Leishmaniasis, depending on whether the lesions are in the viscera or in the skin.

VISCERAL LEISHMANIASIS

(Indian Kala-Azar—Infantile Kala-Azar)

In the Indian kala-azar, which is found in Assam, Madras, Ceylon, China, Indo-China, Dutch East India, Arabia and Sudan, the patients are generally older children and adults. Mackie reported 195 cases from Assam, of which 100 cases were in children from six to ten years old.

In the infantile kala-azar, which prevails around the Mediterranean—in Tunis, Algiers, Italy, Greece, Malta, Trieste, Portugal and probably the entire Mediterranean region—90 per cent of the patients are children under four years old.

Clinically, both forms of kala-azar are characterized by an acute or chronic febrile course, with anemia, enlargement of the spleen and later the liver, a tendency to hemorrhages, gangrene and dysenteric symptoms, and tending to end fatally.

The spleen enlarges early, and later reaches the midline and down to the crest of the ilium, or larger. At times the liver is enlarged and there is ascites, due, according to Rogers, to a special form of cirrhosis of the liver.

Epidemiology.—In India there is evidence that kala-azar is a house disease, and a number of persons in a house may have the disease. In the same way, it appears that sleeping in a house where there is a case of kala-azar frequently leads to infection. On the other hand, there are instances where a person with the disease has associated with other persons for a long time without anyone contracting the disease from him. Neither does the infection spread in hospitals, where vermin are not present. All of this indicates that the infection is spread by some biting arthropod, and not by contact; and the bedbug is strongly suspected of being the transmitter.

The usual history is that an infected person came into a village and that the disease spread from the house in which he lived.

The organisms are found in the nasal mucus of a fair percentage of the cases; Forkner and Zia found the organisms in the nasal secretion of 12 of 22 cases; and in smears from the tonsils in 3 of 10 cases. Intraperitoneal injection of nasal secretion, saliva, and material from the tonsils, into hamsters showed that living parasites were present in a fair number of cases.

The investigations of Archibald and Mansour confirm the findings of Forkner and Zia. Leishmania were found in nasal smears of 7 of 35 cases examined; and they transmitted the infection to two monkeys by the nasal material of one of their cases: one by intradermal inoculation and one by nasal swabbing. They also carried out contact experiments with monkeys. Four healthy monkeys were kept in an insect-proof room with four monkeys inoculated intraperitoneally with kala-azar material: all of the inoculated animals developed kala-azar, as did two of the uninoculated ones. On repeating the experiment, three of the uninoculated animals developed kala-azar.

The organisms are present in the intestinal ulcerations, but there is no evidence to support the suggestion that they are spread in the urine and feces.

In regions where infantile kala-azar is found, the dogs are infected with Leishmania; but the greatest incidence of the disease in the human does not necessarily correspond with the greatest incidence of infection in the dogs. While there are experiments which tend to show that the dog flea and the human flea transmit the infection, all recent work has failed to confirm that view. Giraud says the infection is transmitted by dog ticks in the Marseilles district.

Mechanism of the Disease Process.—In the present state of our knowledge it is not possible to explain the entire disease process in leishmaniasis. The organism, introduced into the body, probably by a biting arthropod, enters the endothelial cells and multiplies there by simple fission. The infected cell breaks down and the liberated parasites invade other endothelial cells, polymorphonuclear leukocytes, endothelial leukocytes and sometimes eosinophils. The parasites are especially numerous in the endothelial cells in the spleen and liver, and less numerous in the bone marrow, where they are found mainly in the mononuclear cells. The organisms are found in smaller numbers in various other tissues. Some of the parasites, escaping from the ruptured endothelial cells, are taken up by the polymorphonuclear leukocytes and appear in the peripheral circulation.

Maggiore considers that the anemia of kala-azar is due to alterations in the tissue of the bone marrow; that is, the anemia is due to injury to the blood-forming tissue, and is not due to destruction of the red cells. It may well be that the leukopenia, due to reduction of the polymorphonuclear leukocytes, is a result of the same action on the bone marrow, while the increased endothelial leukocyte count is due to the involvement of the endothelial cells in different parts of the body. The ulceration of the intestinal mucosa and the skin is in all probability due to shutting off of the blood supply from plugging of the capillaries by the proliferation and swelling of the endothelial cells. The hemorrhages are probably due to the degeneration of the endothelium of the capillary walls and to the lowered coagulability of the blood. The secondary infections and gangrene are undoubtedly favored by the decrease in the number of the polymorphonuclear leukocytes.

Symptomatology.—CLINICAL HISTORY.—The incubation period is, according to Rogers, from three weeks to several months. Manson saw a case in which the incubation period was apparently not over ten days.

The first symptom is an irregular fever, which usually shows two remissions in the twenty-four hours—the "double quotidian" fever of Rogers. In some cases there is a low-grade continuous fever. After three to six weeks of this irregular fever there are periods of freedom from fever, but the condition progresses and later there is a continuous fever to the end.

Gastro-intestinal symptoms appear early; nausea and vomiting are not common; but the bowels are irregular, with a tendency to diarrhea.

The spleen enlarges, and later fills the abdomen, so the outline of it can be seen through the abdominal wall. The liver does not enlarge so early or so much; the spleen and liver may be painful and tender.

The skin becomes dry and furfuraceous, and dark or earthy in color. The hair is brittle and falls out. A papular eruption frequently appears on the forearms, lower part of the body and legs. The eruption may itch at times; there may be areas of edema in the skin; and there may be small ulcers in the papules, or there may be large ulcers, especially on the foot or leg.

Hemorrhages are common in kala-azar. Hemorrhages in the skin may appear as purpuric spots, especially on the face and body; or there may be extensive ecchymoses, especially where there is pressure. There may be nosebleed, and hemorrhage from the gums or any part of the gastro-intestinal tract. There may be hemorrhage on the serous surfaces, as peritoneum, pleura and the meninges.

The early gastro-intestinal disturbances continue; and from being a simple diarrhea, the stools later consist of blood and mucus, and a dysenteric attack may end the process.

Gangrene is common, especially about the mouth, and Christophers saw gangrene of the vulva and the colon. This may well be associated with the great reduction in polymorphonuclear leukocytes, which may amount to an agranulocytosis, and may be acute.

As the disease progresses, the patient becomes emaciated, until he is a skeleton, the abdomen being protuberant as a result of the enlarged spleen.

The patient gradually becomes more and more emaciated; there are great weakness and exhausting diarrheal attacks. The course of the disease may be rapid and the patient may die in three or four months; or the disease may be more chronic and the patient may live for one or two years. It is common for some intercurrent affection, as pneumonia and septic conditions, or the dysenteric attacks, to bring the case to a close.

LABORATORY FINDINGS.—The blood shows an anemia, the red cells being as low as two million, and the hemoglobin being reduced in proportion. There is marked leukopenia, the reduction being at the expense of the polymorphonuclear leukocytes; and there is a relative, and at times an absolute, increase in the number of endothelial leukocytes and lymphocytes. There is a decreased coagulability of the blood, and Archibald found a decrease in the alkalinity of the blood in cases of kala-azar in Sudan.

Diagnosis.—CLINICAL DIAGNOSIS.—The principal reason for considering the clinical diagnosis is to point out the necessity for a laboratory diagnosis.

The disease is frequently confused with malaria, the only points being the double daily rise in the temperature, and the absence of constitutional symptoms in keeping with the fever, in kala-azar. Later in the disease the dysenteric attacks have to be differentiated from amebic and bacillary dysentery. The infantile form has to be differentiated from leukemia and various anemias.

LABORATORY DIAGNOSIS.—The blood in kala-azar shows a decrease in the number of red cells, down to two million, with a corresponding decrease in the hemoglobin percentage. There is a leukopenia; the total leukocyte count being below 3,000 often down to 1,000, or even down to 625 per cubic millimeter. This leukopenia is due to a decrease in the polymorphonuclear leukocytes, which are as low as 20 per cent, or even down to 5 per cent, of the total leukocytes. There is a relative increase in the mononuclears; and often an absolute increase, especially in the endothelial leukocytes.

The diagnosis is definitely made only by finding the parasite. Examination of the peripheral blood should be made first, as the parasites can usually be found there on careful search. Patton examined the peripheral blood of 84 kala-azar patients, many of them in the early stage of the disease. He found Leishmania in 42 of the cases on the first examination, and the organisms in the blood of more cases on repeated examination, until, on the twentieth examination, he found the organisms in the blood of the 84th case. The organisms are found in the polymorphonuclear leukocytes and also in the endothelial leukocytes. Examination of the peripheral blood will also rule out leukemia.

40101

The superficial lymph glands are frequently enlarged and Leishmania may be found by puncture of one of these enlarged glands.

The organisms can be found in the juice obtained by splenic puncture; but splenic puncture is contraindicated when there are ascites, marked anemia, jaundice, strong tendency to hemorrhage, or severe complication as pneumonia. When puncture is to be done on such cases, Rogers gives 20 grains (1.3 Gm.) of calcium lactate on the evening before and repeats it shortly before the puncture. The needle should be as small as can be used; a pad is bound over the splenic area after the operation, and the patient is kept in bed for twenty-four hours.

The organisms are found in the liver and bone marrow. The bone marrow may be punctured by drilling into the sternum or head of the tibia. Liver puncture is not as good as splenic puncture for diagnosis.

Leishmania are found in the papules and ulcerations of the skin, in blisters produced by the application of a vesicant to the skin, and in the feces, free or in shreds of mucus.

Blood culture on Nicolle's modification of the Novy-MacNeal medium is frequently positive.

Complement fixation and various serum reactions have been tried but give questionable results. Formol-gel reactions have been reported as of value, as have skin tests.

Animal inoculation is of value, about in the following order: hamster, rhesus monkey, dog, ground squirrel, mole rat, and even the guinea pig and the mouse.

Complications.—Secondary septic infections are common, especially cancrum oris, pneumonia and pleurisy. Apparently part of the diarrhea and dysentery is due to secondary infection of the ulcers in the intestine. Cystitis is not uncommon. As might be expected, tuberculosis is not an infrequent complication.

While the decrease in the number of polymorphonuclear leukocytes probably accounts for the frequency of secondary infections, which so commonly prove fatal, on the other hand there are cases where a secondary infection, as cancrum oris, seems to have increased the resistance of the body to such an extent that there is improvement or even cure of the kala-azar.

Treatment.—Prophylaxis.—In India the best results are obtained by abandoning infected villages and putting the village on a new site. At times it may be sufficient to abandon infected houses. The evidence now is that bedbugs are the transmitter, and it is to be remembered that these bugs will live for months in a house without feeding; so it is practically necessary to destroy an infected house.

The results of treatment at Shillong led Knowles to suggest that it may be easier to thoroughly treat all cases than to carry out household removals over long periods of time.

Around the Mediterranean, it seems advisable to direct prophylactic measures toward the dog as the reservoir of the infection. Children especially should not be allowed to associate closely with a dog, and infected and stray dogs should be destroyed.

Curative Treatment.—Since the various compounds of antimony have come into use in the treatment of leishmaniasis, it appears that the drug is very nearly specific for the disease. **Antimony and potassium tartrate** has commonly been used in 1 or 2 per cent aqueous solution, injected intravenously. Di Cristina and Caronia treated cases of infantile kala-azar in this way, with satisfactory results. Knowles advised that physiologic salt solution be used instead of water in making the solution. Rogers preferred **sodium antimony tartrate,** for the reason that the sodium salt is less irritating if any of the solution escapes into the tissues about the vein. The first dose is 5 cc. (1.35 fl.dr.) of this solution. If the first dose is well borne, 10 cc. (2.70 fl.dr.) of the solution are given every other day.

Rogers refers to three deaths that followed the intravenous use of potassium and antimony tartrate, and calls attention to the fact that at times the solution is cloudy, and there is a heavy precipitate in the flasks. The solution must not be used unless it is clear. Almenara says the solution of potassium and antimony tartrate must be filtered sterile, as it cannot be sterilized by heat.

Antimony and potassium tartrate has been pretty generally replaced by the organic antimony compounds; yet Laurinsich considers that potassium and antimony tartrate is a more active remedy than the organic compounds, and has not found it necessary to abandon the potassium and antimony tartrate.

Of the organic salts of antimony, both the trivalent and the pentavalent salts have been used. **Fuadin** is the trivalent salt commonly used. The pentavalent salts of antimony are most comonly used today. **Neostan, neostibosan, urea stibosan** and **solustibosan** are the ones used. **Solustibosan** the most commonly used of these salts, is a sterile stable solution suitable for intravenous or intramuscular injection. It is not irritating, the solution remains clear, and it is of low toxicity. Struthers, using solustibosan intravenously, gave 2 cc. the first day, and 6 cc. on alternate days or daily, to a total of 59 to 84.5 cc. Yates, using neostibosan, gave a total dosage of 60 cc. for each 100 lb. of body weight; one case received 94 cc. per 100 lb. of body weight in 26 injections. In 9 cases he gave the course in five days, and several adults were given injections of 20 cc. without any toxic effects.

The injections of the antimony salt are continued for some weeks after the leukocyte count is normal and there is no fever.

For the complication of agranulocytosis, which may occur at the end of a course of antimony treatment, the usual treatment of agranulocytosis is advised.

For the prevention of the complication of noma, Fan and Scott advise a large blood transfusion before the injection of antimony is instituted where the hemoglobin is below 50 per cent.

Before antimony came into use in the treatment of kala-azar, quinine was the common drug used in treatment. Frías treated a number of cases of infantile kala-azar with **quinine, arsenic and iron,** and some of the cases recovered and remained well after three or four years.

The ulcers on the skin are to be kept clean, as it is very important to prevent secondary infections. Intestinal parasites should be eliminated, and the patient's strength should be built up with good food and tonics.

Prognosis.—In untreated cases the prognosis is bad, the mortality being about 95 per cent. With quinine and tonic treatment the mortality is reduced to about 75 per cent. Since the introduction of antimony treatment, the mortality has been reduced to a low figure: during 1917, 20 cases were treated by intravenous injections of antimony and potassium tartrate at the King Edward Institute at Shillong, with 15 recoveries and 5 deaths. The complications are usually fatal; though there may be improvement, or apparent cure, after some secondary infection, as cancrum oris.

Pathology.—MACROSCOPIC.—There is great emaciation and edema is often present. The enlarged spleen partly fills the abdomen and its outline can be seen through the abdominal wall. There may be ulcerations and gangrene of the skin. There may be ascites. The enlarged spleen is firm, dark red in color, and the capsule may be thickened. The liver is often, but not constantly, enlarged, and the surface is smooth. The marrow in the long bones is red to dark red in color. There are frequently ulcerations in the large and small intestine. Hemorrhages may occur into the skin, any organ, meninges or bone marrow. When complicated by secondary infection, as noma, there may be infarcts in various organs; and there may be pneumonia and pleurisy as terminal conditions.

MICROSCOPIC.—Visentini has described the microscopic changes in the organs in infantile kala-azar, and Christophers has described the microscopic changes in the organs in Indian kala-azar.

In the spleen the trabeculae are enlarged and there is an increase in the fibrous tissue throughout the organ. The sinuses are enlarged and the whole organ is filled with blood, at times in the form of hemorrhagic infiltration. There is at times fatty degeneration in the cells of the reticulum and in the endothelial cells. The endothelial cells are enormously enlarged and are packed with the parasites. As the cells are destroyed, some of the parasites lie free or in masses of cytoplasm.

In the liver there is atrophy, and at times fatty degeneration, of the parenchyma cells, with enlargement of the sinuses. There is a perivascular round-cell infiltration, with increase of fibrous tissue. Rogers has described a diffuse, intralobular type of cirrhosis of the liver. The endothelial cells in the blood sinuses are enlarged, and are filled with parasites, the same as the endothelial cells in the spleen. The parasites are not found in the parenchyma cells.

The bone marrow contains the parasites, often in great numbers, in the large mononuclear cells.

Scordo found fatty degeneration in the kidneys and adrenals.

In the large and small intestine there is infiltration of the mucosa, followed by necrosis of the epithelium, this ulceration extending as deep as the muscular coat. Parasites are found in the tissues about the ulcers.

The parasites are found in the lymph glands, lung endothelium, capillaries in the testicles, where they may be numerous, in the capillary tufts of the glomeruli in the kidneys, and in the papules and ulcerations of the skin. They have been found in the meninges and the brain, especially when there is hemorrhage into those tissues. Christophers made a thorough examination of the muscles and did not find parasites. Visentini found the parasites in the muscles.

CUTANEOUS LEISHMANIASIS

(Oriental Sore—American Leishmaniasis)

Cutaneous leishmaniasis appears in somewhat different forms in different parts of the world and there has been great confusion with the various ulcerative conditions of the skin. But with the findings of

Leishmania in the lesions, a great part of the confusion has been corrected. The lesions may ulcerate or not, and the South American form tends to involve the mucous membrane more than does the oriental sore.

Epidemiology.—In the tropics, cutaneous leishmaniasis generally is most common in the cool season; and in the subtropical regions, it is most common in the late summer and fall. In some regions, as Bagdad, it is not possible to remain for even a few days without contracting the infection.

It is generally agreed that oriental sore is transmitted by some biting arthropod, as houseflies, mosquitoes or phlebotomus; but in no case has such transmission been proved. The fact that oriental sore can be transmitted by direct inoculation, that it is so constantly associated with some biting arthropod, and that it usually occurs on an uncovered part of the body, is strong circumstantial evidence that some biting arthropod is the transmitter. There is some indication that the infection may be transmitted by bathing in contaminated water, as well as through contaminated clothing.

The South American cutaneous leishmaniasis is constantly associated with the bite of some bug or fly, and Tabanidae are generally incriminated. The usual history is that the lesion followed a fly bite, received while in the forest. There is no proof that flies transmit the infection, and it is to be remembered that the first appearance of the lesion resembles a fly bite and frequently itches intensely: the supposed fly bite may be the beginning of the lesion resulting from inoculation some weeks before.

The lesions are auto-inoculable. The multiplicity of the lesions may be due to multiple primary inoculations, or to auto-inoculation from scratching a single primary inoculation.

The suggestions that the dog or a lizard may be the reservoir for the virus, and that the infection may be transmitted from the reservoir to man by some biting arthropod, as phlebotomus, have no experimental evidence in their favor.

Mechanism of the Disease Process.—Unna considers that the parasites enter the hair follicles and from there penetrate the surrounding corium. It can well be that the parasite is inoculated directly into the corium by the biting arthropod and that the process starts from there. The organism is a parasite of the endothelial cells and is found in enormous numbers in these large cells in the affected area. The endothelial cells of the capillaries are swollen and proliferated and may cause blocking of the vessels. This blocking of the capillaries, together with the abundance of endothelial leukocytes, plasma cells, and the smaller number of polymorphonuclear leukocytes collected at the site of the lesion, causes destruction of the tissue with the resulting ulcer formation. There is some evidence that the enlargement of the lymph glands is due to presence of parasites and that fever corresponds to parasites in the blood.

The tendency of the lesion is to recovery—by what mechanism is not clear—and the ulcer heals, leaving a thin, soft scar, that is often brownish in color and may shrink considerably, causing disfigurement if on the face. There is immunity of some duration, possibly for life, following recovery.

40101

The mucous membrane involvement may be by direct extension from a lesion on the neighboring skin, or may result from infection from a sore on some distant part of the body, either by auto-inoculation or through the blood. The mucous membrane involvement may not appear for months after the primary sore on the skin has healed. Caution is necessary in interpreting the relation of the mucous membrane involvement and the skin lesion, on account of the danger of confusion of other lesions, especially blastomycosis, with cutaneous leishmaniasis.

Symptomatology.—CLINICAL HISTORY.—The incubation period varies from two weeks to three or more months, the average being about two months. The patient frequently connects the lesion with the bite of some arthropod, often a fly; and, especially in South America, the bite is frequently received in the forest.

The lesion is almost always on an uncovered part of the body, as the foot and leg, hand, arm or face. At first there is a small red fleck, like a mosquito bite, and this soon develops a papule in the center and may itch intensely. This papule enlarges gradually, without there being any inflammatory reaction around it. The epidermis becomes smooth and covered with thin scales from the hyperkeratosis; after some weeks it breaks and a serous secretion escapes and dries to form a hard crust on the surface. This crust may heap up, and appear like a syphilitic rupia. If the crust is removed the chronic ulcer, with a yellowish secretion, remains. There may be only one ulcer; but more commonly there are several—up to twenty—partly from multiple primary inoculations, and partly from repeated auto-inoculation from the primary sore. The ulcer continues for a number of months to a year and then heals by the formation of healthy granulations in the floor.

At times the nodule does not ulcerate, but appears as a nodule in the cutis, as large as a pea, not adherent to the underlying tissues. The nodule gradually disappears, with or without any desquamation over the surface where the nodule was located. The keloid-like nodules appear as cystadenomas of the skin and do not ulcerate.

At other times, the ulcer appears as any ordinary chronic ulcer.

At times the lymph glands, especially in the region of the ulcers, are enlarged; but it is not possible to determine how much this may be due to secondary bacterial infection.

In South America there is a frequent involvement of the naso-oral mucous membrane, either by direct extension of a lesion on the neighboring skin, from auto-inoculation from an ulcer on some other part of the body, or through the blood stream. The lesions of the mucous membrane sometimes do not appear until as much as eighteen months after the ulcer on the skin is healed. The patient's voice is changed, and is finally lost as the involvement of the pharynx and larynx progresses. These naso-oral lesions are very chronic, often lasting a number of years, and are usually fatal.

During the progress of the condition it is not uncommon for the patient to have attacks of fever, malaise and headache; but it is not possible to say how much of this may be due to secondary bacterial infection. Mild fever and malaise are not uncommon during the incubation period and before the appearance of a new boil.

The duration of the various forms of leishmaniasis of the skin is usually a number of months to a year; and it is sometimes known as "year's boil."

Diagnosis.—CLINICAL DIAGNOSIS.—There has been a great amount of confusion of the various chronic ulcerations of the skin; and it is difficult to say whether some of the older cases are cutaneous leishmaniasis, yaws, syphilis, tuberculosis, blastomycosis or some of the milder skin affections. It is very important to differentiate cutaneous leishmaniasis from blastomycosis, especially as both conditions are apt to involve the mucous membranes of the nose and mouth. With the finding of the specific parasite in the lesions, the diagnosis becomes possible; and it is not possible to make a diagnosis in any other way.

LABORATORY DIAGNOSIS.—Remove the crust, and make smears from scrapings from the floor and edges of the ulcer, and stain with one of the Romanowsky stains. The parasites may not be numerous, especially in the mucous membrane lesions.

The blood may show an increase in the number of endothelial leukocytes. At times, when there is secondary infection of the ulcer, there may be a leukocytosis.

At times it is possible to obtain a culture of the parasites from scrapings from the ulcer, when inoculated onto Nicolle's modification of the Novy-MacNeal medium. Very rarely it may be possible to obtain a culture of the parasite from the peripheral blood.

Treatment.—PROPHYLAXIS.—The belief that the infection is transmitted by the bite of a fly indicates that one should protect himself against such bites; and, in South America at least, this would seem to be important when going into the forest. As it has been shown that infection can take place through inoculation of the infectious material onto a scarified area of the skin, or through a bleb on the skin, it is important to protect such abrasions from flies. The **lesions** should early be **protected with a dressing,** as the infection is inoculable and auto-inoculable.

CURATIVE TREATMENT.—It was in the treatment of cutaneous leishmaniasis in South America that the excellent results of antimony were first shown; and the use of the drug in other forms of leishmaniasis has given equally good results.

Machado and Vianna, in 1913, treated cases of cutaneous leishmaniasis with **intravenous injections** of a 1 per cent solution of **potassium and antimony tartrate,** and obtained excellent results. Since that time, the antimony treatment has practically supplanted all other methods of treatment in all forms of leishmaniasis. The method of treatment is the same as given under kala-azar. In spite of the developments in the use of the organic antimony salts, Goodall still thinks that potassium and antimony tartrate is the mainstay in the treatment of cutaneous leishmaniasis, and considers this of importance in view of the low cost of the drug.

Savon Salaberry had the best results with **fuadin** intravenously and intramuscularly in cutaneous and mucosal leishmaniasis in Argentina.

Some authorities apply a solution of **potassium and antimony tartrate** to the ulcer, in addition to the intravenous injection of the solution. A 1 to 2 per cent solution may be applied at intervals of one to three days; and a saturated solution is applied every four to eight days. The ulcer receives mild antiseptic dressings in the intervals. This treat-

40101

ment causes a slough to form and healthy granulations then appear in the floor of the ulcer.

Mitchell treated a number of cases by freezing with **carbon dioxide snow.**

Prognosis.—The prognosis in uncomplicated cutaneous leishmaniasis is good. There may be secondary infection with bacteria, which may lead to a fatal termination. Erysipelas may result from secondary infection of the ulcers. The mucous membrane involvement is more serious and, until the introduction of antimony in treatment, was almost uniformly fatal.

Pathology.—MACROSCOPIC.—The developed ulcer is circular or oval, an inch or more in diameter, with a raised skin margin; and covered with a thick hard crust, brownish-yellow in color, and raised above the surface. On lifting the crust the ulcer is seen to have a steep, jagged margin, with the floor covered with pale, unhealthy granulations. There is little induration around the margin of the ulcer.

Thomson and Balfour describe the nonulcerating, keloid-like lesions as resembling the mountains on a relief map, looked at from above. There are a parent lesion and connected secondary growths. The lesions are pink in color, smooth and shiny, with no scaling or evidences of breaking down. They are firm, but soft, and not adherent to the deeper tissue. On puncture, they yield blood and serum or a small amount of cheesy, sebaceous-like material. The largest lesion was 35 by 15 mm.

In the involvement of the mucous membranes, the earlier appearance is that of granulations, and later there are vegetations and extensive ulceration.

MICROSCOPIC.—The characteristic of the process is the formation of areas of cellular infiltration in the cutis, with marked change in the overlying epidermis.

Jeanselme and Rist describe marked thickening of the rete malpighii, with incomplete keratinization of the corneal layer of the epidermis; while Unna and Wright describe thinning of the overlying epidermis. It is probable that the thinning is merely a later stage of the change in the epidermis, especially as Unna describes thickening and hypertrophy of the rete malpighii and hyperkeratosis with the formation of epithelial pearls around the margin of the ulcer. There is edema of the rete malpighii, with vacuolation of the cells. There is some cellular infiltration in the rete malpighii. When the epidermis is thinned, the hair follicles are atrophied and are transformed into horny masses.

The crust is composed of cornified epithelium mixed with fibrin, red blood cells and leukocytes in all stages of degeneration, and cellular debris.

In the keloid-like lesions the change in the epidermis is marked and there is no evidence of breaking down of the epidermis. There are downgrowths of columns of cells from the rete malpighii, with the formation of cell nests and epithelial whorls.

The infiltrated areas in the cutis consist of edematous masses of lymphocytes, plasma cells, endothelial leukocytes, a few giant cells, red blood cells and fibrin, and polymorphonuclear leukocytes. The endothelial cells of the blood vessels are swollen and proliferated, sometimes occluding the vessel. In the center of the area, the tissue breaks down to a necrotic mass. Around the margin of the infiltrated area the cells are less numerous, being mainly lymphocytes and plasma cells, this infiltration extending especially about the blood vessels and lymph vessels. In the periphery there is multiplication of the fixed tissue cells. When the epidermis breaks down over the areas of necrosis, the ulcer results.

The parasites are generally found in the endothelial cells, but they are also found in the polymorphonuclear cells. Not infrequently parasites are found free, probably from the breaking down of endothelial cells. Flagellated parasites have been reported from ulcers. Vianna found the parasites in plain muscle fibers in the wall of a blood vessel in the tissue near an ulcer on the nose of a dog.

In the lesions on the mucous membranes, the picture is that of granulation tissue, with a rather small number of endothelial leukocytes, but with an abundance of lymphocytes and plasma cells, and some giant cells. The parasites are not abundant in these lesions.

There is nothing characteristic in the microscopic appearance of the enlarged lymph glands. Parasites are found, usually in clumps, at times in polymorphonuclear cells: there is no infiltration with endothelial cells

In the blood there may be an increase in the number of endothelial leukocytes. The parasites have been found in the peripheral blood; but this is generally considered to be an accidental escape of the parasites into the blood from the local lesion, rather than an indication that the ulcer is a local manifestation of a general disease. By some authorities it is held that the mucous membrane involvement may be through the blood from a skin lesion, as the mucous membrane lesion may appear months after the skin ulcer has healed.

BIBLIOGRAPHY

Adeodato, I.: Batão endemico dos Paizes quentes particularmente na Bahia, Thèse de Bahia, 1895.

Almenara, G.: Anatomia patologica de las leishmaniasis dermicas, Crón. méd., 33: 429, 1916.

Archibald, R. G. and Mansour, H.: Some observations on epidemiology of kala-azar in Sudan, Tr. Roy. Soc. Trop. Med. & Hyg., 30: 395, 1937.

Borja, A. and Amaral, A.: Contribução ão tratamento da leishmaniose cutaneomucosa pelas injecoes endophlebicas de emetico, Arch. brasil. de med., 5: 145, 1915.

Breda, A.: Beitrag zum klinischen und bacteriologischen Studium der brasilianischen Framboesie oder "Boubas," Arch. f. Dermatol. u. Syph., 33: 3, 1895.

Brumpt, E.: Précis de parasitologie, Deuxième Édition, Masson & Cie, Paris, 1813.

———— and Pedroso, A.: Récherches epidémiologiques sur la leishmaniose forestière américaine dans l'État de São-Paulo (Brésil), Bull. Soc. path. exot., 6: 752, 1913.

Carini, A.: Leishmaniose de la muqueuse rhino-bucco-pharyngée, Bull. Soc. path. exot., 4: 289, 1911.

————: L'Émetique dans le traitement de la leishmaniose cutanée et muqueuse, Bull. Soc. path. exot., 7: 277, 1914.

———— and Paranhos, U.: Identification de l' "Ulcera de Bauru" avec le bouton d'Orient, Bull. Soc. path. exot., 2: 255, 1909.

Castellani, A. and Chalmers, A. J.: Manual of Tropical Medicine, Ed. 2, New York, William Wood & Co., 1913.

Cathoire: Observation d'un cas de piroplasmose généralisée en Tunisie, Arch. gén. de méd., 1: 1426, 1905.

Chagas, E. and others: Leishmaniose visceral americana (Report of Kala-Azar Commission for 1937), Mem. Inst. Oswaldo Cruz, 33: 89, 1938.

Christophers, S. R.: Trans. Committee for the Study of Malaria in India, No. 3, p. 72, 1911.

Christopherson, J. B.: On a case of naso-oral leishmaniasis (corresponding to the description of espundia); and on a case of Oriental sore, both originating in the Anglo-Egyptian Sudan, Ann. Trop. Med., 8: 485, 1914.

————: Notes on a case of espundia (naso-oral leishmaniasis) and 3 cases of kala-azar in the Sudan, treated by the intravenous injection of antimonium tartaratum, J. Trop. M., 20: 229, 1917.

da Cunha, A. M. and Chagas, E.: Études sur la leishmaniose viscérale du Brésil. Vérification du parasite par ponction de la rate et du foie; culture et aspect morphologique; considérations d'ordre général, Compt. rend. Soc. de biol., 123: 709, 1936.

Cunningham, D. D.: On the presence of peculiar parasitic organisms in the tissue of a specimen of Delhi boil, Scient. Mem. Med. Off., Army of India (1884), Part I, p. 21, 1885.

Da Matta, A.: Tableau synoptique de la classification des leishmanioses, Bull. Soc. path. exot., 9 : 761, 1916.

Darling, S. T.: Oriental sore in Panama, Arch. Int. Med., 7 : 581, 1911.

Da Silva, P.: Tratamento da leishmaniose cutaneo-mucosa, pelo tartaro emetico, Arch. brasil. de med., 4 : 271, 1916.

Di Cristina, G. and Caronia, G.: Sulla terapia della leishmaniosi interna, Bull. Soc. path. exot., 8 : 63, 1915.

Donovan, C.: On the possibility of the occurrence of trypanosomiasis in India, Brit. M. J., 2 : 79, 1903.

———— : Kala-azar; its distribution and the probable mode of infection, Indian J. M. Research, 1 : 177, 1913.

Escomel, E.: La espundia, Bull. Soc. path. exot., 4 : 489, 1911.

———— : Contribution à l'étude de la leishmaniose américaine (Laveran et Nattan-Larrier). Formes et variétés cliniques, Bull. Soc. path. exot., 9 : 215, 1916.

———— : Le traitement actuel de la leishmaniose américaine, Bull. Soc. path. exot., 9 : 699, 1916.

Fan, P. L. and Scott, A. V.: Study of noma complicating kala-azar in children, Chinese M. J., 48 : 1046, 1934.

Fede, N.: Le anemie nei bambini e loro patogenesi, Atti d. Cong. pediat. ital., 4 : 140, 1901.

Firth, R. H.: Notes on the appearance of certain sporozoöid bodies in the protoplasm of an "Oriental sore," Brit. M. J., 1 : 60, 1891.

Flu, P. C.: Die Aetiologie der in Surinam vorkommenden sogennanten Boschyaws, Centralbl. f. Bakt., I Abt., Orig., 60 : 624, 1911.

Forkner, C. E. and Zia, L. S.: Further studies on kala-azar; Leishmania in nasal and oral secretions of patients and bearing of this finding on transmission of disease, J. Exper. Med., 61 : 183, 1935.

Frías, A: El kala-azar infantil en Reus y su Comarca, Arch. Españ. de pediat., 2 : 321, 1918.

Giraud, P.: Epidémiologie du kala-azar dans la région marseillaise, Marseille-méd., 2 : 81, 1936.

Gonder, R.: Experimentelle Übertragung von Orientbeule auf Mäuse, Arch. f. Schiffs- u. Tropen-Hyg., 17 : 397, 1913.

Gonzales Rincones, R.: La esponja y la pacada de pito. (Una o dos leishmaniosis), Gac. méd. de Carácas, 24 : 176, 1917.

Goodall, J.: Clinical study of 63 cases of Oriental sore, Indian M. Gaz., 72 : 3, 1937.

Hoare, C. A.: Early discoveries regarding parasite of Oriental sore (with English Translation of memoir by P. F. Borovsky: "On Sart Sore," 1898), Tr. Roy. Soc. Trop. Med. & Hyg., 32 : 67, 1938.

Iturbe, J.: Primer caso de leishmaniosis cutanea en Venezuela, Gac. méd. de Carácas, 24 : 20, 1917.

Jeanselme, E. and Rist, E.: Précis de pathologie exotique, Paris, Masson & Cie, 1909.

Knowles, R.: First annual report of the King Edward VII Memorial Pasteur Institute, Shillong (Assam), for the year ending December 31, 1917, Printed at the Assam Secretariat Printing Office, Shillong, 1918.

Labbe, M., Targhetta and Ameuille: Le kala-azar infantile en France, Bull. Acad. de méd., 3rd series, 79 : 288, 1918.

Laurinsich, A.: Dati statistico-clinici dal 1916 al 1936 raccolti nell'ambulatorio anti-kala-azarico della R. Clinica Pediatrica di Napoli, Pediatria, 45 : 957, 1937.

Laveran, A.: Les leishmanioses chez les animaux, Ann. Inst. Pasteur, 28 : 823, 885, 1914; 29 : 1, 71, 1915.

———— and Mesnil, F.: Sur un protozoaire nouveau Piroplasma donovani (Laveran and Mesnil), parasite d'une fièvre de l'Inde, Compt. rend. Acad. d. sc., 137 : 957, 1903.

———— and Nattan-Larrier, L.: Contribution a l'étude de la espundia, Bull. Soc. path. exot., 5 : 176, 1912.

Leishman, W. B.: On the possibility of the occurrence of trypanosomiasis in India, Brit. M. J., 1 : 1252, 1903.

Lindenberg, A.: L'ulcère de Bauru ou le bouton d'Orient au Brésil, Bull. Soc. path. exot., 2 : 252, 1909.

Machado, R. and Alexio, A.: Uno caso de leishmaniose mutilante, Brazil-med., 32 : 9, 1918.

Machado, W.: Demonstrated a case of cutaneous leishmaniasis treated with tartar emetic, Bol. d. Soc. brasil. de dermatol., 2 : 17, 28, 1913.

McLeod, J. H.: Demonstrated microscopical preparations of a case of Delhi boil, at meeting of Dermatological Society of London, March 12, 1902, Brit. J. Dermat., 14 : 128, 1902.

Maggiore, S.: Contributio allo studio della patogenese dell'anemia nella leishmaniosi interna, Malaria e malattie dei paesi caldi, 7 : 18, 1916.

Mayer, M.: Leishmanien. Handbuch der pathogenen Mikroörganismen, Kolle und Wassermann, zweite Auflage, Jena, Gustav Fischer, Bd. VII, S. 419, 1913.

Migone, L. E.: Un cas de kala-azar à Asuncion (Paraguay), Bull. Soc. path. exot., 6 : 118, 1913.

Minett, E. P. and Field, F. E.: Notes on a case of dermal leishmaniasis in British Guiana, J. Trop. Med., 16 : 249, 1913.

Miranda, Bueno de: Arch. d. Soc. de méd. et cir. de São Paulo, 1 : 500, 1910.

Mitchell, T. J.: Carbon-dioxid snow with special reference to the treatment of Oriental sores, J. Roy. Army M. Corps, 22 : 440, 1914.

Monge, C.: La leishmaniasis del dermis en el Peru. Espundia, uta, etc., Crón. méd., Lima, 31 : 231, 1914.

Moreira, J.: Existe na Bahia o Botão be Biskra, Ann. Soc. méd.-chir. de Bahia, p. 6, February, 1895.

———— : Du bouton endémique, observé à Bahia (Brésil), J. d. mal. cutan. et syph., Par., 7 : 594, 1895. (The name on this article is M. Juliano, and it is so quoted by Scheube.)

Nattan-Larrier, L., Touin and Heckenroth, F.: Sur un cas de pian-bois de la Guyane. (Ulcère à leishmania de la Guyane), Bull. Soc. path. exot., 2 : 587, 1909.

Nicolle, C.: Sur trois cas d'infection, splénique infantile à corps de Leishman, observés en Tunisie, Arch. Inst. Pasteur de Tunis, p. 3, 1908.

Patton, W. S.: Is kala-azar in Madras of animal origin? Indian J. M. Research, 1 : 185, 1913.

———— : The examination of the peripheral blood of 84 patients suffering from kala-azar at the General Hospital, Madras, during the period from 15th June, 1912 to 15th July, 1913, Indian J. M. Research, 2 : 492, 1914.

Pedrosa, A. M.: Leishmaniose local do Cão, Ann. paulist. de med. e cir., 1 : 33, 1911.

Pianese, G.: Sull'anemia splenica infantile. Reunione dei Patologi in Roma, Gazz. internaz. med.-chir., 8 : 265, 1905.

Pittaluga, G.: El kala-azar infantil (esplenomegalia parasitaria de los miños) en la costa de Levante de España, Rev. clín. de Madrid, 8 : 265, 1912.

Pupo, J. de A.: Dos casos de blastomycosis, Ann. paulist. de med. e cir., 5 : 148, 1915.

Rogers, L.: Preliminary note on the development of trypanosoma in cultures of the Cunningham-Leishman-Donovan bodies of cachexial fever and kala-azar, Lancet, 2 : 215, 1904.

———— : The conditions affecting the development of flagellated organisms from Leishman bodies, Lancet, 1 : 1484, 1905.

———— : Chronic splenomegaly in lower Bengal with special reference to the prevalence and clinical differentiation of kala-azar, Indian M. Gaz., 52 : 7, 1917.

———— : Dangers of tartar emetic solutions, Indian M. Gaz., 53 : 161, 1918.

Ross, R.: Notes on the bodies recently described by Leishman and Donovan, Brit. M. J., 2 : 1261, 1401, 1903.

Row, R.: Leishmania donovani and L. tropica, Brit. M. J., 1 : 717, 1912.

———— : Some experimental facts re kala-azar (Indian), J. Trop. Med., 15 : 327, 1912 ; 16 : 1, 1913.

———— : Generalized leishmaniasis induced in a mouse with culture of Leishmania tropica of Oriental sore, Bull. Soc. path. exot., 7 : 272, 1914.

Russell, A.: Natural History of Aleppo, London, p. 266, 1756.

Savon Salaberry, J.: Leishmaniosis tegumentaria y mucosa americana. (Estudio de algunos casos. Tratamiento), Prensa méd. argent., 23 : 2427, 1936.

Scheube, B.: Die Krankheiten der warmen Länder, Vierte Auflage, Jena, Gustav Fischer, 1910.

Seidelin, H.: Leishmaniasis and babesiasis in Yucatan, Ann. Trop. Med., 6 : 295, 1912.

Spagnolio, G.: Die Leishmaniose bei Menschen und Hunden. Studium des Krankheitsgebietes, Centralbl. f. Bakt., 1 Abt., Orig., 75 : 294, 1915.

Splendore, A.: Buba-Blastomicosi-Leishmaniosi, Arch. f. Schiffs- u. Tropen-Hyg., 15 : 105, 1911.

Stitt, E. R.: Diagnostics and Treatment of Tropical Diseases, Ed. 2, Phila., P. Blakiston's Son & Co., 1917.

Struthers, E. B. and Lin, L. C.: Treatment of kala-azar with solustibosan, new antimony compound, Chinese M. J., 52 : 355, 1937.

Sun, C. J. and Wu, C. C.: Notes on study of kala-azar transmission; further observations on natural infection of Phlebotomus chinensis with Leptomonas donovani, Chinese M. J., 52 : 665, 1937.

Susu, B. J.: Espundia in the Anglo-Egyptian Sudan, J. Trop. Med., 20 : 146, 1917.

Tejera, E.: Varios casos de leishmaniosis americana en el Estada Julia. Nota preliminar, Gac. méd. de Carácas, 24 : 145, 1917.

Thomson, D. B. and Balfour, A.: Two cases of non-ulcerating "Oriental sore," better termed "Leishman nodules," J. Roy. Army M. Corps, 14 : 1, 1910.

Tropical Diseases Bulletin: Published monthly by Tropical Diseases Bureau, Imperial Institute, S. W. 7. Gives excellent abstracts of all current literature on tropical diseases.

Vianna, G.: Demonstrated case of oral leishmaniasis treated with tartar emetic, Bol. d. Soc. brasil. de dermatol., 2 : 17, 28, 1913.

———— : Leishmania brasiliensis als Parasit glatter Muskelfasern, Mem. Inst. Oswaldo Cruz, 6 : 40, 1914.

Visentini, A: Studi interno ad alcune malattie trop. in Sic. e Calabria, fasc. 1, 1910.

Wenyon, C. M.: Kala-azar in Malta, with some remarks on the various leishmaniases, Tr. Soc. Trop. M. & Hyg., 7 : 97, 1914.

Wright, J. H.: Protozoa in a case of tropical ulcer ("Delhi sore"), J. Med. Research, 10 : 472, 1903.

Yates, T. M.: "Sdt. 561" in treatment of kala-azar, Chinese M. J., 52 : 339, 1937 (abstr., Trop. Dis. Bull., 35 : 181, 1938).

Young, T. C. M.: Annual sanitary report of the province of Assam for 1916, abstr., Trop. Dis. Bull., 10 : 326, 1917.

Zia, L. S. and Forkner, C. E.: The syndrome of acute agranulocytosis and its occurrence as a complication of kala-azar, Am. J. M. Sc., 188 : 624, 1934.

CHAPTER XXIX

RELAPSING FEVER

By Eugene R. Whitmore, B.S., M.D.

Synonyms.—Febris recurrens, Tick fever, Famine fever.

Definition.—The term "relapsing fever" is applied to a group of specific fevers which closely resemble each other clinically, caused by blood spirochetes, and characterized clinically by one to four or more paroxysms of fever, each lasting five to six days, with an afebrile interval of about six days.

Etiology.—Predisposing Causes.—Relapsing fever occurs epidemically, endemically and sporadically. It prevails especially under conditions of filth and overcrowding, and during times of privation and famine. In India, it is common in jails and police hospitals; while Rabinowitsch, who studied relapsing fever in Russia, finds that typhus fever is more commonly favored by conditions such as exist in asylums.

Season.—It is generally found that relapsing fever prevails more in winter; probably as a result of greater crowding, privation and insanitary conditions at that season of the year. Rabinowitsch studied an epidemic in Russia in 1906. The epidemic began in January, 1906, and gradually increased to December of that year: the number of cases fell in January, 1907, rose again in March and had decreased slightly by May, 1907. Robledo says the disease in Colombia is most frequent in March and April; and that it is not rare in October and November.

Age and Sex.—Rabinowitsch found that relapsing fever was more common among persons from 15 to 30 years of age; and that it was over three times as common among men as among women. However, he is of the opinion that this prevalence among young men is due to the fact that these are the persons who would be crowded together, under unhygienic conditions, as laborers; and that there is no difference in age or sex susceptibility.

EXCITING CAUSE: THE ORGANISM.—Relapsing fever is caused by organisms which are commonly classed as protozoa and placed in the flagellata; or they are classed as transition forms between the bacteria and the flagellata of the protozoa; or they are classed with the bacteria. Whether the spirochetes causing relapsing fever in different parts of the world are different species or are varieties of one species is difficult to say. For the present, the different morphological and biological differences make it advisable to consider them as different species. It is useless to discuss genera in the spirochetes until there is agreement as to whether they belong to the bacteria, to the protozoa, or are separate groups.

Morphology.—The spirochetes of relapsing fever are 8 to 40 μ, usually 17 to 30 μ, long, and 0.3 to 0.5 μ in diameter, the Central African relapsing fever spirochete being generally considered as larger than the others. In stained preparations it is not possible to make out any structure, though there are irregularities of staining in the interior that are considered by some observers to represent granules of chromatin. There is no evidence of an undulating membrane. The ends are pointed, and a flagellum on one end is described by most observers. The flagella described along the sides of the organism are considered to be artefacts. There are 3 to 6, or even 10, curves in the body.

In the living preparation, the spirochetes are seen to have three kinds of motion: (1) a corkscrew-like motion, (2) a wave-like forward and backward movement, and (3) lateral bending and looping movements. The movement of the spirochetes is most active at the height of the fever attack.

Resistance to Physical and Chemical Conditions.—The spirochetes remain alive for a day or more under the cover glass when sealed, and they remain alive for weeks in the ice-box. Novy and Knapp kept them alive for 40 days in blood drawn in the beginning of the attack of fever, and they lived 30 days on blood agar without multiplying. They remain alive for some days in the blood of leeches.

They are killed in the blood in half an hour at 45° to 48° C. They are quickly killed by chemical agents.

Development.—(a) *In the Vertebrate Host.*—The spirochetes appear in the peripheral blood in large numbers during the attack of fever. Whether multiplication is by longitudinal or transverse division is disputed. Shortly before the crisis the spirochetes roll up, and part of them are taken up by the endothelial cells of the spleen, liver and bone marrow. Others assume a cyst-like form, and are seen to break up into fine granules. By some authorities, it is considered that this cyst-like form is a resistant stage; and that the granules are the forms which develop the new generation for the relapse, and can also pass through a bacterial filter. Todd and Wolbach showed that *Spirochæta duttoni,* in the blood-serum of a rat, would pass through a Berkefeld filter that took out *Bacillus prodigiosus* and *Staphylococcus aureus,* at over 50 pounds pressure; but not at atmospheric pressure. However, Todd doubts whether spirochetes are filtrable in the usual sense of the term.

Spirochetes are found in the peripheral blood at each relapse, but not during the interval between relapses.

(b) *In the Arthropod Host.*—I. Ticks: The development of *Spirochæta duttoni* in the tick, *Ornithodorus moubata*, was studied by Dutton and Todd, and by R. Koch. Dutton and Todd found motile spirochetes in the stomach and malpighian tubes of infected ticks for five weeks after feeding; and they found that ticks, hatched from eggs laid by infected ticks, could transmit the infection to monkeys. Koch found that, four days after feeding, the spirochetes had disappeared from the stomach of the tick, and had collected in the ovaries; and that the spirochetes enter the eggs and multiply there, being visible up to the twentieth day of development of the embryo. Koch did not find spirochetes in the embryos after twenty days; but they are present, as the young ticks transmitted the infection to monkeys.

While the infection of the ovaries accounts for the transmission of the infection to the next generation of ticks, the adult tick itself is also infectious after feeding on infected blood. The form in which the spirochetes exist in the body of the tick has been a subject of discussion.

Leishman studied the development of the spirochete in the tick, and only occasionally could he find the spirochetes in the eggs. He found that the spirochetes were not present longer than ten days in the stomach of the tick; but that they broke up into small coccus-like or ovoid granules of chromatin. These granules pass to the malpighian tubes and to the ovaries, entering the unripe egg and infecting the embryo that develops in that egg. These bodies in the malpighian tubes and in the coxal glands are deposited on the skin when the tick bites.

A number of workers have studied the granules in the various organs of ticks; and some have found granules in the organs of ticks which had not been infected. Wittrock found granules in the tissues of unfed offspring of uninfected ticks. Most workers are of the opinion that the granules found in ticks are not a phase in the life-cycle of spirochetes; but Leishman has recently reaffirmed his belief that these granules are such a phase.

Marchoux and Couvey state that the spirochetes do not disappear from ticks, but that they are fine and are difficult to see. They consider that infection takes place through inoculation of spirochetes as such. Kleine and Eckard found spirochetes in the ovaries, coxal glands, malpighian tubes, cephalic glands, stomach and salivary glands of ticks; and they found spirochetes in the eggs laid by infected ticks. They found comma-shaped bodies in ticks, but infection was not produced by injecting these bodies; and they conclude that spirochetes as such are necessary for the tick to transmit the infection.

Regardless of the form in which the spirochetes exist in the body of the tick, it seems definitely agreed that infection is from contamination with the secretion of the coxal glands and feces of the tick when it

is biting. If there is a period during which the tick is not infectious,
it is only the time necessary for the infectious form of the spirochete
to reach the feces and coxal glands in sufficient number to produce infection. Wittrock found that emulsions of the organs of ticks were
infectious at all times from one hour to ninety-six days after feeding
on infected blood; and concludes that there is no cycle of development
in the tick. The ticks remain infectious for eighteen months; and
there is evidence that the infection may be transmitted hereditarily as
far as the third generation of ticks.

II. Lice: Nicolle and Blanc have studied the development of
Spirochæta berbera in the clothes louse. They find that the spirochetes
disappear rapidly from the body of the insect, and no spirochetes are
visible. The louse is not infectious until about the fifth or sixth day;
but still no spirochetes are visible. On the seventh to tenth days,
slender spirochetes appear in the body cavity of the louse, and the louse
is still infectious. After the tenth day, the spirochetes are adult, and
the louse is not infectious. No spirochetes are found after the nineteenth
day. The spirochetes are in the body cavity of the louse, and infection
takes place through crushing the louse on the skin. In the course
of their experiments, a man was bitten 15,500 times by infected lice without becoming infected; then an infected louse was crushed and placed
on his conjunctiva, and he developed relapsing fever. They got evidence of hereditary transmission only occasionally.

Rabinowitsch failed to transmit the infection with clothes lice in
Russia; and Robledo failed to transmit the infection with head lice in
Colombia.

III. Bedbugs: Nothing is known of the development of spirochetes
in the bedbug. Tictin and Rabinowitsch found that the spirochetes remained alive in the intestine of the bugs for 5 to 7 days after feeding
on infected blood; but they did not find any further development in the
bug. Tictin transmitted the infection to monkeys by crushing bugs as
soon as they had gorged on infected blood, and injecting the blood from
the intestine of the bugs into monkeys. But when he waited 48 hours
after the bug had fed on infected blood, he was not able to transmit
the infection to monkeys by injection of the intestinal contents of the
bugs; though he found living spirochetes in the intestine of bugs as
long as 77 hours after feeding on infected blood.

Rabinowitsch is of the opinion that Tictin's experiments do not indicate that the spirochetes undergo any development in the bedbug, as
the immediate injection of blood from the intestine of the bug amounted
to the same thing as injecting the blood direct from the infected person. He does not accept Tictin's explanation of his failure to transmit
the infection with bugs 48 hours after feeding as due to the small number (6) of bugs used. Rabinowitsch tried to transmit the infection to
himself by allowing bugs to bite him immediately after, and five days
after feeding on infected blood; the bugs failed to transmit the infection.

Cultivation.—Noguchi cultivated *Spirochæta duttoni, Spirochæta
kochi, Spirochæta obermeieri,* and *Spirochæta novyi* on his spirochete

medium. Hata used a simplified medium in the cultivation of *Spirochæta obermeieri*. Some observers have described branching forms in cultures of the spirochetes, and have held this as an indication of the vegetable nature of the spirochetes.

Transmission to Lower Animals.—*Spirochæta obermeieri* can be transmitted to monkeys very readily; and it can be transmitted to rats, mice and guinea pigs by intraperitoneal injection. Rats, mice and guinea pigs usually have a mild infection.

Spirochæta duttoni is readily transmitted to monkeys, either by injection of blood or by the bite of infectious ticks. Rats, mice, rabbits and guinea pigs are readily infected by *Spirochæta duttoni*. The dog, pony, sheep and goat develop light infection.

Spirochæta berbera is readily transmitted to monkeys by the injection of blood; or by injecting crushed infectious lice. The infection is not transmitted to monkeys by the bite of infectious lice. Rats, mice, guinea pigs and rabbits are susceptible to infection with *Spirochæta berbera*.

Spirochæta novyi and *Spirochæta carteri* are both readily transmitted to monkeys, rats and mice.

Relation of the Spirochetes in Relapsing Fever in Different Regions. —While there are minor differences in the morphology and animal susceptibility of the different relapsing fever spirochetes, it is not possible to separate them into species on those differences; and it is not possible to separate them by cross immunization. But they can be separated by their reactions with sera which are specific against the different spirochetes. Thus, a highly immune serum, prepared by injecting a rabbit with *Spirochæta obermeieri*, will agglutinate and destroy *Spirochæta obermeieri*; but it has no effect on any of the other relapsing fever spirochetes.

Epidemiology.—It is generally agreed that the spirochetes of relapsing fever are transmitted by biting arthropods in different countries; but it does not appear that the spirochetes are specifically adapted to any particular arthropod in a given locality. Nuttall points out that a number of arthropods can carry the same spirochete, and that the same arthropod may carry a number of different spirochetes.

The bedbug (Fig. 1) has long been considered as the transmitter of *Spirochæta obermeieri*; but Tictin's work is the only experimental evidence in favor of such transmission. The clothes louse has also been suspected; but there is no experimental evidence that the infection is transmitted by this arthropod. Authorities have reported outbreaks of relapsing fever accompanying outbreaks of typhus, and considered that both were transmitted by lice. Hagler saw relapsing fever and typhus together in Serbia. Typhus stopped when lice disappeared; but relapsing fever continued until the wards were fumigated to get rid of bedbugs. Kuelz saw relapsing fever in Serbia, and found it impossible to prevent the disease by eradicating lice.

In Central African relapsing fever, the tick has long been considered as the transmitter of this condition; and all experimental work confirms that opinion. The infection follows caravan routes; and the rest houses along the routes seem to be great sources of infection. Koch noted that the infection remained attached to a house for years; and he suggested that, in the absence of the human, the ticks bite the rats and mice, and so keep up the infection in the house. It is a little difficult to know how such an abandoned house is infected with rats and mice, unless the human frequents it enough so that there will be food for rats

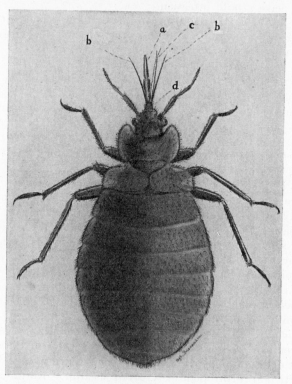

FIG. 1.—CIMEX LECTULARIUS (Female). (× 13.)

The mouth parts are turned forward, and the cutting parts are drawn out of the groove in the dorsal surface of the labium (a). The double-grooved mandibles (b) are drawn widely apart; the maxillæ, with their serrated tips, lie close together (c). The distal segment of the labrum (d) is visible.

and mice; in that case it may well be man himself that keeps up the infection in such abandoned houses.

Spirochæta berbera is transmitted by the clothes louse (Fig. 2).

It is generally considered that *Spirochæta carteri* is transmitted by clothes lice. In Persia, miana fever, which is relapsing fever, is transmitted by a tick, *Argas persicus* or *Ornithodorus savignyi*. In addition to his experience in Serbia, Kuelz saw considerable relapsing fever in Macedonia and Persia; and he is of the opinion that some other arthropod than lice transmits the infection, and he suggests fleas as the transmitter.

Mouzels, in Tonkin, found spirochetes in the stomach of mosquitoes in houses where there were cases of relapsing fever, while lice and bugs were often absent. Mouzels thinks any blood-sucking arthropod may transmit the infection.

It is not known how *Spirochæta novyi* is transmitted. Robledo is of the opinion that it is transmitted by *Argas persicus (americanus)* in Colombia; while Franco and his co-workers are of the opinion that it is transmitted by *Ornithodorus turicata* or possibly by *Argas reflexus*.

The spirochetes can pass through the unbroken skin or mucous membrane. It is generally agreed that the infection is not transmitted by biting; but that the organisms are deposited on the skin, in the feces or

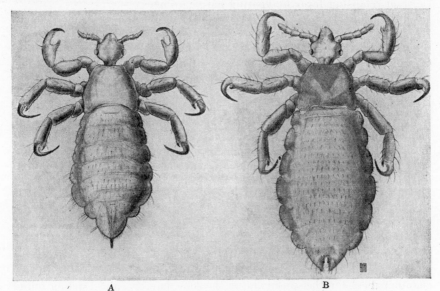

A   B

FIG. 2.—PEDICULUS HUMANUS CORPORIS.

A, male; B, female. (× 35.)

in the gland secretions of the arthropod, and are rubbed into the bite wound or pass directly through the unbroken skin. In the case of louse transmission, it seems that the important way of infection is from the crushing of lice on the skin.

Infected blood, as from the menstrual flow, or from childbirth, rubbed on the unbroken skin, will transmit the infection. The possibility of infection through sexual intercourse should be borne in mind.

Spirochetes are found in the blood from hemorrhages, as from nosebleed; in the bloody stools; in the saliva; and they have been found in the sweat and in the tears, when they are numerous in the blood. Since the spirochetes are present in the saliva, it does not appear that their presence in the sputum of cases of complicating pneumonia is of special significance.

Rabinowitsch is of the opinion that bedbugs are not the only means of transmission of the relapsing fever spirochete in Russia. He failed to transmit the infection by the bite of bedbugs and lice; and he says that bedbugs were so numerous in some places that no one could have escaped the infection if it was transmitted by the bugs. He also points out that physicians and nurses are rarely infected, though they frequently get bugs on their clothing. From these considerations, together with the fact that the spirochetes are found in the secretions and discharges, Rabinowitsch is of the opinion that infection may take place by way of the mouth in persons who live in the insanitary conditions under which relapsing fever is found.

Darling is of the opinion that persons in the Panama Canal zone contract relapsing fever by visiting native villages.

Mechanism of the Disease Process.—The parasite, entering through the unbroken skin or mucous membrane, or rubbed into the wound produced by the bite of the arthropod, undergoes some unknown form of multiplication. After a few days an attack of fever sets in. The spirochetes do not appear in the blood for some hours, or even until the second or third day after the onset of the fever. The fever is considered to be due to a toxin produced by the spirochetes. After a few days' fever, the parasites disappear from the blood; and some hours later the temperature falls to normal. Just before the attack of fever stops, the blood contains antibodies which kill and dissolve the spirochetes.

After the temperature becomes normal, no spirochetes can be found in the blood; but the blood is still infectious for another animal, and it remains infectious after being passed through a Berkefeld filter. There is discussion as to the form in which the spirochetes exist in the peripheral blood during the interval after the attack of fever. It is generally held that the spirochetes exist at this time in the "infective granule" form of Balfour, as described in the development of the spirochete in the human host. Numerous workers have found the spirochetes in the endothelial cells in the spleen and in the bone marrow; and Darling found them in the endothelial cells in the liver. This finding of spirochetes in the endothelial cells has led to discussion as to whether it is a part of the mechanism of recovery in relapsing fever; and there are numerous authorities on both sides of the question. Darling considered that the spirochetes in the endothelial cells in the liver were an indication that this was a mechanism of defense; though he noted that emulsion of a liver that contained only a trace of blood was more infectious than was heart's blood. Rabinowitsch found spirochetes free or in the cells, and is of the opinion that phagocytosis plays no part in relapsing fever; he also holds that it is a strong argument against Metchnikoff's phagocytic theory.

After a few days, in which there are no symptoms, whatever form of the organism exists in the body develops into spirochetes which are resistant to the antibodies which have been elaborated against the original strain, and multiply to produce another attack of fever. The same process is repeated, until finally the antibodies overcome the spirochetes, and the disease process is at an end.

It has been suggested that the spirochetes continue to live in the body of man for some time, as a labile infection; but there is no evidence that this happens. It is interesting that the spirochete, at each relapse, has different biological reactions than it had at the previous or the subsequent relapse, and these reactions remain fixed on transmission to other animals; but they are lost when the organism is passed through an arthropod host.

A small number of cases have no relapse. Cassaux reports that one-fourth of his patients had no relapse, and two-thirds of them had only one relapse. In Rabinowitsch's tabulation of 3,464 cases, 29.01 per cent. had no relapse; 64 per cent. had one relapse; 6.29 per cent. had two relapses; 0.59 per cent. had three relapses; 0.17 per cent. had four relapses; and 0.03 per cent. (one case) had five relapses.

Immunity.—There is immunity following an attack of relapsing fever, but the immunity is of short duration, infection being possible within forty days to six months. In Serbia, Walko saw one person have relapsing fever eleven weeks after recovery from an attack. Jarussow reports that, in the Moscow epidemic in 1908, one-third of all the cases had second attacks.

Nicolle and Blaizot report experimental work in which a monkey had relapsing fever, was infected with the same virus in less than six weeks after recovery, and was again infected with the same virus, seventy-four days after recovery from the second attack.

Apparently there is more marked immunity after infection with *Spirochæta duttoni*. Koch was of the opinion that natives in the endemic region had the disease in youth and were immune. This is not borne out, though the attack in youth may cause the succeeding attacks to be milder.

The anemia is due to the destruction of the red cells by the toxin; and this destruction of red cells, with the disturbed function of the liver, leads to the hematogenous jaundice. The leukocytosis is due to the toxin, and is polymorphonuclear: at times it may be mononuclear, but it is suggested that this is due to malaria or amebiasis.

Rabinowitsch considers the cause of the pathologic changes is the spirochetes and their products of metabolism. Thus, he says, the infarcts and hemorrhages in the spleen are due to injury of the endothelium by the toxin. Mühlens is of the opinion that further study along this line is necessary.

Death from the disease itself usually occurs in collapse during or following the crisis; or death may be due to suprarenal deficiency. Death more commonly results from some complication, as rupture of the spleen, pneumonia or myocarditis.

Symptomatology.—Clinical History.—*Period of Incubation.*—There is an incubation period of two to twelve days, usually five to eight days, during which there are no symptoms; or there may be a prodromal stage of a few hours to two or three days, consisting of headache, loss of appetite and lassitude.

Mode of Onset—Symptoms during Progress of Disease.—The attack begins suddenly, with a chill and aching in the head, back and joints.

The temperature rises rapidly to 103° to 104° F. (39.4° to 40° C.) ; the pulse is rapid—110 to 120; the face is flushed; there is epigastric pain; nausea and vomiting are frequently present.

The temperature remains high for five to six days, often with irregular fluctuations amounting to as much as four degrees. During this time there is nausea and vomiting; the skin is usually dry and hot, but there may be light perspiration, and the skin is yellow tinged. There may be constipation, but diarrhea is frequent in some epidemics. Nosebleed is frequent, also hemorrhages from the gastro-intestinal tract, the gums, into the conjunctiva, and from the ears. Hematuria is rare; there may be hemorrhages into the skin, and metrorrhagia. There is bronchitis, with cough, rapid pulse and respiration, and pains in the joints and muscles. There may be delirium—sometimes abrupt and violent, and rarely stupor. There may be a rose-red, macular eruption on the thorax, abdomen and legs, lasting for a day or two. Herpes is common. The spleen and liver are enlarged and tender; the urine is high colored and contains albumin. There is a rapidly developing anemia; a moderate leukocytosis, the increase being due to increase in the polymorphonuclears, and spirochetes are found in the blood.

About the sixth or seventh day the patient breaks out in a profuse perspiration, the temperature falls to normal in one to two hours, and the patient is apparently normal. The spleen and liver return rapidly toward normal in size, and the patient gains in strength.

Rarely there is recovery after one attack of fever. More commonly, after about six or seven days of freedom from fever, the *relapse* sets in with a chill, as with the first attack of fever, and the entire attack is repeated. At times the relapse is more severe than the first attack of fever, but more commonly the relapse lasts only three or four days, ending by crisis just as the first attack of fever. In about two-thirds of the cases, this relapse ends the course of the disease, and the patient returns to normal. A second relapse is not uncommon; a third and fourth relapse are much less common, and very rarely are there more than four relapses.

At times instead of the rapid rise of the temperature, there may be a gradual onset, with rheumatic-like pains, headache and constipation. The temperature curve may be irregular, or it may show a tertian or quartan intermittency. The temperature may fall by lysis, over six hours to three days. There may be a pseudocrisis on the third or fourth day, the temperature going up again for three to five days. In the crisis the temperature may fall, then rise to or above the original temperature and fall again—all in a few hours. There may be a chill at the crisis.

The spleen may not be markedly enlarged, and Robledo speaks of this in the relapsing fever of Colombia.

Meningeal symptoms may be prominent: severe headache, stiffness of the muscles of the neck and body, hyperesthesia, clouded mental condition and Kernig's sign may be present.

Reinfection during the same epidemic is not uncommon. The second attack is generally marked by shorter attacks of fever and fewer relapses.

Diagnosis.—DIFFERENTIAL DIAGNOSIS ON CLINICAL HISTORY.—Malaria, dengue, small-pox, influenza and yellow fever have to be differentiated from relapsing fever, and this is very difficult from the clinical picture alone. The early stages of plague may be confused with relapsing fever. Franco and his co-workers draw a parallel between the clinical picture in yellow fever and relapsing fever, and suggest a relationship in the etiological agent in the two diseases. The enlarged spleen speaks against small-pox, influenza, yellow fever and dengue. When the meningeal symptoms predominate there may be confusion. Weil's disease may cause confusion, especially with the bilious form of relapsing fever. Typhus may cause confusion, the stupor and the dark, macular eruption being points in favor of typhus.

LABORATORY FINDINGS.—There is a polymorphonuclear leukocytosis in relapsing fever, which speaks against *dengue*.

Agglutinins and spirillicidal substances appear in the serum of the patients late in the course of the disease: these substances may be of assistance in diagnosis late in the course of the disease or during convalescence.

The finding of the spirochetes in the blood is the one definite diagnostic sign. It is to be remembered that the spirochetes are not numerous in the peripheral blood in some forms of relapsing fever, especially in the early days of the Central African form, and that the spirochetes are not found in the blood from a short time before the crisis to the beginning of the relapse.

The blood may be examined direct in a smear between slide and cover-glass, with the condenser well lowered; or it may be examined by dark-field illumination. Smears may be made in the usual way, as for examination for malaria, and stained with any of the Romanowsky stains. As the parasites may not be numerous, the thick drop method may be used. The hemoglobin may be washed out and the smear fixed and stained with a Romanowsky stain; or, what is simpler, the thick drop preparation, as soon as dry, is placed in Giemsa's staining solution for half an hour, then removed and carefully rinsed in distilled water—but not flushed with it—and dried in the air. The hemoglobin is washed out of the unfixed smear by the Giemsa solution, and only leukocytes, blood platelets and spirochetes stain in the smear. The blood may be dropped into acetic acid solution to dissolve the red cells, then centrifuged to collect the spirochetes and leukocytes in the sediment.

Even if the spirochetes are not found in the blood, as during the interval, they are present in an infectious form, and the blood will produce infection when injected into a susceptible animal. Monkeys are the most satisfactory, but if monkeys are not available, some of the blood should be injected intraperitoneally into a mouse or rat. Rats and mice are readily infected with *Spirochæta duttoni*, *Spirochæta berbera* and *Spirochæta novyi*, when injected intraperitoneally with infected blood. Rabinowitsch found that very young rats and mice—a few days old, without hair—were very susceptible to infection with *Spirochæta obermeieri*.

In *Weil's disease,* though the spirochetes are in the peripheral blood in the first six or seven days of the disease, they are rarely found on direct examination, and they are smaller than the spirochetes of relapsing fever. The spirochete of Weil's disease produces characteristic lesions in guinea pigs, on intraperitoneal injection of blood, in the first week of the disease, and later appears in the urine and feces.

Complications.—Complications of the respiratory tract are the most important. Pneumonia is a severe complication. Bronchitis and pleurisy are fairly common. Marked icterus is hardly to be considered as a complication, but it makes for a bad prognosis. Dysentery is fairly common. There may be rupture of the spleen, at times spontaneously, more commonly from trauma, as from getting out of bed during the delirium. Splenic abscess has been reported. The frequent hemorrhages into any of the tissues are hardly to be considered as complications; they are more common in cases with jaundice. There may be cerebral hemorrhage. Angina is fairly common during the attacks of fever. There may be edema from heart failure or from nephritis. Kuelz says that the so-called relapsing fever edema is not peculiar to relapsing fever, but is due to deficient diet—lack of vitamins. Iridocyclitis is fairly common. Pregnant women abort almost without exception.

There is a difference of opinion as to whether the bilious typhoid fever in Egypt is a severe form of relapsing fever, with marked jaundice, or there is an added septic infection, or there are two different diseases. Rabinowitsch thinks that bilious typhoid fever is not relapsing fever. It is probable that some of these cases are Weil's disease, and Rabinowitsch saw two cases of Weil's disease in the epidemic of relapsing fever studied by him.

Clinical Varieties.—The clinical picture of relapsing fever varies a great deal, and in addition to the ordinary form, as just described, Casaux describes ambulatory, typhobilious, typhoid-like and bilious forms. When the liver is seriously affected there is a bilious form.

Treatment.—PROPHYLAXIS.—The conditions under which relapsing fever flourishes—filth and famine—should be corrected, if they exist.

Prophylaxis is aimed directly at removing the spirochetes from man as the source of infection, by curing the cases promptly, and at protecting persons from the bites of bedbugs, lice and ticks. In Africa it is necessary to avoid the native houses; and Darling is of the opinion that relapsing fever in Panama is contracted by visiting the native houses. It is worthy of note that the tick, *Ornithodorus moubata,* will not come into moist earth or where there is moisture. Stitt says the ticks bite only at night, and that a night-light will keep them away. Mosquito nets protect from adult ticks as well as from mosquitoes. As *Ornithodorus moubata* does not travel more than thirty yards away from the house, it is advised to sleep in the open, at least that distance away from the houses. Lice and bedbugs are more difficult to avoid, and the eradication of those insects is discussed in the section on Parasitic Arthropods.

Rabinowitsch advises measures to prevent infection by mouth. It is to be borne in mind that the infection is in the discharges and secretions, and that it will pass through the unbroken skin and mucous membranes. A number of laboratory infections have resulted in this way.

GENERAL MANAGEMENT.—**Salvarsan** or **neosalvarsan** is a specific in relapsing fever. It is not necessary to give large doses, and there is some evidence that relapsing fever patients do not stand large doses of salvarsan well. Protocalis recommends two doses of 0.2 gram of salvarsan: one dose during the first attack; the second dose four or five days after the temperature has fallen. Even with this treatment, he got relapses in 25 per cent. of his cases. Levaditi found that the best time to give salvarsan was just before the crisis, as it took less of the drug to produce a cure at that time.

Brault and Montpellier found **neosalvarsan injections in oil** unsatisfactory, as the absorption was too slow; rapid absorption is necessary in order to kill the spirochetes. **Antimony preparations** have not given satisfactory results in the treatment of relapsing fever.

Cool sponging may be given for high temperature, and **aspirin** for the pain in the head, back and joints. A **hypodermic injection of morphin** may have to be given. When there are meningeal symptoms and the headache is due to intracranial pressure, **lumbar puncture** will relieve the pain. The cough may require **sedative cough mixtures**.

The vomiting may be allayed by **hot fomentations or counterirritation** over the epigastrium and by **cracked ice**. The thirst is relieved by **acid drinks,** as lemonade and cracked ice or soda water. Constipation or diarrhea may require treatment.

Complications are treated as they arise.

It is necessary to watch the patient, as he may develop delirium and get out of bed, and there is danger of death from heart failure or collapse, or from rupture of the spleen spontaneously or on slight exertion.

At the time of the crisis it is necessary to support the patient with **stimulants,** as **camphorated oil,** and to apply **external heat.**

During the attack, the **diet should be liquid.** *After the attack* is over, it is necessary to **feed the patient well,** as the anemia is marked. **Fresh air and rest** complete the recovery.

Prognosis.—Before the introduction of salvarsan treatment of relapsing fever, the mortality was from 2 to 5 per cent. In China and Indo-China the mortality was often as high as 25 to 40 per cent.; and in the epidemics in India and China in 1912-1913, the mortality was as high as 70 to 80 per cent. Alcoholic liver and weakened heart muscle are apt to be badly affected in relapsing fever. Severe jaundice makes for a bad prognosis, as the mortality is about 40 per cent. in such cases. Of the complications, pneumonia is severe, the mortality being 35 to 40 per cent., or even as high as 70 per cent. As most of the deaths are due to complications, death is not very common in children on account of the rarity of complications. Persons living in the conditions under which relapsing fever thrives are apt to be lowered in general resistance, and this makes for a bad prognosis, as well as for the frequency with which other diseases are found with relapsing fever. The long course of the disease is one of its worst features.

Pathology.—Rabinowitsch has made an extensive study of the pathology of relapsing fever.

MACROSCOPIC.—The skin is frequently jaundiced, especially in the African relapsing fever, and all the organs may be bile stained. The appearance of the organs will vary with the stage of the disease in which death takes place.

The spleen is enlarged, Rabinowitsch reporting one case in which it weighed 1700 grams. The capsule is tense and thin. On section, the spleen is soft and diffluent, dark red in color, filled with blood, the follicles are enlarged, and infarcts are numerous. The kidneys are enlarged and congested. The liver is enlarged and congested, the capsule is tense, the lobules are indistinct: there may be a layer of fibrin over the surface of the liver. The heart is soft and flabby. There is congestion of the lungs and brain.

Metastatic abscesses may be found in the liver, kidneys, spleen and various parts of the body.

MICROSCOPIC.—Early in the attack the vessels in the spleen are intensely congested and there are some hemorrhages in the spleen pulp. The follicles are enlarged, and there is an increase in the lymphocytes throughout the spleen pulp, with macrophages containing red blood cells and lymphocytes.

As the attack progresses the hemorrhages increase and amount to infarcts; at the same time the follicles become less prominent and the lymphocytic infiltration less marked.

At the time of the crisis, or two or three days after it, the hemorrhagic areas show considerable change: the red cells are in all stages of disintegration, there are homogeneous areas of fibrin, the endothelium of the vessels is swollen and lost, the macrophages are filled with cells and cellular débris, and karyorrhexis is marked in the areas of lymphocytes. The spleen rapidly returns to normal in microscopic appearance after this time.

Spirochetes are not found in the spleen in the beginning of the attack, but they are numerous shortly before the crisis, partly free and partly in the endothelial cells.

In the kidneys the epithelium of the tubules is swollen and cloudy, and as the condition progresses the change in the epithelium becomes more marked until the outline of the cells is lost and there is nothing but granular débris. There is not infrequently infiltration of red cells in the interstitial tissue; more rarely an abundance of red cells between the layers of Bowman's capsule.

The liver parenchyma is swollen and cloudy: the blood sinuses are filled, and there is pigment in the endothelial cells as well as in the parenchyma cells. There may be round cell infiltration about the portal vessels. Rabinowitsch considers the increase in interstitial tissue and the fatty change in the parenchyma cells as due to a previous chronic condition, as alcoholism. Darling found spirochetes in the endothelial cells of the liver.

The heart muscle always shows marked changes. Frequently the striations are lost; the nuclei are pale or do not stain, and the cell shows marked vacuolation, or is reduced to a mass of granular débris. The muscle cells often contain pigment and at times there is pigment and red cells between the muscle fibers.

There are areas of softening in the bone marrow. There is nothing characteristic in the mucosa of the gastro-intestinal tract.

The metastatic abscesses appear throughout any of the organs.

History.—Hippocrates described an epidemic of relapsing fever in Thasos. Fever with relapses was known in London and Ireland in the eighteenth century, and during an epidemic of fever in England, in 1826 and 1827, it was recognized that there were two types of fever that had been included in "typhus fever." There were repeated epidemics of the milder type of typhus fever, and in 1843, Henderson recognized that this mild fever was not typhus. In 1868, during an epidemic in Berlin, Obermeier found "fine motile threads" in the blood of relapsing fever patients, and he published his findings in 1873, giving the name "Spirillum febris recurrentis" to the organism. Obermeier's finding was confirmed in other countries of Europe; but relapsing fever came to be more and more rare in Europe, and the organism did not receive any great attention. Cohn gave the name *Spirochæta obermeieri* to the organism of relapsing fever in Europe. Hindle says *Spirochæta recurrentis* is the proper name for this spirochete.

In North America, relapsing fever was observed in Philadelphia in 1844 and was supposed to have been brought in by Irish immigrants, so the disease was considered to be identical with European relapsing fever. During the next thirty years, the disease was pretty well known in the eastern states, and in 1874 an epidemic was observed among some Chinese laborers in California. Since that time the disease has been reported from Central and South America, and the West Indies. In 1906 a number of workers studied the spirochete of American relapsing fever and considered it different from the spirochetes of relapsing fever in Europe, Asia and Africa. Shellack gave the name *Spirochæta novyi* to the spirochete of American relapsing fever.

In 1857 Livingston described "human tick disease" from Portuguese South Africa, and stated that the natives considered the disease was transmitted by the bite of ticks. From 1901 to 1904, a number of observers studied and described the tick fever of Central Africa. Novy and Knapp gave the name *Spirochæta duttoni* to the organism of relapsing fever in Central Africa. Some authorities separate the spirochetes of relapsing fever of East and West Africa, giving the name *Spirochæta duttoni* to the spirochete in West Africa, and the name *Spirochæta rossii* to the spirochete in East Africa. *Spirochæta kochi* is a synonym of *Spirochæta rossii*.

In 1853 Griesinger described a "bilious typhoid" fever in Egypt, and since that time there has been confusion as to whether bilious typhoid is a severe form of relapsing fever that is found in North Africa, or there are two diseases; one of them relapsing fever, and the other bilious typhoid of unknown cause. Sergent and Foley considered the spirochete of relapsing fever in North Africa to be a distinct species, and named it *Spirochæta berbera.*

Relapsing fever had been known in India since the eighteenth century. Lyall studied an epidemic in the Punjab in 1852 to 1853; and Carter found spirochetes in the blood of cases in Bombay in 1877. Hill described relapsing fever in China in 1904; Imbert described it in French Indo-China in 1910; and Schneider described it from northern Syria in 1912. Mackie gave the name *Spirochæta carteri* to the spirochete of relapsing fever in India.

Geographical Distribution.—There have been extensive epidemics of relapsing fever in Ireland, and there were severe epidemics in Russia in 1865 and in 1881. There have been lesser epidemics in England, Scotland, Germany, Denmark, Norway and the Balkan States. The disease has not been so common in Europe in recent years; but it was fairly prevalent on the eastern front during the recent war.

The disease is constantly present in India, French Indo-China and China. The cases reported from the Philippines seem to have been in persons who came from an endemic area, and the infection may have originated outside the Philippines. It is endemic in Syria and Arabia.

The disease is endemic in Portuguese South Africa and German East Africa; and there was an extensive epidemic along the caravan route from Dar-Es-Salaam to Muanza in 1903-1904. It is endemic in the Sedan. Other endemic centers in Africa are Uganda, Congo Free State, Nyassaland and Rhodesia.

In former years there was confusion regarding bilious typhoid fever in Egypt, but it is certain that relapsing fever is prevalent in Egypt, Tunis and Algiers.

The disease has not prevailed in epidemic form in the United States since 1869; but it is endemic in the southwestern part of the United States, in Mexico, Panama, Colombia, Venezuela, Cuba, Peru, Bolivia and Chili.

BIBLIOGRAPHY

ASHBURN, P. M., VEDDER, E. B., AND GENTRY, E. R. A spirillum in the blood of a case of blackwater fever. Bull. Manila Med. Soc., 1912, iv, 198.

BRAULT, J., ET MONTPELLIER, J. Essai de traitement de la fievre recurrente Nord-Africaine par des injections intramusculaires d'Olarsol. Bull. Soc. path. exot., 1914, vii, 473.

BRUMPT, E. Précis de parasitologie. 1913, 2d Ed., Masson & Company, Paris.

CARTER, H. V. Spirillum fever. London, 1882.

CASAUX, J. Considerations cliniques sur la fièvre récurrente en Indochine. Rev. de méd. et d'hyg. Trop., 1912, ix, 97.

CASTELLANI, A., AND CHALMERS, A. J. Manual of tropical diseases. 1913, 2d Ed., Wm. Wood & Company, New York.

CONSEIL, E. La fièvre récurrente Nord-Africaine. (Étude clinique sur cent soixante cas.) Arch. Inst. Pasteur, Tunis, 1913, No. 12, 37.

DARLING, S. T. The relapsing fever of Panama. Arch. Int. Med., 1909, iv, 150.
—— Relapsing fever in Panama. Trans. Seventeenth Internat. Cong. of Med., 1913, Sect. xxi, Trop. Med. and Hyg., Part 2, p. 279.

DOBELL, C. Researches on the spirochetes and related organisms. Arch. f. Protistenk., 1912, xxvi, 119.

FANTHAM, H. B. Spirochetes and their granule phase. Brit. Med. Jour., 1916, 409.

FRANCO, R., TORO, G., AND MARTINEZ, J. Fiebre amarilla y fiebre espiroquetal. Sesiones científicas del Centenario, Academia nacional de medicina, Republica de Colombia, Tomo I, Parte iv, Seccion iii, Medicina tropical—Bacteriologia, p. 169. Imprenta Nacional, Bogotá, 1911.

HAGLER, F. Relapsing fever. Mil. Surg., 1916, xxxix, 36.

HATA, S. A contribution to our knowledge of the cultivation of Spirochæta recurrens (recurrentis). Centralbl. f. Bakt., I Abt., Orig., 1913, lxxii, 107.

JEANSELME, E., AND RIST, E. Précis de pathologie exotique. 1909, Masson & Company, Paris.

KLEINE, F. K., AND ECKARD, B. Ueber die Lokalisation der Spirochäten in der Rückfallfieberzecke (Ornithodorus moubata). Ztschr. f. Hyg. u. Infektionskrankh., 1913, lxxiv, 389.

KUELZ, L. Beiträge zur Pathologie und Therapie des Rückfallfieber. Arch. f. Schiffs-u. Tropen-Hyg., 1917, xxi, 181.

LEISHMAN, W. B. A note on the "granule-clumps" found in Ornithodorus moubata and their relation to the spirochetes of African relapsing fever (tick fever). Ann. de l'Inst. Pasteur., 1918, xxxii, 49.

LEVADITI, C. Intervention de l'organisme dans la Guérison médicamenteuse des maladies à spirilles. Bull. Soc. path. exot., 1912, v, 524.

MANSON, P. Tropical diseases. 1918, 6th Ed., Wm. Wood & Company, New York.

MARCHOUX, E., ET COUVY, L. Argas et spirochètes. Bull. Soc. path. exot., 1912, v, 796.

—— Ibid. (Premier Mémoire.) Ann. de l'Inst. Pasteur, 1913, xxvii, 450.

MOUZELS, P. La fièvre récurrente au Tonkin et plus particulierement à Hanoï pendant les epidémies de 1911 et 1912. Ann. d'Hyg. et méd. Colonial, 1913, xvi, 249.

MÜHLENS, P. Rückfallfieber—Spirochäten. Handbuch der pathogenen Mikroorganismen. Kolle und Wassermann, 1913, 2d Ed., vii, 864, Gustav Fischer, Jena (with bibliography).

NICOLLE, C., ET BLAIZOT, L. Nouveaux points de l'étude expérimentale du spirochète de la fièvre récurrente Nord Africaine: réceptivité du lapin. Bull. Soc. path. exot., 1912, v, 472.

—— Deuxième note sur la courte durée de l'immunite dans le fièvre récurrente expérimentale. Bull. Soc. path. exot., 1913, vi, 242.

NICOLLE, C., BLAIZOT, L., ET CONSEIL, E. Etiologie de la fièvre récurrente. Compt. rend. Soc. de biol., Paris, 1912, cliv, 1636.

—— Conditions de transmission de la fièvre récurrente par le pou. Ibid., 1912, clv, 481.

NICOLLE, C., AND BLANC, G. Les spirilles de la fièvre récurrente sont-ils virulents aux phases successives de leur évolution chez le pou? Demonstration de leur virulence à un stade invisible. Compt. rend. Acad. d. sc., 1914, clviii, 1815.

NOGUCHI, H. Pure cultivation of Spirochæta duttoni, Spirochæta kochi, Spirochæta obermeieri, and Spirochæta novyi. Jour. Exper. Med., 1912, xvi, 199.

NUTTALL, G. H. F. Herter lectures. 1. Spirochetosis. Bull. Johns Hopkins Hosp., 1913, xxiv, 33.

PINO POU, R. Aclaraciones oportunas. Historia del descubrimiento de la fiebre recurrente en Venezuela (relapsing fever). Gaz. méd. de Caracas, 1918, xxv, 93.

PORTOCALIS, A. Le traitement de la fièvre récurrente. Compt. rend. Soc. de biol., 1918, lxxxi, 273.

RABINOWITSCH, M. Ueber die Rückfalltyphus Epidemie in Kiew. Berl. klin. Wchnschr., 1907, xliv, 1408 and 1458.

———— Ueber die febris recurreis. Virchow's Arch. f. path. Anat., 1908, cxciv, Beiheft, 38.

———— Ueber die Spirochæta pallida und Spirillum obermeieri, Ihre intrazellulare Lagerung und deren Bedeutung. *Ibid.*, 1909, cxcviii, 346.

ROBLEDO, E. Fièvre récurrente de Colombie. Bull. Soc. path. exot., 1909, ii, 117.

RUGE, R., AND ZUR VERTH, M. Tropenkrankheiten und Tropenhygiene. Ph. Bockenheimer (editor), Berlin, 1912.

STITT, E. R. Diagnostics and treatment of tropical diseases. P. Blakiston's Son & Company, Philadelphia, 2d Ed., 1917.

TAUSIG AND JURINAC. Ueber eine Fall von Milzruptur bei Febris recurrens. Wien. klin. Wchnschr., 1917, xxx, 1651.

TICTIN, J. Zur Lehre vom Rückfalltyphus. Centralbl. f. Bakteriol., 1897, I Abt., Orig., xxi, 179.

TODD, J. L. A note on the transmission of spirochetes. Proc. Soc. Exper. Biol. and Med., 1913, x, 134.

———— The relapsing fevers. Osler and McCrae, Modern medicine, 1914, 2d Ed., vol. II, p. 133, Lea & Febiger, Philadelphia.

TODD, J. L., AND WOLBACH, S. B. Concerning the filterability of Spirochæta duttoni. Jour. Med. Research, 1914, new series, xxv, 27.

WALKO, K. Ueber das Rückfallfieber. Wien. klin. Wchnschr., 1915, xxviii, 491.

WITTROCK, O. Beitrag zur Biologie der Spirochæta des Rückfallfiebers. Ztschr. f. Hyg. u. Infektionskrankh., 1913, lxxiv, 55.

WOLBACH, S. B. Distribution and morphology of Spirochæta duttoni and Spirochæta kochi (rossii) in experimentally infected ticks (Ornithodorus moubata). Jour. Med. Research, 1914, n. s., xxv, 37.

TRYPANOSOMIASIS

(*African Trypanosomiasis—American Trypanosomiasis*)

By E. R. Whitmore, M.D.

Under this heading are included two diseases, found in different parts of the world, and having different clinical courses, both caused by trypanosomes.

African trypanosomiasis is an endemic disease in some parts of Africa, while *American trypanosomiasis* is an endemic disease in some parts of South America.

AFRICAN TRYPANOSOMIASIS

Synonyms.—Sleeping sickness; Negro lethargy.

Definition.—A chronic disease caused by *Trypanosoma gambiense* and *Trypanosoma rhodesiense*, characterized anatomically by an inflammatory condition of the lymphatic system, with enlargement of the lymph glands and meningo-encephalitis and meningomyelitis. Clinically the disease is marked by irregular fever, emaciation, lassitude, weakness, tachycardia, erythema and edema of the skin, nervous and mental disturbances; and later, at times dementia, and commonly a protracted lethargy—sleeping sickness.

History.—John Atkins in 1734 described "the sleeping distemper" which he had seen among the natives on the Guinea coast in 1721. In 1803 Winterbottom described the disease on the west coast of Africa, near Sierra Leone. He noted the enlargement of the cervical glands, and says that this enlargement of the glands was known to the slave traders, and when present in a Negro was a sign for refusal of a slave. Other observers described the disease from different parts of Africa; and in 1869 Guerin saw the disease in Martinique, in slaves who had been brought there from Africa. A case was brought to London in 1891, and two cases were brought there in 1900. Several cases have come to the United States and have been studied here.

In 1901 Ford found a parasite in the blood of a patient with a peculiar type of fever from Gambia, and in 1902 Dutton recognized the parasite to be a trypanosome and gave it the name *Trypanosoma gambiense*. In 1902 Castellani found trypanosomes in the spinal fluid of cases of sleeping sickness in Uganda and gave the organism the name *Trypanosoma ugandense*. The findings of Todd and Castellani were confirmed by different observers; and Castellani and Nabarro showed that *Trypanosoma gambiense* and *Trypanosoma ugandense* were the same, and that sleeping sickness was only a stage in the febrile disease in which Todd and Dutton had found trypanosomes in the blood.

In 1903 Bruce and Nabarro showed that *Trypanosoma gambiense* was transmitted by a biting fly, *Glossina palpalis*. Kleine showed experimentally that *Trypanosoma gambiense* undergoes a cycle of development in *Glossina palpalis*.

In 1910 Stephens and Fantham reported that trypanosomiasis in Rhodesia was caused by a trypanosome that was different from *Trypanosoma gambiense,* and they gave the name *Trypanosoma rhodesiense* to the new trypanosome. In 1912 Kinghorn and Yorke showed that *Trypanosoma rhodesiense* was transmitted by *Glossina morsitans*, a biting fly closely related to *Glossina palpalis*. A number of observers, notably Bruce and his coworkers, hold that *Trypanosoma rhodesiense* is a variety of *Trypanosoma brucei;* while a number of other observers, as Laveran, hold that it is a distinct species.

Geographic Distribution.—The disease was first described at Sierra Leone, but it was soon found to extend far south of there. It has been carried by infected men into neighboring regions, until now it is found in a broad strip of territory, extending from 20° north to about 12° south of the equator, on the western coast of Africa, and extending inland to Uganda and Rhodesia. The disease has been carried to the West Indies, but did not spread there, as the arthropod host was missing. It is probable that the focus in Rhodesia has been an endemic focus for some time and that it is not due to the spread of the West Coast disease.

Etiology.—PREDISPOSING CAUSES.—*Race* is not a predisposing factor. *Sex* seems to play no part in predisposition, though Manson notes that females are more liable to infection. In the same way, *age* does not seem to play any part in predisposition, though some observers hold that young children are more liable to infection. The disease is most common in young adults, probably because their occupation and habits lead to greater exposure to infection.

Occupation is of considerable importance, as persons in certain occupations are especially exposed to the bites of infected flies. Fishermen and persons who live or work along the shores of lakes and streams are especially exposed to infection with *Trypanosoma gambiense*, as *Glossina palpalis* lives on the borders of such waters. Porters who travel through the fly zones are especially liable to infection, on account of their great exposure to the bites of infected flies.

EXCITING CAUSE: THE ORGANISM.—(*a*) *Trypanosoma Gambiense.*—*Trypanosoma gambiense* is the cause of African trypanosomiasis, except in Rhodesia. This organism appears the same in the spinal fluid as in the blood of man.

Morphology.—In the blood it is 16 to 30 microns long and 1.5 to 2 microns in breadth, though it varies greatly in size—is polymorphic, short plump forms being 14 to 20 microns long, and long slender forms being 23 to 32 microns long. The anterior end is usually drawn out to a point along the flagellum, but it may be rounded; the posterior end is usually rounded, but it may be drawn out to a point. The undulating membrane is small; the flagellum is well developed. The nucleus is oval and is situated about the middle of the body; the blepharoplast is oval and is situated at the posterior end, often just in front of a distinct vacuole. There is often a number of granules in the cytoplasm about the nucleus.

Cultivation.—*Trypanosoma gambiense* is difficult to cultivate. Thomson and Sinton cultivated it on the Nicolle modification of the Novy-MacNeal medium—the N.N.M medium—using rat's blood. They mixed two parts of rat blood with one part of a 1 per cent citrate solution, and mixed equal parts of agar and citrated blood. The medium was heated to 45° C. for two hours to destroy the complement and was allowed to stand for two days at 25° C. for the water of condensation to collect. The cultures were kept at 22 to 24° C.

Occurrence in Lower Animals.—Spontaneous infection occurs frequently in antelopes. Yorke and Blacklock found one ox infected with *Trypanosoma gambiense*, and Kleine and Eckard found one ox, one sheep and one goat infected. The infected animals are not sick as a result of the infection.

Experimentally, monkeys are readily infected; parasites appear in the peripheral blood in from 18 to 20 days, the animal is quite sick and dies in a few weeks to a few months. White rats are susceptible; the course is usually chronic, and marked by periods of latency when no parasites are found in the blood, and periods when the parasites are numerous in the blood. Mice usually have a chronic infection; but when the strain is carried in rats or mice for some time, it becomes more virulent and kills in three to six weeks. In rabbits and guinea pigs the infection runs a chronic course with few parasites in the blood. Dogs are susceptible and the infection may run a fairly acute course. Horses, cattle, goats, sheep and hogs are susceptible; but the infection is light.

Development in the Vertebrate Host.—The development of *Trypanosoma gambiense* has been studied especially in the blood of the rat. After inoculation the parasites multiply by longitudinal division until they are very numerous in the peripheral blood. Then the parasites undergo a change in structure, becoming less numerous in the peripheral blood, and numerous in the lungs, spleen and bone marrow. The nucleus of the parasite contracts and flattens, a large clear vesicle forms beside the nucleus, and a cytoplasmic sheath forms around both. The other structures of the parasite disappear, and these bodies lodge in the spleen and bone marrow, where they remain during the latent period—ten days or more—when no parasites are found in the peripheral blood. These are the "latent bodies" of Moore and Brienl. At the termination of the latent phase the other structures of the trypanosome are developed anew and the latent body becomes a trypanosome which multiplies by longitudinal division, the parasites reappearing in the peripheral blood.

Fry and Rankin observed extrusion of granules from trypanosomes. When the trypanosomes are about to disappear from the peripheral blood, many of them extrude granules, usually from some point near the middle of the body; and these granules take on the Leishmania form. They may now elongate and form trypanosomes, or they may divide before forming trypanosomes.

Wolbach and his coworkers, working with *Trypanosoma gambiense* in the blood of animals, conclude that it does not pass through bacteria-proof filters. Trypanosomes do not pass through the placenta.

Development in the Arthropod Host.—When *Glossina palpalis* feeds on blood containing *Trypanosoma gambiense*, the trypanosomes pass through the stomach of the fly, and in twenty-four hours lose their infectivity for the vertebrate host and multiply in the posterior part of the midgut. In ten to twelve days slender forms develop, and from the twelfth to the twentieth day they move forward to the proventriculus. From here they pass to the salivary glands, become attached to the walls of the gland ducts, and develop into Crithidia forms which divide and form small trypanosomes similar to those in the blood of the vertebrate host; and these small forms are injected with the saliva into the subcutaneous tissues of the vertebrate host when the fly bites. Just how the trypanosomes get from the proventriculus to the salivary glands of the fly is not quite clear, though it is generally considered that they pass along the hypopharynx into the salivary glands. Trypanosomes are not found in the juice of the body cavity of the fly. The development in the salivary glands requires two to five days.

The development in the fly is favored by high atmospheric temperature—24 to 29° C. (75.2 to 84.2° F.); while low temperature—15 to 21° C. (59 to 69.8° F.)—delays or prevents development, but does not kill the trypanosomes. Under favorable conditions the development in the fly is complete in twenty to thirty-four days, and the fly remains infective the rest of its life.

Trypanosoma gambiense completes its cycle of development in a small percentage of *Glossina palpalis* which feed on infected blood, as only about 6 to 8 per cent of the flies become infective. The infection is not transmitted to the pupa of the fly.

(*b*) *Trypanosoma Rhodesiense.*—*Trypanosoma rhodesiense* is the cause of trypanosomiasis in Rhodesia.

Morphology.—*Trypanosoma rhodesiense* resembles *Trypanosoma gambiense* in size, form and polymorphism. The nucleus is generally situated well to the posterior end, near the blepharoplast; but it may be situated near the middle of the body as in *Trypanosoma gambiense;* and in the short plump forms it may even be behind the blepharoplast. The posterior position of the nucleus is best shown in the blood of rats.

Cultivation.—Thomson and Sinton cultivated *Trypanosoma rhodesiense* in the same way they cultivated *Trypanosoma gambiense.*

Occurrence in Lower Animals.—Spontaneous infection occurs frequently in wild animals, as the antelope, hartebeest, waterbuck, impala and wart hog. Kinghorn and Yorke found one dog infected.

Experimentally, the same animals as given under *Trypanosoma gambiense* are susceptible to infection with *Trypanosoma rhodesiense.* *Trypanosoma rhodesiense* is generally more virulent than is *Trypanosoma gambiense;* and it causes severe disease in sheep and goats, killing them in forty to forty-five days.

Development in the Vertebrate Host.—The development of *Trypanosoma rhodesiense* in the vertebrate host is practically the same as that of *Trypanosoma gambiense.* Fantham has studied the development of the latent forms in the lungs. The blepharoplast moves close to the nucleus, and the rest of the body is lost, leaving a rounded body containing the nucleus and the blepharoplast. This rounded body becomes surrounded by a capsule and becomes a cyst 2 to 4 microns in diameter—the latent body or preflagellar stage. After a time these bodies increase in size and length, and develop into trypanosomes again.

Development in the Arthropod Host.—When *Glossina morsitans* feeds on blood containing *Trypanosoma rhodesiense,* the trypanosome goes through the same cycle of development as does *Trypanosoma gambiense* in *Glossina palpalis.*

The development of *Trypanosoma rhodesiense* is affected by atmospheric temperature in the same way as is that of *Trypanosoma gambiense.* Under favorable conditions *Trypanosoma rhodesiense* completes its cycle of development in *Glossina morsitans* in fourteen days, but only about 5 per cent of the flies become infective.

There is a difference of opinion as to whether *Trypanosoma rhodesiense* is a distinct species or is a variety of *Trypanosoma brucei,* which is the cause of nagana, the tsetse fly disease of horses and cattle in Africa. Both trypanosomes are transmitted by *Glossina morsitans.* Laveran found that sheep immunized to *Trypanosoma brucei* were susceptible to infection with *Trypanosoma rhodesiense.* Chalmers says that animals immunized to *Trypanosoma brucei* are killed by *Trypanosoma rhodesiense,* and vice versa. On this basis, it is held that *Trypanosoma rhodesiense* is a distinct species. Bruce does not consider cross inoculations as reliable for differentiation, and depends on morphology, action on animals, and manner of development in the fly, in the separation of species. On this basis, it is held that *Trypanosoma rhodesiense* is *Trypanosoma brucei.*

(*c*) *Other Trypanosomes.*—Macfie gave the name *Trypanosoma nigeriense* to a trypanosome found in the blood of young persons in Nigeria. This trypanosome is less virulent than is *Trypanosoma gambiense* and is transmitted by *Glossina tachnoides.* Bruce is of the opinion that *Trypanosoma nigeriense* is *Trypanosoma gambiense.*

Castellani and Chalmers express the opinion that more than one species of Trypanosoma is included in the species *Trypanosoma gambiense,* and they note that the Uganda strain appears to be different from the Gambia strain.

Trypanosomes that cause disease in lower animals may cause occasional cases in man. Thus there have been laboratory infections in man with laboratory strains of *Trypanosoma brucei.*

Epidemiology.—(*a*) SOURCE OF INFECTION.—*Man* is an important source of infection. As men may have trypanosomes in the blood for several years without being too sick to go about their usual occupation, it is easily understood that man spreads the disease along caravan routes and from place to place. Mayer gives the following percentages of apparently healthy persons who have *Trypanosoma gambiense* in the blood: 0.6 per cent in Gambia; 4.6 per cent in Congo; and 28.7 per cent in Uganda.

But man is not the only source of infection. Where infected areas have been depopulated, infected flies were still found in the area a year or more later. Wild animals are frequently found infected with *Trypanosoma gambiense* and *Trypanosoma rhodesiense*, and remain in good condition. So it is evident that *lower animals* act as reservoirs for the infection. While domestic animals are occasionally found infected, it does not appear that they play an important part as reservoirs for the infection. Antelopes act as reservoirs for infection with *Trypanosoma gambiense;* while the antelope, waterbuck, hartebeest, wart hog and impala act as reservoirs for infection with *Trypanosoma rhodesiense*.

The relative importance of man and lower animals as sources of infection varies in different regions. Yorke and Blacklock consider man as the chief source of infection with *Trypanosoma gambiense* in Sierra Leone, but they think domestic animals may be of some importance. Human trypanosomiasis may be very chronic in Sierra Leone, and trypanosomes may be found in the blood when examining for some other organism, as malarial parasites. They consider that wild animals are the chief source of infection in South Central Africa. Duke says that antelopes are the reservoir for *Trypanosoma gambiense* on the uninhabited islands of the Victoria Nyanza Lake.

(b) MODE OF TRANSMISSION.—The infection is transmitted by the *bite of infected tsetse flies, Trypanosoma gambiense* being transmitted by *Glossina palpalis,* and *Trypanosoma rhodesiense* being transmitted by *Glossina morsitans*.

The flies may transmit the infection mechanically for a short time after feeding on an infected animal. Then there is a period, corresponding to the length of time necessary for the cycle of developing in the fly, during which time the fly cannot transmit the infection. Following this period, the infection is transmitted by the bite of the fly.

Carpenter studied the habits of *Glossina palpalis* with special reference to its role in the transmission of *Trypanosoma gambiense*. The females live about four months and the males live about eight months. There are no natural enemies; and the pupae are found at the base of trees and under fallen logs, only a few yards from the water's edge and a few feet above it, out of the way of birds. The flies feed on blood, especially on lizards, having a special liking for certain lizards; they also feed on crocodiles and birds. Of mammals, they feed on the antelope, hippopotamus and otter. Lamborn says that some wasps are parasitic on the pupa of glossina and that dragonflies prey on the adult flies.

Tsetse flies also breed in shaded places, in sand along river beds, where the water leaves the sand uncovered in the dry season.

The female tsetse fly gives birth to one large larva at a time; this larva immediately bores a couple of inches into the sand and changes to a pupa. In about a month the adult fly emerges from the pupa.

Tsetse flies bite during the day, even in sunlight, and will follow human beings some distance. Both males and females bite and can transmit trypanosomes.

Sexual intercourse has been considered to be a mode of transmission of the infection. Koch noted infection of fifteen women in a fly-free area and considered that they were infected by their husbands who had returned from working in fly zones. Bernard noted infection of prostitutes in the same way. It is known that trypanosomes can pass through an unbroken mucous membrane; and dourine, a trypanosomiasis of horses, is transmitted by sexual intercourse. Neiva showed that *Trypanosoma equinum, Trypanosoma evansi* and *Trypanosoma equiperdum* can be transmitted from guinea pig to guinea pig by the instillation of a drop of infected blood into the conjunctival sac.

Mosquitoes are suggested as transmitting the infection, as children are often infected though not exposed to the bite of tsetse flies.

Martin and Leboeuf suggest *tattoo wounds* as sources of direct infection.

The all-important mode of transmission is through the *bite of infected tsetse flies.*

(*c*) SUSCEPTIBILITY.—All races and ages and both sexes are susceptible to infection

Symptomatology.—Generally the bite of a glossina leaves only a small papule which itches for a short time and then disappears. At times, possibly due to contamination with pyogenic bacteria, there is an inflammatory area at the site of the bite, with a swelling of the neighboring lymph glands. These infected bites may cause painful furuncle-like swellings on various parts of the body; they are usually single, but there may be as many as five.

It is usual to describe the symptoms under two stages: (1) trypanosome fever, and (2) sleeping sickness. Martin and Leboeuf describe the symptoms under three stages: (1) *incubation,* (2) *invasion* and (3) the *developed disease;* and they divide the third stage into three periods: (*a*) *beginning*—organisms in the blood but not in the spinal fluid; (*b*) *infection of the nervous system*—when the organisms enter the spinal fluid, and (*c*) *terminal period.* The stage of invasion and the first period of the stage of the developed disease, in the Martin and Leboeuf description, correspond to the usually described stage of trypanosome fever; while the second and third periods of the developed disease in the Martin and Leboeuf description correspond to the usually described stage of sleeping sickness.

1. INCUBATION.—The stage of incubation, from the bite of the fly to the appearance of trypanosomes in the blood, is ten to twelve days. The period from the bite to the development of symptoms may be as short as ten days, but more commonly it is two to three months. The inhabitants of some infected regions consider that the incubation period may be long and that a man may develop the disease up to seven years after leaving an infected region.

2. INVASION.—The stage of invasion is represented by the first symptoms of the disease. The resistance of the body has been overcome and the organisms circulate in the blood. This stage begins with irregular remittent or intermittent fever of 39.4 to 40° C. (103 to 104° F.), and in whites is commonly accompanied by an erythematous rash. There are nervous excitement, insomnia and prostration. After about a week the fever and symptoms disappear, though the pulse may remain rapid.

These symptoms may be absent in natives; and they may reach the period of infection of the nervous system without having fever.

3. THE STAGE OF THE DEVELOPED DISEASE.—(*a*) The *first period* is of variable length and trypanosomes are found in the blood but not in the spinal fluid.

After an afebrile period of a few days to two or three weeks the fever returns but is generally not so high as in the first period—38.3 to 38.9° C. (101 to 102° F.). After about a week the fever again disappears, and these febrile and afebrile periods continue to alternate.

Headache is common, and may be persistent, but it is not very severe. There may be neuralgic pains, with cramps in the calves of the legs and pains in the feet. A very common symptom is superficial and deep hyperesthesia, and a slight blow or pressure will produce sharp pain. The patient is very susceptible to cold.

There are insomnia, weakness, anemia and emaciation. Photophobia is not uncommon and there may be iritis and cyclitis.

In the white person there is commonly an erythematous eruption from the beginning of the fever. This eruption appears as poorly defined, pinkish patches, appearing especially on the chest. These patches may be ring-shaped or crescentic, and are frequently seen better at a little distance from the patient.

The erythematous eruption is often not seen in the Negro. Here the skin is often dry and scaly, at times with severe pruritus. There is frequently a papular eruption that may itch considerably. The eruption may be vesicular, or may ulcerate or be pigmented. It is these types of eruption to which Martin and Leboeuf refer as trypanids and compare them to syphilids.

Areas of localized edema are not uncommon, sometimes with a large erythematous patch. These areas of edema often appear over the sternum, on the arms and on the internal surface of the thighs, and are fleeting.

The heart is rapid—about 120 per minute; and this tachycardia commonly continues through the afebrile period.

There is loss of sexual power; the menses may be suppressed or they may continue for almost the entire duration of the disease.

There may be dysenteric crises, which may dominate the picture.

The lymph glands are enlarged and movable, and about the consistence of a ripe plum. The lymph glands in the posterior cervical triangle are very commonly enlarged; other superficial lymph glands less commonly. This enlargement of the lymph glands is an important clinical sign, and the natives recognize that a person with enlarged posterior cervical glands will have sleeping sickness.

The spleen is often enlarged and the liver may be enlarged.

Mental symptoms are not prominent. Whites may be sad or irritable, and may be neurasthenic. They show loss of attention and are apt to make errors in figures and in writing. Natives often show no mental changes; but they may continue to do their work as automatons, may be expansive or morose, and may lose their self-respect and become lax in discipline.

This period lasts from a few months to seven years. Natives may go through the entire period, with trypanosomes in their blood, without being sick.

(b) The *second period* begins with the entrance of the trypanosomes into the subarachnoid space.

All symptoms are increased in severity. The febrile periods are more frequent; there is marked nervousness and the headache increases and may be severe. There may be ringing in the ears, or deafness.

The patient becomes dull and apathetic, and is tired by the least exertion; the gait is weak and shuffling, and the entire figure is relaxed and drooping, thus adding to the appearance of apathy and moroseness. The puffy eyelids tend to fall shut and there is a state of physical asthenia. With this, there is a state of mental and intellectual asthenia; the patient does not enter into conversation, answers slowly when spoken to and even simulates sleep to avoid conversation. He becomes careless in his habits. The appetite is good, but the patient will not go to the trouble of getting food, and he may go to sleep with food in his mouth. The digestive apparatus is undisturbed.

The condition is one of intellectual asthenia and lethargy, rather than actual sleep. When spoken to, the patient is easily aroused, but he will yawn and stretch, as though he had just wakened; and he may even be angry at being disturbed.

Mental symptoms are quite common. At night there may be mental disturbance amounting to delirium or mania. The patient may have fits of excitement or anger, in which he is quarrelsome or destructive; after the fit is over, he returns to the lethargic state. There may be delusions of grandeur; hallucinations of sight, hearing, smell or taste. There may be melancholia, but suicide is rare. There may be amnesia, catatonia, echomimia, echolalia, negativism or mutism. There may be impulse to steal and the patient may collect all sorts of worthless things.

There is a tremor of the muscles, especially noticeable in the tongue, lips and hands. There may be epileptiform attacks. Rigidity and muscular contractions are rather common. There may be hemiplegia or paraplegia. The reflexes are generally normal; though the deep reflexes may be exaggerated early, and lost later. There is loss of coordination in walking and Romberg's symptom is often present. The pupils are equal and react to light and accommodation. Control of the sphincters is retained to near the end. There may be hyperesthesia or anesthesia.

The edemas increase, especially about the face and may extend to the glottis. This period, about 75 per cent of the cases, lasts from three to six months.

(c) In the *third period* the condition is one of complete decrepitude. The general weakness and emaciation increase; there is marked tremor; contractures; and the lethargy is profound. The patient is neglectful and oblivious; will eat dirt; saliva dribbles from the mouth; and there is incontinence of feces and urine. The patient falls when he tries to walk. The blood pressure falls; there is cardiac arrhythmia; the temperature is subnormal; decubitus appears on different parts of the body; the patient passes into a comatose condition and dies.

Death may result from an epileptiform or apoplectiform attack, or from cachexia; but more commonly it results from a complication, as pneumonia, meningitis or dysentery.

This period, about 13 per cent of the cases, lasts from two to three months.

The disease may last from eighteen months to several years. After involvement of the nervous system, the disease usually does not last over four to eight months; though it may be prolonged to two years or more by treatment.

The entire clinical course is variable. Lethargy is the most striking characteristic, and this form is most common; but the disease may resemble general paralysis. About a sixth of Martin and Ringenbach's cases had psychoses. The course may be rapid or slow, and there may be periods of latency followed by relapse.

There may be no enlargement of the glands throughout the disease. While the pulse is usually rapid—100 to 140 per minute—it may be as slow as 50 per minute, probably due to irritation of the vagus as it passes through the subarachnoid space.

The course of the Rhodesian form of the disease is more rapid than that of the Gambian form, often lasting not over four or five months, and the lethargy may not appear.

Diagnosis.—Clinical Diagnosis.—The disease may escape diagnosis for a long time. The history is important, especially a history of residence in an endemic area and of having been bitten by tsetse flies. In the early stage of the fever there is apt to be confusion with *malaria;* but chills and sweats are rare in the fever attacks, and the fever is not affected by quinine. The enlarged lymph glands, erythema and headache may cause confusion with *syphilis;* and the danger of confusion is increased by the fact that the Wassermann reaction is not infrequently positive in the blood of cases of trypanosomiasis—possibly cases of the two diseases together.

While *enlarged cervical lymph glands* are an important sign, it must be remembered that such enlarged glands are frequently met with in persons who are free from trypanosomes. Mayer says that in Uganda, from 50 to 75 per cent of the natives have enlarged lymph glands, but only 28.7 per cent of the healthy persons harbor trypanosomes. There may be no enlargement of the lymph glands throughout the disease.

In an endemic area the irregular fever, the rapid pulse, the asthenia, the headache, the eruption, the enlarged cervical lymph glands (Winterbottom's sign), the deep hyperesthesia (Kerandel's sign), and the tremor of the tongue (Low-Castellani sign) make it possible to arrive at a clinical diagnosis with a fair degree of accuracy.

In addition to malaria and syphilis there may be confusion with *filariasis, dysentery, relapsing fever* or *liver abscess;* and any of these conditions may exist with trypanosomiasis. In *beriberi* the lymph glands are not enlarged, and the heart is involved.

After involvement of the central nervous system, the lethargy, emaciation and edema, and tremors and muscular contractures are of importance in diagnosis.

The various mental states are difficult to differentiate from such mental states due to other causes. The pupils are normal.

In all cases it is important to make a laboratory examination for trypanosomes, and only in this way can a definite diagnosis be made.

LABORATORY DIAGNOSIS.—*Blood.*—Trypanosomes may be found in the peripheral blood, especially during attacks of fever; but trypanosomes are not numerous in the peripheral blood, and long search is necessary—even then it is frequently impossible to find them.

Citrated blood may be repeatedly centrifuged and the sediment examined on the third centrifugalization, or the leukocyte layer may be examined after centrifuging citrated blood in narrow tubes. In obtaining trypanosomes from the blood of cattle, Teague and Clark defibrinated the blood with sticks, strained it through gauze, mixed it with an equal volume of water, allowed it to stand a few minutes, centrifuged and examined the sediment.

Trypanosomes are considered to be more numerous in the erythematous areas on the skin than in the general circulation. The erythematous areas may be scarified and blood films from the scarified area examined.

There is secondary anemia, the red cells falling to as low as two million per cubic millimeter. The leukocyte count is often disturbed by secondary infections. In uncomplicated cases the leukocytes are normal in number or rise to 10,500 per cubic millimeter. There is an increase in the mononuclear elements, the lymphocytes rising to 37 per cent of the total count.

There is auto-agglutination of the red cells, but it is not specific. Various serum reactions—agglutination, precipitin, complement fixation, trypanolysis and attachment—have been tried, but the results are not very satisfactory.

Gland Puncture.—Trypanosomes are especially numerous in the lymph glands. An enlarged lymph gland is punctured with a dry syringe; a small amount of gland juice is aspirated and examined for trypanosomes. This is the most satisfactory method of direct microscopic diagnosis.

Spinal Fluid.—After involvement of the central nervous system, trypanosomes are found in small numbers in the spinal fluid by centrifuging about 10 cc. and examining the sediment.

Dubois and Van den Branden tried the reaction of Boveri on the spinal fluid in cases of trypanosomiasis in the stage of nervous system involvement. The reaction is positive in this stage of the disease, but it is not specific, being due to the presence of proteins.

Early in the disease the spinal fluid is normal. After involvement of the central nervous system it is often slightly turbid and contains serum albumin and serum globulin; lymphocytes are fairly numerous and there are larger vacuolated cells.

Animal Inoculation.—When trypanosomes are not found on direct microscopic examination of the body fluids, 10 cc. of blood or spinal fluid may be injected into a susceptible animal. Monkeys are the most satisfactory animal for the purpose, but may not be available. The most satisfactory of the available animals is the guinea pig, injected intraperitoneally. Dogs are satisfactory. Rats and mice are not satisfactory as they are frequently infected with trypanosomes in nature, and this might lead to confusion.

Complications.—Acute infectious conditions are the usual complications, as pneumonia, purulent meningitis and dysentery. Pleurisy, pulmonary gangrene and tuberculosis are also met with. The secondary bacterial infections produce secondary lesions throughout the body, and these infections have also caused confusion regarding the etiology of the disease.

Iritis and iridocyclitis are quite frequently met with—especially in Rhodesian trypanosomiasis—and in four of Daniels' cases it was the eye lesions which led the patient to seek medical advice. Orchitis is less frequent. These conditions are hardly to be considered as complications, as they are due to the action of the trypanosomes.

Abortion, premature birth, stillbirth, and death a few days after birth are the rule in trypanosomiasis.

Treatment.[*]—GENERAL MANAGEMENT.—If possible, the patient should be removed to a **temperate climate,** should be given **rest** and an **abundance of good food,** placed under **good hygienic conditions,** and **protected from the cold,** as persons suffering from trypanosomiasis feel the cold very keenly.

Atoxyl was the first drug to give good results in the treatment of trypanosomiasis; but the danger of optic neuritis, the need from prolonged treatment, the pain of the injections, and its practical uselessness in advanced cases have brought about its replacement by some of the newer drugs. However, atoxyl and some allied compounds are still used, especially combined with other drugs. Trypanosomes disappear from the blood in six to seven hours after an intramuscular injection of 0.5 Gm. (7½ grains) of the drug: the patient may have a febrile reaction at this time. There are several methods of giving atoxyl, Martin and Leboeuf advising 0.5 Gm. (7½ grains) intramuscularly, to be repeated in 48 hours; after an interval of 10 days the same two doses are to be given, with the 48-hour interval; and treatment is to be continued in this way.

Tryparsamide, a derivative of atoxyl, is the most satisfactory of the arsenicals in use today; it is especially valuable in the more advanced cases in which other drugs have given much less satisfactory results. The dose is 1 to 3 Gm. (15 to 45 grains) for an adult and should not exceed 0.04 to 0.045 Gm. (⅗ to ¾ grain) per kilo of body weight; in excess of this the drug may cause blindness, especially in the advanced cases which are in poor physical condition. This dose should not be repeated at intervals of less than one week. The desired dose is freshly dissolved in 10 cc. (2½ fl.dr.) of sterile distilled water at room temperature, and given intravenously. Fifteen weekly injections are given; then a rest period of one to three months; and the course is repeated, after blood examination, lumbar puncture, gland puncture if indicated, and general physical examination. While the drug must be pushed to the limit of safety, and one must avoid producing arsenic-resistant strains of trypanosomes by the use of small doses, any single dose should not exceed 2 Gm. (30 grains) in cases not under close observation.

Kopp and Solomon list a number of untoward reactions from tryparsamide, in the treatment of syphilis, of which visual disturbances are especially prominent: optic atrophy and toxic amblyopia. They point out that these visual disturbances are most likely to occur during the first 8 to 12 injections of the drug; and, when such disturbances occur, the drug should be discontinued permanently.

Bayer 205 is well borne and is especially good in the first period of the disease; but in the second and third periods, while there may be marked temporary improvement, the cases relapse. The drug is given intravenously in doses of 0.5 Gm. (7½ grains) every three days, for four doses. This usually cures cases in the first period, but tryparsamide had better be used in cases in the second and third periods of the disease. It is well to combine treatment with Bayer 205 and tryparsamide.

* A large number of trypanocidal drugs have been developed; and this, with the number of different names for the same or allied compounds, is often confusing. Henry and Gray discuss these compounds, and they are grouped here; the names under each number are for the same or allied compounds.

Pentavalent arsenic compounds.

1. Atoxyl, soamin, trypoxyl, arsamine, sodium arsanilate, sodium aminarsonate.
2. Tryparsamide, tryparsone, glyphenarsine, tryponarsyl, trypotan, novatoxyl.
3. Etharsonal, proparsonal.
4. Fourneau 270, orsanine.
5. Acetylarsan, acetarsol, acetarsone, kharophen, orarsan, osvarsan, spiricid, stovarsol.
6. Formyphenarsine, treparsol.
7. Troposan.

Symmetrical ureas (carbamides).

1. Bayer 205, germanin, Fourneau 309, moranyl, belganyl, antrypol. Naganol is a form for veterinary use.

Tartar emetic has proved to be a valuable drug in the treatment of trypanosomiasis; trypanosomes disappear from the blood in five to ten minutes after an intravenous injection of 50 mg. (¾ grain) of the drug. Tartar emetic is given intravenously in doses of 50 to 100 mg. (¾ to 1½ grains) dissolved in 75 to 150 cc. (2½ to 5 oz.) of water. One difficulty with tartar emetic is the severe pain and inflammation that is caused by the escape of the solution into the tissues around the veins. Van den Branden undertook to overcome this difficulty by giving the tartar emetic intravenously in oil: he could give 150 mg. (2¼ grains) of tartar emetic (3.75 cc. [1 fl.dr.] of oil) this way; but there were severe symptoms—especially violent coughing (possibly fat embolism)—when 200 mg. (3 grains) of tartar emetic (5 cc. [1¼ fl.dr.] of oil) were given. Antimony salts may produce a fall of blood pressure and dyspnea; so it is advisable to give a **hypodermic injection of caffeine** a few minutes before giving the antimony.

Tartar emetic is usually **combined with atoxyl,** in order to prevent the formation of drug-resistant strains of the trypanosome. A series of ten daily injections of tartar emetic is given, with an interval of a month before the next series. Atoxyl is given in doses of 0.5 Gm. (7½ grains) every five or six days, or 0.2 Gm. (3 grains) every three days.

Daniels and Newham had difficulty in treating Rhodesian trypanosomiasis with atoxyl and tartar emetic, and they obtained satisfactory results from the subcutaneous injection of **antimony oxide** in a case in which atoxyl and tartar emetic had failed.

Masters recommends antimony oxide alone or combined with **soamin.** He dissolves antimony oxide in equal parts of glycerin and water by heating it gently, 1 cc. of the solution containing 0.65 mg. (1/100 grain) of antimony oxide. He gives 2 to 3 cc. of the solution intramuscularly every other day until 26 mg. (⅖ grain) are given. If trypanosomes do not disappear from the blood he gives 0.77 Gm. (12 grains) of soamin every five days, continuing the antimony oxide injections. Masters considers that soamin given in large doses is more effective than when given in numerous small doses. Antimony may be given with tryparsamide, especially in cases with concomitant schistosomiasis.

Numerous other drugs have been used, but have not given satisfactory results, or have not been used in enough cases to determine their value.

Treatment must be continued until the patient's pulse, temperature and weight are normal and until at least two animal inoculations prove negative. If treatment is discontinued too soon, the patient will relapse; and relapse is serious and increases the danger of involvement of the nervous system. Treatment can do no more than prolong life.

PROPHYLAXIS.—Prophylaxis is based on the premises that (1) man is an important source of infection, spreading it from place to place, and that certain wild animals serve as reservoirs of the infection and keep it up in endemic areas; that (2) the infection is spread from man to man or from reservoir to man by the bites of tsetse flies; and that (3) both sexes and all ages and races are susceptible to the infection.

1. *Source of Infection.*—**Early diagnosis and treatment** of cases is important. Persons ill with trypanosomiasis should be **segregated** in treatment camps, or treated in localities where they are not exposed to the bites of flies.

Many persons have trypanosomes in their blood for years without being sick. These persons are a very important source of infection, as they continue at their occupation and travel from place to place. In order to detect such cases it is necessary to make **systematic examinations of persons exposed** and of all suspects coming into a locality. Lester reports on surveys in northern Nigeria: up to the beginning of 1938, the survey had examined 2,200,200 natives; 300,000 cases of trypanosomiasis had been discovered. In order to carry out these examinations it is necessary to have segregation camps in which exposed persons, suspects and travelers are held until they can be examined. Servants are given health certificates and travelers are given medical passports.

42101

It is important that all infected persons found be given **prompt treatment** in order to free their blood of trypanosomes as soon as possible.

Depopulation of infected districts has not resulted in eradication of the infection, as the wild animals in the district served as reservoirs and kept up the infection in the flies.

Destruction of the wild animals that act as reservoirs in a district has not given satisfactory results.

2. *Mode of Transmission.*—**Destruction of the tsetse flies** has given good results, where it could be carried out, satisfactorily. Various traps have been tried, but without much success. Some success has been obtained in catching flies by men wearing white clothes and having on their backs a square of black cloth covered with birdlime. In their work in the island of Principe, Da Costa and his coworkers caught 470,000 flies in this way in three years. Shircore has suggested revolving screens, like the ordinary revolving exit and entrance door, covered with birdlime and set up along caravan routes, for the catching of *Glossina morsitans* as they follow the porters through the screens.

Koch advised killing crocodiles and destroying their eggs, as an attack on the fly through its food supply. But the flies feed on the blood of other animals, so that this method is not satisfactory.

The best results follow **destruction of the breeding and resting places of the fly.** The flies require considerable moisture and a temperature not above about 25° C. (77° F.). They breed in a narrow strip of ground, well covered by vegetation, close to the edge of the water. Clearing a strip about fifteen feet wide along the edge of the water will to a great extent prevent breeding. But the trees and stumps should be removed, as Lamborn has shown that the flies breed in the decaying vegetation around fallen trees and under logs. As the flies rest in the shade of the forest and will follow humans some distance, it is advisable to clear a strip 100 yards wide along the water, especially at crossings, and 300 yards wide around villages. Da Costa and his coworkers eradicated the disease from the island of Principe by clearing and draining and by catching flies.

As the pupae are one or two inches in the ground, among roots or under logs, they are difficult to destroy. Minchin suggested the breeding of jungle fowl for the destruction of the pupae.

3. *Personal Prophylaxis.*—It is necessary to instruct the people regarding the disease, and to secure their cooperation in any preventive work that is to be undertaken. Misery and famine are to be relieved. **Occupations which expose to fly bites should be avoided, also areas in which the flies live. Travel in the fly regions should be undertaken at night. Whites should live at a distance from natives, and persons in occupations where they are specially exposed should live at a distance from other people.**

White clothes should be worn, as white does not attract the flies. The face, hands and ankles should be protected from the bites of flies by **nets, gloves and boots or leggings,** in spite of the discomfort from the heat.

Repellants, as **citronella oil,** are of some value.

Vaccination does not offer much hope. There is no evidence of immunity after trypanosomiasis, such as there is after some bacterial diseases. Schilling and Rondini allowed suspensions of trypanosomes to stand for some hours at incubator temperature, and then injected the suspensions into animals. These animals were protected against infection on injection of infective blood seven days later. Laveran could not confirm this work, and considers that in general there is not satisfactory evidence of protection.

Prognosis.—With the use of Bayer 205 and tryparsamide, the prognosis is good, even when the patient cannot be removed from the endemic area. Kesselberger finds that 75 per cent of the cases can be cured; and with early diagnosis and proper treatment under favorable conditions, up to 80–90 per cent of the cases can be cured. He notes that the results in the treatment of even far-advanced cases may be remarkably good.

When the patient can be removed to a temperate climate early in the disease, and can be given good food, rest and proper treatment, the prognosis is better.

Relapse occurs if treatment is discontinued too soon.

Mechanism of the Disease Process.—The trypanosomes injected into the subcutaneous tissues by the bite of the fly, multiply and circulate in the peripheral blood.

Schuberg and Böing injected trypanosomes (*Trypanosoma lewisi* and *Trypanosoma brucei*) into the skin of animals and studied the manner in which the trypanosomes entered the tissues. The trypanosomes very quickly enter the lymph spaces of the corium and then pass through the connective tissue to the neighboring lymph glands. Here they multiply enormously and are found in large numbers in the glands on the same side of the body before they are found in the peripheral blood.

In the human, the trypanosomes probably multiply and travel in the lymphatics, and the toxin causes inflammatory reaction in the lymph vessels, glands and follicles. The trypanosomes enter the blood stream early, producing a general infection, and later they enter the cerebrospinal fluid.

Wolbach and Binger conclude that the lesions in trypanosomiasis are due to the trypanosomes which invade the connective tissue structures of all organs, the reticular tissue of lymph glands and the spleen, and the substance of the brain. Martin and Leboeuf draw the following parallel between syphilis and trypanosomiasis: (1) local lesions; (2) eruption, etc. (trypanids); (3) nervous system. They consider the early lesions due to toxin from the trypanosomes and the later lesions due to changes in the tissues.

Early in the disease there is round-cell infiltration of the tissues and organs, and later there is an increase in the connective tissue. The round-cell infiltration about the blood vessels in the central nervous system compresses the vessels and causes anemia of the brain. This, with the presence of trypanosomes in the brain tissue, gives rise to the cerebral changes which give the clinical picture of lethargy, or sleeping sickness.

The course of the disease caused by *Trypanosoma rhodesiense* is the same as that caused by *Trypanosoma gambiense*, except that the Rhodesian disease is generally more severe than is the disease caused by *Trypanosoma gambiense*.

IMMUNITY.—Recovery appears to be the result of the general resistance of the body, rather than any specific immunity. It is not known whether persons who recover are immune, but there does not appear to be immunity in recovered animals.

Schilling doubts whether there is spontaneous recovery in human trypanosomiasis, but there may be long periods of latency. There are antibodies—precipitins, trypanolysin, opsonins and substances which produce agglomeration of trypanosomes—in the blood of infected animals, and these antibodies prevent superinfection.

Heckenroth and Blanchard found that the serum of infected animals is almost always protective, and that it very exceptionally produced agglutination, rarely produced attachment, and frequently produced lysis, of the trypanosomes.

Todd reports that of twelve cases of trypanosomiasis in natives of Gambia in 1911, four were living and in good condition at the end of 1918; the others had died at irregular intervals. Todd considers that this proves there is some immunity to human trypanosomiasis, but it is not determined whether it is a sterilizing immunity or a tolerance immunity.

CAUSES OF DEATH.—The disease may run a rapid course and cause death from inanition in a few months.

Secondary bacterial infection is very common, and death is often due to purulent meningitis, pneumonia or dysentery.

Pathology.—MACROSCOPIC.—The body is emaciated and the enlarged lymph glands are visible in the neck and groins.

On opening the body there is nothing markedly abnormal. The bronchial and mesenteric glands are enlarged; all of the lymphatic glands are congested and they may be hemorrhagic. The organs are pale; the heart is soft and flabby; the liver and spleen may be slightly enlarged; the kidneys show nothing.

The important lesions are in the brain. The cerebrospinal fluid is increased in quantity; the meninges are congested and there is diffuse pachymeningitis with adhesions. The arachnoid is cloudy and the subarachnoid space contains a yellowish, turbid exudate. The brain tissue is usually firmer than normal, is congested, and may be edematous. The gyri are flattened and there is excess of fluid in the ventricles.

Lesions of complications are very common; especially pneumonia and dysentery, and, less frequently, purulent meningitis.

MICROSCOPIC.—The main change is the round-cell infiltration around the blood vessels in the meninges and brain, the so-called coat-sleeve infiltration. The infiltrating cells are mainly plasma cells, but lymphocytes are numerous and mast cells are also present. There are isolated areas of plasma cells in the nervous tissue. The nerve cells show chromatolysis. Later there is increased formation of fibrous tissue with thickening of the meninges and the adventitia of the blood vessels. Mayer says that the change in the brain resembles that in paresis, but the genesis of the change is just the reverse: in trypanosomiasis, the interstitial inflammatory change is primary, and the parenchymatous changes result from this; while in paresis the primary change is the degeneration of the parenchyma.

The changes are less marked in the spinal cord; the lining of the central canal often shows proliferation of its cells. There are no changes in the peripheral nerve fibers.

All organs show the round-cell infiltration, the condition being well marked in the lymph glands, the spleen and the heart muscle. In the lymph channels the infiltrating cells are in more or less dense clumps; while they lie singly or in small groups in the stroma of the organs. In the lymph glands the cellular infiltration leads to formation of connective tissue.

Trypanosomes are found in the lymph glands from the beginning of the disease and are usually fairly numerous there. As soon as the disease is established, trypanosomes are found in the blood, though not in great numbers. When the central nervous system becomes involved, trypanosomes are found in the cerebrospinal fluid, but they are always very scarce there. Wolbach found trypanosomes in the neuroglia cells in the brain. Vianna found cysts, like those of *Trypanosoma cruzi*, in the muscles of cases of sleeping sickness and in animals infected with *Trypanosoma gambiense*. Trypanosomes disappear from the tissues and fluids in a few hours after the death of the host.

AMERICAN TRYPANOSOMIASIS

Synonyms.—Chagas' disease; Opilaçao (in part).

Definition.—An acute or chronic disease, caused by *Trypanosoma cruzi*, and characterized anatomically by enlargement of the thyroid gland and of the lymph glands, and by meningo-encephalitis. It is characterized clinically by symptoms of thyroid and suprarenal insufficiency.

History.—In 1909 Chagas was on a malaria expedition in the northern part of the state of Minas Geraes, Brazil, and he found there a conenose bug that was known as "barbeiro" by the natives. This bug lived in the houses, and at night, after the lights were out, would come out and bite the occupants. Chagas recognized the importance of studying such a bug as to its possible role in the transmission of disease; and on studying the bugs he found in the hindgut, flagellates of the Crithidia form. It was a question whether this was a flagellate limited to the intestine of the bug, or was a stage in the cycle of development of some flagellate from a vertebrate host.

He sent some of the bugs (*Triatoma megista*) to the Oswaldo Cruz Institute in Rio de Janeiro, where the bugs were allowed to bite monkeys, whereupon the monkeys developed trypanosomes in their blood. Chagas studied the trypanosomes and found that the bugs were actually the intermediate host of the trypanosome, and that it was eight days from the time bugs were fed on the monkey until the bugs could transmit the infection.

Chagas then returned to Minas Geraes to search for the disease transmitted by this bug. He found that the people in whose houses the bugs lived were in poor health, and some of them had physical findings that are known to indicate trypanosomiasis—enlarged lymph nodes, edemas and a peculiar puffiness of the face. He remembered that he had seen similar cases which did not yield to quinine. But he could find nothing in the blood of these persons. Finally he saw a child with fever, enlarged lymph nodes, puffiness of the face and enlargement of the thyroid gland; and he found numerous trypanosomes in the peripheral blood, identical with the ones which the bugs had transmitted to the laboratory animals. Then he was able to produce trypanosomiasis in guinea pigs by the injection of blood from the chronic cases in which he had not found trypanosomes in the patients' blood. Chagas named the trypanosome *Trypanosoma cruzi*.

In 1919 Tejera found cases of the disease in Venezuela, and showed that *Rhodnius prolixus*, a reduviid bug related to Triatoma, was the transmitter of the disease there.

Geographic Distribution.—The disease was first described from the state of Minas Geraes, Brazil, and is fairly common there; it also occurs in São Paulo and at Bahia. It has been found in the states of Trujillo and Zulia, Venezuela; it occurs in Argentina, Uruguay and the eastern part of Peru. Brumpt found five species of Triatoma, and one species of Rhodnius, infected in Mexico; and he reports two cases of the disease studied in Mexico.

Etiology.—PREDISPOSING CAUSES.—The disease is more severe in children than in adults. It appears to be more common in children, possibly because the bugs have a better opportunity to bite them.

EXCITING CAUSE: THE ORGANISM.—*Trypanosoma cruzi* is the cause of the disease. This organism is 18 to 20 microns long and about 1.5 microns in breadth. The flagellum is not much longer than the body; the undulating membrane has few undulations; the anterior end is pointed; the posterior end is usually pointed, but may be rounded; the blepharoplast is large and is situated close to the posterior end; the nucleus is situated about the middle of the body.

Trypanosoma cruzi appears in the peripheral blood of the human in two forms: (1) Small, slender forms, with a large blepharoplast, and an oval nucleus. This form is actively motile and moves rapidly across the microscopic field. (2) Larger forms, with a smaller spherical blepharoplast and a spherical nucleus. This form has an active motion, in the form of the letter S, but scarcely changes its position in the microscopic field. Chagas considers the first form as neutral and the second form as sexual, but Brumpt considers the first form as young and the second form as adult trypanosomes.

Virulence.—The virulence varies. Guinea pigs die in from five to ten days when bitten by infected Triatoma, but on repeated passage the virulence is lowered until the duration of the disease is about two months. Passage through monkeys raises the virulence again. The virulence is raised by passage through mice.

Cultivation.—Chagas cultivated *Trypanosoma cruzi* on Novy-MacNeal medium. The culture grew readily and developed Crithidia forms which lived two months. The first and second subcultures grew, and guinea pigs were infected by injection of cultures. The organism grows readily in the beginning but is difficult to carry in culture, and no one seems to have obtained growth beyond the second subculture.

Occurrence in Lower Animals.—Armadillos commonly have *Trypanosoma cruzi* in their blood, even when they are far from human habitations; and Chagas found 40 to 50 per cent of armadillos infected in regions where Chagas' disease is found. The animals are not sick. Cats are occasionally found infected in houses where there are cases of the disease.

Experimentally, monkeys are susceptible, but the susceptibility is commonly limited to young monkeys and to certain species: marmosets are susceptible. The incubation period is from 10 to 14 days, and the monkey dies in from 3 to 4 weeks.

Mice are susceptible, the incubation period at first being from 10 to 14 days; but with repeated passage through mice the virulence is raised and the incubation period is reduced to about 6 days. In the beginning the mice generally recover, but after the strain has become more virulent the mice die in from 2 to 4 weeks.

In rats the incubation period is from 6 to 18 days and the animals usually recover. In rabbits the incubation period is about 2 weeks and the infection is transient. The disease is usually chronic in guinea pigs and recovery is frequent, but the infection may be acute and cause death. Dogs are susceptible.

Development in the Vertebrate Host.—When blood containing *Trypanosoma cruzi* is injected into a susceptible animal, part of the trypanosomes circulate in the blood as trypanosomes, and part of them enter the muscle fibers and the neuroglia cells and there develop the Leishmania form. When the trypanosomes from the digestive tract of the invertebrate host are injected into a susceptible animal, all of the trypanosomes enter the muscle fibers and neuroglia cells and there develop the Leishmania form. These Leishmania forms multiply until the cells containing them are converted into cysts containing these forms. In four or five days the Leishmania forms begin to assume the trypanosome form; the cysts formed of the muscle fiber or neuroglia cell rupture, and the trypanosomes gain access to the blood, appearing in the peripheral blood as long, slender, actively motile trypanosomes. About the eighth day the larger trypanosomes appear in the peripheral blood.

Development in the Arthropod Host.—The cycle of development in *Triatoma megista* is typical of the development in other arthropods. The large trypanosomes taken into the stomach of *Triatoma megista* in any stage of its development (larva, nymph or adult) pass to the intestine, assume the Crithidia form, lose the flagellum and become spherical in about twenty hours, and divide. They then develop a flagellum and, in about forty-eight hours, appear as Crithidia forms in the midgut, and multiply rapidly. In ten days to several weeks they develop into metacyclic trypanosomes in the hindgut. These metacyclic trypanosomes persist in the intestinal contents of the bug for a long time, probably throughout the life of the bug. In bedbugs the infection lasts only about two months.

In keeping with his belief that there are sexual and neutral forms of the trypanosome in the blood of the vertebrate host, Chagas describes two methods of development in the arthropod host: (1) the asexual method as described above, giving rise to parasites in the hindgut; and (2) a sexual method of development, giving rise to parasites in the hindgut, in the body cavity, and in the salivary glands.

Twice Chagas saw flagellates in the body cavity, and three times in the salivary glands of bugs he caught. The infection is not transmitted to the young through the egg.

Epidemiology.—(*a*) SOURCE OF INFECTION.—*Man* is a source of infection, especially children during acute attacks of the disease when trypanosomes are fairly numerous in the peripheral blood. In the chronic cases, trypanosomes are scarce in the peripheral blood, though they are present in 5 or 10 cc. of blood.

Chagas found trypanosomes in the blood of a *cat*, in a house in which there were triatomes; and Torres considers that the cat acts as a reservoir for the infection.

Chagas considers that the *armadillo* serves as a reservoir for the infection. Armadillos are common around human habitations; and Chagas found 40 to 50 per cent of armadillos, caught in regions where Chagas' disease is found, infected with *Trypanosoma cruzi*.

(*b*) MODE OF TRANSMISSION.—Chagas found *Triatoma megista* to be the transmitter of the infection in Minas Geraes; and Torres says that larvae and adults of *Triatoma megista,* feeding on man and cats, is the only way in which *Trypanosoma* is transmitted in Brazil.

The triatomes live in the houses which have cracks in the walls; they also live in outbuildings, especially chicken houses, where they live on the blood of chickens. *Triatoma megista* may live in the burrows of armadillos, but *Triatoma geniculata* is the bug usually found in such burrows. The larvae of *Triatoma megista* are about the size of an ordinary bedbug; and larvae, nymphs and adults bite and spread the infection. The bugs do not bite until night, after the lights are out, when they come out and bite the sleeping people. The bite is not painful; and Chagas saw about twenty larvae, nymphs and adult bugs biting a child that was sleeping calmly. The bugs do not come out in the day, but they will bite if a person leans against the wall for any length of time. They spread very rapidly from house to house, and from town to town.

Tejera found *Rhodnius prolixus* to be the transmitter of the infection in Venezuela. This bug has very much the same habits as *Triatoma megista*. It lives in the grass houses, and especially in the grass roofs of houses, where it multiplies abundantly; but it is rarely found in houses with tile roofs. It comes out at night, after the lights are out, to bite. It is frequently found in the burrows of armadillos and other animals.

Chagas showed that the infection can be transmitted by the *bite* of *Triatoma megista*. Torres transmitted the infection to kittens by the bite of *Triatoma megista,* the bugs being confined in tubes, and biting through the gauze covering the end of the tube, so that soiling with feces was prevented. Of 35 bugs tested in this way, 19 transmitted the infection and 13 failed to transmit it. Torres failed to get infection by depositing the feces of infected bugs on the unbroken skin of animals and he is of the opinion that the infection is transmitted in nature by the bite of the bug.

Brumpt is of the opinion that the usual mode of infection is through the *dejections* of the bug. The bugs defecate freely when biting and, as they commonly bite on the lips and cheeks (hence the native name ''barbeiro,'' the barber), the dejections of the bug may soil the buccal mucosa, although there may be no evidence of it. Brumpt considers that the infection may also pass through the unbroken skin or through the wound made by the bite. He failed to transmit the infection to monkeys by the bite of infected bugs or by placing the feces of infected bugs on the skin, but a monkey was infected by placing the feces of infected bugs in the conjunctival sac. In another set of experiments there was one infection through the unbroken skin. Mayer and da Rocha-Lima could not determine experimental transmission of the infection through the bite of infected bugs or ticks.

Tejera succeeded in infecting mice by allowing infected *Rhodnius prolixus* to bite them; but of four mice bitten, only one became infected, and that mouse had only a few trypanosomes in its blood. He infected mice by the instillation of intestinal contents of infected bugs into the conjunctival sac, into the anus, and on the genital mucosa.

While *Triatoma megista* is the transmitter of the infection in Brazil, and *Rhodnius prolixus* is the transmitter in Venezuela, *Trypanosoma cruzi* is not strictly adapted to these two arthropod hosts, but may complete its cycle of development in a number of other arthropods, and they may transmit the infection. In nature, it completes its cycle of development in *Triatoma megista, Triatoma geniculata* and *Rhodnius prolixus; Triatoma megista* and *Rhodnius prolixus* transmitting the infection to man, and *Triatoma geniculata* transmitting the infection in armadillos. Brumpt succeeded in infecting other species of Triatoma, including *Triatoma sanguisuga* from Texas; bedbugs; and a tick, *Orni-*

thodorus moubata. Neiva transmitted the infection to dogs, through the dog tick, *Rhipicephalus sanguineus,* from experimentally infected dogs. Brumpt considers that the common bedbug, *Cimex rotundatus,* of Brazil, may be as important as *Triatoma megista* in the transmission of the infection.

The distribution of *Trypanosoma cruzi* does not correspond to the distribution of Chagas' disease. In Brazil, armadillos are infected, though far from human habitations, and *Triatoma geniculata* transmits the infection from armadillo to armadillo. Kraus and Rosenbusch found triatomes infected with *Trypanosoma cruzi* in the mountainous regions of Argentina, but they did not find any cases that they could be sure were Chagas' disease. Maggio did not find Chagas' disease, but he found triatomes infected with flagellates which behaved in every way as *Trypanosoma cruzi* when injected into animals.

Brumpt discusses this difference in the distribution of *Trypanosoma cruzi* and Chagas' disease. Bugs, living on lower animals, may become adapted to life on man; so, some bugs (*Triatoma megista* and *Rhodnius prolixus*) can keep the infection going in man. Other bugs do not become adapted to life on man, but keep the infection going in lower animals (as with *Triatoma geniculata* and armadillos; and probably the bugs in Argentina transmit the infection in some lower animal).

(c) SUSCEPTIBILITY.—There is no difference in sex or race susceptibility. Young children are more susceptible than are adults; and the disease commonly runs an acute course in children, while in adults the disease is commonly chronic from the beginning.

Symptomatology.—Chagas divides the disease into two clinical forms: acute and chronic. In the acute cases the symptoms are severe and the parasites are found on direct examination of the blood.

ACUTE FORM.—This form of the disease generally affects children under one year of age, and it is seen in children only a few months old.

The period of incubation is about ten days. The disease begins with fever, the temperature going as high as 40° C. (104° F.); the fever is continuous, with a slight morning remission at times. There is a peculiar puffiness of the face; and, early in the disease, on palpation, the skin of the face gives a characteristic crepitation, which has been likened to that produced by rubbing sheets of gelatin together. The thyroid gland is enlarged, also the lymph glands, especially in the axillary and inguinal regions. The liver is somewhat enlarged and the spleen can be felt below the border of the ribs. There may be serous effusion into the pleural, pericardial and peritoneal cavities.

Trypanosomes are found in fair number in the peripheral blood during the fever.

Chagas divides the acute form into two groups: (1) the meningo-encephalitic form, in which there is nervous system involvement with resulting idiocy, paralyses or imbecility; and (2) a group in which the nervous system is not involved.

The acute form lasts ten to thirty days, and the child may die—at times with the clinical picture of meningo-encephalitis—or the disease may pass into the chronic form. Chagas says that spontaneous recovery does not occur at this time.

CHRONIC FORM.—The acute form may pass into the chronic form, or in adults the disease may be chronic from the beginning.

Chagas divides the chronic form into five clinical forms, according to the predominant symptoms: (1) the *pseudomyxedematous form;* (2) the *myxedematous form;* (3) the *cardiac form;* (4) the *nervous form,* and (5) chronic forms with *persistent acute and subacute manifestations.*

1. In the *pseudomyxedematous form* there is a slight mucous infiltration of the subcutaneous tissue, without the solid edema and parchment-like skin, or skeleton changes of myxedema. There is a violet—or blue—bronzing of the skin. The thyroid and lymph glands are enlarged. Convulsions are common.

2. In the *myxedematous form* there are the solid mucous infiltration of the subcutaneous tissue, the mental deterioration or arrested development, and the skeletal changes of myxedema. The parchment-like, dry skin pits on pressure. The lymph glands are enlarged and the thyroid gland is atrophied. Inflammations of the eyes, as conjunctivitis, are common.

3. The *cardiac form* is an important one; and Chagas considers that the symptoms are due to the presence of the parasites in the muscle fibers, with the inflammatory reaction when the parasites escape from the muscle fibers, and the resulting myocarditis. Marked arrhythmia is an important symptom, especially in children; while extrasystole is common in older persons. Heart block, with the pulse below 30 per minute, is not uncommon. Sinus irregularity is common in children, possibly due to vagus disturbance or to the myocarditis. Mackenzie's rhythmus nodalis may occur.

There is danger of death in asystole in cases of the cardiac form.

4. In the *nervous form* there is great variation in the localization of the symptoms, on account of the irregular scattering of the foci of parasites in the brain. Diplegias are the most common. There may be paralysis or a spastic condition of the lower extremities, with athetosis in the upper extremities; there may be choreiform movements, or contractures in the lower extremities may be present. The reflexes may be increased. There may be disturbances of speech, amounting to aphasia, or pseudobulbar paralysis. There may be paralysis of the ocular muscles. There may be convulsions when there is extensive involvement by foci in the cerebral cortex. Other convulsions appear to be due to hypothyroidism, and thyroid extract relieves them; these cases are in children or older persons with arrested development (infantilism).

5. In the *form with acute and subacute exacerbations* there are fever and other acute symptoms in addition to the symptoms of any one of the chronic forms. In adults it is usually the cardiac form, and there are enlarged thyroid and evidences of suprarenal insufficiency. There are few parasites in the blood.

The exacerbations are not like severe acute attacks, and Chagas thinks they may be due to reinfection.

Under the name of *metaschizotrypanotic manifestations* Chagas includes the cases of infantilism with long-standing goiter and other sequelae of the disease.

Diagnosis.—Clinical Diagnosis.—In the endemic area the physical findings of enlarged thyroid, with a myxedematous condition of the skin, irregularity of heart action, bronzing of the skin and paralysis, would lead one to suspect Chagas' disease. The acute cases may be mistaken for *malaria,* while the chronic cases may be mistaken for *uncinariasis;* examination of the blood and feces is necessary for differentiation.

The chronic cases may be mistaken for *goiter,* which is common in many parts of South America; and the question has been raised whether the thyroid changes are a part of Chagas' disease, or are endemic goiter in persons with Chagas' disease. While Kraus and Rosenbusch found triatomes infected with *Trypanosoma cruzi* in the mountainous regions of Argentina, they did not find any acute cases of Chagas' disease, but they found cases of cretinism and goiter.

Chagas holds that the thyroid involvement is characteristic of the disease. He saw the disease, with thyroid involvement, in four children, all less than three months old and exclusively breast-fed, thus ruling out goiter due to drinking water. Thyroid involvement is always present; and the thyroid is always enlarged, except in the myxedematous form, where the thyroid is atrophied and the symptoms of thyroid insufficiency are very marked. Thyroid enlargement is found in children and adults in Triatoma-infested houses, and not in houses free of Triatoma.

The nervous form must be differentiated from *syphilis.*

A definite diagnosis is possible only on the finding of the trypanosome.

Laboratory Diagnosis.—In the acute cases trypanosomes are found in the blood in fair numbers. When brain symptoms develop, the number of trypanosomes increases in the peripheral blood until death. When the disease goes on to the chronic form the number of trypanosomes decreases in the peripheral blood, until they are no longer found except during acute or subacute exacerbations.

Trypanosoma cruzi is very fragile and it is difficult to make a smear in which the trypanosomes are not torn. Tejera mixes a few drops of blood with some 10 per cent sodium citrate solution to prevent coagulation, then puts a small drop of the citrated blood on a clean slide, exposes it one-half minute to the vapor of a 2 per cent osmic acid solution, and then smears out in the usual way. He stains fifteen minutes by Pappenheim's panoptic method.

Trypanosomes may not be found in the peripheral blood longer than two to three weeks after the onset of fever, but they can be demonstrated in the blood of chronic cases by the injection of 5 to 10 cc. of blood into a guinea pig or a young monkey. Mice and rats are suitable for demonstrating the trypanosome by injection of blood, but mice may have *Trypanosoma duttoni* in their blood, and rats frequently have *Trypanosoma lewisi* in their blood; and these trypanosomes might lead to confusion.

The guinea pig is the most satisfactory of the available animals for demonstrating *Trypanosoma cruzi* by the injection of blood. At times the trypanosomes are so scarce in the peripheral blood of the pig that they cannot be found on direct examination of the blood. Chagas advises examining for parasites in the endothelial cells of the capillaries in the lungs of the pig. Brumpt suggests xeno-diagnosis, that is, allowing *Triatoma megista* to bite the pig, and, as the digestive tract of the bug is a good culture tube for the parasites, they will multiply there and can be found by examining the intestinal contents of the bug.

When parasites are not found in the blood, a postmortem diagnosis may be made by examining for the parasites in the tissues, especially the heart muscle, the muscles of the legs, arms and back, and the brain.

The blood shows secondary anemia. In the acute cases there is a slight leukocytosis, with an increase in the percentage of mononuclears; in the chronic cases there is no change in the leukocyte count. The Wassermann reaction is negative.

Complications and Sequelae.—There are no special complications. The sequelae are important, as so many of the cases occur in young children. The sequelae are enlarged thyroid with hyperthyroidism, infantilism, cretinism, paralysis, idiocy and aphasia.

Treatment.—No very satisfactory treatment has been found. Mazzi and Govi report an acute case of Chagas' disease in a four-year-old child. They gave **sulfarsenol,** starting with a dose of 0.06 Gm. (1 grain). At 4-day intervals they gave 0.06 Gm. (1 grain), 0.12 Gm. (2 grains), 0.12 Gm. (2 grains), 0.18 Gm. (3 grains), 0.18 Gm. (3 grains). The case cleared up.

Mazzi used Bayer 7602 in two cases, and Torrealba used it in one case; they believe it had some favorable effect. Herr and Brumpt used it in a laboratory infection, from getting the feces from an infected bug from Mexico into the eye. The temperature gradually subsided and was normal on the thirtieth day (Yorke does not consider there was much evidence that the drug had any favorable action in this case).

Symptomatic treatment, especially for the hyperthyroidism, may lessen the severity of some of the symptoms.

PROPHYLAXIS.—(*a*) *Source of Infection.*—Persons suffering with the disease should be **protected from the bites of Triatoma and Rhodnius.**

Armadillos (and possibly other wild animals) and cats act as reservoirs for the infection, but no practical results can be expected from destruction of these animals.

(*b*) *Mode of Transmission.*—The best results are obtained by **preventing Triatoma and Rhodnius from living in the houses and feeding on the people.** Tejera's finding that *Rhodnius prolixus* lives and breeds in the grass roofs of houses—but not in houses with tile roofs—and the finding of *Triatoma megista,* especially in the poor houses in Minas Geraes, indicates that **better construction of houses** would go far toward eliminating the bugs from human habitations. Triatoma is said to be attracted by articles made of leather.

Sulfur fumigation and whitewashing of the houses have been recommended for the destruction of the bugs.

(c) *Susceptibility of the Population.*—The bugs bite at night and the adults can fly; so it is necessary to **sleep under nets,** as well as to **prevent the bugs coming up the legs of the bed or along the hammock ropes.**

Nothing is to be expected from vaccination.

Prognosis.—In the acute cases the prognosis is bad, as they die or pass into the chronic form. The prognosis is bad in the cardiac form and sudden death may occur. The sequelae are permanent.

Mechanism of the Disease Process.—The trypanosomes inoculated by the bug—either by the bite, or from the feces through the mucous membranes or skin—enter the tissue cells, especially the muscle and neuroglia cells, lose their flagellum and assume the Leishmania form. These Leishmania forms multiply by simple fission until the infected cells come to have the appearance of cysts filled with the parasites. After a time the cells rupture and trypanosomes appear in the peripheral blood. The multiplication of the parasites in the muscle fiber simply separates the fibrils and bulges the sarcolemma, without other damage to the fiber. There is no inflammatory reaction about the infected cell until it ruptures or the parasite dies, the inflammatory reaction being due to the toxin set free.

The toxin causes the early symptoms of the acute form, and it causes the fatty degeneration of the liver, the meningitis, and the changes in the thyroid and suprarenal glands. The myocarditis is due to the damage done to the heart muscle by the development of the parasites in it, and the waxy degeneration of the muscle fibers caused by the toxin. The changes in the brain substance are due to the localization of the parasites in the brain, as well as to the toxin.

Immunity.—Nothing is known regarding immunity in man. Mayer and da Rocha-Lima found that rats, guinea pigs and rabbits were immune after recovery from infection; and Brumpt found that recovered mice were immune eight months after recovery. Serum from Mayer and da Rocha-Lima's immune animals did not protect other animals against infection when injected twenty-four hours before or at the time of inoculation. Mayer and da Rocha-Lima found that relapse occurred; and one guinea pig relapsed after a latent period of eight months.

Causes of Death.—Failure of the heart is a common cause of death. In the acute cases death may result from asthenia or from meningo-encephalitis.

Pathology.—Macroscopic.—There may be bronzing of the skin and there is often a myxedematous condition of the subcutaneous tissues. The axillary and inguinal lymph glands are considerably enlarged, the cervicals less so. The thyroid gland is generally enlarged and hard, but it may be atrophied.

There is a yellowish serous fluid in the pleural, pericardial and peritoneal cavities. The mediastinal lymph glands are enlarged; the pericardium is congested and may be hemorrhagic; the heart shows an intense myocarditis.

The liver is enlarged and fatty; the spleen is moderately enlarged, congested and soft. The mesenteric lymph glands are enlarged; the suprarenal glands are congested.

The most marked changes are in the meninges and the brain. The cerebro-spinal fluid is increased in amount; the dura is congested and is adherent to the bone. The pia is thickened and edematous, and there may be a gelatinous exudate in the subarachnoid space. There are areas of meningitis. There may be areas of chronic encephalitis. There may be adhesions over the spinal dura.

Microscopic.—In the *heart* the parasites are abundant in the muscle fibers, many of the fibers forming cysts filled with the parasites. When a cyst ruptures, some of the parasites are found free; others in phagocytes. In acute cases there is diffuse inflammatory reaction in the interstitial tissue; in chronic cases there are localized areas of inflammatory reaction. The small blood vessels of the heart show perivascular round-cell infiltration. There may be pericarditis or endocarditis, but no parasites are found in the lesions.

The *thyroid gland* shows sclerosis and round-cell infiltration, the acini being small or dilated to form cysts; and there are frequently areas of calcification. There is increase in the number of cells in the interstitial islands of cells. No parasites are found in the thyroid.

The *liver* shows marked fatty degeneration and in acute cases the degeneration may be as marked as in yellow fever. The *suprarenals* are congested and fatty, and show inflammatory reaction; later they show degeneration. The parasites are not usually found in the suprarenal glands, but they may be found either in the cortex or the medulla. The *kidneys* may show inflammatory reaction.

In the *central nervous system* the meninges and blood vessels show a mild perivascular round-cell infiltration, of the same type as is seen in African trypanosomiasis. In the brain there are scattered foci, seen with low magnification, in which the parasites are collected. The neuroglia cells are packed with parasites, and swell to form cysts, without any reaction around the cell. When the cell ruptures there is a collection of mononuclear and polymorphonuclear cells which take up the parasites. No parasites are found in the nerve cell.

The *skeletal muscles*, especially of the legs, arms and back, are commonly invaded by the parasites. As long as the parasites remain in the muscle fibers there is no inflammatory reaction. When the fiber ruptures, and the parasites escape, there is inflammatory reaction around the area, and the inflammatory cells pass into the ruptured muscle fiber. There is round-cell infiltration about the blood vessels in the muscles.

The *testicles* show inflammatory reaction, and the epithelial cells lining the seminal tubules are infected with the parasites; and parasites may be found in the spermatozoa. There is round-cell infiltration of the interstitial tissue and about the blood vessels. Vianna found trypanosomes in the semen of two of six infected guinea pigs.

The *ovaries* are sclerotic and contain cysts, but no parasites are found.

The parasites are found in the endothelial cells in the capillaries of the *lungs*. Da Rocha-Lima found the parasites in fatty and connective tissues, the spleen, bone marrow, lymphatic glands, and in the unstriped muscle in the walls of the *intestine* and the *arteries*.

Secondary infections are not common.

BIBLIOGRAPHY

Bayma, T.: Un caso de mixedema congenito. Apontamentos sobre la Distribuição do "Triatoma" Estado de S. Paulo, Rev. med. de S. Paulo, 16 : 103, 1913.

Bruce, D.: The Croonian lectures on trypanosomes causing disease in man and domestic animals in Central Africa, Lancet, 1 : 1323; 2 : 1, 55, 109, 1915.

————, Harvey D., Hamerton, A. E., Davey, J. B. and Lady Bruce : The trypanosomes found in the blood of wild animals living in the sleeping-sickness area, Nyasaland, Proc. Roy. Soc., London, 86 : 269, 1913.

————, Hamerton, A. E., Watson, D. P. and Lady Bruce : The trypanosome causing disease in man in Nyasaland. Part III. Development in Glossina morsitans, Proc. Roy. Soc., London, 87 : 516, 1914.

Brumpt, E.: Pénétration du Schizotrypanum cruzi à travers la Muqueuse Oculaire Saine, Bull. Soc. path. exot., 5 : 723, 1912.

————: Immunité partielle dans les infections à Trypanosoma cruzi. Transmission de ce Trypanosome par Cimex rotundatus. Rôle regulateur des hôtes. Passage à travers la peau, Bull. Soc. path. exot., 6 : 172, 1913.

Brumpt, E.: Le xénodiagnostic. Application au diagnostic de quelques infections parasitaires et en particulier à la Trypanosomose de Chagas, Bull. Soc. path. exot., 7 : 706, 1914.

————: Réduvides de l'Amerique du Nord capables de transmettre le Trypanosoma cruzi, Bull. Soc. path. exot., 7 : 132, 1914.

————: Maladie de C. Chagas au Brésil. Môde de transmission, origine, conditions qui determinent sa repartition actuelle, Bull. Acad. de méd., Paris, 81 : 251, 1919.

———— and Gonzalez, L.: Présentation d'un Réduvide du Vénézuela, le Rhodnius prolixus chez lequel évolue Trypanosoma cruzi, Bull. Soc. path. exot., 6 : 382, 1913.

————, Mazzotti, L. and Brumpt, L. C.: Epidemiological inquiries on Chagas' disease in Mexico. Reduviid vectors, animal reservoirs, and human cases, Ann. de parasitol., 17 : 299, 1939.

Carpenter, G. D. H.: Second report on the bionomics of Glossina fuscipes (palpalis) of Uganda. Rep. Sleeping Sickn. Comm. Roy. Soc., No. 14, p. 1, 1913.

Castellani, A. and Chalmers, A. J.: Manual of Tropical Medicine, Ed. 3, London, Baillière, Tindall & Cox, 1919.

Chagas, C. : Ein neu-entdeckter Krankheitsprozess des Menschen, Mem. Inst. Oswaldo Cruz, 3 : 219, 1911.
———— : Thireoidite parasitaria, Rev. med. de S. Paulo, 15 : 337, 1912.
———— : Tripanosomiase americana, Forma aguda da molestia, Mem. Inst. Oswaldo Cruz, 8 : 37, 1916.
———— : Processos patojenicos da tripanosomiase americana, Mem. Inst. Oswaldo Cruz, 8 : 5, 1916.
———— : Host of Trypanosoma cruzi, Rev. med.-cir. do Brasil, 26 : 220, 1918 (J. A. M. A., 71 : 1015, 1918).
Chalmers, A. J. : The classification of trypanosomes, J. Trop. Med., 21 : 221, 1918.
Da Costa, B. F. B., Sant' Anna, J. F., Santos, A. C. D. and Alvareo, M. G. de A. : Sleeping sickness : a record of four years war against it in Principe, Portuguese West Africa. Published in Portuguese in Arch. de hyg. e path. exot., March 30, 1915. Translated by permission of the Lisbon School of Tropical Medicine by J. A. Wyllie, F. R. G. S., London, Baillière, Tindall & Cox, 261 pp., 1916.
Daniels, C. W. : Eye lesions as a point of importance in directing suspicion to possible trypanosome infection, Ophthalmoscope, 13 : 595, 1915.
———— and Newham, H. B. : Treatment of trypanosomiasis, Lancet, 1 : 102, 1916.
Delanoe, M. and Mme. P. : A propos du Schizotrypanum cruzi, Bull. Soc. path. exot., 5 : 599, 1912.
Dubois, A. and Van den Branden, F. : La reaction de Boveri dans la Trypanosomiase humaine, Bull. Soc. path. exot., 7 : 261, 1915.
Duke, H. L. : The wild game and human trypanosomiasis ; with some remarks on the nomenclature of certain Pan-African trypanosomes, J. Trop. M. & Hyg., 18 : 13, 1915.
Ehrlich, P. : Schlafkrankheit. IV. Internat. Kong. z. Fürsorge f. Geisteskr., Berlin, Oct., 1910, Offizieller Bericht, Halle, p. 644, 1911.
Escomel, E. : La trypanosomiase humaine existe dans les forêts orientales du Péron, Bull. Soc. path. exot., 12 : 723, 1919.
Fry, W. B. and Rankin, H. S. : Further researches on the extrusion of granules by trypanosomes and on their further development, with a note on methods by H. G. Plimmer, Proc. Roy. Soc., London, 86 : 377, 1913.
Guerreiro, C. : Urologische Untersuchungen bei der Krankheit von Carlos Chagas, Mem. Inst. Oswaldo Cruz, 4 : 66, 1912.
Hartmann, M. : Ueber die Schizogonie von Schizotrypanum cruzi, Arch. f. Protistenk., 38 : 113, 1917–18.
Heckenroth, F. and Blanchard, M. : Récherches sur les propriétés du serum des malades atteints de trypanosomiase au Congo français, Bull. Soc. path. exot., 6 : 444, 1913.
Henry, T. A. and Gray, W. H. : Trypanocidal and anti-malarial drugs, Trop. Dis. Bull., 32 : 385, 1935.
Herr, A. and Brumpt, L. : An acute case of Chagas' disease acquired accidentally from Mexican triatomata, Bull. Soc. path. exot., 32 : 565, 1939.
Kellersberger, E. R. : African sleeping sickness : a clinical study, South. M. J., 29 : 239, 1936.
Kinghorn, A. and Yorke, W. : Further observations on the Trypanosomes of game and domestic stock in North Eastern Rhodesia, Ann. Trop. Med., 6 : 483, 1912.
Koch, H. : Bericht über einen Versuch, Glossina palpalis durch Fang zu beseitigen, Arch. f. Schiffs- u. Tropen-Hyg., 18 : 807, 1914.
Kofoid, C. A. and McCulloch, I. : On Trypanosoma triatomae, a new flagellate from a hemipteran bug from the nests of the wood rat Neotoma fuscipes, Univ. Calif. Pub. Zool., 16 : 113, 1916.
Kopke, A. : Notes sur la maladie du sommeil et sa médication, Bull. Office Internat. d'hyg. pub., 6 : 1722, 1914.
Kopp, I. and Solomon, H. C. : Untoward reactions of tryparsamide, Am. J. Syph., Gonor. & Ven. Dis., 24 : 265, 1940.
Kraus, R. and Rosenbusch, F. : Kropf, Kretinismus und die Krankheit von Chagas. 2. Mitteilung, Wien. klin. Wchnschr., 30 : 1104, 1917.

Kraus, R., Rosenbusch, F. and Maggio, C. : Kropf, Kretinismus und die Krankheit von Chagas, Wien. klin. Wchnschr., 28 : 942, 1915.
Lamborn, W. A. : Second report on glossina investigations in Nyasaland, Bull. Entomol. Research, 6 : 249, 1915.
———— : Third report on glossina investigations in Nyasaland, Bull. Entomol. Research, 7 : 29, 1916.
Lankester, E. R. : The Kingdom of Man. Nature's Revenges ; the Sleeping Sickness, New York, Henry Holt & Company, Inc., 1907.
Laveran, A. : Surra, nagana ferox, nagana de l'Ouganda et infections dues au Trypanosoma rhodesiense, Bull. Soc. path. exot., 9 : 731, 1916.
Lester, H. M. O. : 7 (Tryp.), Trop. Dis. Bull., 37, 1940.
Maggio, C. and Rosenbusch, F. : Studien über die Chagaskrankheit in Argentinien und die Trypanosomen der "Vinchuchas" [Wanzen, Triatoma infestans Klug], Centralbl. f. Bakt., l. Abt., Orig., 77 : 40, 1915.
Marie, A. and Darré, H. : La maladie du sommeil. IV. Internat. Kong. z. Fürsorge f. Geisteskr., Berlin, Oct., 1910, Offizieller Bericht, Halle, p. 695, 1911.
Martin, G. : Trypanosomiase Americaine. Grall et Clarac's traité du pathologie exotique, clinique et therapeutique, Paris, J. B. Baillière et fils, Vol. III, pp. 394, 1912.
———— and Leboeuf : Trypanosomiase Africaine, ou maladie du sommeil. Grall et Clarac's traité du pathologie exotique, clinique et therapeutique, Paris, J. B. Baillière et fils, Vol. III, pp. 302, 1912.
———— and Ringenbach : Troubles psychiques dans la maladie du sommeil, Encéphale, 1 : 625 ; 2 : 97, 149, 1910.
Martin, L. and Darré, H. : Formes cérébrales de le maladie du sommeil, Bull. et mém. Soc. méd. d. hôp. de Paris, 27 : 599, 1909.
Masters, W. E. : The symptomatology and treatment of human trypanosomiasis in the Lusanga area, District Dukwango, Belgian Congo. A report based upon 370 recorded cases and 6,200 intravenous and intramuscular injections, J. Trop. Med. & Hyg., 21 : 13, 25, 1918.
———— : The treatment of human trypanosomiasis by injectio antimonii oxidi, J. Trop. Med. & Hyg., 21 : 146, 1918.
Mayer, M. : Trypanosomen als Krankheitserreger. Handbuch der pathogenen Mikroörganismen. Kolle und Wassermann, Ed. 2, Jena, Gustav Fischer, 7 : 321, 1913.
———— and da Rocha-Lima, H. ; Zum Verhalten von Schizotrypanum cruzi in Warmblutern und Arthropoden, Beiheft z. Arch. f. Schiffs- u. Tropenhyg., 18 : 101, 1914.
Mazza, S. : The first hundred cases of the acute form of Chagas' disease in Argentina, Prensa méd. argent., 23 : 1979, 1936.
———— and Govi : Trop. Dis. Bull., 33 : 208, 1936.
Minchin, E. A. and Thomson, J. D. : The rat trypanosome, Trypanosoma lewisi, in its relation to the rat-flea, Ceratophyllus fasciatus, Quart. J. Micr. Sc., 60 : 463, 1915.
Mott, F. W. : Sleeping sickness. IV. Internat. Kong. z. Fürsorge f. Geisteskr., Berlin, Oct., 1910, Offizieller Bericht, Halle, p. 659, 1911.
———— : Comparative neuropathology of trypanosome and spirochete infections, with a résumé of our knowledge of human trypanosomiasis, Proc. Roy. Soc. Med. (Path. Sect.), 4 : 1, 1910–11.
Neiva, A. : Infecção de cobayas pela passagem do Trypanosoma equinum através da conjunctiva sã. Nota prévia, Brasil-med., 27 : 333, 1913.
———— : Transmissão do Trypanosoma cruzi pelo Rhipicephalus sanguineus (Latr.). Nota prévia, Brasil-med., 27 : 498, 1913.
Schilling, C. : Immunität bei Protozoöninfektionen. Handbuch der pathogenen Mikroörganismen. Kolle und Wassermann, Ed. 2, Jena, Gustav Fischer, 7 : 565, 1913.
Schuberg, A. and Böing, W. : Ueber den Weg der Infektion bei Trypanosomen und Spirochätenerkrankungen, Deutsche med. Wchnschr., 39 : 877, 1913.
Shircore, J. O. : A method for the trapping of Glossina morsitans suggested for trial, Tr. Soc. Trop. M. & Hyg., 9 : 101, 1915–16.

Spielmayer, W. : Schlafkrankheit und progressive Paralyse, München. med. Wchnschr., 54 : 1065, 1907.

Stitt, E. R. : Diagnostics and Treatment of Tropical Diseases, Ed. 2, Philadelphia, P. Blakiston's Son & Company, 1917.

Teague, O. and Clark, H. C. : A trypanosome of Panamanian cattle and a method for concentrating trypanosomes in peripheral blood, J. Infect. Dis., 22 : 154, 1918.

Tejera, G. : La Tripanosomosis americana, o enfermedad de Chagas, en Venezuela, Gac. méd. de Caracas, 26 : 104, 1919.

Thomson, J. G. and Sinton, J. A. : The morphology of Trypanosoma gambiense and Trypanosoma rhodesiense in cultures : and a comparison with the developmental forms described in Glossina palpalis, Ann. Trop. Med., 6 : 331, 1912.

Torres, M. : Molestia de "Carlos Chagas." Transmissão do T. cruzi pela Picada do T. megista, Brasil-med., 27 : 321, 1913.

———— : Algunos fatos que interessan a epidemiolojia da molestia de Chagas, Mem. Inst. Oswaldo Cruz, 7 : 120, 1915.

———— : Estudo do miocardia na molestia de Chagas (fórma aguda). I. Alteraçoes da fibra muscular cardiaca, Mem. Inst. Oswaldo Cruz, 9 : 114, 1917.

Tropical Diseases Bulletin. Published by Tropical Diseases Bureau, Hospital for Tropical Diseases, Endsleigh Gardens, Euston Road, London, N. W. 1. Contains excellent abstracts of all literature on Trypanosomiasis.

Valladares, P. : Polyorrhomenosis e cruzi-trypanose, Brasil-med., 30 : 362, 1916.

Van den Branden, F. : Essais de trâitement de la trypanosomiase humaine par l'émétique huileux, Bull. Soc. path. exot., 11 : 379, 1918.

Vianna, G. : Beitrag zum Studium der pathologischen Anatomie der Krankheit von Carlos Chagas, Mem. Inst. Oswaldo Cruz, 3 : 276, 1911.

Villela, E. : Fórma aguda da doença de Chagas. Primeira verificação no Estado de S. Paulo, Brasil-med., 32 : 65, 1918.

Wolbach, S. B. and Binger, C. A. L. : A contribution to the parasitology of trypanosomiasis, J. Med. Research, 22 : 83, 1912.

———— : A contribution to the pathological histology of trypanosomiasis, Brit. M. J., 2 : 1188, 1912.

————, Chapman, W. H. and Stevens, H. W. : Concerning the filterability of trypanosomes, J. Med. Research, 33 : 107, 1915.

Yorke, W. and Blacklock, B. : The reservoir of the human trypanosome in Sierra Leone, Ann. Trop. Med., 9 : 383, 1915.

CHAPTER XXXI

AMEBIASIS

By Charles F. Craig, M.D., M.A. (Hon.), F.A.C.P., F.A.C.S., Colonel,
U. S. Army Medical Corps (Retired), D.S.M.

Synonyms.—Amebic dysentery, entamebic dysentery, endamebic
dysentery, amebic colitis, amebic enteritis, amebic abscess of liver and
other organs.

Definition.—By the term "amebiasis" is meant the invasion of the
tissues of the body of man by the protozoan organism known as *Endamoeba histolytica* and includes all of the clinical pictures caused by such
invasion. Thus it embraces the signs and symptoms present in mild
infections in which vague gastro-intestinal symptomatology is present;
those present in infections accompanied by severe enteritis, or amebic
enteritis; those present in acute dysentery, or amebic dysentery; and
those present in abscess of the liver, brain or other organs, or caused by
the invasion of the skin. In most of our textbooks, even those of recent
date, amebiasis is considered under the general title of "amebic dysentery," but this is entirely incorrect, as amebic dysentery is simply part
of the clinical picture of infection with this organism, or amebiasis.
Amebic dysentery is not a disease entity, but is merely one stage in the
development of amebic infection and to consider the entire subject of
amebiasis under this heading would be like considering the entire subject
of malaria under the title "pernicious malarial fever."

It is also most important that the physician realize that only a small
proportion of the individuals suffering from amebiasis ever develop
amebic dysentery and that the term "tropical," as connected with this

type of dysentery, is erroneous, as many cases of amebic dysentery occur in temperate and cold climates. In fact, as is well known, the first case of amebic dysentery was described by Lösch, in St. Petersburg, Russia, and it was in this patient that he discovered and described the causal parasite, *Endamoeba histolytica.*

History.—Although the clinical symptoms connected with amebiasis, especially those occurring when dysentery accompanied the infection, were well known for many years prior to the discovery of the causative organism, there was no clear distinction made between dysentery of such origin and other forms of dysentery occurring in the tropics and elsewhere. In 1875 Lösch studied a patient in St. Petersburg, Russia, suffering from severe dysentery and in his stools found an ameba which was undoubtedly that now known as *Endamoeba histolytica.* The patient died and at autopsy the same ameba was found in the material removed from the ulcerations present in the large intestine, and rectal injections of such material in a dog were followed by an attack of dysentery. However, Lösch did not consider the ameba as the cause of the dysentery either in the man or dog but believed that the bacteria present were the real cause of the dysenteric symptoms. For this reason his work did not attract much attention.

The first investigator to consider this ameba as the cause of a distinct form of dysentery was Kartulis, who in 1886 published his researches upon amebic dysentery in Egypt and stated his belief that the ameba was the cause of a form of dysentery occurring in that country. In 1891 Councilman and Lafleur published their classical monograph upon amebic dysentery, describing its peculiar pathology and confirming Kartulis' statement that the ameba discovered by Lösch, which he called "Amoeba coli," was responsible for a distinct type of dysentery especially prevalent in tropical countries. In 1893 Quincke and Roos first described the morphologic differences between the ameba found in dysenteric stools and those found in the stools of healthy individuals and in those suffering from other diseases, and concluded that there existed a pathogenic ameba, causing dysentery, and a harmless ameba which may be present in the intestine of man in both health and disease.

Although the work of Quincke and Roos pointed to the existence of pathogenic and nonpathogenic amebae in the intestine of man, the credit of first giving a clear description of the morphology of such amebae belongs to Schaudinn, who in 1903, in a careful study of the question, showed definitely that there live in the intestine of man two amebae, one identical with that described by Lösch as "Amoeba coli," and causing ulceration of the intestine, and one which had been previously described by several observers, notably by Casagrandi and Barbagallo, which lives in the lumen of the bowel without invading the tissues or producing other lesions. Schaudinn called the pathogenic ameba, *Entamoeba histolytica,* and the nonpathogenic ameba *Entamoeba coli.* The writer confirmed Schaudinn's work in 1905, and Walker and Sellards in 1913 demonstrated by experiments upon man that Schaudinn's results were correct so far as the existence of a pathogenic and nonpathogenic ameba in the intestine of man is concerned. At the time that Schaudinn established the genus Entamoeba for the parasitic amebae of man he described, he was apparently unaware of the fact that in 1875 Leidy established the genus Endamoeba to include an ameba occurring in the cockroach which has not yet been proved to differ sufficiently in morphology from *Endamoeba histolytica* or *Endamoeba coli* to justify placing the latter organisms in another genus. As the generic name given by Leidy has priority over that given by Schaudinn, it follows that *Endamoeba histolytica* and *Endamoeba coli* are the proper names of these amebae rather than *Entamoeba histolytica* and *Entamoeba coli*. The generic name "Endamoeba" has been accepted by the International Commission on Zoological Nomenclature and should be used by all zoologists.

Besides the two species of ameba mentioned above, three other species are now known to exist in man's intestine, all of which are nonpathogenic so far as known. In 1911–1912 Prowazek described a species which is now known as *Iodamoeba buetschlii;* in 1917 Wenyon and O'Connor described a species they called *Endolimax nana,* and in 1918 Jepps and Dobell described still another species which they named *Dientamoeba fragilis.* All of these species have been abundantly confirmed and we now know that man may harbor in his large intestine no less than five species of amebae; i.e., *Endamoeba histolytica, Endamoeba coli, Endolimax nana, Iodamoeba buetschlii* and *Dientamoeba fragilis,* but only one, *Endamoeba histolytica,* has been proved to be a pathogenic organism.

The most important advance made in the study of amebiasis after the differentiation of the pathogenic ameba from the harmless species, was the cultivation of *Endamoeba histolytica,* first accomplished by Cutler in 1918, but placed upon a practical basis by the observations of Boeck and Drbohlav in 1924–1925. These observers were the first to demonstrate that this ameba could be cultivated for an indefinite period upon simple culture media upon which the organism can be easily grown.

In 1927 the writer described a complement fixation test which has proved of value in the diagnosis of amebiasis, and also demonstrated the presence of hemolytic and cytolytic substances in cultures of *Endamoeba histolytica,* thus proving the correctness of the generally accepted opinion that this organism depended for its pathogenic activity, in large part, upon the action of such substances secreted by the ameba.

Geographic Distribution.—The geographic distribution of *Endamoeba histolytica* is world-wide, as proved by the fact that a certain proportion of the people of every locality in which surveys have been made for its presence have been found infected. While this is true, it is also true that it occurs much more frequently in the subtropics and tropics, probably not because of climatic conditions so much as because sanitary conditions in such regions are usually far below those of temperate regions. The severe phases of amebiasis, as amebic dysentery and amebic abscess of the liver, are much more frequently seen in the tropics than in temperate regions, but it should be remembered that both these conditions are present in temperate and cold regions and are frequently overlooked because of the prevalent opinion among the profession that they are tropical diseases and do not occur in colder climates. Indeed, it is probable that if one could know of the many cases of both of these conditions that have been wrongly diagnosed in all parts of the temperate zones, one would be amazed at their number. The writer has frequently observed both severe amebic ulceration of the intestine and amebic abscess of the liver in patients in the United States who have come to the autopsy table without these conditions being diagnosed by the attending physician.

38111

While amebiasis has a world-wide distribution, the symptom-complex known as amebic dysentery and amebic abscess of the liver, which are a part of the clinical picture of amebiasis, occur most frequently in tropical and subtropical regions, and the common distribution of these conditions is of importance, but recognizing the fact that they do occur throughout the world less frequently. In North America such types of amebiasis are observed most frequently in the Southern United States, as in Louisiana, Alabama, Georgia, Florida, Mississippi and Texas, but numerous cases have been reported from California, Tennessee, the Carolinas and Virginia. In Central and South America these conditions are prevalent in Colombia, Chile, Brazil, the Argentine Republic, Ecuador, Guatemala, Honduras, Nicaragua, Panama, Peru and Venezuela, and in the islands of the West Indies, as Cuba, Haiti, San Domingo, Puerto Rico and other islands of this group. In Europe, amebic dysentery is common in the southern portion of Russia, in Poland, Greece, Spain, Italy, Sardinia and Malta, while in Asia it is frequently encountered in Palestine, Syria, Mesopotamia, India, China, the East Indies, Cochin China, the Malay States, Siam, Korea, Formosa and Japan. It is often seen in the islands of the Pacific, especially in the Philippine Islands, although in these islands it has shown a steadily declining morbidity and mortality rate since the American occupation with the consequent improvement in general sanitation, especially the installation of properly guarded general water supplies. In Africa, amebic dysentery and amebic abscess of the liver are frequently observed throughout the tropical and subtropical regions of the continent but are especially prevalent in Algeria, the Congo basin, Egypt, British East Africa, Togo, Tripoli, Tunis and the Ivory Coast.

It should be distinctly understood that while amebic dysentery and its most important complication, amebic abscess of the liver, have the general geographic distribution mentioned in the preceding paragraph, infection with *Endamoeba histolytica,* or amebiasis, occurs in all parts of the world and may be followed by dysentery and liver abscess in any locality. The reason that these latter conditions are more frequently observed in the countries mentioned are, in all probability, a lessened resistance on the part of the human host and constant reinfection because of poor sanitary conditions.

Etiology.—The cause of amebiasis is an ameba, *Endamoeba histolytica,* an animal organism consisting of a single cell, and hence belonging to the Protozoa, class Rhizopoda. In addition to this ameba, the intestine of man may be parasitized by four other amebae, all of which are harmless parasites of man. The names of these five species of amebae found in the human intestine, and their *zoological classification,* are shown in thé following tabulation:

Class RHIZOPODA v. Siebold, 1845.
    Order AMOEBIDA Calkins, 1902.
        Family AMOEBIDAE Bronn, 1859.
            Genus Endamoeba Leidy, 1879.
                Species *Endamoeba histolytica* (Schaudinn, 1903), Hickson, 1909.
                    Endamoeba coli (Grassi, 1879), Hickson, 1909.
            Genus Endolimax Kuenen and Swellengrebel, 1917.
                Species *Endolimax nana* (Wenyon and O'Connor, 1917), Brug, 1918.
            Genus Iodamoeba Dobell, 1919.
                Species *Iodamoeba buetschlii* (v. Prowazek, 1912), Dobell, 1919.
            Genus Dientamoeba Jepps and Dobell, 1918.
                Species *Dientamoeba fragilis* Jepps and Dobell, 1918.

The *morphology* of these various amebae differs and their diagnosis is based upon morphologic differences which will be discussed under Diagnosis.

Endamoeba histolytica is the only pathogenic ameba so far differentiated in man and it lives in the lumen and in the tissues of the intestinal tract, preferably in the large intestine but not infrequently in the lower portion of the ileum and in the appendix. It is a true tissue parasite, and there is not sufficient evidence now available demonstrating that it can live for any great length of time in the intestine of man without penetrating the tissues. Some authorities have tried to prove that this ameba, like the other amebae living in the human intestine, can multiply indefinitely in the lumen of the bowel without producing lesions, but the evidence they have brought forward to the date of writing is inconclusive and the consensus of opinion at present is that *Endamoeba histolytica* does not live in man's intestine without penetrating the tissues and producing lesions, even though the latter may be microscopic in size. It has been the writer's experience, in studying infection with this parasite both in man and the dog, that in every instance in which it has been possible to study autopsy material, the parasite has penetrated the tissues and produced lesions, although in some instances such lesions were almost microscopic in size. In such instances sections of the affected area have invariably shown the parasite within the mucous, submucous or muscular coats of the intestine. Furthermore, a study of sections of apparently healthy intestines showed nests of these amebae beneath the mucous membrane, in several instances. Such findings explain the absence of clinical symptoms in many cases of amebiasis, but they do not support the theory that this ameba lives for long periods of time within the lumen of the bowel without penetrating the tissues.

Endamoeba histolytica occurs in the intestine in two forms, the motile or trophozoite form, and the immotile or cystic form. A third form is usually described, the precystic form, which consists of the rounded up, motionless trophozoite, prior to the development of a cyst membrane. The motile forms are found in fluid or semifluid stools, while the cysts are found in solid or semisolid stools, although rarely motile forms may be found in formed stools in mucus which has been scraped off an ulcer during the passage of the stool through the intestine. The cysts are the infective stage of the parasite, being swallowed by man in food or drink contaminated by feces containing them, but infection may occur through swallowing the motile forms if such forms should reach material ingested by man, as it has been shown by Craig (1903), Wagner (1935) and Swartzwelder (1937) that infection of cats and dogs may occur by feeding motile trophozoites, thus proving that the generally accepted statement that the trophozoites cannot pass through the stomach without being killed by the acidity of the gastric juice is erroneous.

The *life cycle of Endamoeba histolytica* is briefly as follows: The cysts are swallowed in contaminated food or drink and after reaching the lower portion of the ileum and the upper portion of the large intestine, the cyst liberates a motile ameba containing 4 nuclei. After liberation from the cyst this ameba eventually divides into 8 young amebae, according to Dobell and others, or into 4 young amebae, according to Swartzwelder and others. Dobell (1928) described a complicated series of divisions of the four-nucleated amebae after leaving the cyst in cultures, the end product being 8 young amebae; but Swartzwelder (1937), working with dogs, was unable to confirm this observation and never observed any metacystic amebae with more than 4 nuclei or the division of the amebae into 8 young amebae.

After excystment, the young amebae, or trophozoties, resulting from division of the excysted ameba, invade the tissues of the intestine by virtue of their ameboid motility and the softening and cytolysing of the tissue through a cytolytic substance which they excrete. In the tissues the trophozoites divide by simple fission into two amebae and thus nests of the parasites are formed and from these foci the amebae penetrate farther into the intestinal coats.

The amebae remaining in the lumen of the bowel and which do not succeed in penetrating the tissues, may perhaps multiply for a limited period of time, but conditions for such multiplication soon become unfavorable and they then round up, lose their motility, and become the precystic forms, which eventually secrete a cyst wall and become cysts. The latter are the usual infective agents, are passed from the bowel with the stools, and are swallowed in food or drink contaminated with the feces containing the cysts. We know nothing about the usual time consumed in excystment or encystment but there is sufficient evidence available to demonstrate that cysts occur in the stools in large numbers at certain intervals and are scarce at other times. In cultures it has also been noted that multiplication of the motile forms, or the trophozoites, also occurs at uncertain intervals, cultures at one time showing few trophozoites, while at another time multitudes are found to be present.

The cysts observed in evacuated feces may contain 1, 2, 3 or 4 nuclei, the fully developed cyst containing 4 nuclei, although cysts of this species of ameba have been seen containing 8, or even more, nuclei. Hegner, Johnson and Stabler (1932) and Tsuchiya (1932) have apparently demonstrated that under favorable conditions the uninucleate and binucleate cysts may develop into quadrinucleate cysts after the feces containing them have left the bowel, while Swartzwelder (1937) has shown that excystment of cysts formed in the host never occurs while the cysts are in the host's intestine.

The *cultivation of Endamoeba histolytica* was first accomplished by Cutler (1918), but his observations were not confirmed and the media he employed were too complex for general use. To Boeck and Drbohlav (1924–1925) we owe the development of simple culture media for this parasite upon which it is possible to cultivate the organism outside the body of man for months and years. Their observations have been abundantly confirmed and numerous other media have been found satisfactory in the cultivation of *Endamoeba histolytica*. Although cultivation is possible, pure cultures, while they have been obtained, are of little value, as the ameba requires bacteria in the cultures in order to exist, and it has not been maintained in pure cultures for more than a few days.

The experimental infection of some of the lower animals, by feeding cysts and trophozoites, or inoculating these per rectum, has been repeatedly accomplished, and the infection is followed by symptoms and lesions more or less resembling those seen in human infections. Of the animals so far experimented with, the dog exhibits symptoms and lesions which most resemble those found in man. The dog has been experimentally infected by Lösch (1875), Hlava (1887), Harris (1901), Dale and Dobell (1917) and Faust (1930); the cat by numerous investigators, especially by Marchoux (1899), Craig (1905), Wenyon (1912), Martin (1930), and Meleney and Frye (1932–1933); the monkey by Musgrave (1906), Dobell (1931), Hegner, Johnson and Stabler (1932), and Swartzwelder (1937); the rat by Lynch (1915), Brug (1919), Kessel (1928), Chiang (1925), Tanabe (1934) and others; the guinea pig by Baetjer and Sellards (1914) and Chatton (1918). Amebic abscess of the liver has occurred in kittens and in dogs after experimental infection of the intestine with this ameba.

Natural infections with *Endamoeba histolytica* have been observed in dogs, monkeys, the domestic pig and rats. To just what extent any of these animals act as reservoirs of infection for man is unknown, but it is doubtful if any of them are of much importance in the transmission of human infection.

The *causative relationship of Endamoeba histolytica* to disease in man is now undoubted and there is ample evidence available to prove that this parasite is the cause of ulceration of the intestine with the production of characteristic lesions and the symptoms of a severe type of dysentery in man, and that abscesses of the liver, brain, lung and other organs as well as lesions in the skin, are produced by this parasite. Space forbids the enumeration of the very numerous experiments by scientific observers in all parts of the world which demonstrated many years ago that *Endamoeba histolytica* produced pathologic lesions in experimental animals, and it is sufficient here to review briefly the work of Walker and Sellards (1913), who were able to demonstrate that in human volunteers the feeding of cysts of this ameba produced typical amebic dysentery and that, in some of the volunteers, a "carrier" condition developed unaccompanied by definite symptomatology.

Walker and Sellards experimented upon volunteers, who were prisoners in Bilibid Prison in Manila. Twenty volunteers were fed with material containing cysts of *Endamoeba histolytica*, of whom 18 showed the parasite in their stools in from 1 to 44 days after feeding, the average period after feeding being 9 days. Of these 18 men who became infected, 4 (22.2 per cent) developed typical dysenteric symptoms, the period of incubation, from the time of feeding to the appearance of symptoms, being 20, 57, 87 and 95 days, with an average of 64.8 days. These observers also fed human volunteers material containing the cysts of *Endamoeba coli*, the common nonpathogenic ameba, and while they showed this ameba in their stools at varying periods after feeding, no symptoms of the infection occurred in any case. Walker and Sellards fed cysts from so-called healthy "carriers" of *Endamoeba histolytica* to volunteers, and in all of the men who developed amebic dysentery the cysts fed were from such "carriers," thus proving that the amebae found in symptomless individuals were capable of producing amebic dysentery in other individuals. However, it should be remembered that the absence of symptoms in infection with this parasite does not prove that lesions are also absent from the intestine, for severe ulceration may be present without the occurrence of symptoms. In 1891 Dock demonstrated that this could occur and since his observations Councilman and Lafleur (1891), Musgrave (1910), Bartlett (1917), James (1928) and

Craig (1932) have all described cases in which marked ulceration of the intestine was found at autopsy in patients dying of other conditions than amebiasis and in whom no symptoms of the infection had been noted.

Epidemiology.—The transmission of *Endamoeba histolytica* from man to man depends upon the ingestion of food or drink contaminated with the cysts of this parasite. While motile forms may pass through the stomach unharmed and produce infection, such an occurrence would be almost impossible in nature, as the fecal material would have to be swallowed very soon after passage and contamination of food with freshly passed feces from acute amebic enteritis or dysentery would be practically impossible. Drying kills the motile forms instantly and liquid feces would have to reach food or drink in order for infection to occur from such forms.

As infection occurs through the ingestion of the cysts, the resistance of these forms to various physical and chemical agents is important in the understanding of the epidemiology of the infection. The cyst wall protects the cyst from many injurious agents and for this reason infection with the cysts is possible for a considerable period of time after the passage of feces containing them. It has been found that if the feces are kept in a shady, moist place, at room temperature, the cysts may remain alive for from 9 to 21 days, while if the temperature is lower they may remain alive for as long as 3 months. Stone, in a personal communication, informed the writer that he has kept cysts in cultures for as long as 14 months in the icebox, at 32° F., and they were still viable. In water the cysts may remain alive for from 1 to 5 weeks, at ordinary temperatures, if bacterial contamination is not excessive, but they die out rapidly in badly polluted water. In distilled water they remain alive for 10 to 20 days. The thermal death point of the cysts is about 50° C. (122° F.) and drying kills the cysts almost instantly.

It has been shown that the cysts are quite resistant to various chemicals. Thus they will withstand a 1:2500 dilution of bichloride of mercury for 30 minutes; a 0.5 per cent solution of formalin for 30 minutes; a 1 per cent solution of carbolic acid for 30 minutes, and a 2 per cent solution of potassium permanganate for as long as 3 days. Chlorination of water, as applied to public water supplies, has no effect upon the cysts of *Endamoeba histolytica*, as it has been repeatedly shown that almost 100 times the amount of chlorine usually used in the bacterial purification of water is necessary in order to kill the cysts of this parasite. This is a most important fact to be remembered as many sanitarians and physicians believe that chlorination of water renders it safe so far as the transmission of amebiasis is concerned. Filtration through sand filter beds, or other filter beds used in public water supplies, removes the cysts from the water and thus filtered water is safe as regards transmission of amebiasis. This is also true of domestic filters that remove bacteria from water.

As flies are intimately concerned in the transmission of amebiasis, the length of time that the cysts of *Endamoeba histolytica* remain viable in the intestine of the fly is of practical interest. Thomson and Thomson (1916) were the first to demonstrate that the cysts of this parasite could be found in the droppings of flies, in a viable condition, and in

1917 Wenyon and O'Connor found that they may remain alive in the intestine of the fly for 24 hours and in the feces for at least 16 hours. In 1918 Roubaud demonstrated viable cysts of this ameba in the feces of flies for as long as 48 hours after they had fed upon contaminated material, while Root (1921) found living cysts in the fly's intestine for 49 hours after feeding. Other authorities, as Wenyon and O'Connor (1917), Buxton (1920) and Frye and Meleney (1932), have found cysts of this ameba in flies caught in human habitations.

Cockroaches may also transmit amebiasis as it has been demonstrated by Tejera (1926) and Meleney and Frye (1936) that viable cysts of *Endamoeba histolytica* may be found in the feces of these insects for as long as 48 hours after passage.

The *usual methods of transmission of amebiasis* are through the ingestion of the cysts of *Endamoeba histolytica* in contaminated water; by food contaminated while being handled by "carriers" of the ameba; by the use of human excrement for fertilization purposes; or through the droppings of flies and, probably, cockroaches, that have fed upon material containing the cysts.

The *transmission of amebiasis by water* contaminated with fecal material containing the cysts is of frequent occurrence in rural or other localities where there is no impounded and filtered general water supply, and has been regarded as important ever since amebiasis has been a recognized clinical condition. The experience of the soldiers of the United States Army while campaigning in the Philippine Islands, during the Philippine Insurrection, is an excellent illustration of transmission by water. During this campaign the men drank water from wells and springs throughout the localities covered by active operations, and amebiasis, and especially its serious stage, amebic dysentery, was exceedingly common among our soldiers and one of the principal causes of morbidity and mortality in our army. With the cessation of active military operations, and the return of the troops to posts in which the water supply was carefully controlled, amebiasis and amebic dysentery ceased to be of much importance as a cause of disease. A similar decline in the occurrence of amebic dysentery in Manila was noted after the introduction of a filtered public water supply and this has been true in every locality where amebiasis was common, following the establishment of a properly constructed and guarded water supply.

While water is seldom of great importance in the transmission of amebiasis in towns or cities having a filtered general water supply, it may become contaminated after leaving the point of distribution, as was well illustrated in the extensive epidemic of amebic dysentery originating in certain Chicago hotels, in which a cross-connection between the sewer and the water supply of one of the hotels, and the consequent back siphonage and backing up of the sewage owing to floods, resulted in excessive pollution of the water distributed to the hotels and consequent infection of hundreds of the guests. Thus, improper plumbing of hotels or other public buildings may result in contamination of the local water supply even in otherwise perfectly sanitated towns or cities.

It is unnecessary to stress the danger of the contamination of food or water in localities where human excrement is employed for the fertilization of garden produce. This practice is widespread in many Oriental countries and amebiasis is frequently transmitted in this manner.

The *transmission of amebiasis by food handlers* who are passing cysts of *Endamoeba histolytica* is of frequent occurrence, both in public eating places and in the home. It has been conclusively demonstrated that at least 50 per cent of individuals harboring this ameba continually pass cysts although no definite symptoms of the infection may be noted. Many of these individuals are food handlers and undoubtedly often contaminate the food they handle owing to faulty personal hygiene. Anyone who has watched the preparation of salads, as lettuce and tomato salad, and observed how much the ingredients are handled by the salad makers, can easily understand how such food may be contaminated by the food handler unless proper sanitary precautions are observed, and it is undoubtedly true that transmission of amebiasis frequently occurs in this manner. Likewise, in the home, if the member of the family who prepares the food is infected with *Endamoeba histolytica*, transmission of the infection to other members of the family is liable to occur. The writer has records of several instances in which a cook who was a carrier of this parasite infected other members of the family, and the very frequent occurrence of familial infection confirms this method of infection where the possibility of other methods has been eliminated.

Transmission through the droppings of flies and cockroaches that have fed upon fecal material containing the cysts of this parasite is of importance under certain conditions. In military camps when flies are numerous and fecal material available to them, amebiasis may be thus transmitted and the same is true of civilian camps where large numbers of men are crowded together, as in various commercial projects. Flies and cockroaches may also be of importance in the home as transmitters of amebiasis if they gain access to fecal material. In rural regions, where indiscriminate defecation is permitted in close proximity to the dwelling house, this method of transmission may be responsible for many infections.

The public swimming pool, as a possible source of infection, should also be considered, for although the water in such pools may be chlorinated, the amount of chlorine that can be employed is insufficient to kill the cysts of *Endamoeba histolytica*.

The question of the possible existence of strains of *Endamoeba histolytica* which are nonpathogenic, or of an ameba identical with this parasite in morphology which is a harmless commensal in man, must be considered. Brumpt (1928) described an ameba in man which is identical in morphology with *Endamoeba histolytica* but which is only slightly pathogenic for kittens and produces no symptoms or lesions in man, and his observations have been supported, especially by Simic (1931–1933). These observers believe that this nonpathogenic ameba is usually mistaken for *Endamoeba histolytica* and that it explains the large number of symptomless carriers supposedly infected by the latter organism. On the other hand, English and American students of the subject have been unable to confirm the existence of this harmless counterpart of *Endamoeba histolytica*, which Brumpt named *Entamoeba dispar*, and the consensus of opinion today is that such a species does not exist. On the other hand, there is good evidence available that *Endamoeba histolytica* strains do vary somewhat in virulence, although no strain has yet been found that is nonpathogenic to kittens and dogs, and, presumably, to man. Sellards and Baetjer (1915) were apparently the first to demonstrate that strains of *Endamoeba histolytica* vary in virulence, and Meleney and Frye (1933–1937) have added very valuable evidence demonstrating that certain strains of this parasite vary in their virulence for kittens, although they were unable to find any strain that did not produce lesions in these animals. Faust and Swartzwelder (1935) found that passing a single strain of *Endamoeba histolytica* through 60 dogs resulted in a marked shortening of the period of incubation before dysentery was produced in these animals, and that the severity of the lesions increased with passage, thus demonstrating that it is possible to raise the virulence of a strain by passage through animals.

As regards the relative pathogenicity of strains of this ameba present in symptomless carriers and those suffering from dysentery, there is no evidence that there is any difference and much evidence that there is not. Thus, Kessel (1928), experimenting with kittens, found that practically as large a percentage of the animals became infected with amebae from symptomless carriers as with those from cases of acute amebic dysentery, that the incubation periods were similar, that the average length of life in the two groups did not vary, and that the spontaneous recovery occurred in individual kittens in both groups. His work has been confirmed by others and there is little reason to believe that the amebae from symptomless carriers are less apt to produce serious lesions than those from cases of amebic enteritis or dysentery.

Some authorities have also claimed that certain strains of *Endamoeba histolytica* that produce smaller cysts than the average are less pathogenic, but this question is still undecided. In our own experience, strains that have been employed in our laboratories which produced small cysts were just as virulent to dogs as the strains producing large cysts.

The writer believes that the evidence now available demonstrates that there is no such thing as a nonvirulent strain of *Endamoeba histolytica*, but that there are strains of this ameba which do vary in virulence, and that the virulence of a strain may be raised by rapid passage through suitable animal hosts.

The natural *infection of certain of the lower animals* with *Endamoeba histolytica* has been well established. Kessel (1926), Dobell (1926), Hegner and Chu (1930) and Dobell (1931) have all found this ameba in naturally infected monkeys, and Knowles and Das Gupta (1934) were able to produce severe diarrhea in man by feeding material containing the cysts of *Endamoeba histolytica* obtained from a naturally infected monkey. Kessel in 1928 found pigs in China naturally infected with this ameba and was able to produce dysentery in kittens with the ameba from the pigs. The rat has been found naturally infected with this ameba by Lynch (1915), Chiang (1925), Andrews (1932) and Awakjan (1936), while dogs have been found naturally infected by Faust (1930), Andrews (1932) and Kubo (1936). How important any of these animals may be in the transmission of amebiasis to man remains to be determined.

The *incidence of infection* with *Endamoeba histolytica* varies greatly in different localities, for, while this parasite has a world-wide distribution, it is very common in some localities and absent or rare in others. It may be stated as a fact that wherever it has been carefully searched for it has been found in a certain proportion of the inhabitants of the surveyed locality, but the percentage of infections varies exceedingly and

largely depends upon the sanitary conditions present in various localities.
In the writer's work *Amebiasis and Amebic Dysentery* (1934) there are
given tables containing the results of surveys made for *Endamoeba histolytica* in all parts of the world, but especially in the United States,
and the reader is referred to that work for statistical details, but it may
be stated that, so far as the United States is concerned, surveys have
been made in practically all portions and it has been found to date
that of 67,911 individuals who have been examined, 6869 were found to
be infected with this ameba, or 10.1 per cent.   These results justify the
writer's estimate, published in 1926, that approximately 10 per cent of
the population of the United States were infected with *Endamoeba histolytica*.

While this percentage is a fair estimate of the total incidence of
amebiasis in this country, it should be remembered that the incidence
varies very greatly in different localities, being much higher in the
Southern States than in other parts of the country, and varying considerably in different localities in these states.   For instance, the percentage of infections in Tacoma, Washington, was found by Cresswell
and Wallace to be less than 1 per cent, while in New Orleans, Faust and
Headlee (1936) found the percentage of infection to be 9.8 per cent.
In certain regions in Tennessee, Milam and Meleney (1931) found over
30 per cent of the individuals examined infected, and in 20,237 individuals in this state examined by Meleney, Bishop and Leathers (1932),
2305 (11.4 per cent) were infected with *Endamoeba histolytica*.   These
figures well illustrate how much the incidence of infection with the
parasite varies in different localities, and much more work remains to be
done before we will have reliable statistics regarding the real incidence
of this infection.   It is certainly true that we probably have but little
conception of the amount of sickness caused by this parasite throughout
the world, but we do know enough to demonstrate that it is frequently
the cause of disease and that all infections with it should be promptly
and properly treated.

The *epidemic occurrence* of amebiasis and amebic dysentery is possible if conditions are favorable to the transmission of the infection, although amebic dysentery is usually observed only sporadically.   That
epidemics of amebic dysentery may occur has been abundantly proved,
although some authorities have denied the possibility of the epidemic
spread of this infection.   The writer has frequently called attention to
our experience in the Philippines during the Philippine Insurrection,
where our troops operating in the field repeatedly suffered from epidemics
of amebic dysentery, as proved by bacteriologic and protozoological investigations, but perhaps the most classical example of such an epidemic
is furnished by that originating in Chicago, in 1933, during which more
than 1000 cases of amebic dysentery with more than 60 deaths were
reported within a period of approximately three months.   This epidemic
was remarkable in that it was caused by transmission of the infection by
water in a city having a filtered water supply, and was due to the contamination of the stored water supply of a certain hotel, which had
become contaminated with sewage through cross-connections in the
plumbing between the sewer and the water supply pipes of the hotel.
Under these conditions those infected swallowed many cysts of *Endamoeba histolytica* and the consequent infections were of rapid incubation
and unusual virulence.   The fact that a large proportion of the food

handlers in this hotel were also carriers of the ameba added fuel to the flames, and resulted in the greatest epidemic of amebic dysentery that has ever been studied and recorded. In all, 1050 cases of amebic dysentery have, to date, been traced to this hotel infection, and over 70 deaths have occurred, a mortality of 6.66 per cent.

Hardy and Spector (1935) report a second epidemic of amebiasis in Chicago, in 1934, due to a polluted water supply. This occurred in persons who had drunk known polluted water during a fire in the stockyards in May of that year. An investigation showed that of 300 men in the fire companies who drank this water, 35 suffered from mild diarrhea, 49 from severe and more lasting diarrhea, and 158 had still more severe symptoms, consisting of severe colic and violent diarrhea, while typical amebic dysentery occurred in 6 of the 158 severe cases. *Endamoeba histolytica* was present in the stools in 42.4 per cent of the cases with mild diarrhea, 51.2 per cent of those with moderate diarrhea, and 62.1 per cent of those with severe diarrhea, the total number in each class being 33, 43 and 140 respectively. Of 161 control individuals who had not partaken of the polluted water, 25, or only 15.5 per cent, were positive for *Endamoeba histolytica*. The authors rightly conclude that epidemics of amebiasis and amebic enteritis and dysentery may occur coincidently with epidemics of other water-borne infections, when such conditions are present, for 69 cases of typhoid and 2 of paratyphoid fever also occurred among the individuals drinking this polluted water.

Other observers have recorded epidemics of amebic dysentery caused by a polluted water supply, and it is now well established that infections with *Endamoeba histolytica* may occur in epidemic form if conditions are favorable.

The *general factors* influencing the incidence of amebiasis are climate, race, sex, food and occupation.

Climate has a profound influence upon the incidence and severity of amebiasis. It has long been known that the severe clinical pictures of this infection, as amebic dysentery and amebic abscess of the liver, are much more frequently observed in the tropics and subtropics than in temperate regions. While much of the greater prevalence of such symptoms is undoubtedly due to poorer sanitation in such regions which favor reinfections and larger doses of the infective cysts, it cannot be denied that a hot climate, per se, does favor the occurrence of virulent infections, probably by reducing the resistance of the infected individual. Removal of severely infected individuals from a tropical climate, where they contracted their infection, to a temperate one is invariably followed by great improvement in the clinical symptoms and frequently by complete recovery from such symptoms. The writer has frequently observed soldiers suffering from severe amebic dysentery and carried on board transports at Manila in litters, walk ashore at San Francisco, having recovered from the symptoms of dysentery without any other treatment than proper diet, rest, and change from the humid, hot climate of the Philippines to the cool, bracing temperatures of the ocean voyage, which apparently so increased the patient's resistance as to result in the disappearance of symptoms. While the incidence of amebiasis in the tropics is largely due to insanitary conditions there can be no question that the depressing climate has much to do not only with the severity of the symptoms but with the actual incidence, by greatly reducing the normal resistance of the individual to the infection.

Race is of importance only in that native races living in insanitary surroundings apparently develop some immunity to the effects of the parasite and, perhaps, to actual infection, although the latter has not been proved. The influence of race is shown by the fact that symptomless carriers of *Endamoeba histolytica* are much more frequently encountered in natives living in regions where the infection is widespread, while in the same regions the white population, not native to the region, suffers from severe symptoms and symptomless carriers among them are much less frequently found in such regions. In other words, while the native races are not immune to infection they have developed enough resistance to enable them to escape the severe symptomatology so often seen in the "stranger within the gates." It is certainly true that no race is immune to infection with this parasite, but, as in the malarial infections, natives living in infected localities do develop a resistance to the effects of the infection.

Sex is of some importance in the epidemiology of amebiasis and it is generally stated that infections are less common in females than in males. Thus, Strong (1925) found the ratio of males to females in 217 cases to be 180 males to 37 females, and Tao (1931) found 11.45 per cent of males infected to 8 per cent of females in China, several thousand individuals being included in his survey. On the other hand, Andrews (1934) at Fresnillo, Mexico, examined 525 Mexican females, finding 74 infected (14.1 per cent), while of 1686 males, 218 were infected (12.9 per cent). The writer believes that there is little, if any, difference between males and females as regards susceptibility to infection with *Endamoeba histolytica*, and that the differences that are noted can probably be explained by differences as regards chances of exposure to infection. However, it must be admitted that amebic abscess of the liver is certainly much less common in women than in men, and the reason for this has never been demonstrated.

Food supply is of importance in that an insufficient, or improper, food supply favors infection because of reducing the normal resistance of the individual to the infection. Starvation predisposes to infection by reducing resistance and a long-continued diet deficient in vitamins and minerals also favors infection with this parasite for the same reason. It is also probable that certain food substances, if taken in too-large quantities, or too often, also favor infection and the production of severe symptoms. Thus, Hegner believes that a carbohydrate diet favors infection and the development of symptoms, while the experiments of Faust (1932) and of Faust, Scott and Swartzwelder (1935) have demonstrated unquestionably that certain food substances have a profound effect upon the course of an amebic infection in dogs. This subject has not been investigated as thoroughly as it deserves to be, but enough has been done to indicate that not only the quantity but the kind of food may have a marked effect upon the incidence and development of infection with *Endamoeba histolytica*.

The subject of *immunity in amebiasis* has been touched upon in discussing the racial differences noted in infection with this parasite, and it has been stated that there is no evidence that any race is immune to infection with *Endamoeba histolytica*, and, in fact, there is not sufficient evidence available to demonstrate that real immunity, either natural or acquired, ever occurs. While a certain proportion of the inhabitants of localities where the infection is endemic apparently escape infection, it is impossible to be sure whether such freedom from infection is due to an immunity or to lack of exposure. Certainly there is no evidence that recovery from infection with this parasite confers immunity, for reinfections have been frequently observed within a few weeks after recovery. It has already been stated that natives of endemic localities show a certain amount of tolerance to the infection, as evidenced by the absence of the more severe symptoms, as diarrhea or dysentery, but this tolerance to the infection is not evidence of anything but a partial immunity to the results of infection rather than to infection.

That certain so-called "immune bodies" do develop in the blood of individuals suffering from infection is shown by the presence of complement-fixing bodies in the blood serum of the infected, as demonstrated by the writer and confirmed by many others, as well as precipitins, first shown to be present by Wagener (1924), but that these are real immune bodies remains to be demonstrated.

Pathology.—The pathology of amebiasis varies greatly in different individuals and the lesions are due to the cytolysis of the tissues and, in most instances, to the action of bacteria that may be present. Thus the pathology of amebiasis is usually caused by the combined action of the ameba and bacteria, although the lesions of pure amebic infection are often present and are characteristic. It is impossible to say how much of the pathology of advanced amebic infection of the intestine is due to the ameba alone, as in all cases pathogenic bacteria are invariably present in the lesions and presumably have something to do with the pathologic picture.

The lesions in amebiasis vary with the extent and virulence of the infection, and lesions microscopic in size and involving only the superficial layer of the mucous membrane may be present in the mildest infections, while in the most severe numerous large ulcers, penetrating to the muscular or even the peritoneal coat of the intestine, may be present. Owing to this wide variation in the pathologic lesions encountered in this infection, it is best to describe the pathology as it is observed in symptomless "carriers," in those presenting definite intestinal symptomatology short of actual dysentery, and in those presenting the symptoms of classical amebic dysentery.

PATHOLOGY IN SYMPTOMLESS CARRIERS OF ENDAMOEBA HISTOLYTICA. —The pathology observed in carriers of this ameba is important, for the impression prevails that unless symptoms of the infection are present, lesions are not being produced in the intestine and the infection can be ignored. The pathology in carriers of *Endamoeba histolytica* has been studied by Dock (1891), Musgrave (1910), Bartlett (1917), Craig (1934) and others, and it has been demonstrated that microscopic lesions existed in all the cases studied, and macroscopic lesions in practically all. Thus there is no such thing as a "healthy carrier" of this parasite, if by that term we mean one in whom no lesions are present in the intestine. In most carriers the lesions are undoubtedly minute and heal almost as rapidly as they are produced, but it has been found that in many a considerable amount of ulceration may exist without any symptoms of the infection being noticed by the individual.

The minute lesions consist simply in small areas of cytolysis affecting the superficial layer of the mucous membrane, which, upon proctoscopic examination, are seen as minute areas of inflammation, or as very

small definite ulcers, scrapings from which show numbers of motile
Endamoeba histolytica. In many of these cases pin-point pigmented
areas may be seen which indicate the site of minute healed ulcers. In
still other carriers the characteristic ulcers observed in cases of amebic
dysentery may be present, the morphology of which will be described
in considering the pathology of that symptom-complex of amebiasis.
Bartlett, as the result of his study of the pathology of amebiasis in symptomless carriers, concluded that when symptoms do occur there is already marked ulceration of the intestine and that large ulcers may exist
in the intestine without producing any symptoms whatever, and the
writer is in full accord with his conclusions. It should also be remembered that amebic abscess of the liver may occur in individuals who
have never suffered from amebic enteritis or amebic dysentery, thus
proving that the amebae may be carried in the circulation to the liver
in cases where the intestinal lesions were insufficient in number or severity to cause symptoms.

PATHOLOGY IN INDIVIDUALS HAVING INTESTINAL SYMPTOMS OF MILD
CHARACTER.—In patients suffering from repeated attacks of mild diarrhea alternating with periods of constipation, the pathologic lesions
present are those already described for symptomless carriers, but ulceration is much more marked and the ulcers have the characteristic
morphology observed in cases of amebic dysentery. In many of these
cases numerous ulcers may be present, varying in size from those just
visible to the naked eye to those as large as a dime, the intervening
mucous membrane being normal in appearance.

PATHOLOGY OF AMEBIC DYSENTERY.—The pathology of uncomplicated amebic dysentery is absolutely characteristic and one who has had
even a limited experience in the autopsy room with this and other forms
of dysentery should be able to diagnose the amebic type by a mere inspection of the diseased intestine, so typical are the lesions of this form
of dysentery. While this is true, it should be remembered that sometimes a combined infection with both bacillary and amebic dysentery
may occur, and in such instances the pathology may be very confusing
and one or the other of the infections may be overlooked.

The *location of the lesions* in amebic dysentery, as well as in amebiasis of the intestine in general, is important, and it will always be
found that the oldest and most advanced lesions are found either in the
ileocecal region or the rectum, and frequently in both. Next in frequency are the flexures of the large intestine or any portion of the intestine where stasis has occurred from any reason. In some cases of
amebiasis the lesions are confined to the ileocecal region but in most
cases of amebic dysentery lesions are found elsewhere in the colon, and
especially in the rectum. In some instances, ulcers are found in the
lower portion of the ileum and in the appendix, and invasion of the
latter organ by *Endamoeba histolytica* has been reported by numerous
observers. In 78 fatal cases of amebic dysentery reported by the author (1934), lesions were observed in the ileocecal region, the descending
colon just above the rectum, and in the rectum in 57 cases; in 12 cases
the lesions were distributed throughout the colon but most severe and
numerous in the rectum and ileocecal region; and in 9 cases ulcerations
were found only in the rectum but healed lesions were present just
below the ileocecal valve. Bartlett (quoted by Thomson and Robertson, 1929) in 56 fatal cases of amebic dysentery found lesions through-

out the large intestine in 29; throughout the colon but absent from the rectum in 9; in the descending colon and rectum only, in 6; in the colon only, in 2; in the cecum, ascending colon and sigmoid in 6, and in the cecum and ascending colon in 4. While the rectum is involved in most cases of amebiasis and amebic dysentery, the ulcerations are not infrequently limited to the ileocecal region, especially in patients presenting mild diarrhea or indefinite intestinal symptomatology. Thus, Woolley and Musgrave (1904) in 25 symptomless carriers of *Endamoeba histolytica* found the lesions limited to the cecum and ascending colon in 11 cases, to the descending colon, sigmoid flexure and the rectum in 8 cases, and distributed throughout the large intestine in 6 cases, while Rogers (1922) observed at autopsy no less than 13 cases in which the ulcerations were limited to the cecum in a total of 36 cases of amebiasis.

It is true that the longer an infection with this parasite has lasted, the more general the distribution of the lesions, and that the regions most frequently showing ulceration are the ileocecal region, ascending colon, the sigmoid and the rectum.

The *location of amebic ulceration in the appendix* is of special interest to the clinician, as invasion of this organ frequently causes symptoms of appendicitis. In 1928 James stated that the appendix showed lesions in 33.3 per cent of cases of amebiasis autopsied in Panama, while Bannerji, Chopra and Ray (1936) state that the appendix was found infected in 5 per cent of 475 appendectomies performed in Calcutta. Clark (1925), in a series of 186 autopsies upon patients dying of amebic dysentery in Panama, found amebic ulcers present in the appendix in 76 cases, or over 40 per cent, and perforation of such ulcers had occurred in 9.2 per cent. It is thus evident that the appendix is frequently the seat of amebic ulceration and invasion of this organ probably occurs in the majority of infections that have become well established and have existed for some time.

The *macroscopic appearance of the large intestine* varies with the distribution of the amebic lesions. Usually it is of a grayish-white color externally with brownish areas scattered along the gut, marking the site of ulcerations that have penetrated to the muscular coat of the intestine, and if gangrene has occurred, black areas may be observed externally. Adhesions of the intestine to surrounding structures may be present, and if the infection has persisted for a long time, the intestine is often greatly thickened, due to fibrous scar formation following the healing of ulcerations. In very acute cases the intestine may show no definite pathology externally, even though marked ulceration may be present, or there may be large gangrenous areas visible externally.

When opened, the large intestine presents the lesions that are characteristic of amebic dysentery, lesions varying in size from minute superficial areas of necrosis to ulcers measuring sometimes several centimeters in diameter. The minute, superficial lesions already described as occurring in symptomless carriers are always present as pinhead necrotic areas surrounded by a small area of edema and inflammation, but in amebic dysentery cases numerous much more advanced lesions are present and color the picture of the pathology.

Succeeding the minute lesions just mentioned in order of severity are small nodular elevations of the mucous membrane, situated at the

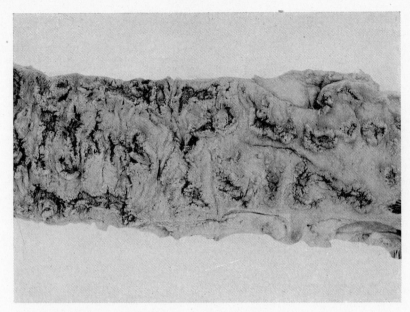

Fig. 1.—Acute Amebic Dysentery. Appearance of Colon in an Acute Amebic Dysentery Case. Note irregular, ragged-appearing ulcers, many of which communicate with one another by sinuses through the mucous and submucous coats of the intestine.

summits of the folds of the mucous membrane, which present a minute opening at their apex from which mucus may be seen to be exuding. Upon incising such nodules it is found that a flask-shaped cavity is opened containing glairy yellowish or bloodstained mucus which, upon examination, is found to consist largely of cytolysed tissue containing numerous motile trophozoites of *Endamoeba histolytica*. These nodular elevations are situated in the mucous and submucous coats of the intestine and are surrounded by a small area of edema but little evidence of inflammation. It is apparent that the amebae have cytolysed the tissues of the intestine, the cytolysis proceeding downward and laterally. When definite ulceration is present the tissues surrounding the minute opening at the apex of the nodule disintegrate and disappear, leaving an ulcer with overhanging edges which extends in a flask-shaped manner beneath the mucous coat of the intestine. At first the floor of the ulcer is formed by the submucous coat of the intestine, but as cytolysis and necrosis proceeds, it may be formed by the muscular or even the peritoneal coat of the gut. These ulcers spread not only downward but laterally, and may communicate one with another beneath or through the mucous or submucous coats by sinuses which are filled with cytolysed tissue and mucus containing many motile amebae, while similar material removed from the floor of the ulcers also shows the presence of motile trophozoites of *Endamoeba histolytica*. In some instances the ulcers, instead of being circular in shape, are elongated, having long, narrow openings, the so-called "buttonhole ulcers." These ulcers and the sinuses extending between ulcerations and beneath the mucous mem-

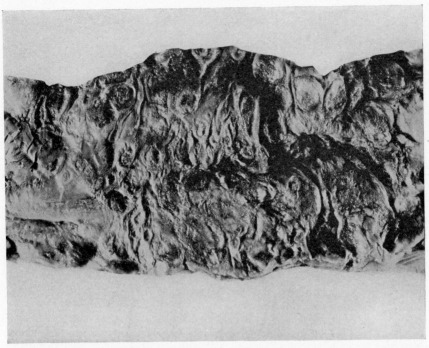

FIG. 2.—CHRONIC AMEBIC DYSENTERY. APPEARANCE OF COLON IN A CASE OF
CHRONIC AMEBIC DYSENTERY. Note active and healed ulcerations and the large
areas of mucous membrane which have been replaced by fibrous scar tissue. (Preparation by Duval. Tulane University.)

brane are characteristic of amebic dysentery, and in the most severe
infections the extension of the ulcers, the undermining of the mucous
and submucous coats, and the occurrence of profound cytolysis and
necrosis results in the entire interior of the affected portions of the
large intestine resembling an old buffalo skin, hence the term frequently
encountered in the older descriptions of the pathology, the "buffalo
skin" appearance of the intestine.

Besides the type of ulceration described above, ulcers may be observed which begin as superficial areas of cytolysis and necrosis and
gradually enlarge and deepen without the occurrence of nodular thickening of the intestinal coat. These ulcers are not so numerous as those
beginning as nodular elevations of the mucous and submucous coats of
the intestine but are quite numerous and always present along with the
more typical type of ulceration.

There is a very great variation in size and extent of amebic ulcers
even in marked cases of amebic dysentery. Minute ulcers just visible
to the naked eye, larger ulcers, round or oval in shape, with rounded or
overhanging edges, and still larger ulcers with irregular, sharply cut,
overhanging edges, sometimes so large as to encircle the intestine, usually
occur together in the average case of amebic dysentery, although dysen-

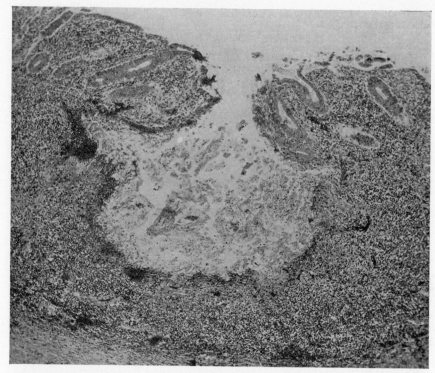

Fig. 3.—Typical Flask-shaped Ulceration of Amebic Dysentery. Section Through the Colon Showing Destruction of Mucous and Submucous Coats and Production of a Flask-shaped Cavity Containing Cytolysed Material and Amebae. (Army Medical Museum Collection.) (From Craig's Amebiasis and Amebic Dysentery, Charles C. Thomas, Springfield, Ill.)

teric symptoms may be present in individuals having few and small ulcerations, so far as can be determined.

As the writer has stated elsewhere (1934), "There are three types of lesions present in amebic dysentery that the writer regards as absolutely diagnostic of the condition: (1) The nodular thickenings situated at the summits of the folds of the mucous membrane which, when incised, are found filled with a viscid gelatinous material containing motile trophozoites of *Endamoeba histolytica*; (2) ulcers having thickened walls and presenting shaggy yellowish-brown edges which are always undermined. These ulcers are often covered in with a necrotic membrane which, on removal, reveals the interior of the ulcer filled with brownish-yellow material or pus, the floor being formed by the submucous or muscular coat. In advanced cases when many of these ulcers are present the interior of the intestine resembles the rough yellowish-brown, shaggy appearance presented by old buffalo skins; (3) the almost invariable presence of sinuses connecting ulcers and situated beneath, or in, the mucous membrane."

In very rare instances the invasion of the coats of the intestine by *Endamoeba histolytica* is followed by the development, especially in the rectum, of granulomatous masses resembling papillomata or small tumors. Such amebic granulomata may be mistaken for malignant disease, but the ameba may be easily demonstrated in scrapings from the small tumors, while typical amebic ulcerations are also present along with these atypical lesions.

In fulminant cases of amebic dysentery, in which death may occur within a few days, the interior of the large intestine may present marked evidences of acute inflammation, much of the mucous membrane being edematous, thickened, and covered with necrotic tissue or mucus, while certain areas are gangrenous and others present the lesions typical of amebic dysentery. It is the writer's belief that practically all such infections are mixed infections with *Endamoeba histolytica* and pathogenic bacteria, especially the dysentery bacilli or streptococci. Such infections, fortunately, are comparatively rare and when they do occur are invariably fatal.

In healing, the smallest ulcerations, just visible to the naked eye, usually leave a minute pigmented area surrounded by a minute amount of fibrous scar tissue. Frequently the only evidence of amebiasis shown by the proctoscope are such tiny pigmented areas interspersed with similar-sized areas of superficial necrosis. Ulcers of larger size, which have involved the mucous and submucous coat, when healed, leave a definite area of scar tissue, while still larger ulcers, involving the muscular coat of the intestine, are evidenced by a large fibrous scar which may cause contraction of the gut and partial obstruction. In cases of chronic amebic dysentery, in which there have been many acute and severe exacerbations, large areas of the mucous and submucous coats of the intestine are found to be replaced by dense scar tissue, and the writer has observed cases at autopsy in which practically all of the coats of the large intestine were so thickened by connective tissue as to cause the gut to resemble a piece of rubber hose, the caliber at the same time being greatly diminished, in some places so much so as to permit only of the passage of a lead pencil.

The *appendix* when invaded by *Endamoeba histolytica* may present little macroscopic evidence of such invasion, or it may be edematous, increased in size, and show more or less evidence of acute inflammation. When there is no secondary bacterial complication there is little or no evidence of inflammation, but after the development of ulceration secondary bacterial infection almost invariably occurs and then the usual pathologic picture of acute appendicitis may be present. The ulcers in the appendix are usually small in size but typical in morphology of amebic ulceration.

The *microscopic pathology* of amebiasis and amebic dysentery is just as characteristic as the macroscopic pathology, the typical findings being the occurrence of numerous amebae lying in nests within cytolysed tissue, and the absence of the round-cell infiltration so characteristic of bacterial infections.

While such round-cell infiltration does occur in many instances, it is always an indication of mixed infection with *Endamoeba histolytica* and pyogenic bacteria, for in a pure amebic infection there is absolutely no round-cell infiltration, the cytolysis of the tissue by the amebae apparently attracting no leukocytes to the involved area.

38111

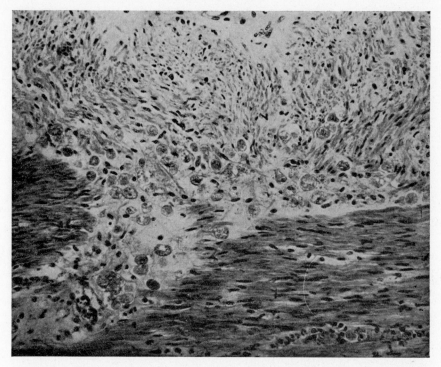

Fig. 4.—Section of Colon Showing Invasion of the Submucosa and the Muscular Coat of the Intestine by *Endamoeba histolytica*. (Preparation by James and Getz, Panama. Army Medical Museum Collection.) (From Craig's Amebiasis and Amebic Dysentery, Charles C. Thomas, Springfield, Ill.)

Cysts of *Endamoeba histolytica* have not been observed in tissues in man, the trophozoites only being found in the lesions. According to the severity of the infection the amebae may be found lying in cytolysed areas in the mucous, submucous, muscular, or even the peritoneal coat. They are frequently present within the glands or in the interglandular tissue, and, if the muscular tissue is involved, may be seen lying in groups within the muscular tissue, surrounded by cytolysed material, or singly between the muscular fibers with little or no evidence of cytolysis. Sometimes the entire muscular coat of the intestine is destroyed in places and hemorrhagic areas may be seen produced by the cytolysis of the capillaries and consequent hemorrhage. Such lesions of the muscular coat may be observed with no evidence that they have resulted from extension of ulcers into the invaded area, and are undoubtedly due to the migration of the amebae from portals of entry in the mucous and submucous coat without the production of ulceration. Thus it is not necessary to have ulcer formation in order for the submucous or muscular coats of the intestine to become involved, a fact generally overlooked in the description of the pathology of amebiasis and one most important from the clinical standpoint, for such involvement may occur in individuals in whom macroscopic lesions cannot be

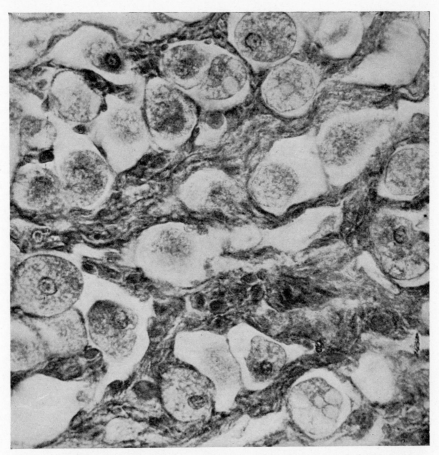

FIG. 5.—*Endamoeba histolytica.* NUMEROUS TROPHOZOITES LYING WITHIN THE SUBMUCOUS COAT OF THE COLON. Note lack of inflammatory reaction in the tissue. (Preparation by James and Getz, Panama. Army Medical Museum Collection.)

demonstrated in the mucous membrane of the large bowel. Ulceration of the intestine begins by invasion and breaking down of the mucous membrane, followed by gradual cytolysis of the submucous and muscular tissue, but amebic abscesses of the coats of the intestine may be present without visible ulceration of the interior of the bowel covering such abscesses.

The amebae multiply within the tissues by binary division. Thus, nests of these parasites are formed and from these nests amebae wander off into the surrounding tissues and form new nests, cytolysis of the invaded tissue occurring with the consequent development of the amebic lesion. In this manner, in some infections, all of the coats of the intestine may become involved and the clinical symptom-complex known as amebic dysentery may be produced, while in others, and the vast

38111

majority, healing takes place rapidly, and the lesions do not become so extensive as to give rise to dysenteric symptoms.

PATHOLOGY OF THE BLOOD IN AMEBIASIS.—While the blood does not present a characteristic picture in amebiasis, certain changes do occur as the result of infection with *Endamoeba histolytica* which are of importance. In *carriers without symptoms* the blood often is normal but many such individuals have a slight degree of anemia, the red blood corpuscles numbering about 4,000,000 per c.mm., the hemoglobin being slightly reduced, while the leukocyte count is normal. In patients having rather severe and repeated attacks of diarrhea there is almost always considerable anemia, the blood count averaging 3,500,000 erythrocytes per c.mm., with a reduction of 20 to 25 points in the hemoglobin reading, and sometimes a slight leukopenia. In acute attacks of dysentery the blood count for erythrocytes may be above normal if bowel movements are numerous and profuse, but usually the count approaches normal, while the hemoglobin reading and leukocyte counts are also about normal, unless the acute dysenteric attack has been preceded by attacks of diarrhea when the blood may show the same changes as already described for such infections. In chronic amebic dysentery there is almost always a considerable degree of anemia, the erythrocyte count averaging slightly over 3,000,000 cells per c.mm., the hemoglobin reading about 60 per cent, and there is a slight increase in the number of neutrophilic leukocytes. In such cases, however, any marked degree of leukocytosis should lead one to investigate very carefully the possibility of the presence of an amebic hepatitis or abscess of the liver. Eosinophilia does not occur in uncomplicated amebic infections.

The pathology of the blood in amebic abscess of the liver will be discussed in the consideration of that subject.

PATHOLOGY OF AMEBIC ABSCESS OF THE LIVER.—The most frequent and important of the complications of intestinal amebiasis is abscess of the liver, usually produced by the organisms reaching the liver through the portal circulation. The gross and microscopic pathology of this lesion is just as characteristic, in most instances, as the gross and microscopic pathology of the intestinal infection, but, despite this, the condition is not infrequently incorrectly diagnosed, even upon the autopsy table. The incidence, predisposing causes and clinical features of this complication are discussed under Complications.

Macroscopically the liver is usually somewhat enlarged but if only a single abscess is present, and that one deeply situated within the organ, enlargement may not be apparent. The abscess may be single or multiple, the most typical picture being that of a large, single abscess situated in the upper portion of the right lobe of the liver, but it should be remembered that multiple abscesses frequently occur and these may be distributed throughout the organ. The excellent analysis of Clark (1925) of 95 cases of amebic liver abscess observed by him, shows that in 55 there were multiple abscesses, and in 24 cases studied by the writer (1934) multiple abscesses occurred in 15 cases. On the other hand, in a series of 73 cases reported by Ochsner and DeBakey (1935) a single abscess was observed in 45, or 61 per cent.

While the most typical location of an amebic abscess of the liver is in the dome of the right lobe, the abscess may be located anywhere within this organ. In the analysis of Clark (1925), referred to above, including

95 cases, 53, or 55.7 per cent, occurred in the right lobe of the liver; 16, or 16.8 per cent, in both the right and left lobes; 15, or 15.7 per cent, in all lobes; and 8, or 8.4 per cent, in the left lobe. In the writer's experience the majority of amebic liver abscesses are limited to the right lobe of the liver, but any portion of the organ may be involved, the smallest number occurring in the left lobe.

Externally the liver usually shows some evidence of hepatitis and fatty degeneration, and the abscess may be visible as a large one situated near the dome of the right lobe, frequently connected by adhesions to the diaphragm, or there may be several visible abscesses scattered over the organ, or no abscess may be visible externally. The cut surface usually shows venous congestion and areas of fatty degeneration, and abscesses may be exposed which were invisible externally. The writer has observed several instances in which the liver appeared practically normal externally but which, when sectioned, showed the presence of one or more typical amebic abscesses internally.

The *macroscopic* appearance of amebic liver abscesses varies greatly with the age of the abscess. The earliest evidence of abscess formation is the occurrence of whitish, oval or circular areas in the substance of the organ, caused by beginning cytolysis of the tissue in such areas. No trace of an abscess wall is visible at this time. Slightly older abscesses are evidenced by similar areas which now have a brownish-yellow color, the beginning of an abscess wall being evidenced by a narrow, white border composed of more or less fibrous tissue. Still older and larger abscesses have a more or less well-defined fibrous outer layer surrounding a mass of cytolysed and necrotic liver tissue, brownish-red in color, while the fully developed abscess has a well-defined wall and is filled with chocolate-colored cytolysed and necrotic material in uncomplicated amebic infections. If secondary bacterial infection is present the abscess wall is thicker and the contents are yellow or greenish in color and many pus cells are present. In uncomplicated amebic infection the interior of the abscess wall frequently presents a ragged appearance due to fibers of uncytolysed connective tissue and frequently bands of such tissue stretch across the abscess cavity, the remains of the connective tissue framework of the liver. In many large abscesses there is no actual abscess cavity, but the entire interior of the abscess is composed of partly cytolysed and necrotic tissue supported by the still partially intact connective tissue in the involved area.

The contents of a fully developed amebic liver abscess, in cases uncomplicated by a secondary bacterial infection, consist of a cholocate-colored, grumous material which microscopically is seen to be composed of cytolysed and necrotic liver cells, partially cytolysed connective tissue, red blood corpuscles and a few leukocytes. The abscess contents usually contain motile trophozoites of *Endamoeba histolytica* but usually few in number, and repeated examination is almost always necessary in order to detect them. If there is a secondary bacterial infection present the abscess contents lose their characteristic features and may consist of yellowish or greenish pus and show the usual morphology of a pyogenic abscess. In such instances amebae will not be found in the contents of the abscess, and the amebic nature of the lesion will be discovered only by sectioning the abscess wall in which the amebae will be found to be present. It has been the writer's experience, as well as that of others, that from 40 to 50 per cent of amebic liver abscesses are complicated by a secondary bacterial infection.

The *microscopic pathology* of amebic liver abscesses varies with the age of the abscess. In the beginning abscess sections usually show a central area of cytolysed liver tissue surrounded by a narrow area of capillary congestion in which trophozoites of *Endamoeba histolytica* are generally present. At first there is no evidence microscopically of an abscess wall but in more advanced abscesses there is a well-defined layer of connective tissue surrounding the cytolysed material, in which trophozoites of the ameba are present. Large, old abscesses, upon section, show a well-marked abscess wall composed of dense connective tissue, the inner side of which is covered with cytolysed and necrotic material, with, here and there, fibrous strands of connective tissue, while most internally occurs the chocolate-colored contents of the abscess, composed as described above. It is often impossible to demonstrate the amebae in the wall of the older abscesses, but they are usually easily demonstrated in the smaller abscesses near the border of the connective tissue zone and in the cytolysed material in the youngest abscesses in which there is little evidence of connective tissue proliferation.

As already stated, the amebae usually reach the liver from the intestine through the portal circulation, but there is evidence supporting the belief that in some instances they reach this organ through the lymphatics or the peritoneal cavity.

THE PATHOLOGY OF AMEBIC ABSCESS OF THE LUNG.—Next to amebic abscess of the liver, abscess of the lung is the most frequent complication of amebiasis and amebic dysentery. The lung abscess is almost always secondary to abscess of the liver, following rupture of the latter through the diaphragm into the lung, although a primary amebic abscess of the lung may occur, the amebae reaching the lung through the blood stream.

The lower right lobe of the lung is usually the site of the abscess and always so if it has been produced by rupture of an amebic abscess of the liver. In such instances the diaphragm is usually adherent to the lung and the base of the abscess is formed by the adherent diaphragm, while in other instances the abscess cavity may involve both the liver and the lung. The contents of the abscess are usually chocolate-colored and consist of degenerated cells, red blood corpuscles, cytolysed material and motile trophozoites of *Endamoeba histolytica*. Usually the abscess cavity communicates with a bronchus and the patient coughs up the characteristic chocolate-colored material from the abscess cavity mixed with the elements of the sputum. In those rare instances in which a primary amebic abscess occurs in the lung, it may be situated in either lung, but usually in the lower or middle lobe of the right lung. If there is no secondary bacterial infection the contents of lung abscesses are similar to those of amebic abscess of the liver, but if secondary bacterial infection is present the abscess may contain yellowish or greenish pus, as in bacterial abscesses in general.

In the great majority of cases amebic abscess of the lung occurs singly, but multiple abscesses are sometimes encountered, and this is very frequently the case when secondary bacterial infection is present. They vary in size but are usually large, as abscess of the lung is not recognized usually until it has become of considerable size. When secondary bacterial infection is present many small abscesses, metastatic in character, are usually present, besides the large amebic abscess originally present.

Microscopically the structure of the abscess wall is similar to that of amebic abscess of the liver, and in the abscess contents, the inner surface of the wall of the abscess, and in the area of newly formed connective tissue surrounding the abscess trophozoites of *Endamoeba histolytica* may be demonstrated.

THE PATHOLOGY OF AMEBIC ABSCESS OF THE BRAIN.—Amebic abscess of the brain is a very rare complication of amebiasis and amebic dysentery and in the cases reported the abscess has been single almost invariably, but has varied in location, although in all cases reported the cerebrum alone has been involved. The abscess usually follows amebic abscess of the liver or lung but may, very rarely, occur primarily in the brain. The invasion of the brain occurs through the blood either from lesions in the intestine or from pre-existing foci in the liver or lung. In the brain, *Endamoeba histolytica* produces cytolysis very rapidly with rapid abscess formation, followed by the death of the patient usually within two weeks.

Macroscopically the involved region of the brain appears edematous and inflamed externally and the abscess wall is thin or may be absent, the abscessed area appearing as a softened, brownish-red, oval or round area, surrounded by a slightly inflamed area. If the abscess wall is developed it is always thin and surrounds a mass of chocolate-colored, cytolysed material, the abscess contents. In all of the cases of amebic abscess of the brain that have been reported in which bacteriologic examinations have been made, the abscesses have been found bacteriologically sterile.

Amebic abscess of the spleen, kidneys, ovaries, testicles and other organs have been reported but are so exceedingly rare as to be of little practical importance.

PATHOLOGY OF AMEBIASIS OF THE SKIN.—Under certain conditions *Endamoeba histolytica* may invade the skin and cause extensive ulcerative lesions. Such invasion is always by direct continuity from some foci of infection, as in the skin surrounding the drainage tract of an amebic liver abscess or extension of the amebic infection from the rectum to the skin surrounding the anus. So far as the writer is aware there have been no instances reported in which there was an invasion of the skin by this parasite through the blood stream.

In cases in which the edge of a drainage wound only is involved, the tissue of the edge is edematous, of a dusky red color, while necrotic areas may be present or actual ulceration may have occurred. Engman and Meleney (1931), who have studied this form of amebiasis very thoroughly, thus describe the usual appearance of the lesions in the skin: ''(1) A rapidly spreading ulcerative process, the activity of which varies in different portions of the margin; (2) a border that presents as a whole an irregular outline as a result of the varying rapidity of the process; (3) an overhanging edge of dying epidermis from under which pus may be expressed; (4) an advancing halo beyond the margin of the ulcer which varies in color from a dusky red through various shades until it merges gradually with the color of the normal skin; (5) pain and extreme tenderness on pressure; (6) the floor of the ulcer composed of indolent granulation tissue covered irregularly with debris and pus.''

Symptomatology.—The symptomatology of amebiasis, as would be inferred from a study of the pathology of this infection, is of protean character, varying all the way from slight, indefinite intestinal irrita-

38111

tion to the severe symptoms of fulminant amebic dysentery, or those
which characterize amebic abscess of the liver or other organs.   There
are no pathognomonic symptoms of intestinal amebiasis and the diagnosis must rest upon the demonstration of the parasite, but certain symptoms do occur in all stages of this infection that are suggestive and, in a
few instances, almost diagnostic.   The popular conception that the symptom-complex, amebic dysentery, is a tropical or subtropical condition
should be abandoned, as typical cases of amebic dysentery occur throughout the temperate zones and are frequently mistaken for bacillary dysentery.   These severe symptoms of intestinal amebiasis are undoubtedly
much more frequently encountered in warm countries and this has given
rise to the erroneous conception of amebic dysentery as a tropical disease.
It should also be remembered that dysentery is but one symptom of
amebiasis and that it occurs only after much ulceration has already taken
place in the intestine.   Contrary to the usual opinion, constipation is
by far a more common symptom of intestinal amebiasis than is diarrhea
or dysentery, especially in temperate regions.

The *period of incubation of amebiasis* varies so greatly that one can
hardly regard this infection as having a distinct period of incubation in
the usual conception of that term.   In speaking of the period of incubation we mean the period elapsing from the time of infection to the
development of symptoms of the infection.   As a matter of fact, one
very seldom can be sure just when an infection with *Endamoeba histolytica* occurred, and the infection may exist so long without any
definite symptomatology that it would be almost impossible, without
experimentally infecting human beings and then carefully guarding their
food supply, to ascertain accurately periods of incubation.   The only
experiments upon man which are on record are those of Walker and
Sellards (1913), in which 20 men were fed material containing the cysts
of this ameba, of whom 18 became parasitized and 4 developed amebic
dysentery.   Of the 4 developing dysentery, the periods elapsing between
the feeding and the occurrence of symptoms of dysentery were 20, 57, 87
and 95 days respectively, although the average period after feeding
before amebae were found in the stools was only 9 days.

Under certain conditions it is possible to arrive at a rough estimate
of the usual period of incubation in intestinal amebiasis.   Thus, in an
epidemic of amebic dysentery that the writer observed at El Paso, Texas
(1916), 100 cases were studied with reference to the period of incubation
before symptoms appeared.   All of these individuals were soldiers coming from northern states and, while a previous infection could not be
eliminated, it is probable that not more than a very small percentage had
such an infection.   It was found that in 30 of these patients symptoms
of dysentery developed within 30 days after reaching the camps at El
Paso; 66, or 66 per cent, within 60 days after arrival; and 90, or 90 per
cent, within 90 days after arrival.   If the number of cysts ingested is
excessive it is probable that the period of incubation is much shortened,
for in the Chicago epidemic incubation periods as short as 4 to 7 days
were observed and the average incubation period is stated by O'Connor
(1934) to have been from 10 to 18 days in the cases that he studied.

The period of incubation, therefore, in intestinal amebiasis is most
variable and would appear to depend upon the number of cysts ingested,
the resistance of the individual and, perhaps, upon the virulence of the
strain of *Endamoeba histolytica*.   At any rate, it is usually impossible to

ascertain accurately the exact period of incubation and this is not, consequently, of as great practical importance in the diagnosis of this infection, as it is in many other diseases. When one remembers that one may be infected with this ameba for months and years without any definite symptomatology being noted, it is unreasonable to speak of a period of incubation of amebiasis.

The symptomatology of intestinal amebiasis varies so greatly that it is best to consider the symptoms that occur during various stages of the infection, and it is believed that for this purpose it is wise to divide the cases into several classes, remembering that the infection is a progressive one and that there may be no very sharp line of demarcation between certain classes.

Individuals infected with *Endamoeba histolytica* may be divided into the following classes: Class 1, the so-called "healthy carriers" or cyst passers, in whom there are no appreciable clinical symptoms; Class 2, those individuals presenting mild and indefinite intestinal and nervous symptomatology; Class 3, those having attacks of severe diarrhea in addition to the symptoms present in Class 2 patients; and Class 4, those actually suffering from acute or chronic amebic dysentery.

SYMPTOMS IN SO-CALLED "HEALTHY CARRIERS" OR CYST PASSERS.—As a rule there are no symptoms noted in this class of individuals and the infection is discovered during surveys for the ameba or accidentally while examining the stools for some other parasite. It is estimated that at least 30 per cent of individuals infected with *Endamoeba histolytica* will be found in this class during any survey for the infection, but while no symptoms may be noted by the infected individual or any evidence of the infection be found except the presence of the ameba in the stools, active symptoms may develop in such individuals at any time, and it is probably true that they all do present symptoms at some time if the infection persists. In fact, the writer has observed several individuals in whom the first definite symptoms of amebiasis consisted of those associated with amebic abscess of the liver, no evidence of the intestinal infection having been noted. It is certainly true that while symptoms may be absent in these so-called "healthy carriers" of *Endamoeba histolytica,* the parasites are continually attacking the mucous membrane of the intestine and some of them are penetrating it and producing lesions, even though such lesions may be microscopic in size, so that, strictly speaking, there can be no such thing as a "healthy carrier" if by that term is meant one in whom no lesions of the infection are being produced.

SYMPTOMS IN CLASS 2 INFECTIONS.—In at least 50 per cent of infections with *Endamoeba histolytica,* the infected individuals present mild symptoms connected with the intestinal tract and the nervous system. Often the symptoms are not noted by the patient but can only be ascertained upon questioning, as they may have existed for so long a time and caused so little discomfort as to be considered a matter of course and of no significance.

The symptoms most commonly observed which are *connected with the intestinal tract* are constipation, abdominal distention and colic, a capricious appetite, nausea and anorexia; while those *connected with the nervous system* are headache, insomnia, somnolence, mental depression and mental sluggishness. In addition, many patients note an irregular action of the heart, an easily accelerated pulse and flushing, attended by sweating of the palms of the hands and the soles of the feet.

Constipation is a very common symptom and may alternate with short periods of diarrhea but, more commonly, the constipation is of a chronic type. It is most important that it be remembered that constipation is much more frequently present in these mild infections with *Endamoeba histolytica* than diarrhea and that an absence of a history of diarrhea is no indication that amebiasis is not present. If diarrhea does occur in these cases it is usually of only a few hours' duration at most and very frequently consists of but one profuse, diarrheal stool accompanied by more or less abdominal colic. Such slight attacks of diarrhea commonly occur at night, the patient being awakened by abdominal colic which is followed by a large stool, free from blood or mucus, but containing numerous motile trophozoites of *Endamoeba histolytica*. Complete relief is experienced after the passage of the stool and an attack may not occur again for weeks or months. In other cases the stools may number from two to four and the diarrhea may persist for a day or two, but such cases belong rather to Class 3 than to Class 2, as regards symptomatology. If the diarrhea persists for a day or two the stools may contain mucus, but blood is absent. In these mild amebic infections indiscretions in diet, or the use of alcohol, may precipitate a diarrheal attack, and the patients usually blame something eaten for the condition, especially as it clears up so promptly, and thus the amebic infection is not suspected.

Abdominal distention and colic are frequent symptoms in this class of cases. The distention usually becomes noticeable shortly after eating and the patients complain of an uncomfortable feeling of fullness in the gastric region, followed an hour or so later by general distention of the abdomen and the passage of considerable gas. Eructations of gas are commonly present and more or less abdominal colic may also occur, although sometimes there is no pain in the abdomen in these mild infections. Usually, however, pain in the abdomen is present and may vary from slight colicky pain in the epigastric region or lower in the abdomen, to attacks of acute pain, frequently simulating that of appendicitis and situated in the region of the appendix. Many of these patients actually have an invasion of the appendix by the amebae and the symptoms are those of a subacute or chronic appendicitis, but the same symptoms may be present when the appendix is not involved. The writer has observed many cases in which a diagnosis of chronic appendicitis had been made and operation decided upon, but in which an examination of the feces, or a complement fixation test, demonstrated an infection with *Endamoeba histolytica*, and proper treatment resulted in the disappearance of the symptoms. The symptoms of cholecystitis may also be closely simulated by amebiasis, and in both suspected appendicitis and cholecystitis a careful examination should be made of the feces before operative procedures are undertaken.

A type of pain that is very common in mild intestinal amebiasis is a dull, aching feeling in either the right iliac region or low down on the left side of the abdomen. Frequently this type of pain is almost constant and, while not severe, is most annoying to the patient, constantly attracting his attention to his intestinal tract and causing much worry and mental depression.

A *capricious appetite* is a common symptom in mild infections and periods of days occur in which the appetite is poor, while other periods occur in which the patient has a voracious appetite. At other times there may be almost complete *anorexia* or slight *nausea* may occur after eating or between meals. *Vomiting* seldom occurs in these mild infections unless it follows some dietary indiscretion.

Among the symptoms connected with the nervous system, *headache* is the most common and varies in character. In most mild amebic infections, if it is present, it consists of a dull boring ache most frequently located over the eyes or the upper frontal portion of the head, although it may be situated at the vertex or be occipital in location. The headache is most frequently noted upon awaking in the morning and disappears toward evening but it may be constant throughout the day. It may occur day after day for weeks or disappear and return at two- or three-day intervals. The headache is always more noticeable and more constant in constipated individuals than in those having daily bowel movements. After cessation of the headache the scalp frequently is hyperesthetic or a heavy feeling persists between the attacks. Many individuals complain of a *poor memory* and *nervous irritability* is frequently a prominent symptom. *Muscle ache* is a common symptom, especially in the muscles of the legs upon awaking in the morning. Usually muscle ache disappears after slight exercise but in many cases the muscles feel sore upon pressure and muscle ache may persist, especially if the muscles of the arms, back or abdomen are involved. It is probable that this muscle ache is a type of mild neuritis produced by the absorption of toxic material through the intestinal lesions produced by the amebae. In fact, all of the nervous symptoms in amebiasis are those common to a low-grade toxemia and are not difficult of explanation if one remembers the pathology of the condition.

Insomnia may be present but is rare in mild infections, but sleepiness is a common symptom. Many patients complain of this symptom occurring during the day, especially after the noon meal, and a dull listless mental condition, accompanied by lack of desire for the daily task, is of common occurrence in mild infections with this ameba. *Mental depression* is also a common symptom and many of these patients become more or less hypochondriacal owing to their abdominal symptomatology and the worry that it causes them.

The *heart* is not infrequently affected, even in mild infections with *Endamoeba histolytica*. A weak heart action is frequent, the pulse being more rapid than normal and of small volume, while arrhythmias are not uncommon and exertion produces palpitation, localized flushing of the skin, and perspiration especially of the palms of the hands. The best study of the heart in infections with *Endamoeba histolytica* has been made by Wilson (1923), who states his belief that the symptoms referable to this organ are caused by the absorption of toxins which act directly upon the cardiac vagus, which results in the organ accelerating upon slight exertion or mental excitement, with the occurrence of palpitation, dyspnea, dizziness and pain.

In this class of amebic infections, and often in carriers without appreciable symptoms, *underweight* is a common finding. It may be confidently stated that in practically every amebic infection there is some loss of weight, but individuals presenting symptoms are often much

38111

underweight and the elimination of the infection almost invariably leads to a gain in weight and a return to normal in this respect. Periods of loss of weight often alternate with periods in which there is a gain, and it will usually be found that the loss-of-weight periods coincide with the presence of definite symptomatology caused by the amebic infection.

In this class of patients there is often considerable *tenderness of the abdomen*, especially in the right inguinal region, at the sigmoid flexure, or low down in the lower right quadrant. It is in these regions that ulceration most often occurs and this probably accounts for the tenderness. *Tenderness over the liver* may be present and indicates amebic hepatitis or abscess formation, and *amebic abscess* of the liver not infrequently occurs in this class of infections. Here, again, it must be stressed that an amebic abscess of the liver may occur in an individual who has never suffered from diarrhea or dysentery.

Fever is rarely noted in mild infections with *Endamoeba histolytica*, although during attacks of diarrhea a mild degree of fever may be present, the temperature usually being between 37.5 and 38° C. (99.5 and 100.4° F.). In some cases an evening temperature of 37.5° C. (99.5° F.) is observed lasting for days or weeks but even this is unusual, and, when it occurs, the question of a possible amebic hepatitis or beginning abscess formation in the liver should be carefully considered. A *subnormal* temperature is very commonly observed in the morning, the temperature varying between 35.5 and 36° C. (95.9 and 96.8° F.), the latter temperature being that commonly noted. During the day the temperature usually rises to normal but in many cases the highest temperature observed during the 24 hours is 36.5° C. (97.7° F.) and this may persist for weeks and months.

SYMPTOMS IN CLASS 3 INFECTIONS.—In this class of infections the patients suffer from repeated attacks of diarrhea which may be severe in character and last for several weeks, or less severe and lasting for only a few days. The general symptomatology in these cases is similar to that already described in Class 2 infections, but usually more pronounced and debilitating. The chief difference between the symptomatology of these infections and those in the preceding class is the occurrence of very definite attacks of diarrhea which may last for several weeks, alternating with periods of constipation. The diarrheal attack usually begins suddenly, frequently at night, but there may be prodromal symptoms characterized by the occurrence of several mushy stools per day before the actual diarrheal attack begins. The diarrhea is accompanied by colicky pains in the abdomen and the number of stools varies between 3 and 10 or more, the feces being semifluid or fluid in consistence and containing much bile and usually a considerable amount of mucus. Blood is absent macroscopically, but microscopically blood corpuscles are often present and motile trophozoites of *Endamoeba histolytica*, some containing red blood corpuscles. Attacks of diarrhea may occur at frequent intervals or may be separated by weeks or months of constipation, or the diarrhea may be continuous for weeks. In the most severe cases a small amount of blood may be present in the stools macroscopically and such infections are really very mild cases of amebic dysentery, the number of bowel movements not exceeding 4 to 6 a day, accompanied by slight tenesmus and the passage of much mucus containing numerous amebae. If untreated, many of the patients belonging in Class 3 will eventually develop the typical picture of amebic dysentery, and severe dysenteric symptoms may develop suddenly and at any time in these individuals.

A mild degree of fever, ranging from 37.5 to 38° C. (99.5 to 100.4° F.), is sometimes observed during the diarrheal attacks, and even higher temperatures have been reported, but it is probable that if much fever is present there is a complication caused by bacterial or coccal infections, and it should be remembered that the bacilli of bacillary dysentery and other organisms causing diarrhea are not infrequently the cause of the diarrhea and that the amebae are simply coexisting organisms in the intestine. If there is continued fever and the blood shows a slight leukocytosis, amebic hepatitis or beginning abscess formation in the liver should be suspected.

SYMPTOMS IN CLASS 4 INFECTIONS (AMEBIC DYSENTERY).—In patients in this class there are definite symptoms which are described in all of our textbooks as those of amebic dysentery, and which have given the name to this type of dysentery. Usually the impression is given by medical writers that amebic dysentery is a disease *sui generis,* but such an impression is absolutely erroneous, as amebic dysentery is simply a part of the clinical picture of amebiasis, and it is often most difficult to classify many patients so far as this symptom-complex is concerned. If we classify all patients who pass small amounts of blood and mucus in their stools as cases of amebic dysentery, then many patients will be so placed who are practically free from any other symptom usually connected with our clinical conception of amebic dysentery, and who are more properly placed in Class 3, while if a more strict rule be applied the question arises as to where we will draw the line between amebic dysentery and the more severe forms of amebic diarrhea. In the following description of the symptomatology of acute amebic dysentery, the writer has included all individuals who pass several bloody stools a day, accompanied by tenesmus and the other symptoms which are connected with what we consider typical acute amebic dysentery, while in the discussion of chronic amebic dysentery is included patients who have suffered from repeated attacks of dysentery characterized by the symptom-complex of acute amebic dysentery. Even so classified, the severity of the symptoms varies greatly, from patients passing a few bloody mucoid stools a day to those presenting the picture of fulminant infection in which very numerous bloody stools are passed and prostration is rapid and severe, death following within a few days after the onset of the dysenteric symptoms.

The *incubation period* of amebic dysentery has already been considered and will not be further discussed, beyond stating that it is very rarely possible to determine the date of infection and hence the period elapsing between that date and the onset of dysenteric symptoms. To the writer, it is foolish to speak of a period of incubation for this symptom-complex because of the impossibility of determining such a period and because it does not mean what the period of incubation does in bacterial, rickettsial and virus diseases.

The onset of dysenteric symptoms in intestinal amebiasis may be sudden or there may have been a history of diarrheal attacks preceding the appearance of blood in the stools and the typical dysenteric symptom-complex. When the onset is sudden, the first symptom noted is abdominal pain which is quickly succeeded by the passage of a semifluid or fluid bloody stool, these symptoms being repeated several times, the stools finally consisting almost entirely of mucus and blood and having a peculiar musty, albuminous odor. *Abdominal pain* may be slight in the milder cases of dysentery or very severe in those in which many stools occur, and is of a cramplike character in most cases. Sometimes quite severe dysentery may be present with little or no abdominal pain but this is rare. Tenderness of the abdominal muscles and, in severe infections, rigidity of these muscles occur, and in fulminant infections there may be so much tenderness and rigidity that peritonitis may be suspected.

The onset may be initiated by a *chill*, or chilly sensations, while fever may be present at the onset and persist during the dysenteric symptoms or may be entirely absent. Temperatures varying between 37.5 and 39° C. (99.5 and 102.2° F.) are not infrequently observed in the more severe cases of amebic dysentery and even higher temperatures are rarely encountered. However, the writer's experience has shown that fever is not so generally present in amebic dysentery as it is in bacillary dysentery, but the general belief that fever never occurs in amebic dysentery is erroneous, as is the statement that if fever is present it must be due to a secondary bacillary infection. While such combined infections undoubtedly occur, fever is not an uncommon symptom in uncomplicated amebic dysentery, during the acute attack. In long-continued chronic amebic dysentery, fever is generally absent during the acute exacerbations and in many such infections there may be a subnormal temperature.

In fulminant infections with *Endamoeba histolytica, prostration* is very rapid due to the excessive number of bowel movements and toxemia. In the usual case there is little prostration for several days and in some cases the patient may be up and about although passing several dysenteric stools a day.

The *number of bowel movements* varies markedly, mild cases averaging from 6 to 8 a day, and in temperate regions many such cases occur and the diagnosis is missed because of the relatively slight character of the symptoms. In more severe attacks the bowel movements vary from 8 to 15 a day, while in the tropics such cases usually have from 15 to 20 movements a day. Fulminant cases may have as many as 40 bowel movements a day, but in such attacks the stool consists of a small amount of bloody mucus. *Tenesmus* is present to some extent in all cases of amebic dysentery but is usually much less marked than in bacillary dysentery. In the more severe infections, especially in fulminant cases, tenesmus is usually very intense and practically constant. Tenesmus is always greater if rectal ulceration has occurred, and if there are no ulcers in the rectum, tenesmus may be so slight as to cause little discomfort to the patient. The greater the number of the bowel movements, the greater the tenesmus even though rectal ulceration be absent. In uncomplicated cases of amebic dysentery the *stool* consists largely of bloodstained mucus and contains no pus. Trophozoites of *Endamoeba histolytica* are always present and can be easily demonstrated. The differential characteristics of amebic and bacillary dysentery stools will be discussed under Diagnosis.

In the vast majority of cases the acute attack of amebic dysentery disappears in a few days, even without treatment, and the patient appears normal except for a loss of weight and strength. *Emaciation* is not marked unless several acute attacks have been experienced. In chronic cases that have suffered from many acute exacerbations, emaciation may be extreme. In severe acute attacks, emaciation may be marked due to the excessive number of bowel movements and the inability to take a proper amount of food.

Loss of appetite, gaseous eructations, distention of the abdomen, headache, muscular aching, insomnia, nervous irritability, mental depression, a rapid, irregular and weak pulse, are all common symptoms during acute amebic dysentery, and in fulminant infections toxic symptoms are very marked. In such infections it is undoubtedly true that many of the symptoms of toxemia are due to a combined infection with the bacilli of dysentery or streptococcus infections.

The duration of an attack of amebic dysentery varies greatly, but it may be stated that in the mildest cases the usual duration of dysenteric symptoms does not exceed a week and sometimes the attack may cease within three or four days. More severe attacks may last for several weeks and in the fulminant cases death may occur within a few days.

SYMPTOMS OF CHRONIC AMEBIC DYSENTERY.—Some authorities recognize a group of cases to which the name of subacute amebic dysentery has been applied. The writer believes this classification to be an unnecessary refinement, as such infections are really milder forms of chronic amebic dysentery, and they will be included in the description of the latter.

Following the primary acute attack of amebic dysentery the symptoms may wholly disappear or may continue in a modified form. Usually the stools become normal in consistence and appearance, the acute symptoms disappear, and constipation may be present or the bowels may move in a normal manner. In other cases a diarrheal condition persists for some time, to be succeeded by another acute attack of dysentery. Whichever condition may be present, it is true that almost invariably, unless the infection is eliminated by treatment, or disappears spontaneously, the primary dysentery attack is succeeded within a variable period by another acute attack, during which the symptoms may be milder, as severe, or more severe, than those of the primary attack, and succeeding attacks of dysentery may occur for months or years. The clinical picture of chronic amebic dysentery is that of repeated acute attacks of dysentery with intervals in which the dysenteric symptoms disappear and the patients enjoy fairly good health, or suffer from the symptoms described in Class 2 and 3 infections.

In the chronic amebic dysentery cases the symptoms usually become less and less severe with each attack, although death may occur at any time, especially if the condition has lasted for many months and the patient is weakened and emaciated. Fever may or may not be present during the acute dysentery attacks, and if present, especially if it persists after the cessation of the attack, is usually caused by an amebic hepatitis or liver abscess. Most individuals suffering from chronic amebic dysentery have a sallow complexion, are more or less emaciated, and complain of the symptoms common in Class 2 and 3 infections. In addition there is always present an anemia which may be severe and lead to profound weakness and disability.

38111

Due to the repeated attacks of dysentery, most patients with a chronic amebic dysentery which has persisted for months become helpless invalids. The invasion of the coats of the large intestine by *Endamoeba histolytica* in these patients has led to extensive ulceration and the healing of many ulcers has caused large areas of the mucous membrane to be replaced by dense fibrous scar tissue, resulting in thickening of the wall of the intestine and lessening of its caliber. The replacement of the normal mucous membrane by scar tissue leads to nonabsorption of fluids and to a condition of chronic diarrhea which persists between the actual dysenteric attacks. Even after the elimination of the amebic infection more or less diarrhea may persist, especially noticeable in hot weather when the fluid intake is greatest, and this often leads patients to believe that the amebic infection has not been eliminated.

Complications and Sequelae.—Amebiasis may be complicated by a number of important conditions and followed by sequelae which are the result of the amebic infection.

Complications.—The most important complications of amebiasis are amebic abscess of the liver, amebic abscess of the lung, amebic abscess of the brain and amebic appendicitis. More rarely amebiasis is complicated by invasion of the skin, perforation of the intestine, intestinal hemorrhage, peritonitis, invasion of the gallbladder or urinary amebiasis. In addition, long-continued amebic infection may be complicated by any acute or chronic disease or by a subacute or chronic nephritis, sometimes a sequela of the amebiasis. Chronic gastritis or enteritis is frequently present as a result, rather than a complication.

Amebic Abscess of the Liver.—The most frequent and most important of the complications of amebiasis is abscess of the liver. It is difficult to ascertain the exact incidence of this complication, for it varies greatly in different localities. It is much more frequently encountered in the tropics and subtropics than in temperate regions, but in the latter many cases are overlooked or wrongly diagnosed, so that it is impossible to estimate the incidence of this complication in temperate countries, as the United States. Again, the incidence as given in works upon the subject is sometimes based upon the number of cases observed at autopsy or upon the number observed at both the autopsy table and diagnosed and operated upon with a successful result. The incidence when based upon autopsy reports will naturally be higher than if based upon the total number of cases of amebiasis observed. Thus, Strong and Musgrave (1900), in the Philippines, found 23 per cent of 100 autopsied cases of amebic dysentery having abscess of the liver, while Clark (1925), in Panama, found 51 per cent of 186 cases of amebic dysentery presenting abscess of the liver. In the writer's experience 33 per cent of cases of amebic dysentery coming to autopsy have shown this complication. If, however, we estimate the incidence of this complication upon the total number of infections with *Endamoeba histolytica* it is at once evident that it must be very small and even if we base the estimate upon the number of cases of amebic dysentery observed it is much smaller than one would at first believe. Thus Tao (1931) found this complication in only 18 of 1000 cases of amebiasis, or 1.8 per cent, his figures being based upon all cases of amebic infection observed, whether with or without symptoms, while Ochsner and DeBakey (1935) in 388 cases of amebic dysentery observed at Charity Hospital, in New Orleans, found amebic abscess of the liver in 59, or 15.2 per cent. The writer in 745 cases of amebic dysentery observed this complication in but 5 per cent of the cases.

Among the *predisposing causes of amebic abscess* of the liver may be mentioned sex, age, exposure and starvation, the use of alcohol, traumatism to the liver, and diet.

Sex is apparently an important predisposing cause as this complication is much less common in females than in males. Strong (1925) states that the statistics of India show that the ratio of males to females is as 7 to 1, and Ochsner and DeBakey (1935), in an analysis of 73 cases of liver abscess, found that 65 were in males and only 8 in females, a ratio of 8 males to 1 female. The reason for this great difference in the occurrence of amebic abscess of the liver in males and females has never been satisfactorily explained.

Age is also a predisposing factor as few instances are on record of this complication occurring in childhood. Rogers (1930), studying almost 400 cases of liver abscess in Calcutta, found that 70 per cent occurred between the ages of 21 to 40 years, 5 per cent below 20 years of age, and 5 per cent after 50 years of age. Only 2 cases in children less than 10 years of age were observed by Rogers, while Ochsner and De-Bakey (1935) found that the average age in 73 cases showing this complication was 44 years, the youngest patient being 8 years of age and the oldest 70 years of age.

Exposure and starvation are predisposing causes in that they reduce the resistance of the indivdual, and if amebae are present in the liver favor their rapid multiplication. The same is true of the use of alcohol and of traumatism to the liver. The writer has observed the development of an amebic liver abscess after traumatism to the liver in individuals who had never suffered from symptoms of amebiasis, but were carriers of *Endamoeba histolytica*.

(*a*) *Relationship of Dysentery to Amebic Liver Abscess*.—The old belief that an amebic abscess of the liver could develop only in those suffering from dysentery must be abandoned, for we now know that this complication may occur in individuals who have never suffered from recognizable symptoms of amebiasis. While it is true that a majority of the patients suffering from this complication have also suffered from attacks of dysentery, it is also true that a very considerable proportion of such patients give no history of such attacks. Thus, Futcher (1903) obtained a history of dysentery in only 5 of 21 cases; Elliott (1915), in only 47 of 116 cases; and Ochsner and DeBakey (1935) in 52 cases found no history of dysentery in 21, or 40.3 per cent. Leiva (1934) reported a case in which there were amebic abscesses in the liver, lung, kidney and brain in a patient chronically constipated and with no history of diarrhea or dysentery; Freund (1934), 3 cases in which amebic abscess of the liver occurred in individuals who had no history of any gastro-intestinal disturbance; while Armitage (1919) reported a carrier without any symptoms or history of symptoms of amebiasis who developed a liver abscess and later an abscess of the brain. The writer has observed this complication in carriers without symptoms and it is now evident that absence of symptoms of intestinal amebiasis does not indicate that an amebic abscess of the liver, or other organs, may not develop.

An amebic abscess of the liver may develop in individuals who have suffered from amebic dysentery months or years before, and in whom the intestinal infection has been eliminated. Durand (1913) has described a case occurring 29 years after the dysenteric attack; Low (1916), one occurring 20 years after, and Mallory reported (1920) one occurring 30 years after an attack of acute amebic dysentery. While such cases may be instances of reinfection and the occurrence of the abscess in individuals without intestinal symptoms, it is true that an abscess of the liver may occur long after the cessation of dysenteric symptoms.

The *absence of Endamoeba histolytica* from the stools is not evidence that an amebic abscess of the liver is not present, for a considerable number of patients having amebic liver abscess have shown negative stool examinations. Thus Chen, vanGorder and Yuan (1931) found no amebae in the stools of 65.9 per cent of their cases of amebic liver abscess, and Ochsner and DeBakey (1935) in 131 cases of amebic abscess of the liver found that the stools were reported negative for amebae in no less than 63.9 per cent. It will thus be seen that a negative stool report should not be taken very seriously if symptoms are present that indicate a liver abscess.

From what has been said it is evident that the period of incubation of a liver abscess cannot be ascertained, as there is no way of knowing when the liver became infected. Amebic abscess of the liver may develop during an acute attack of amebic dysentery or not for months or years afterward and it may develop in individuals who have never suffered from diarrhea or dysentery.

Rupture of the Liver Abscess.—The most common and important of the complications that may attend an amebic abscess of the liver is the rupture of the abscess into surrounding cavities or organs. It is surprising how often this accident occurs and its frequency demonstrates how often liver abscess is undiagnosed in the early stages, as rupture of such an abscess occurs only after it has attained a large size. The frequency of rupture of amebic abscess of the liver and the site of rupture are well shown in the following data:

Waring, in 300 cases of amebic abscess of the liver, found that rupture had occurred in 68, of which 28 had ruptured into the right pleural cavity; 14 into the pericardium; 15 into the right lung; 2 into the colon; 3 into the vena cava; 2 into the kidney; 2 into the lumbar region, and one each into the stomach and the bile ducts. Dutroulau in 66 cases observed rupture of the abscess in 25, of which 10 ruptured into the right pleural cavity; 7 into the right lung; 2 into the pericardium; 1 into the colon; 1 into the stomach, and 4 into the right lumbar region. Clark, in 95 cases of liver abscess, observed rupture in 25, of which 9 ruptured into the greater peritoneal cavity; 5 into the lesser peritoneal cavity; 8 into the diaphragm; 1 into the diaphragm and body wall; 1 into the stomach, and 1 into the vena cava. Ochsner and DeBakey, in 73 cases of amebic liver abscess, found that 14 had ruptured, 7 into the right lung, 1 into the right pleural cavity, and 6 into the peritoneal cavity. The writer in 28 cases observed rupture in 10, 6 into the right pleural cavity, 2 into the pericardium, 1 into the right lung, and 1 into the right kidney.

From these observations it will be seen that rupture of an amebic abscess of the liver is of frequent occurrence and that the rupture is most apt to occur into the pleural cavity, the lung or the pericardium. If rupture occurs into the pleural cavity an empyema follows, while if it is into the lung an amebic abscess of this organ develops. Rupture into the pericardium produces a purulent pericarditis followed by death, while rupture into the peritoneal cavity may be followed by a general peritonitis; although in some cases the contents of the abscess, if bacteriologically sterile, may become walled off and absorption occur, or a lumbar abscess may follow eventually.

The gross and microscopic *pathology* of amebic abscess of the liver has already been considered under Pathology.

Symptoms of Amebic Abscess of the Liver.—Prior to abscess formation in the liver there is a period of variable duration in which the organ is inflamed and tender. This period has been termed by Rogers the "presuppurative" stage of amebic liver abscess and its recognition is most important as proper treatment will prevent abscess formation. Rogers (1935) has well described this condition, which is best termed "amebic hepatitis," and has divided it into two types, an acute and chronic type. In the *acute type* fever and leukocytosis are present and the liver is enlarged and tender. The fever may reach as high as 40° C. (104° F.) but is usually a degree or two lower. It is remittent in type and daily in occurrence, the highest temperature occurring in the evening. It declines toward morning accompanied by profuse perspiration. The leukocytes number between 15,000 and 30,000 per c.mm., the increase being in the neutrophiles. In the *chronic form* of amebic hepatitis the fever is usually only a degree or two above normal, while there may be only a slight leukocytosis present. The duration of the acute type is from two weeks to over a month, while the chronic type may last for several months and may disappear without abscess formation. However, the occurrence of fever and leukocytosis, together with tenderness over the hepatic region, should always be regarded as indicating an amebic hepatitis.

The *symptoms of liver abscess* of amebic origin vary much, and sometimes are so slight that the patient does not consult a physician until the abscess is of considerable size. Usually, however, the symptoms are definite and attract the patient's attention early in the development of the condition. The onset of symptoms may be acute but it is usually gradual, the first symptom noted being *pain and tenderness* over the liver area. The pain is usually of a dull aching or boring type, but may be acute and occur in paroxysms. Usually the pain is in the liver area but may be referred to the right shoulder, right axillary region or to the back. In some cases the first symptom of a liver abscess noted by the patient has been a sudden, stabbing pain in the liver region produced by the rupture of an abscess but this is very unusual. The pain in some cases is referred to the right inguinal region and may very closely simulate that of an acute attack of appendicitis.

Fever usually accompanies the pain, but pain may be present for some time before fever occurs. The fever may occur daily or it may occur for a few days and be succeeded by an apyrexial period. Cases have been observed in which fever apparently did not occur during the development of the abscess, but the writer believes that such cases were probably not carefully checked as to the possible occurrence of fever at some time. The temperature range varies greatly in different cases, but usually is between 38 and 39° C. (100.4 and 102.2° F.), is highest at night, remitting toward morning with marked perspiration, sometimes so profuse as to weaken the patient greatly. The fever is often septic in type and always so if there is a complicating secondary bacterial infection. Continuous temperature curves have been noted in some cases of amebic abscess of the liver, only slight remission occurring during the morning hours.

Leukocytosis is always present in amebic abscess of the liver after the abscess is well developed and a high leukocytosis may be present in the presuppurative stage, or amebic hepatitis, as already noted. The increase in the number of leukocytes is in the neutrophiles and the average number of leukocytes per c.mm. varies in different individuals and in the same individual from day to day. Futcher found that the average leukocyte count in 15 cases of amebic liver abscess was 18,500 per c.mm. and the highest count was 53,000 leukocytes per c.mm. Elliott (1915), in an analysis of 116 cases of amebic abscess of the liver, found that the average count was from 15,000 to 20,000 leukocytes per c.mm. Higher counts than these are sometimes observed and the writer believes that if a secondary bacterial infection is present, the leukocyte count is always higher than in a pure amebic infection of the liver. A high leukocyte count does not always mean the presence of abscess of the liver, as cases of amebic hepatitis may have high counts, but, in conjunction with other symptoms of liver abscess, a marked leukocytosis is of great diagnostic importance. On the other hand, a low leukocyte count does not mean that an abscess of the liver is not present, for large amebic abscesses of this organ have been found in patients with counts as low as 10,000 or 12,000 leukocytes per c.mm.

The *facial appearance* of patients suffering from abscess of the liver is often very suggestive. The *skin* is sallow and there is usually slight jaundice, while the expression is one of weariness and apathy. The *eyes* are lusterless, the *cheeks* sunken, and there is usually considerable *loss of weight*. The *pulse* is weak and may be irregular, there is almost constant *headache,* and *prostration* may be extreme if the abscess has persisted for some time. *Nausea* and *vomiting* may be present and *anorexia* is a common symptom. Many patients suffering from this condition present an appearance very similar to that of malignant disease of the liver and have been so diagnosed, the real condition being discovered upon the autopsy table.

Chronic Amebic Hepatitis.—It is probably a fact that the liver is affected in the majority of cases of amebiasis as the amebae are continually reaching this organ through the portal blood stream, as evidenced by the finding of these organisms in the capillary vessels in sections of the intestine from cases of intestinal amebiasis. In a comparatively few individuals this invasion of the liver is followed by an acute form of hepatitis, the symptoms of which have already been described, and some of these cases eventually develop an abscess of the liver. In addition to this form of hepatitis there occurs a chronic form of the condition which persists for months and even for years and which is rarely recognized by the practitioner as due to *Endamoeba histolytica*. Indeed, in many of these cases the original intestinal infection has disappeared, so that the stools may be negative for the parasite, although amebae may still be present in the liver.

Patients suffering from this condition usually are underweight and have a sallow complexion. They are subject to attacks of so-called ''biliousness'' during which they suffer from nausea, anorexia, vomiting of bile-stained material, and constipation or diarrhea. The tongue is thickly coated with a yellowish fur, and there is frontal or occipital headache and a sense of discomfort or dull aching in the hepatic region, and there may be tenderness over this region. Fever is absent and the blood count is usually normal or there may be a slight leukocytosis, caused by an increase in the neutrophiles. Almost invariably these patients give a history of having suffered from attacks of amebic dysentery and most of them have lived in the tropics or subtropics. Between attacks the health is fairly good and the attacks may occur often or there may be long intervals between them. The amebic origin of this form of hepatitis is demonstrated by the fact that a few injections of emetine hydrochloride will result in its disappearance and a return to health. This form of hepatitis should always be thought of in individuals presenting the symptoms mentioned and who give a history of amebic infection.

Empyema and Abscess of the Lung.—Due to the fact that a considerable proportion of amebic abscesses of the liver rupture into the pleural cavity, *empyema* is a frequent complication of the latter condition. It is frequently undiagnosed and discovered only at autopsy, as there may be no very definite clinical symptoms unless there is a secondary bacterial infection, when the symptomatology will be that of a bacterial empyema.

Abscess of the Lung.—This may be either primary or secondary to rupture of an amebic abscess of the liver into the lung. The *incidence* of abscess of the lung varies considerably as recorded in the literature. Kartulis observed this complication in about 8 to 10 per cent of his cases; Strong in but 1 of 100 cases of amebic dysentery; while Futcher observed it in 9 of 119 cases of dysentery. The incidence is much higher when abscess of the lung occurs as a complication of amebic abscess of the liver. Thus, in 95 cases of amebic abscess of the liver admitted to Charity Hospital and the Touro Infirmary in New Orleans, and reported by Ochsner and DeBakey (1936), 15 (15.7 per cent) were complicated by pleuropulmonary extension; in 7 the liver abscess perforated into the lung, in 5 into the pleural cavity, and in 3 there existed a bronchopleural fistula.

A *primary amebic abscess of the lung* is very rare and is caused by invasion of the organ through the blood stream. The writer has observed but one case of primary abscess of the lung and in this case the diagnosis of pulmonary tuberculosis was made by the attending physician despite the absence of tubercle bacilli from the sputum, the amebae that were present being mistaken for epithelial cells.

The symptoms of primary abscess of the lung are similar to those of abscess of the liver and closely simulate those of pulmonary tuberculosis. Fever, pain in the affected lung, chills and a hacking cough are present, and there is expectoration of a more or less chocolate-colored sputum which contains motile trophozoites of *Endamoeba histolytica*. The symptoms mentioned develop gradually and become more pronounced with the development of the abscess. The *physical signs* are dullness over the affected area, diminished breath sounds, and, if the abscess is of some age, coarse or bubbling râles over that area. There is gradual loss of weight, the patient has a sallow skin, anorexia and nausea may be present, while a secondary anemia may occur. In some cases spontaneous recovery occurs, the abscess emptying itself eventually through a bronchus.

The symptoms of a *lung abscess due to rupture of a liver abscess into the lung* are similar to those occurring in a primary abscess of the lung but are often of sudden onset, rather than gradual as in the latter condition. This condition can occur only when there are adhesions between the tissues overlying the liver abscess and the lung, the rupture actually occurring through the diaphragm and pleura directly into the lung. In rare instances the patient may notice a severe pain in the affected area at the time of rupture but usually there is no history of such pain. Pleurisy may be present and an empyema may complicate the clinical picture in those instances in which the liver abscess has also ruptured into the pleura. The symptomatology may thus be the combined symptomatology of amebic abscess of the liver, the lung, and amebic or bacterial empyema. A cough always develops, either suddenly or gradually, and the sputum is of a brownish-yellow or chocolate color and contains motile trophozoites of *Endamoeba histolytica*. The sputum may also contain Charcot-Leyden crystals, and red blood corpuscles and elastic fibers are usually present. Fever, chills and sweating are common symptoms of a lung abscess and often lead to a diagnosis of pulmonary tuberculosis. The blood usually shows a leukocytosis, the leukocyte count varying between 16,000 and 25,000, with an increase in the neutrophiles and sometimes a slight increase in the eosinophiles.

Amebic Abscess of the Brain.—This complication is a very rare one and the writer has never observed a case. A search of the literature has resulted in finding records of 53 cases in which the diagnosis was justified. The *pathology* of this condition has already been considered and the *symptomatology* has varied greatly, depending upon the location of the abscess in the brain. Usually the location is in the cerebrum, only one case being reported in the cerebellum, and the symptoms have been those usually associated with abscess of the brain caused by bacteria. Thus, convulsions, nausea and vomiting, epileptiform seizures, severe headache, hallucinations, mania and localizing symptoms have been observed. The cerebrospinal fluid appeared normal and fever was usually absent, unless the abscess ruptured into the ventricle when fever developed rapidly. The amebae reach the brain through the blood stream and there has been almost invariably a history of an amebic abscess of the liver or this condition has existed at the time of the development of the abscess in the brain. Amebic abscess of the brain terminates fatally within a short time, death occurring usually in from one to two weeks.

Amebiasis of the Skin.—Invasion of the skin by *Endamoeba histolytica* sometimes occurs, usually as the result of the invasion of the tissues by the amebae in operation wounds upon amebic liver or lung abscesses, or in the region of the anus in cases of amebic dysentery. There are many reports in the literature upon this complication, and Engman and Meleney (1931) have reviewed the literature and reported additional cases. The pathology of this complication has been described. The most common symptoms are tenderness and pain in the ulcerated region, with chills, fever, headache and general malaise in most of the cases reported. Usually the invasion of the skin follows operative procedures for intestinal amebiasis or liver abscess, but primary amebic infection of the skin has been reported rarely, and Crawford (1933) has reported a case in which amebic ulceration of both buttocks followed an amebic abscess of the perineum.

Intestinal Hemorrhage.—In every case of amebic dysentery there is some hemorrhage from the intestine, the stools containing bloodstained mucus and, more rarely, clotted or fresh blood, but severe intestinal hemorrhage is fortunately of rare occurrence, although one would expect to encounter it more frequently in patients who have numerous and large amebic ulcers in the intestine. Fatal hemorrhages have been reported by some observers and repeated attacks of severe hemorrhage by others, but the writer has never observed a case in which death was due to hemorrhage or in which the hemorrhage was severe enough to call for transfusion. However, such cases have been reported and it should be recognized that severe and even fatal hemorrhages may complicate intestinal amebiasis.

Perforation of the Intestine.—This serious, and usually fatal, complication of intestinal amebiasis is comparatively rare, although it has frequently been the cause of death in patients suffering from amebic dysentery. The writer has found this complication present at autopsy in a considerable proportion of fatal cases of amebic dysentery and generally as an unrecognized condition by the attending physician. Perforation is usually followed by peritonitis but sometimes the area in which the perforation has occurred has been walled off by adhesions and a localized abscess results which later may rupture into the peritoneal cavity. Pericolic and pericecal abscesses may follow perforation and the perforation may occur in any part of the affected intestine, but usually the perforating ulcer has been situated in the cecum, sigmoid or rectum. Perforation of an ulcer situated in the appendix sometimes occurs, followed by symptoms of appendicitis, and such cases are generally considered as of bacterial origin and the amebic infection is not suspected by the surgeon.

Amebic Appendicitis.—The invasion of the appendix by *Endamoeba histolytica* is not infrequent and such invasion may be followed by the symptoms of an acute or chronic appendicitis or there may be no symptoms present, the condition being discovered at autopsy. There are two forms of appendicitis which are caused by invasion of the appendix by this parasite, an acute and chronic form, the latter being by far the most common. The pathology of amebic appendicitis has already been considered and it will be remembered that lesions may be present varying all the way from those just visible to the naked eye to ulcers of considerable size which may even perforate the organ.

The *incidence* of involvement of the appendix in amebiasis is undoubtedly much greater than statistics would indicate as many cases are overlooked, especially in individuals who have had no history of diarrhea or dysentery, and because often the symptoms disappear following healing of the lesions or are overshadowed by others connected with the intestinal infection.

In the *acute form* of amebic appendicitis the symptoms are like those associated with a bacterial appendicitis and in this type there is probably often a mixed infection with some pyogenic bacterium. The onset may be sudden with severe pain in the region of the appendix, fever, nausea and vomiting, and a marked leukocytosis. This acute form of amebic appendicitis may be the first intimation that the patient has of the infection, but, more often, acute symptoms suddenly develop in the

38111

chronic type of amebic appendicitis, following several attacks in which the symptoms have been less severe.

In the *chronic form* of amebic appendicitis the symptoms are similar to those occurring in chronic forms of bacterial appendicitis. There are recurring attacks of dull pain in the appendicular region accompanied by slight tenderness and rigidity of the muscles, together with anorexia or slight nausea. The attacks of pain may occur at irregular intervals and last but for a short time, or there may be a constant feeling of discomfort in the right iliac region with recurring attacks of pain. The pain may be colicky in character and quite severe, such attacks lasting for but a few moments or persisting for hours. There may be intervals of days or weeks between the attacks, during which time the patient feels well, but usually there are other intestinal symptoms present due to the amebic infection. Constipation is the most frequent bowel condition in this chronic form of amebic appendicitis, but diarrhea may be present at irregular intervals in some cases. The writer has observed scores of cases in which the surgeon had diagnosed chronic appendicitis and an operation was about to be done, when stool examinations and a positive complement fixation test demonstrated the presence of *Endamoeba histolytica,* and proper treatment was followed by complete recovery. *Except in emergencies the writer believes that a careful examination of the stools for this parasite should be made in every case of appendicitis before resort to operation.*

It should be remembered that symptoms simulating appendicitis may often occur in patients suffering from intestinal amebiasis without the appendix being involved, but in many cases the symptoms are due to actual invasion of the appendix by the parasite.

Peritonitis.—This complication may follow the perforation of an ulcer of the intestine into the peritoneal cavity or the rupture of a liver abscess into that cavity. Areas of local peritonitis are usually observed at autopsy in old chronic cases of amebiasis, the coils of the intestine being adherent in the involved areas and covered with fibrin or old adhesions may be present, due to preceding local area of peritonitis. A fatal result usually follows a general peritonitis of amebic origin.

Amebiasis of the Gallbladder.—Rarely the gallbladder may be invaded by *Endamoeba histolytica* with symptoms simulating those of chronic cholecystitis. Nichols (1922) has described a case in a carrier of this parasite, in which the gallbladder was enlarged and, upon removal, was found to contain purulent material in which many motile trophozoites were found and sections of the wall of the organ also contained amebae. Smithies (1928) reported 12 cases in which this ameba was found in drainage from the gallbladder and 4 in which it was found in the contents of the bladder removed at operation. Such observations demonstrate that *Endamoeba histolytica* may invade the gallbladder, but that, as Smithies suggested, the gallbladder acts as a source of infection for the intestine, or that the gallbladder is the source of the amebae found in the intestine in symptomless carriers, is certainly not supported by any evidence of value.

Urinary Amebiasis.—There are few records of real value which demonstrate that this species of ameba invades the urinary bladder. Baelz (1883), Fischer (1914) and Walton have each reported one case in which this parasite was found in the urine and in which the bladder may have been infected, and the writer saw a case in which the ameba occurred in the urine, reaching the bladder through a fistula between the intestine and the bladder. In the cases reported it is probable that the urinary infection followed that in the intestine, although infection of the bladder might result from a primary amebic abscess of the kidney, if such ever occurs.

Other Complications.—In an infection which persists for as long as does infection with *Endamoeba histolytica* it is evident that any disease occurring during such persistence might be regarded as a complication, but there are some conditions so frequently encountered with this infection that they deserve consideration as real complications. Chronic gastritis and chronic enteritis are very frequently observed and, in long-continued cases of chronic amebic dysentery, a bronchopneumonia or lobar pneumonia may develop during an acute exacerbation or between the attacks of dysentery, and lead to a fatal issue. A form of chronic nephritis may also develop in patients suffering from chronic amebic dysentery, and acute nephritis may also occur. Myocarditis may complicate amebiasis but there is no proof that it is the result of amebic infection. Cirrhosis of the liver has been reported as a complication of chronic amebic dysentery, and pyelonephritis has also been found as a complication in a few recorded cases. Amebic abscesses of the kidney, spleen, ovaries, pancreas and testicles have also been reported but so very rarely as to be "medical curiosities." Gastric and duodenal ulcer sometimes complicate intestinal amebiasis and the latter infection is usually overlooked in such cases because of the more typical symptomatology of the former. The same is true of cholecystitis, which is not an infrequent complication.

SEQUELAE.—Whether any sequelae result in the long-continued mild infections with *Endamoeba histolytica* is unknown, all the sequelae that have been noted having followed acute or chronic amebic dysentery, usually the chronic form. In very severe acute amebic dysentery the extensive destruction of the mucous membrane of the intestine may result in fibrous scar tissue causing contractures, or adhesions may form which may cause kinks in the intestine, and favor obstruction. Such sequelae, however, are much more frequently found in patients who have suffered from repeated attacks of dysentery. It has already been stated that in such patients a frequent sequela is the occurrence of a chronic diarrhea due to the replacement of the normal mucous membrane of the intestine by scar tissue, and the consequent inability of the individual to absorb fluid, so that a diarrheal condition persists which is especially apt to be severe in hot weather when the fluid intake is increased. In such individuals a condition simulating sprue may occur, the stools being semi-fluid in consistence, very light yellow in color, large in amount and containing much gas. The tongue may become sore, thus leading to a diagnosis of probable sprue in its early stages. Many such cases have been observed by the writer and most of them have proved to be sequelae of chronic amebic dysentery.

Contracture of the intestine, due to scar formation, may be a sequela and adhesions are frequently found following long-continued amebic infection. Obstruction of the intestine may result from such contractures or adhesions, usually incomplete, but complete obstruction may be a sequela.

In long-continued amebic infections, in which there have been many acute attacks of diarrhea or dysentery, a severe secondary anemia may occur as a sequela. Myocarditis has been reported as a sequela, as well as chronic nephritis.

Diagnosis of Amebiasis.—The demonstration of *Endamoeba histolytica* in the exudates, feces or tissues of the suspected individual is essential for the diagnosis of amebiasis. While, in the most typical cases of acute amebic dysentery, or the acute exacerbations in chronic cases, a clinical diagnosis might be made with some degree of accuracy, it should not be accepted unless the parasite has been demonstrated in the stools, and in the vast majority of cases of amebiasis the symptoms are either so indefinite or so lacking in specificity that little reliance can be placed upon them in diagnosis. However, certain clinical conditions do occur which are very apt to be confused with various types of amebiasis and should be considered.

DIFFERENTIAL DIAGNOSIS OF AMEBIASIS.—Among the conditions that are most apt to be confused with that phase of amebiasis known as amebic dysentery are other forms of dysentery, i.e., balantidial, schistosomal and bacillary dysentery.

Balantidial Dysentery.—The form of dysentery caused by the invasion of the large intestine of man by the ciliate organism, *Balantidium coli*, resembles amebic dysentery in its symptomatology and cannot be distinguished except by the demonstration of the ciliate in the stools or, after death, in sections of the intestine.

Schistosomal Dysentery.—In infections with the flukes, *Schistosoma mansoni* and *Schistosoma japonicum,* a dysenteric condition is present in which the intestinal symptomatology is indistinguishable in many cases from that of amebic dysentery. However, infection with *Schistosoma mansoni* is accompanied by general symptoms that serve to distinguish it from amebiasis, as urticaria, fever and chills, which occur for a considerable period before the appearance of dysentery and are caused by the migration and growth of the worms, while there is usually enlargement of the liver and spleen and the occurrence in the rectum of papillomatous growths and sinuses leading into the adjacent tissues. In *Schistosoma japonicum* infections the dysentery is usually indistinguishable from that caused by *Endamoeba histolytica* and cannot be distinguished clinically.

Bacillary Dysenteries.—The most common and most important infections with which amebiasis is often confused are the various types of bacillary dysentery. Amebic dysentery and many cases of bacillary dysentery are clinically indistinguishable, contrary to the general opinion that marked clinical differences exist between them. The bacillary dysenteries differ greatly in symptomatology, according to the organism which causes these infections, and while it may be possible in rare instances to differentiate bacillary dysenteries upon clinical symptoms alone, the writer has observed so many mistaken diagnoses when this has been attempted that he believes *a clinical diagnosis of either bacillary or amebic dysentery, based entirely upon symptomatology, is usually worthless.* There are so many cases of bacillary dysentery that present the symptomatology of amebic dysentery, and vice versa, that the only manner in which they can be differentiated is by the demonstration of *Endamoeba histolytica* or one of the dysentery bacilli in the stools, or by serologic reactions as agglutination in bacillary dysentery and complement fixation in amebic dysentery. While this is true it is well to remember that certain symptoms do occur in these types of dysentery that are most suggestive and these will now be considered.

In bacillary dysentery the onset is usually sudden, while in amebic dysentery there is usually a history of attacks of intestinal irritation or diarrhea for some time before the dysenteric attack. However, when the infective dose of the cysts of *Endamoeba histolytica* has been excessive, as in the Chicago epidemic of amebic dysentery, the onset of this form may be very sudden and accompanied by chills and fever. Fever is much more common in bacillary dysentery than in amebic, but many cases of the latter have fever, contrary to the usual belief. Arthritic symptoms are more common in bacillary dysentery and tenesmus is more marked as a rule. Relapses are much more common in the amebic form than in bacillary dysentery, and prostration is usually more severe in the bacillary dysenteries caused by the Shiga and Flexner organisms than it is in amebic dysentery. The period of incubation in amebic dysentery is unknown in the vast majority of cases but is usually less than a week in the bacillary forms. Bacillary dysenteries are essentially epidemic while amebic dysentery is endemic, but exceptions to this rule have occurred. Liver abscess is not a complication of bacillary dysenteries but is characteristic of a small proportion of cases of amebic dysentery.

The types of bacillary dysentery occurring in this country very commonly simulate amebic dysentery in their symptomatology, and while many such cases have been incorrectly diagnosed as amebic in origin, the writer believes that much more frequently attacks of amebic dysentery have been diagnosed as bacillary, where no bacteriologic or microscopic examination of the stools has been made. In his experience, no less than one third of the dysentery cases he has observed, in which the diagnosis of bacillary dysentery had been previously made, were later shown to be of amebic origin, and this common error in diagnosis is largely responsible for the idea which is prevalent in the medical profession that amebic dysentery does not occur in this country, or is a medical curiosity. This mistake in diagnosis is especially liable to occur in those so-called bacillary dysentery infections in which relapses have occurred, as such infections have almost invariably proved to be amebic in origin in the writer's experience.

Chronic Ulcerative Colitis.—In many instances the diagnosis of chronic ulcerative colitis has been made in cases of amebic colitis, and vice versa, for the reason that the symptomatology of these two conditions is so frequently indistinguishable. Not infrequently the diagnosis of ulcerative colitis is based entirely upon the appearance of the ulcerations through the proctoscope, no effort being made to make a bacteriologic or protozoological diagnosis of the cause of the ulceration. This method of diagnosis is based upon the assertion of certain gastrointestinal specialists that the ulcers of ulcerative colitis are morphologically so characteristic that they can be easily distinguished from amebic ulcerations. This is not true, for the writer has not infrequently observed cases in which a proctoscopic diagnosis had been made of ulcerative colitis based upon the appearance of the ulcers present which proved to be amebic, the organism being found in material removed from the ulcers. In long-standing cases of either condition the symptoms and proctoscopic findings are indistinguishable, and while in chronic ulcerative colitis the ulcers are usually more superficial and of more general distribution, as well as more uniform in size, than those caused by *Endamoeba histolytica,* so many variations occur that a diagnosis based upon the type of ulcer present is not reliable in many cases. In the more acute cases of ulcerative colitis the general inflammatory appearance of the mucous membrane between the ulcers is most suggestive and it is in this type of case that the proctoscopic diagnosis is most apt to be correct, but even in these cases a careful search should be made for *Endamoeba histolytica* before the possible amebic origin of the condition is eliminated. It should also be remembered that patients with chronic ulcerative colitis may also have an amebic infection and the discovery and treatment of the latter condition very frequently greatly benefits the colitis. In fact, it has been suggested by Kieffer and others that a primary amebic infection of the intestine may precede the chronic ulcerative colitis, certain bacteria finding their way into the amebic lesions with resulting production of the colitis.

Chronic Mucous Colitis.—Many cases of chronic mucous colitis have been diagnosed as amebic colitis, and amebic colitis has sometimes been diagnosed as mucous colitis. The general symptoms of chronic mucous colitis may be like those of an amebic colitis, but the passage of long strings, shreds, or casts composed of mucus does not occur in amebic colitis unless there is a complicating mucous colitis. Both conditions may coexist, so that in every case an examination should be made for *Endamoeba histolytica.*

DIAGNOSIS OF AMEBIC HEPATITIS AND OF AMEBIC ABSCESS OF THE LIVER.—It has already been stated that amebic abscess of the liver is frequently overlooked and only discovered at the autopsy table. In this country this is due quite largely to the impression in the profession that this type of abscess does not occur in temperate, but only in tropical regions. The resemblance of the symptoms of amebic hepatitis to those which accompany any inflammatory condition of the liver, and the fact that an amebic abscess of the liver may occur in individuals who have had no history of dysentery, also lead the practicing physician astray unless he is well acquainted with the subject and is upon the lookout for such conditions.

The occurrence of a daily rise of temperature, a leukocytosis, and tenderness in the liver area in any individual showing *Endamoeba histolytica* in the stools indicates an amebic hepatitis and probable beginning abscess formation, while an increase in the temperature, accompanied by chills and sweating, an increase in the number of leukocytes, and definite pain in the liver area are almost conclusive of the presence of a liver abscess in such patients. Cholecystitis may cause the same symptoms and must be excluded if possible, and the differential diagnosis may be very difficult unless the roentgen ray shows the presence of an abscess. The absence of *Endamoeba histolytica* from the stools does not negative the presence of an amebic abscess of the liver, for the liver abscess may develop after the intestinal infection has spontaneously disappeared or been eliminated by proper treatment. In all suspected cases of amebic liver abscess a complement fixation test for amebasis should be made, if possible, as this test gives a four-plus reaction in most cases, in the writer's experience.

The physical signs in amebic abscess of the liver have already been considered, but the fact that such abscesses are frequently single and located in the upper portion of the right lobe of the organ, is often of great assistance in the diagnosis and a roentgenogram showing bulging of the upper border of the liver is often diagnostic. If the abscess is deep seated the diagnosis is most difficult and can be made only by the most careful consideration of the history, symptoms, the coexistence or not of an intestinal amebiasis, and as a last resort, the result of treatment with emetine hydrochloride. As the writer has said elsewhere (*Amebiasis and Amebic Dysentery*, p. 177), "A small treatise could be written upon the distinction of amebic liver abscess from syphilis, tuberculosis, or tumors of that organ; from gall stones, catarrhal and suppurative cholangitis and pyemic abscesses of the liver; from hepatic coccidiosis, hydatids, schistosome infections, kala-azar and enteric fever; and from numerous other conditions that will suggest themselves to the clinician. A careful survey of the entire situation, including the clinical history, the symptomatology and physical signs, and recourse to the laboratory aids available in the differentiation of each of the conditions mentioned, should result in a correct diagnosis."

In patients presenting symptoms or signs suggesting a liver abscess, the most careful examination should be made of the stools for *Endamoeba histolytica.*

DIAGNOSIS OF AMEBIC ABSCESS OF THE LUNG.—The differential diagnosis of an amebic abscess of the lung must be based upon the demonstration of *Endamoeba histolytica* in the sputum, as the symptoms and physical signs may be indistinguishable from those of tuberculosis with cavity formation, pyemic abscesses, tumors or parasitic infections. If a brownish expectoration is present the condition may be suspected, and if amebic in origin motile amebae will be found in the sputum. The sudden development of a cough and pain in the chest, with the expectoration of much anchovy-sauce-like sputum, usually indicates the rupture into the lung of an amebic abscess of the liver, and motile amebae will be found in the expectorated material. A primary amebic abscess of the lung is impossible to differentiate clinically and the diagnosis must rest upon the finding of the amebae in the sputum. As the vast majority of lung abscesses due to *Endamoeba histolytica* are secondary to amebic abscess of the liver, the presence of such an abscess is of great value in the interpretation of symptoms and signs occurring in the lung.

DIAGNOSIS OF AMEBIC ABSCESS OF THE BRAIN.—The clinical diagnosis of an amebic abscess of the brain, without the aid of laboratory methods, is impossible, as the symptoms and signs are not different from those present in abscesses of other causation. Fortunately, amebic abscess of the brain is a very rare complication of amebiasis, and almost invariably occurs in individuals having an amebic abscess of the liver, so that the presence of such an abscess is of value in determining the character of the lesion in the brain.

DIAGNOSIS OF CUTANEOUS AMEBIASIS.—While there may be some clinical features that suggest cutaneous amebiasis, the diagnosis must rest upon the demonstration of the trophozoites of *Endamoeba histolytica* in the involved tissues. Ulcerative or suppurative lesions developing at the edge of a drainage wound following operation upon an amebic abscess of the liver are most suspicious and the same is true of such lesions around the anus in amebiasis of the rectum. A careful examination of material obtained from such lesions usually will show the presence of the ameba and the diagnosis will thus be established.

USE OF THE ROENTGEN RAY IN THE DIAGNOSIS OF INTESTINAL AME-BIASIS.—Some authorities believe that characteristic changes which are rendered visible by the x-ray occur in the intestine in infections with *Endamoeba histolytica*. Vallarino (1925), Smithies (1926), Ikeda (1934) and Bell (1936) have all described such changes and regard the roentgen ray as of distinct value in the diagnosis of intestinal amebiasis. Ikeda, who has studied this subject very thoroughly, states that the roentgenologic picture is not actually diagnostic but very suggestive, does not resemble that found in chronic colitis or tubercular colitis, and does determine the location, extent and degree of ulceration in the intestine, and regards it as a reliable and accurate method of demonstrating active lesions. He found that no distinct changes are noted in the early stages of the infection but that later fine saw-tooth-like projections along the wall of the colon are observed, while still later fine feathery or thorny filling defects occur. In subacute or chronic intestinal amebiasis he observed a shortening or contraction of the colon, together with filling defects. His findings are, in general, in agreement with the other authors mentioned and it is apparently true that in many cases of intestinal amebiasis characteristic changes are visible in the roentgenogram. However, the diagnosis of invasion of the intestine is so much more easily and accurately made by fecal examinations for the parasite that the method should never be relied upon in diagnosis, although it may be of some value in locating the lesions produced by the ameba.

THE PROCTOSCOPE IN THE DIAGNOSIS OF INTESTINAL AMEBIASIS.—It is unfortunate that many gastro-enterologists appear to rely almost entirely upon proctoscopic examinations in the diagnosis of intestinal amebiasis. The proctoscope is not necessary in diagnosis, as a microscopic examination of the feces for *Endamoeba histolytica* should demonstrate the organism in every case of infection if properly made. It has already been stated that one who relies upon the appearance of lesions revealed by the proctoscope in differentiating amebic lesions from those present in other conditions is very apt to be mistaken, and, in addition, it should be remembered that amebic lesions do not occur in the rectum in a large percentage of cases of amebiasis, especially in the early stage of intestinal amebiasis, when a diagnosis is most important. Certainly the proctoscope should never be used for the purpose of diagnosing intestinal amebiasis until several examinations of the feces have been negative for the ameba and the complement fixation reaction has also been negative. As Simon (1934) has well said, "The character of the ulcerative lesions in amebiasis, as viewed through the proctoscope, can in no manner be considered pathognomonic. Moreover, in the vast majority of individuals who harbor *Endamoeba histolytica,* no visible evidence of the infection can be found by rectal examination."

The use of the proctoscope, as a *diagnostic* instrument in intestinal amebiasis, should be abandoned, for it has been the writer's experience that *Endamoeba histolytica* can always be found in the stools if properly searched for, and if one is not capable of recognizing this organism and therefore resorts to the proctoscope, the results will never be conclusive and practically every infection in carriers and those presenting

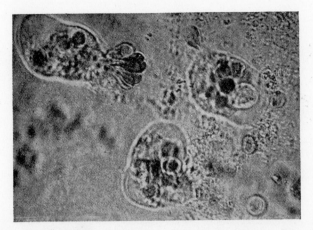

Fig. 6.—*Endamoeba histolytica.* Unstained Motile Trophozoite. Note material adhering to posterior end of the trophozoite in the upper left-hand corner of the photomicrograph, a common occurrence in the feces and in cultures. × 750. (Army Medical School Collection.)

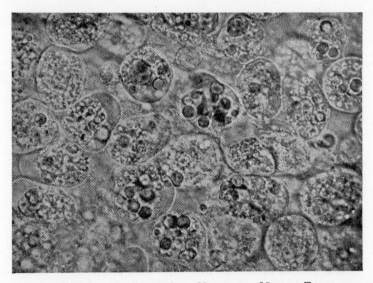

Fig. 7.—*Endamoeba histolytica.* Numerous Motile Trophozoites, Some Containing Red Blood Corpuscles. (After Westphal, Arch. f. Schiffs- u. Tropen-Hyg.)

mild symptomatology will go unrecognized, just at the time when their recognition is most important from a therapeutic standpoint.

Laboratory Diagnosis of Amebiasis.—It has already been stated that no diagnosis of amebiasis is reliable unless *Endamoeba histolytica* has been demonstrated in the stools, exudates or tissues of the individual suspected of harboring this parasite. Such demonstration depends

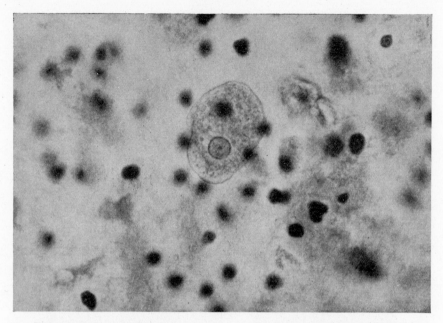

FIG. 8.—*Endamoeba histolytica* IN FECES. HEMATOXYLIN-STAINED PREPARATION SHOWING THE TYPICAL NUCLEAR STRUCTURE, I.E., THE DELICATE NUCLEAR MEMBRANE LINED WITH MINUTE CHROMATIN GRANULES AND THE MINUTE, CENTRALLY PLACED KARYOSOME. × 680. (Army Medical Museum Collection.) (From Craig's Amebiasis and Amebic Dysentery, Charles C. Thomas, Springfield, Ill.)

upon laboratory methods and is complicated by the fact that there occur in the human intestine four other amebae which may be confused with *Endamoeba histolytica* and which are harmless, so far as is known. It is necessary, therefore, to consider the morphology of all of these amebae and the differential characters upon which we must depend in making a diagnosis of *Endamoeba histolytica*.

The following amebae may live in the intestine of man and will be considered, i.e., *Endamoeba histolytica*, *Endamoeba coli*, *Endolimax nana*, *Iodamoeba buetschlii* and *Dientamoeba fragilis*.

Endamoeba Histolytica.—This ameba, often called *Entamoeba histolytica*, the only pathogenic ameba living in the human intestine, has two stages in its life cycle, the motile or trophozoite stage, and the immotile or cystic stage of development, in each of which the morphology differs.

(a) *The Trophozoite (Motile Stage of Development).*—This form, found in semifluid or fluid stools, measures from 20 to 25 microns in diameter in dysenteric stools but may be smaller in the stools of carriers. Motility is marked, clear, glasslike pseudopodia composed of the ectoplasm being extruded from the periphery of the organism, into which the endoplasm flows, resulting in the type of motility known as ameboid motility. In freshly passed stools the motility is progressive in type, the ameba moving across the microscopic field in a definite

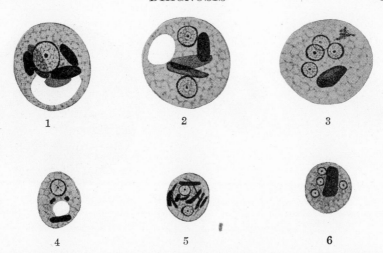

FIG. 9.—CYSTS OF *Endamoeba histolytica* STAINED WITH IRON-HEMATOXYLIN. *1, 2, 3.* Medium-sized cysts, measuring about 12.6 microns in diameter. *4, 5, 6.* Small cysts, measuring about 6 microns in diameter. After Dobell. In Practice of Medicine in the Tropics, Byam and Archibald, Oxford University Press, London.)

direction. The pseudopodium is finger-shaped and the endoplasm often flows so rapidly into it that sometimes it can be distinguished only with difficulty, the entire organism flowing in a sluglike manner across the microscopic field. Ingested material, as crystals, bacteria, etc., is not present in this species *with the exception of red blood corpuscles, which the ameba ingests* with avidity in stools containing blood. Tissue cells and leukocytes may also be ingested by this species, but the ingestion of red blood corpuscles is of great diagnostic importance as the other species of amebae in the intestine do not ingest these cells. A nucleus is not visible in the vast majority of living amebae of this species.

In preparations wet-fixed and stained with hematoxylin, the nucleus and ingested red blood corpuscles are the structures that are of diagnostic importance. The nucleus has a very delicate nuclear membrane stained black upon the inner side of which are very fine granules of chromatin. At the center of the nucleus is a minute chromatin granule, the karyosome, which also stains black, as do the chromatin granules upon the inner side of the nuclear membrane. If red blood corpuscles are present they appear as yellowish-green bodies within the endoplasm of the organism.

In either the unstained or stained trophozoites of *Endamoeba histolytica*, the presence of red blood corpuscles is sufficient evidence upon which to base a diagnosis of the species, but in unstained preparations caution should be used not to mistake the large phagocytic endothelial cells common in bacillary dysentery for this ameba, as such cells often contain red blood corpuscles, and *it is best not to diagnose any cell containing red blood corpuscles as Endamoeba histolytica unless motility is present.*

Prior to encystment the ameba rounds up, rids itself of ingested material and becomes motionless. In this so-called *precystic stage* of de-

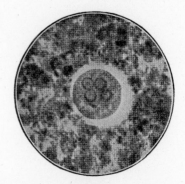

Fig. 10.—Cysts of *Endamoeba histolytica*. Photomicrograph of Cysts Stained with Iron-hematoxylin. (Army Medical Museum Collection. Preparation by Craig. From Craig and Faust's Clinical Parasitology, Lea & Febiger.)

velopment the differentiation of this species from others occurring in the human intestine is more difficult but fortunately either motile forms or fully developed cysts are usually present in addition to precystic forms and we do not have to depend upon the latter in diagnosis.

(*b*) *The Cyst (Immotile Stage of Development).*—The precystic forms mentioned above gradually secrete a cyst wall and become cysts. Cysts are found in semiformed or formed stools and have a very characteristic morphology. They are spherical in shape and vary in size from 5 to 15 microns in diameter, some strains of the ameba producing small cysts and others large ones. Surrounding the cyst is a cyst wall, appearing as a delicate double-outlined refractile membrane, the entire cyst being refractive and hyaline. In unstained preparations the nuclei within the cyst cannot usually be well differentiated but in preparations stained with the iodine they are clearly visible, each presenting a delicate refractive, hyaline nuclear membrane and a central refractive dot, the karyosome. The number of nuclei varies in the vast majority of the cysts from 1 to 4, but cysts containing 8 nuclei are very rarely observed. Hyaline, oval or rounded masses may often be seen within the cysts, most often in cysts containing 1 or 2 nuclei, and these are known as chromatoidal bodies and are of diagnostic importance.

In cysts *stained with any of the hematoxylin methods* the nuclei are clearly differentiated, the cytoplasm of the cysts staining a dull gray and the chromatoidal masses, if present, a jet black. The nuclei in such preparations have a delicate, black-stained nuclear membrane and a central minute black dot of chromatin. In diagnostic practice, the iodine stain is all that is necessary in order to differentiate the cysts of this and the other amebae occurring in the intestine of man except in very exceptional cases when hematoxylin-stained preparations may have to be employed.

The important diagnostic features of the cysts of *Endamoeba histolytica* are the number of the nuclei and their structure and the structure of the chromatoidal bodies, if present.

Endamoeba Coli.—This is a common species of ameba occurring in the intestine of man and is often confused with *Endamoeba histolytica*. The average incidence of this species varies from 30 to 40 per cent in

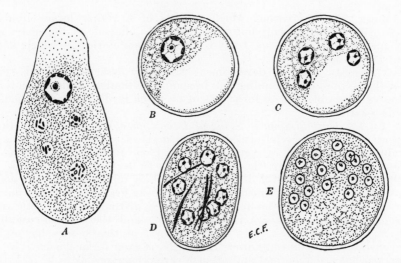

FIG. 11.—*Endamoeba coli.* *A,* Trophozoite. *B, C, D,* Cysts of *Endamoeba coli.* Note chromatoid bodies in *D.* *E,* Unusual cyst of *Endamoeba coli* containing 16 nuclei. × 1600. (After Faust, J. Lab. & Clin. Med.)

most surveys that have been made, and there is no evidence that it is pathogenic either to man or the lower animals. Experiments in feeding human volunteers, made by Walker and Sellards (1913) and others, have never resulted in any evidence that this ameba produces lesions or symptoms, although the organism continued to live for months and years in the intestinal tract of the individuals used in the experiments. Like *Endamoeba histolytica,* this ameba has a motile, or trophozoite, and a cystic stage of development in the intestine of man, in each of which the morphology varies.

(a) *The Trophozoite (Motile Stage of Development).*—As in the · case of *Endamoeba histolytica,* the motile ameba or trophozoite occurs almost entirely in semifluid or fluid stools. In *unstained preparations* the size usually varies between 20 and 30 microns, and the organism appears hyaline and granular. Motility is sluggish, the pseudopodia being broad and blunt and often projected from different parts of the periphery of the organism and withdrawn without resulting motion. The motility is not so progressive and directional as in *Endamoeba histolytica* and the pseudopodia are less glasslike in appearance. Ingested material is usually present in the form of crystals and numerous bacteria, but *this ameba does not ingest red blood corpuscles,* a most important differential feature between it and *Endamoeba histolytica.* A nucleus is usually clearly visible, consisting of a refractile ring of coarse granules enclosing a refractive mass situated to one side of the center of the nucleus.

In *hematoxylin-stained preparations* of this ameba the differential feature of importance is the nucleus. In this species the nuclear membrane is thick, stained black, and has upon its inner surface collections of black-stained chromatin, irregular in contour or consisting of coarse

38111

granules. The karyosome, which consists of a rather large circular mass of black-stained chromatin, is situated to one side of the center of the nucleus, thus differing from *Endamoeba histolytica* in which it is centrally situated.

A precystic stage of development is usually described for this species, the trophozoites rounding up, becoming motionless, and eliminating ingested material. These forms are of no value in diagnosis and should be disregarded.

(*b*) *The Cyst (Immotile Stage of Development)*.—The cysts of this species are found in semiformed or formed stools. They are refractive, hyaline, spherical bodies, varying in size from 10 to 20 microns, and are usually larger than those of *Endamoeba histolytica*. There is a well-defined, double-outlined cyst wall which is refractile, and the contents of the cyst in unstained specimens appear granular and the number and structure of the nuclei cannot be distinguished. With the *iodine stain* the nuclei are rendered visible and the number usually varies from 1 to 8, the fully developed cyst of this species having 8 nuclei. Rarely cysts containing 12, 16, 24 or even 32 nuclei have been observed but are abnormal and of such rare occurrence as to be of little value in diagnosis. The large chromatoidal bodies seen in the cysts of *Endamoeba histolytica* do not occur in the cysts of this species. The nuclear structure is well differentiated, the nuclear membrane appearing as a rather thick refractive hyaline ring surrounding the nucleus, while the karyosome consists of a refractive, rather coarse mass, situated to one side of the center of the nucleus, instead of centrally, as in *Endamoeba histolytica*.

In *hematoxylin-stained preparations* the structure of the nuclei in the cysts of *Endamoeba coli* is distinctive, the nuclear membrane, which stains black, being thicker than in *Endamoeba histolytica*, while the karyosome appears as a large black mass situated to one side of the center of the nucleus. Rounded or oval chromatoidal masses, like those occurring in the cysts of *Endamoeba histolytica*, are absent, but threadlike or filamentous chromatoidal structures may be present, staining black, and sometimes arranged about the periphery of the cyst.

The important diagnostic features of the cysts of *Endamoeba coli* are the number of nuclei, their structure, and the character of the chromatoidal bodies.

Endolimax Nana.—This common species of ameba living in the intestine of man occurs in from 15 to 30 per cent of individuals, as shown in most surveys, and is of great importance in diagnosis because the cysts of this species contain 4 nuclei, as in *Endamoeba histolytica*, and are frequently mistaken for those of the latter organism.

Endolimax nana occurs in the human intestine as a motile trophozoite and in the cystic stage, the latter being preceded by a precystic form which is of little value in the diagnosis of the parasite. This species of ameba is not pathogenic to man so far as known.

(*a*) *The Trophozoite (Motile Stage of Development)*.—The trophozoites, or motile forms, of *Endolimax nana* are found in semifluid and fluid stools and appear in the unstained preparations as hyaline, refractive organisms, usually measuring from 6 to 12 microns in diameter when immotile, thus being smaller than either the trophozoites of *Endamoeba histolytica* or *Endamoeba coli*. The motility of this species may

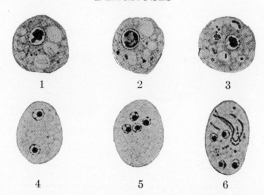

FIG. 12.—*Endolimax nana*. *1, 2, 3*. Trophozoites showing different types of nuclear structure. *4*. Two-nucleated cysts. *5, 6*. Four-nucleated cysts. Stained with iron-hematoxylin. (After Dobell and O'Connor.)

be said to be intermediate in character between the two species above mentioned, as it is somewhat more rapid and progressive than that of *coli* but less so than that of *histolytica*. The pseudopodia are broad and rather short and are frequently projected from the periphery and withdrawn without resultant motility. Ingested material, as starch granules and bacteria, are present but *this species does not phagocyte red blood corpuscles*. A nucleus, having a thin refractile membrane and a large refractile karyosome, may usually be seen in the living specimen.

In *hematoxylin-stained preparations* the structure of the nucleus easily differentiates this species from other amebae living in man. The nuclear membrane is rather thick in well-stained specimens, but no chromatin is seen upon the inner surface of this membrane. The karyosome may be situated at the center, or to one side of the center of the nucleus, appearing as a black, rather large mass; or it may be situated to one side of the center, near or actually in contact with the nuclear membrane; or it may be divided, one portion lying at or near the center, the other near the nuclear membrane or against it, and connected by a delicate filament of chromatin. The cytoplasm appears of a grayish color and is granular in structure and homogeneous in appearance.

(b) *The Cyst* (*Immotile Stage of Development*).—In *unstained preparations* the cysts of *Endolimax nana* appear as ovoid or spherical, hyaline bodies, having a double-outlined cyst wall and measuring from 5 to 10 microns in diameter, usually about 7 microns, or the diameter of a red blood corpuscle. The nuclei are not visible, as a rule, in the unstained preparation, but in the *iodine-stained preparation* the cysts are seen to contain from 1 to 4 nuclei, having a quite thick refractive nuclear membrane and a large karyosome situated centrally or to one side of the center, sometimes in contact with the nuclear membrane.

In *hematoxylin-stained preparations* the nuclear structure is well differentiated, there being a rather thick, black nuclear membrane free from chromatin granules upon its inner surface, and a large black karyosome situated centrally, or to one side of the center, which is sometimes divided into a larger and a smaller portion. Chromatoidal bodies may be present within the cytoplasm in the form of granular or bacilliform small masses, staining black.

38111

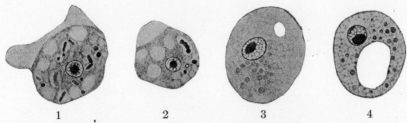

1   2   3   4

FIG. 13.—*Iodamoeba buetschlii.* STAINED WITH IRON-HEMATOXYLIN. *1, 2.*
Trophozoites, showing nuclear structure, vacuoles and inclusions. *3.* Precyst. *4.*
Cyst, showing large glycogen vacuole. (After Dobell and O'Connor.)

The important diagnostic features of the cysts of *Endolimax nana*
are the small size, frequently oval contour, the structure of the nuclei
and of the chromatoidal bodies.

Iodamoeba Buetschlii.—This is a rather rare species of intestinal
ameba, occurring in from 3 to 6 per cent of the individuals examined
in various surveys. It has a motile or trophozoite stage, and an immotile
or cystic stage of development, and is not pathogenic to man or the lower
animals so far as is known.

(*a*) *The Trophozoite (Motile Stage of Development).*—In *unstained
preparations Iodamoeba buetschlii* appears as a hyaline, refractile cell,
measuring from 5 to 20 microns in diameter, the average being from 10 to
15 microns. It is sluggishly motile, the pseudopodia being broad,
rounded and hyaline in appearance. Motility is progressive in type in
freshly passed stools but is quickly lost upon exposure of the stool to the
air. Bacteria, vegetable cells, starch granules and granular debris may
be observed within the cytoplasm, but *this species does not ingest red
blood corpuscles.* A nucleus is not visible in the unstained specimen in
the vast majority of organisms but may rarely be seen as a large, refractile mass surrounded by a hyaline halo.

In *hematoxylin-stained preparations* the peculiar structure of the
nucleus in the trophozoite of this species of ameba is well shown. The
nuclear membrane, staining black, is somewhat thicker than that of
Endamoeba histolytica and small black granules of chromatin may be
observed upon its inner surface. The karyosome is usually situated at
the center of the nucleus, stains black, and is composed of granules
loosely arranged within a filamentous network, the whole lying in a more
dimly stained material. If overstained the entire karyosome may stain
a deep black and appear as a large, more or less irregular mass, lying
near or at the center of the nucleus. The cytoplasm may contain bacteria and there is usually present a large body resembling a vacuole,
called the glycogen mass, which takes a deep mahogany color with the
iodine stain.

(*b*) *The Cyst (Immotile Stage of Development).*—The cysts of this
species are peculiar among those of the amebae living in the intestine of
man in that *normally but one nucleus is present.* In *unstained preparations* the cysts appear as refractile, hyaline bodies, measuring from 6 to
16 microns in diameter, and of various shapes, being ovoid, elliptical,
rhomboidal, almost square, or spheroidal, and are characterized by the
presence of a very large, round body resembling a vacuole, which with
the iodine stain is colored a deep brown or mahogany, and is composed of

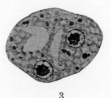

1   2   3

Fig. 14.—*Dientamoeba fragilis.* Stained with Iron-hematoxylin.
1. Single-nucleated trophozoite. *2, 3.* Typical double-nucleated trophozoite. (After Dobell.)

glycogen. This body, sometimes called the iodophilic body, is very
characteristic of this species, for while small glycogen masses do occur
in the other amebae they are not comparable with the glycogen mass of
this species, either in size or the intensity of the iodine stain. The
nucleus in the unstained preparation is not well differentiated, but with
the iodine stain its structure is diagnostic, there being a very large refractile karyosome surrounded by a hyaline zone, and a delicate refractile nuclear membrane. There is a well-defined cyst wall, appearing as
a hyaline double outline surrounding the cyst. More than one glycogen
body may be present and very rarely a cyst is seen in which there are two
nuclei, but this is evidently abnormal.

In *hematoxylin-stained preparations* the glycogen body appears as a
large unstained area within the cyst and the structure of the nucleus is
well shown. The nuclear membrane is thin and the karyosome often
appears to be lying within a vacuole in the cytoplasm of the ameba,
usually situated to one side of the center of the nucleus and sometimes in
contact with the nuclear membrane. The karyosome consists of dark
brown or black-stained granules of chromatin surrounded by one or
more layers of black-stained granules or by more isolated black granules,
giving a very characteristic appearance to the nucleus of this species.

The differential features of the cyst of *Iodamoeba buetschlii* are the
variation in the shape of the cysts, the presence of but one nucleus, the
peculiar structure of the latter, and the large iodine-stained glycogen
body. These cysts for many years were known as "iodine cysts" and
are still referred to by that name in some textbooks.

Dientamoeba Fragilis.—This ameba is a rare species in man and is
characterized by having no cystic stage of development. It has occurred
in from less than 1 per cent to 10 per cent in different surveys and in the
writer's experience, less than 1 per cent of individuals he has examined
have been positive for this species. It is not a pathogenic species so far
as is known.

(*a*) *The Trophozoite* (*Motile Stage of Development*).—This is the
only form of *Dientamoeba fragilis* that has been demonstrated with certainty either in man or in cultures. In the *unstained preparation* the
average diameter is about 10 microns, the motility is active and progressive in freshly passed stools, and the pseudopodia have a characteristic
broad, leaflike shape with the margin indented or serrated. The entire
organism is hyaline and refractile, especially the pseudopodia, and the
nuclei are not usually visible in the unstained specimen. The cytoplasm
may contain bacteria and other ingested material, but *red blood corpuscles are not ingested by this species.*

38111

In *hematoxylin-stained preparations* it will be noted that the majority of the trophozoites of this species contain *two nuclei,* which is diagnostic. In the writer's experience about 80 per cent of the amebae in a preparation will be binucleated and the structure of the nuclei is also characteristic. The nuclear membrane is very delicate and often invisible, the karyosome appearing to lie within a vacuole within the cytoplasm. If visible, the inner surface is free from chromatin granules. The karyosome is almost always situated at the center of the nucleus and varies in structure but is composed of isolated granules varying in number and lying in a dimly staining matrix. The arrangement of the karyosome granules is interesting, the most frequent arrangement being in the form of a tetracoccus, but the granules may be arranged in a circular or crosslike manner or heaped up in a round mass at the center of the nucleus.

Kofoid is the only authority who has described cysts of this species and his observations have not been confirmed.

The diagnostic features of *Dientamoeba fragilis* are the presence of two nuclei in the majority of the organisms, the peculiar structure of the karyosome of the nucleus, and the absence of a cystic stage in the life history of the species.

The most important features in the differential diagnosis of *Endamoeba histolytica, Endamoeba coli* and *Endolimax nana* are given in Table I. These three species are those most commonly encountered in examinations of stools from man and are most frequently confused, *Iodamoeba buetschlii* and *Dientamoeba fragilis* being comparatively rare species and less apt to be confused with *Endamoeba histolytica.*

DIAGNOSTIC IMPORTANCE OF THE CHARACTER OF THE FECES IN AMEBIC AND BACILLARY DYSENTERY.—While the differential diagnosis between amebic and bacillary dysentery should rest upon the demonstration of either *Endamoeba histolytica* or one of the dysentery bacilli in the feces, it is possible to make a differential diagnosis based upon the character of the fecal exudate in these types of dysentery. Willmore and Shearman (1916) were the first to call attention to the marked differences in the cellular exudate in amebic and bacillary dysentery, and the importance of these differences in differential diagnosis has since been stressed by Bahr and Willmore (1917), Manson-Bahr (1919), Anderson (1921), Haughwout (1921) and Callender (1925–1934). The writer is in agreement with the findings of these authorities and believes that a study of the cellular exudate in dysentery is of great importance in the differential diagnosis between amebic and bacillary dysentery. The value of this method of distinguishing these types of dysentery consists in the fact that any physician capable of using a microscope, but who may not be familiar with the morphology of the various amebae living in the human intestine, or so placed as to be unable to make bacteriologic examination of the feces, may, in the majority of cases, make an accurate diagnosis between amebic and bacillary dysentery by a microscopic examination of a freshly passed stool, noting the character of the cellular exudate that may be present. Callender (1925) has well said that "with only a microscope and slides, a relatively inexperienced man can make a presumptive diagnosis (of bacillary dysentery) which will be correct in 90 per cent of the cases without the use of stained preparations, a much higher proportion of positive results than one may ever hope to obtain by bacterio-

TABLE I

DIAGNOSTIC POINTS IN THE DIFFERENTIATION OF ENDAMOEBA HISTOLYTICA,
ENDAMOEBA COLI AND ENDOLIMAX NANA

VEGETATIVE OR TROPHOZOITE STAGE.   UNSTAINED

	ENDAMOEBA HISTOLYTICA	ENDAMOEBA COLI	ENDOLIMAX NANA
Size.........	18 to 60 microns; average 20 to 35 microns	15 to 50 microns; average 20 to 30 microns	6 to 12 microns; average 8 microns
Motility......	Actively progressive and directional	Sluggish; rarely progressive; not directional	Sluggishly progressive
Pseudopodia...	Finger-shaped, clear and glasslike	Shorter and more blunt; less glasslike in appearance	Broad and blunt; not glass-like
Inclusions.....	Red blood corpuscles when feces contain blood; no bacteria in fresh specimens	Numerous bacteria, crystals and other materials; no red blood corpuscles	Numerous bacteria; no red blood corpuscles
Nucleus......	Invisible	Visible	Visible

VEGETATIVE OR TROPHOZOITE STAGE.   STAINED

Nuclear membrane ..	Delicate; inner surface has single layer of minute chromatin dots	Thicker; inner surface lined with coarser chromatin dots	Intermediate in thickness; chromatin rarely seen on inner surface
Karyosome....	Very small; usually in center of nucleus	Twice as large, situated eccentrically	Large and may be divided into one large and one small mass, situated at one side or in center of nucleus
Intranuclear chromatin...	No chromatin between karyosome and membrane	Chromatin grains between karyosome and nuclear membrane	No chromatin between kary-osome and membrane
Inclusions.....	Red blood corpuscles; no bacteria in fresh specimens	No red blood corpuscles; many bacteria and other material	No red blood corpuscles; many bacteria

CYSTIC STAGE OF DEVELOPMENT.   IODINE STAIN

Size.........	6 to 20 microns; average 7 to 15 microns	10 to 20 microns; average 12 to 18 microns	5 to 10 microns
Shape........	Generally spherical; may be oval and rarely irregular	Spherical; rarely oval or irregular	Spherical, oval or ellipsoidal
Nucleus......	One to four; minute karyo-some in center	One to eight; eccentric kary-osome	One to four; large karyosome central or to one side

HEMATOXYLIN-STAINED CYSTS

Size.........	As in iodine-stained spec-imens	As in iodine-stained spec-imens	As in iodine-stained spec-imens
Nuclear structure....	Delicate membrane, minute central karyosome, no chromatin between karyo-some and membrane, mi-nute grains on nuclear membrane	Thicker membrane, larger eccentrically located karyo-some, chromatin grains be-tween nuclear membrane and karyosome, and large granules of chromatin on nuclear membrane	Thick nuclear membrane, large central or divided karyosome
Chromatoidal bodies......	Bar, oval or thick rodlike masses; present in about 50 per cent of the cysts	Filamentous or spicular with square or pointed ends; present in less than 10 per cent of cysts	Small granular or bacilliform masses, not comparable with those seen in the other species
Nuclei, number of...	One to four	One to eight	One to four

logical methods, to say nothing of the delay and uncertainty involved
in arriving at a bacteriological diagnosis.''

The cellular exudate in cases of bacillary dysentery is composed of
innumerable pus cells, while in amebic dysentery there are very few pus
cells. In bacillary dysentery the nuclei of most of the leukocytes show

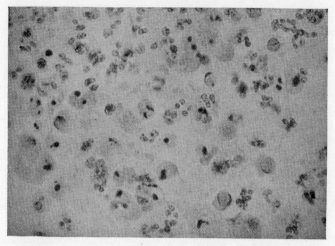

1

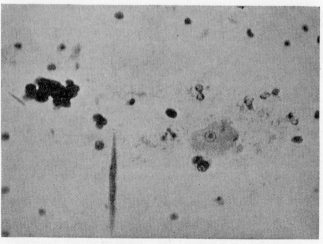

2

Fig. 15.—Exudates in Bacillary and Amebic Dysentery. *1.* Exudate in bacillary dysentery showing numerous leukocytes and macrophages. *2.* Exudate in amebic dysentery showing few neutrophilic leukocytes, the pyknotic nuclei of the leukocytes that are present, a Charcot-Leyden crystal, agglutinated red blood corpuscles, and a small trophozoite of *Endamoeba histolytica.* × 850. Stained with iron-hematoxylin. (Army Medical Museum Collection.) (From Craig's Amebiasis and Amebic Dysentery, Charles C. Thomas, Springfield, Ill.)

toxic degeneration, while in amebic dysentery the comparatively few leukocytes present evidences of cytolysis of the cytoplasm, the nuclei having little or no cytoplasm surrounding them. These *pyknotic bodies,* as they are called, are characteristic of the pus cells occurring in amebic dysentery stools.

In the stools in amebic dysentery Charcot-Leyden crystals usually occur, while they are absent in the stools of bacillary dysentery. In the stools of bacillary dysentery there occur large mononuclear cells which may contain red blood corpuscles, but such cells do not occur in amebic dysentery stools. These large mononuclear cells, or macrophages, closely resemble trophozoites of *Endamoeba histolytica* containing red blood corpuscles and have been frequently mistaken for this parasite, and it is a fact that many cases of bacillary dysentery have been diagnosed as amebic dysentery because of the presence of these cells. However, if one remembers that the macrophages are not motile, whereas the trophozoites of *Endamoeba histolytica* are, there should be no trouble in distinguishing them from amebae. It is a safe rule never to diagnose a cell containing red blood corpuscles in a freshly passed specimen of the stool as *Endamoeba histolytica* unless ameboid motility is present.

If blood is present in an amebic dysentery stool the corpuscles are often agglutinated, occurring in clumps throughout the microscopic field, while in bacillary dysentery the corpuscles are more evenly distributed throughout the field. In bacillary dysentery stools there occured the so-called "ghost cells" of Callender, consisting of pus cells and macrophages in which the cytoplasm and nucleus have been destroyed by toxic degeneration and only the cell membrane remains.

By attention to the morphologic data mentioned above it is usually possible to differentiate between amebic and bacillary dysentery, but it should always be remembered that mixed infections may occur and then the only criterion is the demonstration of motile *Endamoeba histolytica* in a stool composed largely of pus cells.

TECHNIC OF LABORATORY EXAMINATIONS FOR DIAGNOSIS OF INFECTIONS WITH ENDAMOEBA HISTOLYTICA.—The demonstration of infection with *Endamoeba histolytica* may be accomplished by microscopic examinations of exudates or tissues, by cultivation of the ameba from suspected material, and by complement fixation. The microscopic examination of the stool is the most valuable method of diagnosis in cases of intestinal amebiasis and should not be replaced by other methods of diagnosis. In the experience of the writer it is always possible to demonstrate this parasite in the feces in intestinal amebiasis if a proper technic is employed and enough examinations are made. A *single negative examination means but little* and at least six careful examinations should be made before a case is considered negative. In rare instances cultures have been positive when the stools have been negative upon one or two examinations, and the same is true of complement fixation reactions, but repeated examinations of the stools after such findings have almost always shown *Endamoeba histolytica* to be present.

Technic of Stool Examinations.—In making stool examinations for this parasite one cardinal principle must be remembered, i.e., that the motile trophozoite does not occur in semiformed or formed stools except very rarely, but in semifluid or fluid stools, while the cysts of this parasite do not occur in semifluid or fluid stools but in semiformed or formed stools. Hence, it is foolish to look for motile amebae in formed stools or for cysts in fluid stools. It is also most important to remember that freshly passed stools must be examined if one is searching for motile amebae, as these forms soon lose their motility after exposure of the stool to the air and undergo degeneration within a short time. It is essential that the stool reach the laboratory within an hour after passage and has been kept at body temperature in the interval, or, better still, that the stool be passed at the laboratory. If cysts are to be searched for, they may be demonstrated in the stools for many hours after passage and specimens may be sent by mail for examination if they will reach the laboratory within two or three days. If specimens are to be sent by mail to distant laboratories for examination, smears of the feces should be made upon microscopic slides and immediately immersed in Schaudinn's fixative (q.v.). Drying should be most carefully avoided as this so shrinks the amebae that they cannot be recognized. After remaining in the Schaudinn solution for at least 15 minutes, the smears are transferred to suitable containers filled with alcohol and mailed in a double tin container to the laboratory. Such smears will keep indefinitely and after receipt should be stained with one of the hematoxylin stains as hereinafter described.

If stools are fluid or semifluid, a small portion of the stool or, if blood and mucus are present, a small portion of bloodstained mucus is placed upon a microscopic slide and immediately covered with a coverglass and examined with the low- and high-power dry lens. The latter is preferable unless one is well trained in the examination of feces for the ameba. The preparation should not be too thick, and it should be possible to read newspaper print through the specimen if it is properly prepared. A mechanical stage is very useful and convenient in such examinations. The most useful combinations of ocular and objective for fecal examinations are ocular 10 ×; objective 16 mm, and ocular 10 ×; objective 4 mm.

If the feces are formed a small portion should be examined from the exterior of the fecal mass, as well as the interior, the material being emulsified in normal saline, placed upon a microscopic slide and covered with a coverglass, care being taken not to make too thick a preparation.

In examining unstained material for *Endamoeba histolytica* the iris diaphragm of the microscope should be shut down as much as possible, as both the trophozoites and cysts are hyaline in appearance and cannot be well seen unless the light is cut down as much as is possible.

If material from an amebic abscess of the liver or other organ, or from other amebic lesions, is to be examined, the same methods for the examination of the unstained material should be employed as just described.

In the examination of material for the motile forms of *Endamoeba histolytica*, the direct microscopic examination of unstained preparations is essential, but for the differentiation of the cysts the use of iodine solutions is necessary.

(a) *The Iodine Stain.*—The employment of a solution of iodine, by mixing it with the material to be examined, for staining the cysts of the amebae of man results in the nuclei within the cysts being rendered distinctly visible so that their number can be ascertained and their morphology studied. By the employment of the iodine stain it is thus possible to differentiate the cysts of the various intestinal amebae and, in the vast majority of instances, a differential diagnosis may be made in this way without resort to the more difficult and time-consuming hematoxylin staining methods.

Numerous iodine solutions have been recommended for staining the cysts of amebae, the most useful being D'Antoni's * standardized iodine stain. But for those who, for any reason, are so situated as to be unable to prepare this stain, the following iodine solution will be found satisfactory:

Iodine .... 2 Gm.
Potassium iodide .... 4 Gm.
Distilled water .... 100 cc.

The potassium iodide is first dissolved in the distilled water and the iodine is then added. Solutions not over a week old give the best results.

The method of using the iodine stain is to place a drop of the stain upon a microscopic slide and then mix with it a minute portion of the feces, cover with a coverglass and allow the mixture to stand for at least five minutes before examining, to allow the iodine to penetrate the cysts. When stained in this manner the cytoplasm of the cysts stains a lemon-yellow color, glycogen bodies stain a dark brown, and the nuclear membrane and karyosome of the nucleus appear as refractile structures, almost devoid of color. The iodine stain is of no value whatever in the examination of material for the trophozoites of any of the intestinal amebae and should not be used in such examinations.

Concentration Methods.—Some authorities have recommended certain concentration methods in the examination of stools for the cysts of amebae, but careful comparisons of the results of such methods and of the simple direct examination of the feces have shown that nothing is gained by these methods as usually employed. The writer was previously much in favor of concentration methods in the examination for *Endamoeba histolytica* cysts, but the results that have been obtained with such methods have convinced him that they are unnecessary and do not increase the chance of finding cysts in the vast majority of instances and, indeed, there is some evidence to prove that certain concentration methods give fewer positive results than the direct microscopic examination of the feces.

Floatation Method.—Recently Faust and his coworkers (1938) have described a centrifugal-floatation method, using zinc sulphate as the levitating medium, for the demonstration of amebae in specimens of stools. This method is now under trial and has given excellent results, but the exact technic has not yet been published so far as routine fecal diagnosis is concerned.

Staining Methods.—In the vast majority of cases a differential diagnosis of *Endamoeba histolytica* may be made, either by the microscopic examination of unstained fecal material for the motile trophozoites, or of the iodine-stained preparation for the cysts of this parasite. In rare instances it may be necessary to resort to permanent stained preparations in diagnosis, or for the detailed study of the structure of the nucleus of the amebae. It has not been the writer's experience that resort to such staining methods is necessary in routine fecal examinations for *Endamoeba histolytica*, although some authorities claim that such methods are essential in differentiating this species of ameba from the other intestinal amebae of man. Without taking into consideration the difficulty of obtaining good stained preparations, and the time consumed in preparing them, it may be that to one unaccustomed to the appearance of the vari-

* D'Antoni, J. S.: Am. J. Trop. Med., 17: 79, 1937.

ous species of amebae in unstained material the structure revealed in stained organisms makes a differential diagnosis much less difficult, but it is not considered that such preparations are at all necessary in routine diagnosis for those well acquainted with the morphology of the amebae in unstained or iodine-stained preparations.

Many staining methods have been recommended but the following simple method (Faust's) is satisfactory. Before staining it is necessary to fix the specimen in order to avoid washing off the fecal material during the process of staining, and for this purpose Schaudinn's fixing solution is excellent.

(*a*) *Schaudinn's Solution for Fixing.*—This consists of a saturated solution of mercuric chloride in warm water, 2 parts; absolute or 96 per cent alcohol, 1 part. These are mixed and 5 cc. of glacial acetic acid are added to the mixture, which should be heated to body temperature before using.

In fixing the preparation, smears are prepared upon microscopic slides as already described and immersed at once in the Schaudinn solution and left for from 15 minutes to one-half hour, after which the smears are stained with the Faust stain. It should be emphasized that the smears must never be allowed to dry from the time they are made until the fixing and staining process is completed, for drying renders them useless for examination, the distinctive morphology of the various species of amebae being destroyed.

(*b*) *Faust's Stain.*—This stain gives good results in the differential diagnosis of the intestinal amebae and is less time-consuming than other stains that have been recommended. The following method of application of this stain should be carefully adhered to in order to secure good results:

1. Fix in Schaudinn's fixing solution for 2 minutes. (Heated to 60° F.; 15.6° C.)
2. Immerse smears in 70 per cent alcohol; 70 per cent alcohol to which enough iodine has been added to give a port-wine color; 70 and 50 per cent alcohol, leaving in each 2 minutes.
3. Wash in running water for 2 minutes.
4. Immerse smears in 2 per cent aqueous iron-alum solution at 104° F. (40° C.) for 2 minutes.
5. Wash in running water 3 minutes.
6. Stain in 0.5 per cent aqueous hematoxylin for 2 minutes.
7. Wash in water 2 minutes.
8. Differentiate in cold aqueous iron-alum solution. (The same as used in Step 4 but not heated.)
9. Wash in running water 10 to 15 minutes.
10. Immerse smears 2 minutes each in 70, 80, 90 per cent and absolute alcohol.
11. Clear in xylol.
12. Mount in xylol balsam.

With this stain the nuclear membrane, chromatin granules, and karyosome of the nucleus of amebae stain black, as well as the chromatoidal bodies.

USE OF CULTURES IN THE DIAGNOSIS OF INTESTINAL AMEBAE.—Since the successful culture of *Endamoeba histolytica* by Boeck and Drbohlav, many investigators have succeeded in cultivating this parasite and many culture media have been devised for this purpose. The relative value of cultures and of the direct microscopic examination of the stool is still a matter of controversy, some authorities having secured better results with one or the other method, but the writer believes that culture methods are not absolutely necessary in the routine diagnosis of amebiasis, although in rare instances, in which the infection is suspected and *repeated* examinations of the stools for the parasite have been negative, culture should be resorted to, as the parasite sometimes is demonstrable in cultures in such cases. However, if only one microscopic examination of the stool can be made, cultures should also be made at the same time, for cultures have given better results under such circumstances. Thus, St. John and the writer (1927), in a survey of 71 individuals for *Endamoeba histolytica*, found only 6 (8.45 per cent) were positive by one direct microscopic stool examination, while 11 (15.45 per cent) were positive by use of cultures. Our results have been confirmed by others, notably by Poindexter (1933) and Nauss and Salinger (1935), so that it is believed that cultures should be employed in diagnosis routinely when it is impossible to make repeated microscopic examinations of the stools for the ameba.

In employing cultures for the diagnosis of the intestinal amebae, the technic used is most important. One should remember that in routine cultures the amebae are never very numerous and never approach the number of bacteria seen in cultures of the latter. If one employs bacteriologic technic in culturing amebae the chance of obtaining a positive culture is practically nil, and most of the negative reports upon culturing this parasite are due to the fact that bacteriologic technic was employed. It should also be remembered that pure cultures of the intestinal amebae are not obtained by the cultural methods now used and that the cultures will contain not only the amebae but many bacteria. Indeed, it has been found that bacteria are apparently necessary as a source of food supply for the amebae in cultures, for while pure cultures of *Endamoeba histolytica* have been obtained, it has been found impossible to maintain the ameba in such cultures for more than a generation or two.

In examining material for *Endamoeba histolytica,* by the culture method, a small amount (about 0.2 cc.) of the liquid material, or a small portion of the solid stool, the size of a pea, should be inoculated. If one of the fluid media is used this material is thoroughly mixed with it, and if one of the solid media is employed, thoroughly emulsified in the fluid covering the slanted solid medium. The tubes should be placed in an incubator at 37° C. (96.8° F.) and examined at the end of 24 and 48 hours. Aseptic precautions are not necessary but should be employed if possible. At the end of the periods mentioned, about 0.1 cc. of the sediment at the bottom of the fluid culture tubes, or at the junction of the fluid and slant in the solid medium, should be pipetted off with a 1-cc. pipette and a drop of the material so obtained placed upon a microscopic slide, covered with a coverglass, and examined with the high dry objective (16 mm.) and the $10 \times$ ocular. As much material should be examined as possible and it is absolutely useless to examine a platinum loopful of material as in bacteriologic examinations, as the result will be negative even though numerous amebae may be present. If it is desired to maintain the ameba in cultures, transfers should be made with the 1-cc. pipette and at least 0.2 cc. of the material from the original culture should be inoculated in each transfer tube. Here, again, the transfer of a platinum loopful of material will not be successful as a much larger inoculum is needed in the transfer.

In examining material from cultures it should be remembered that the amebae are seldom very numerous, three or four to a microscopic field being considered a very satisfactory culture. Sometimes, many microscopic fields are examined before a single ameba is encountered, especially if the examination is made at the end of 24 hours, and a culture should never be discarded as negative until it has been examined both at the end of 24 and 48 hours, and after the entire microscopic preparation has been gone over very carefully. Here, again, the expectation that many amebae should be present in the material obtained from cultures, and lack of patience in making the examinations, account for the many negative reports as to the value of culture methods in the diagnosis of *Endamoeba histolytica.*

In cultures *Endamoeba histolytica* usually occurs as a motile trophozoite and this is always true if 24- to 48-hour cultures are employed, as in routine diagnosis. Therefore, the diagnosis rests upon the demonstration in such cultures of motile trophozoites of this species. When the material from cultures is placed upon the microscopic slide and examined at once, the ameba will be found rounded up and motionless, so that a period of at least 5 minutes should be allowed to elapse before the specimen is examined. If this is done, and the room is warm in which the examination is made, the trophozoites will be found to have begun to move and the characteristic motility and morphology may be determined. All of the other intestinal amebae have been cultivated but do not develop so well in cultures as does *Endamoeba histolytica.* The morphology of the latter species is the same in cultures as in the intestine, and the progressive character of the motility is similar. Red blood corpuscles are ingested by this ameba if they are present in the culture medium. In doubtful cases a little blood may be added to the culture and if the amebae present ingest the red blood cells, one may be sure that such amebae are *Endamoeba histolytica.*

Culture Media for Endamoeba Histolytica.—There have been several media devised for the cultivation of *Endamoeba histolytica* but for routine diagnostic work the following will be found the most useful:

(a) *Craig's Locke-serum and Ringer-serum Media.*—The following very simple culture media have been found useful in routine diagnosis, a pea-sized portion of the feces to be examined, or 0.2 cc. of the fluid stool being shaken up in the media and incubated for 48 hours at 37° C. (98.6° F.) and examined at the end of 24 and 48 hours.

Medium 1. Locke-serum Medium: This medium consists of a mixture of a modified Locke solution and either inactivated human, horse or rabbit blood serum. The serum used should not be over 48 hours old before use in the culture mixture.

The Locke solution employed has the following formula:

Sodium chloride	9.00 Gm.
Calcium chloride	0.24 Gm.
Potassium chloride	0.42 Gm.
Sodium bicarbonate	0.20 Gm.
Distilled water 1000	cc.

This solution is filtered and autoclaved at 15 pounds' pressure for 15 minutes and allowed to cool. There is then added to it 1 part of inactivated serum to each 7 parts of Locke solution. After adding the blood serum the mixture is filtered through a Berkefeld filter and it is frequently necessary to filter through two or more candles before the mixture comes through clear. After filtration the medium is tubed, placing about 10 cc. in each tube, and incubated for 24 to 36 hours to determine sterility. If found sterile the tubes should be kept in an incubator at 37° C. (98.6° F.) until used. The reaction does not need adjusting. The blood serum is inactivated by heating at 56° C. (132.8° F.) for one-half hour. The addition of a minute amount of rice flour or starch adds to the efficiency of the medium and this should be added just before inoculation of the medium.

Medium 2.   Ringer-serum Medium: This medium is similar to the No. 1 medium except that Ringer's solution is used instead of Locke's solution, and the method of preparation is the same. The Ringer solution used has the following formula:

Sodium chloride	8.00 Gm.
Calcium chloride	0.20 Gm.
Potassium chloride	0.20 Gm.
Distilled water 1000	cc.

Medium 3.   Normal-saline-serum Medium: One part of inactivated human blood serum is added to 7 parts of normal salt solution (0.85 per cent), and from 500 to 1000 cc. of such a mixture are filtered through a Berkefeld filter, tubed, and incubated for 48 hours at 37° C. (98.6° F.) to determine sterility. If found sterile the tubes are stored in an incubator at this temperature and inoculated as required.

(*b*) *Cleveland and Collier's Medium.*—This medium is excellent for routine diagnosis and possesses the advantage that it is almost specific for *Endamoeba histolytica*. It is prepared as follows:

Take 30 Gm. of liver infusion agar (prepared by Digestive Ferments Co., Detroit, Michigan) and 3 Gm. of Na_2HPO_4 and add to a liter of distilled water. The mixture is then autoclaved and slants are poured. The slants are then covered with a mixture consisting of fresh horse serum, 1 part, and 0.8 per cent NaCl solution, 6 parts. No adjustment of reaction is necessary. A little sterile rice flour is added to each tube upon inoculation.

(*c*) *Liver Infusion Agar Medium.*—This medium is recommended by Bundesen, Rawlings and Fishbein (1933) and gives excellent results in routine diagnosis by culture. It is prepared as follows:

One pound of fat-free ground beef liver was added to 500 cc. of tap water in a covered receptacle. This was placed in flowing steam for twenty minutes, then boiled for one and one-half hours longer in an Arnold sterilizer, stirring continually. It was then filtered through a wire screen and sterilized.

The liver infusion agar is prepared by taking 500 cc. of this liver infusion; 500 cc. of tap water; 20 Gm. of washed agar; 10 Gm. of peptone; and 5 Gm. of sodium chloride and mixing, first dissolving the agar in the tap water and then adding the other ingredients. After thorough mixing the mixture is heated in the Arnold sterilizer for 30 minutes, allowed to cool, the reaction adjusted to pH 7.0 and then heated in the Arnold for one and one-half hours. Tubes are then prepared and autoclaved for 30 minutes at 15 pounds' pressure, after which they are slanted, and covered with a mixture composed of 1 part of serum diluted with 6 parts of sterile normal saline solution.

The choice of a culture medium for routine diagnostic work is really immaterial as any of the media described above give good results. It is, however, most important that whatever medium is selected one persists in its use until good results are obtained. Experience with any one culture medium is essential to satisfactory results, and when one has become used to a certain medium, his results will be much better than the results of one who is constantly changing media, with consequent lack of experience with any one medium.

COMPLEMENT FIXATION TEST IN DIAGNOSIS OF AMEBIASIS.—In 1927 the writer described a complement fixation test which is specific in infections with *Endamoeba histolytica* and since that time his observations have been confirmed by Spector (1932), Menendez (1932), Sherwood and Heathman (1932), Heathman (1932), Tsuchiya (1932), Weiss and Arnold (1934), Paulson and Andrews (1936), Stone (1935), Shirogawa (1935), Yamamoto (1936), and Meleney and Frye (1937), and it has been demonstrated that the blood serum of individuals infected with this ameba contains complement-fixing bodies which may be shown to be present when an antigen prepared by extracting cultures of *Endamoeba histolytica* with alcohol is employed in the complement fixation test.

The *technic* of the complement fixation test for amebiasis is the same as that employed in the laboratories of the United States Army in making the Wassermann test and described in the writer's *The Wassermann Test*, 2nd edition, 1921, modified, of course, as regards the antigen that is employed. A human hemolytic system is employed instead of the sheep hemolytic system usually used in the Wassermann test; the serums are inactivated for one-half hour at 56° C. (132.8° F.), and the antigen is an alcoholic extract of mucus rich in this organism obtained from the intestine of experimentally infected dogs or cultures of the ameba. Full directions for preparing the various reagents used in the test, the titrations of these substances, and the exact technic of the test will be found described in the writer's *Amebiasis and Amebic Dysentery*, 1934, pages 231–252, to which the reader is referred.

Interpretation of the Complement Fixation Test for Amebiasis.— Owing to the fact that the antigen used in this test is a rather weak one, partial reactions are of no diagnostic significance, although useful in judging the adequacy of various methods of treatment. In the experience of the writer, one should not regard a reaction as positive with this test unless a three- or four-plus reaction is obtained. In my experience about 85 per cent of infected individuals give a four-plus reaction and about 10 per cent a three-plus reaction. Positive reactions are just as frequently obtained in carriers without any symptomatology as in individuals presenting marked intestinal symptoms or the symptoms of an amebic abscess of the liver. A certain number of individuals known to harbor the parasite will give weak or negative reactions, but the percentage of such cases does not exceed 5 per cent at most. From an experience covering nearly 10 years in the use of this test the writer believes that it is specific for infection with *Endamoeba histolytica* and that it does not give positive results in other intestinal infections, either bacterial or protozoal, nor with syphilis or any other infection or disease. In a recent analysis by the writer (1934), of the results of this test in 1000 individuals, positive reactions were obtained in 175, or 17.5 per cent, and of these the stools were positive for *Endamoeba histolytica* in 157, or 89.7 per cent. All of the patients whose stools were negative but the complement fixation test positive had intestinal symptomatology and in over one half of them but a single stool examination was made for the ameba. Of the 825 individuals giving a negative reaction with the test, the stools were found positive for the ameba in but 12, or 1.4 per cent, thus demonstrating that while the test gives a negative result in some infections with this parasite, the number of such instances is small.

A positive complement fixation reaction becomes negative, after the elimination of the infection by treatment, in from two to four weeks, as a rule, and a persistent positive reaction after this period indicates the persistence of the amebic infection somewhere in the body, even though the stools fail to show *Endamoeba histolytica*.

Practical Value of the Test in Diagnosis and as a Control of Treatment.—In a recent paper the writer has summarized the practical value of the complement fixation test for amebiasis and has stated that, ''While the practical diagnostic value of the complement fixation test for amebiasis is great it should never be employed in preference to a microscopical examination of the feces for *Endamoeba histolytica*, when such an examination can be made by one experienced in the differentiation of this ameba from the other intestinal amebae of man. It has been the experience of the writer that repeated examinations of the feces will almost invariably result in the demonstration of this parasite, if it be present, except in those in whom an abscess of the liver or other organ has developed after the intestinal infection has disappeared, as sometimes happens; and repeated examinations of the feces should always be made before resort is had to the complement-fixation test in the diagnosis of amebiasis.''

When it is impossible to obtain accurate fecal examinations the complement fixation test is of great value and should be employed. However, one should be sure that the individual making this test has had experience with it and is well qualified, as the test is a very technical one and mistakes are easily made in its performance and it is difficult to obtain a good antigen for use in the test.

The complement fixation test is especially useful in the diagnosis of amebic liver abscess under certain conditions, and in the control of various methods of treatment. In the diagnosis of carriers it has been found most useful in routine hospital practice and in making surveys when trained personnel in fecal examinations is not available. The routine application of this test in hospital practice has resulted in the discovery of many carriers of *Endamoeba histolytica*, who, because of absence of definite intestinal symptomatology, would not have been suspected of infection with this organism. Likewise, amebic abscess of the liver has been diagnosed by means of this test in patients in whom these symptoms were atypical, or practically absent, or in whom the intestinal infection had disappeared. The complement fixation test for amebiasis is most useful in the judging of the relative efficiency of drugs recommended in the treatment of this condition and in the control of treatment. Its value, in this respect, depends upon the fact that the elimination of the amebic infection in patients giving a positive complement-fixation reaction is followed within a month, as a rule, by the disappearance of the reaction. It has also been found that sometimes the complement-fixation reaction becomes positive in cases that relapse before amebae can be demonstrated in the stools, proving that the parasites are living in the tissues of the intestine although the stools are negative. A permanent negative reaction in individuals who have given a positive reaction before treatment is conclusive as to the elimination of the infection, while a continued positive reaction after treatment, even though the stools are negative for *Endamoeba histolytica,* indicates that further treatment is necessary in order to eliminate the infection. In the control of treatment the complement fixation test should be made immediately after completion of treatment and at least once a month thereafter for a period of four months, and if, during this time, a negative reaction becomes positive, treatment should be resumed.

The finding of *Endamoeba histolytica* in the stools, or a positive complement fixation test, should not be taken as conclusive of the nature of any clinical condition present until a most careful examination has been made by the clinician for other possible disease conditions. It should be remembered that infection with this parasite occurs in from 5 to 10 per cent of individuals in this country and that it must be very frequently a complicating condition in many other infections and diseases, so that a most careful consideration of all of the symptoms and physical signs present should be made before the clinical condition present is diagnosed as due to this ameba. If this is not done, very serious errors in diagnosis may occur. Thus, malignant disease of the stomach or intestine may remain undiagnosed because the symptoms present are believed to be caused by *Endamoeba histolytica,* owing to the presence of this parasite in the stools or a positive complement-fixation reaction. Such mistakes should not occur if a proper study is made of each case for the possible existence of an infection or disease, the amebic infection being simply coincident.

Prognosis.—The prognosis of amebiasis varies with the resistance of the individual to the infection, the length of time that the infection has existed, the presence or absence of serious symptoms, as dysentery, and the dose and virulence of the infecting strain of *Endamoeba histolytica.* The prognosis in carriers without symptoms is quite different from that in acute amebic dysentery or amebic abscess of the liver, and it is therefore necessary to consider the prognosis in the various types of amebiasis separately.

In *carriers and individuals presenting very mild intestinal symptoms,* the prognosis as regards danger to life and the chances of ultimate elimination of the infection with proper treatment is most excellent. In many of these individuals the infection disappears without treatment while proper treatment is followed by the elimination of the infection in practically 100 per cent of the cases. However, it should be remembered that in even these mild infections lesions are being constantly produced in the bowel and there is always some danger of the development of a liver abscess, so that, while the prognosis is excellent in the vast majority of cases, the patient should be given proper treatment as soon as the infection is discovered, and, if treatment is refused, the prognosis should be guarded and the patient informed of the danger of the development of serious complications.

With the development of repeated attacks of severe diarrhea the prognosis becomes less favorable and should always be guarded, for even proper treatment sometimes fails to eliminate the infection if the diar-rheal attacks have occurred for a considerable period of time.

In *acute amebic dysentery*, with proper treatment, the prognosis is excellent as to recovery from the acute symptoms but should be guarded as to the elimination of the infection. In these cases the amebae have penetrated deeply into the bowel wall and even the drugs which have been found practically specific may not reach them for various reasons, and the infection cannot be eliminated. The prognosis as regards the elimination of the infection becomes progressively worse with each re-curring attack of dysentery, and in the old *chronic cases of amebic dysentery* the prognosis as to cure is usually hopeless, although many of these patients live for years but are more or less invalided by the infec-tion. In untreated cases of acute amebic dysentery the prognosis is good so far as recovery from the acute attack is concerned, but in the so-called fulminant cases the prognosis is very bad and death may occur within a few days despite treatment. The occurrence of complications, as severe hemorrhage, gangrene of the intestine, or perforation during the acute dysenteric attack, renders the prognosis very grave and death usually occurs.

The prognosis in *amebic abscess of the liver* is grave, but if such ab-scesses are discovered early, and proper medical treatment adopted, the prognosis is good. In cases in which the preceding amebic hepatitis has been diagnosed and proper treatment with emetine hydrochloride has been given, the prognosis is excellent, and an amebic abscess of the liver is prevented from developing, but after the development of an ab-scess the prognosis depends upon the duration and size of the abscess, the resistance of the patient and the character of treatment. It should always be guarded, for many patients die despite the best treatment. The occurrence of multiple abscesses renders the prognosis exceedingly grave and most of these cases are fatal, in the writer's experience.

The *prognosis of amebic appendicitis* is excellent if proper treatment is administered, but if undiagnosed and operated upon the prognosis is poor. It has been found that many deaths have occurred following an operation upon the appendix in individuals suffering from intestinal amebiasis, so that the early recognition of the involvement of the appen-dix and proper treatment with anti-amebic drugs is essential for a good prognosis.

The *prognosis of amebic abscess of the brain* is hopeless as death has occurred in all reported cases.

The *prognosis of amebic abscess of the lung* depends upon the time of recognition and the treatment administered. Many cases of lung abscess caused by *Endamoeba histolytica* are not discovered until the patient has become greatly exhausted by the toxemia, fever and other symptoms caused by the condition, and the fact that the vast majority of cases of amebic abscess of the lung also suffer from an abscess of the liver, ren-ders the prognosis still more grave. If the condition is discovered promptly and treatment with emetine hydrochloride is instituted, the prognosis is fair but should always be guarded.

Prophylaxis.—As infection with *Endamoeba histolytica* is usually acquired through the ingestion of food or drink contaminated with fecal material containing the cysts of this parasite, prophylaxis depends upon the prevention of such contamination. In discussing the epidemi-

38111

ology of amebiasis it will be recalled that the methods of contamination of food or drink are through a polluted water supply, infected food handlers, the use of human excrement in the fertilization of garden truck, and the droppings of flies, cockroaches and possibly other insects that have fed upon feces containing the cysts of *Endamoeba histolytica*.

PREVENTION OF TRANSMISSION THROUGH WATER.—The prevention of the pollution of water supplies and the sterilization of polluted water are most important in the prophylaxis of amebiasis. In a community which has a filtered general water supply there is little chance of the transmission of this infection unless through the pollution of the water locally by sewage contamination through cross-connections between the general water supply and sewers, as occurred in the hotel epidemic in Chicago. Filtration through sand filters removes the cysts of *Endamoeba histolytica* and it has been invariably noted that in communities where amebiasis and amebic dysentery were very prevalent the installment of a filtered public water supply is followed by a great decrease in amebic infections.

The role of water in the transmission of amebiasis has been recognized for many years and it is in rural communities where the water supply is obtained from wells and springs, and where the practice of indiscriminate defecation is common, that transmission of this infection most often occurs through polluted water. This method of transmission is also common in military operations in the field when the soldiers drink water from any available source despite orders to the contrary, as was well illustrated in our army operating in the Philippines during the Insurrection. Therefore, the **proper disposal of feces** is a most important prophylactic method and the sanitary privy is just as important in the control of amebiasis as in the control of hookworm or any other parasitic or bacterial infection transmitted by water. Every habitation in rural regions should be provided with a sanitary privy and indiscriminate defecation should be avoided. If fecal material is deposited upon the ground about dwellings, the cysts of this parasite are almost sure to be washed into wells or springs from which the drinking water is obtained, resulting in the transmission of amebiasis through the polluted water.

If a water is suspected or known to be subject to fecal pollution, the only methods of rendering it safe for human consumption is filtration through a sand or porcelain filter, or by boiling. Chlorination, as practiced in the sterilization of water for pathogenic bacteria, is useless in rendering water safe if it contains the cysts of *Endamoeba histolytica*, as these cysts are not killed by any amount of chlorine that can be used for this purpose. If proper filters are not available, boiling must be resorted to in order to kill the cysts, for at the present time there is no chemical method of sterilization of water that is effective in destroying the cysts of this parasite. Travelers in regions where amebiasis is present should insist upon using boiled water only for drinking purposes.

In view of the Chicago experience a careful survey of the possible existence of cross-connections between sewers and the water-supply pipes of hotels, public buildings, factories and restaurants is a preventive measure of much importance. While such connections are unlawful they do exist in many buildings and, while usually not harmful, backing up of sewage may occur in times of flood and the water be contaminated. Such surveys should be made by an experienced sanitary engineer and not by an ordinary plumber, for it is often very difficult to locate the cross-connections, if they do exist.

PREVENTION OF TRANSMISSION BY INFECTED FOOD HANDLERS.—It has already been mentioned, in discussing the epidemiology of amebiasis, that food handlers in hotels, restaurants and in the home are frequently infected with *Endamoeba histolytica* and may transmit the infection to others by contaminating food or drink in handling it, if they are careless as regards personal cleanliness. The relative importance of this method of transmission is actually unknown but it is impossible to explain the occurrence of amebiasis to any extent in a community in which there is a filtered water supply and proper disposal of sewage in any other way than by the contamination of food or drink by infected carriers, so that this method of transmission must be of great importance in such places. Many food handlers are very careless as regards personal cleanliness and it has been experimentally demonstrated that the cysts of this ameba will live beneath the finger nails and upon the hands long enough to be transferred to food. Thus, the examination of food handlers for possible infection, and their proper treatment, is important in the prevention of amebiasis and is a practical measure in many localities. The fact that so many individuals are engaged in preparing food and that a considerable proportion of them would be found infected and require treatment is not an argument against doing what is possible in this respect, and while it would be probably impossible to examine all food handlers and treat the infected in large communities, it is possible to do this in many instances, owing to the small numbers involved, and in our smaller villages and towns it is feasible to examine all food handlers in public eating places for this infection and to render them harmless by treatment which will eliminate their infections.

If food handlers are found infected it is not necessary that they be removed from their occupation during treatment, although this would be best, but if they are informed as to their danger to others and how they may render themselves noninfective, they may continue their occupation while undergoing treatment. Likewise, if one member of a family is found infected with *Endamoeba histolytica,* it is perfectly feasible to examine all other members of the family for possible infection and to treat those found infected.

It is notorious that the incidence of infection with this parasite is exceedingly high in public institutions, as insane asylums, orphan asylums, poor houses and hospitals, and one of the most important preventive measures in such institutions consists in examining all who handle food for this organism and treating all who are found infected. If possible, all inmates should also be examined and treated.

If food handlers are discovered to be infected they should be instructed to scrub their hands thoroughly in soap and water after leaving the toilet and before handling food. Indeed, if the simple procedure of washing the hands carefully after visiting the toilet and before each meal were followed by every one, it is certain that a great deal of infection with this, and other intestinal parasites, would be avoided and the incidence of parasitic disease of the intestine in man would be greatly decreased.

38111

The results that have been obtained in surveys for *Endamoeba histolytica* fully demonstrate the value of such surveys in the discovery and control of amebiasis. Thus, Seckinger (1936), in certain villages in rural Georgia, examined the members of 60 families, comprising 290 individuals, and found 162 (55.8 per cent) infected. In several families the infection rate was as high as 90 per cent, and in one family of 11 members no less than 10 were found positive for *Endamoeba histolytica*. Of these individuals, 1 presented the symptoms of amebic dysentery at the time of examination, in 5 others symptoms of amebiasis were present, while in 4 there were no symptoms of the infection. It is perfectly evident that the discovery and proper treatment of the infections in this group of individuals would greatly benefit those infected and also the community in which they lived, and amply justify the time and money consumed in making the surveys. As much as possible should be done in the examination of food handlers, and the elimination of the infection in those found infected, or we fall short in our application of methods for the prevention of amebiasis.

PREVENTION OF INFECTION BY GARDEN PRODUCE FERTILIZED BY HUMAN EXCREMENT.—In many Oriental countries, as China and Japan, and in some areas in other countries, where vegetable gardens are operated by Orientals, the use of human excrement for fertilization purposes is common. It is evident that garden truck grown under such conditions is very apt to be contaminated with the cysts of *Endamoeba histolytica* and a source of infection to those using such vegetables, if they are prepared and eaten without previous cooking. The enforcement of existing laws forbidding the use of human excrement in the fertilization of garden vegetables is an important preventive measure in amebiasis and, if such laws are not in existence, and it is impossible to place them upon the statute books because of economic or other conditions, one should avoid eating any raw garden produce in regions where such a practice exists. The writer has observed several infections with this ameba in individuals who persisted in eating raw garden produce in such localities despite warnings to the contrary, and the traveler in countries where human excrement is used for fertilization purposes (and this practice will be found to be prevalent in gardens operated by Chinese or Japanese) should realize the grave danger from this source of infection and abstain from eating uncooked vegetables in any form, but especially in the form of salads.

PREVENTION OF INFECTION BY FLIES.—It has already been stated that the cysts of *Endamoeba histolytica* may live in the intestine of flies and be voided in a viable condition as long as 48 hours after the insect has fed upon material contaminated by feces containing the cysts. It is thus evident that the prevention of the breeding of flies and the protection of food from these insects is an important prophylactic measure in regions where amebic infection is endemic and flies are numerous. Food offered for sale in such regions should be covered by appropriate screening devices and the utmost care should be taken to prevent the breeding of flies by proper disposal of wastes. What has been said regarding transmission by flies applies equally well to cockroaches, for it has been demonstrated that the cysts of this ameba may live in, and be voided from, the intestine of cockroaches for many hours after the insects have fed upon material containing them.

OTHER METHODS OF PREVENTION.—In many states and countries amebiasis is not a reportable disease and thus the health statistics of such regions give one no accurate information regarding the prevalence of this infection. One of the most important indirect preventive measures against this infection is making it a **reportable** one, so that some idea may be obtained on its relative incidence and importance in different localities. Until this is done one cannot intelligently apply preventive measures in any locality and much time and money will be frequently wasted in preventing an infection that may be of very little practical importance in certain localities, while nothing is being done in other localities where the infection is an important public health problem.

The **training of laboratory technicians and physicians** in the recognition of the various intestinal amebae of man, and the differentiation of *Endamoeba histolytica* from the other species occurring in the intestine, is a most important indirect prophylactic measure, for unless accurate diagnoses are possible little can be accomplished in the prevention of this infection. Such trained technicians should be available in all city, county and state health laboratories and specimens should be sent to such laboratories for diagnosis unless the attending physician has facilities for making the differential diagnosis.

The **education of the public** regarding the importance of infection with *Endamoeba histolytica*, the methods by which the infection is transmitted, and the measures that are effective in preventing such transmission, is an important indirect prophylactic measure. The public should be informed that amebiasis and amebic dysentery are not tropical infections but prevalent throughout the world, and that infection with this parasite may lead to serious complications, especially amebic abscess of the liver, even though intestinal symptomatology may be slight or absent. The part played by symptomless carriers, especially those who are food handlers, should be stressed, and the importance of personal hygiene in the prevention of infection should be emphasized. The instruction of the public would lead to a demand that proper preventive measures be initiated by the proper authorities, and thus funds would be made available and the true importance of amebiasis as a public health problem would be recognized. Public education as regards amebiasis may be accomplished through the issue of pamphlets by the constituted health departments, through information furnished by the family physician, through radio broadcasts by proper authorities and through instruction in schools and colleges during courses in hygiene. Much may be accomplished by the education of the public in the prophylaxis of amebiasis.

Treatment.—DRUGS THAT ARE AVAILABLE IN THE TREATMENT OF AMEBIASIS.—For the treatment of amebiasis we possess several drugs that are practically specific and these will be considered as regards their chemical nature, their toxic properties and their action upon *Endamoeba histolytica*, after which their application in the treatment of the various phases of amebiasis will be discussed.

At the present time the drugs that have proved most useful in the treatment of amebiasis are **chiniofon, vioform, carbarsone** and **emetine hydrochloride.**

Chiniofon.—This drug was introduced by Mühlens and Menk (1921), under the proprietary name of "yatren," as a specific in amebic dysentery. It is also marketed under the name "anayodin." Chemically it is sodium iodoxyquinolinesulphonate, and depends for its amebicidal properties upon iodine, of which it contains from 26 to 28 per cent. It is supplied by several firms in tablets or pills, each containing 0.25 Gm. (4 Gr.), either uncoated or keratin coated.

The *action* of this drug upon *Endamoeba histolytica* is apparently a direct one upon the motile forms, or trophozoites, and its proper administration is followed by the elimination of the infection in most cases. Vogel (1927) found that a dilution of 1:1000 killed all of the trophozoites of the ameba in cultures within 12 hours, while a dilution of 1:100 killed them in 3 hours. Kofoid and Wagener (1925) found that a dilution of 1:1250 killed all the trophozoites in cultures within 24 hours.

The *toxicity* of chiniofon is very low and it is probably the safest of all the drugs that are now employed in the treatment of amebiasis. Under the name of "yatren," it has been used for nearly 18 years in the treatment of amebic dysentery and the writer has failed to find recorded in the literature a single death caused by this drug when given orally, although Maxon (1933) has reported two deaths apparently caused by it after intravenous administration, a method never recommended for the administration of the drug. The writer has employed the drug in the treatment of hundreds of cases of amebiasis and has never observed any serious toxic symptoms following its use or any injurious effect to health even after repeated courses of treatment with the drug.

Some individuals are more susceptible to chiniofon than others and symptoms are not infrequently observed which by some are considered as toxic in nature. When given in full doses chiniofon usually produces considerable diarrhea during the first few days of its administration but usually this diarrhea is not severe in character, but rarely may be so debilitating that the dose of the drug has to be reduced or administration stopped. In some few cases colicky pains in the abdomen follow administration in full doses. These symptoms can hardly be called toxic and are of no consequence in the vast majority of cases, and it is the universal opinion of those who have extensively employed chiniofon in the treatment of amebiasis that it is a nontoxic drug and an efficient amebicide.

The administration of chiniofon in the treatment of amebiasis is usually followed by the elimination of the infection, but, as in the case of most specific drugs, it sometimes fails to accomplish this and resort must be had to the other remedies that have been found efficient. The writer believes, as the result of extended experience with chiniofon, that, all in all, it is the most efficient drug we possess in the treatment of this infection but it does not eliminate all infections with *Endamoeba histolytica* as some would have us believe.

Vioform.—For several years this drug has been upon the market as a dusting powder used in surgery and was introduced to replace iodoform, as it is odorless. In 1931 Anderson and Koch found that vioform was an efficient amebicide in experimental amebiasis in monkeys and in 1933, David, Johnstone, Read and Leake recommended it in the treatment of amebiasis in man. Chemically it is iodochloroxyquinoline, and depends for its amebicidal activity upon iodine, of which it contains from 37.5 to 41.5 per cent, thus being much richer in iodine than is chiniofon. It also contains from 11.5 to 12.2 per cent of chlorine but whether the chlorine has any amebicidal effect is still undecided. It is marketed as a powder and is administered orally in amebiasis in gelatin capsules each containing 0.25 Gm. (4 Gr.) of the drug.

The *action* of this drug, like that of chiniofon, is a direct one upon the trophozoites of *Endamoeba histolytica,* and depends probably almost entirely upon the iodine content of the drug.

The *toxicity* of vioform appears to be greater than that of chiniofon but is slight unless excessive doses be administered. In rabbits the administration of very large doses resulted in fatty infiltration of the liver with areas of necrosis, while the renal tubules were slightly injured, but the doses employed were such as would never be used in the treatment of amebiasis in man. Among the toxic symptoms that have been noted in rare instances in man, after the administration of this drug in therapeutic doses, were diarrhea, abdominal colic, dyspnea, palpitation of the heart, severe headache, and excessive nervousness, while in one case reported by Anderson and Reed (1934), blood and mucus appeared in the stools after the administration of this drug. The writer has never observed any toxic symptoms in patients treated with vioform and believes that it is a safe drug to use in the treatment of amebiasis.

The *efficiency* of vioform in eliminating infections with *Endamoeba histolytica* is not superior to that of chiniofon, as claimed by some authorities, in the experience of the writer. It has failed in his hands in some cases that responded to chiniofon and it is not recommended in preference to chiniofon in treatment. The one advantage that it possesses is its greater content of iodine, which makes it possible to give a smaller number of pills or capsules per day but it is not believed that this advantage compensates for its lesser efficiency in eliminating infection with this parasite.

Carbarsone.—This drug was introduced by Anderson and Reed (1931) as a specific in the treatment of amebiasis. Chemically it is *p*-carbamino-phenyl arsonic acid and depends for its amebicidal properties upon arsenic, of which it contains 28.85 per cent. It is marketed in capsules, each containing 0.25 Gm. (4 Gr.) of the drug, and is administered by mouth and by rectal injections.

The *action* of carbarsone is a direct one upon the trophozoites of *Endamoeba histolytica,* depending upon its arsenic content.

The *toxicity* of carbarsone is greater than that of chiniofon or vioform but it appears to be the least toxic of any of the arsenicals that have been advocated in the treatment of amebiasis. As is well known, many individuals have a marked susceptibility to arsenic, so that it would be expected that toxic symptoms would be more often observed after the administration of this drug than after that of chiniofon, but extensive use of this drug has demonstrated that while unpleasant symptoms do sometimes occur it is a safe drug to use so far as danger to life is concerned.

The toxic symptoms that have been noted after the administration of carbarsone have been severe abdominal colic, diarrhea, puffiness of the face, erythematous skin eruptions, abdominal distention, dyspnea and prostration, with a rapid, thready pulse. Such symptoms are very rarely encountered in the experience of the writer.

38111

Emetine Hydrochloride.—The use of emetine hydrochloride, one of the alkaloids of ipecacuanha, was initiated by the discovery by Vedder, in 1912, that this drug was a powerful amebicide to free-living amebae when added to cultures of the latter. This discovery impelled Rogers in 1912 to employ it in the treatment of amebic dysentery and amebic hepatitis, with excellent results. The powdered root of ipecacuanha had been used in India for the treatment of dysentery since 1660, but the discovery of the alkaloid, emetine, and its effect upon free-living amebae has resulted in the complete abandonment of ipecacuanha as a remedy in amebiasis.

Emetine hydrochloride has been very extensively employed in the treatment of amebiasis and for many years was regarded as a specific, but more recent studies have shown that while it is most efficient in controlling the symptoms of amebic dysentery it is not capable of eliminating amebic infection when employed alone, except in a comparatively small proportion of cases. For this reason, **emetine hydrochloride should not be employed in the treatment of amebiasis to eliminate the infection but only to control the symptoms of severe diarrhea or dysentery,** after which either chiniofon or carbarsone should be administered. Emetine hydrochloride is given by subcutaneous injection, not to exceed 0.065 Gm. (1 Gr.) per day, for not over 12 days.

The *action* of emetine hydrochloride is directly upon the motile forms, or trophozoites, of *Endamoeba histolytica.* James (1915) has shown that definite degenerative changes occur in the trophozoites after the administration of emetine, consisting in granular disintegration of the nucleus and a fibrillar disintegration of the cytoplasm, and many authorities have shown that this drug is capable of destroying the trophozoites of this ameba in cultures in high dilutions.

Although emetine hydrochloride is capable of destroying the trophozoites of *Endamoeba histolytica* in cultures it is not an efficient amebicide in eliminating infection with this parasite, in the experience of the writer. In the treatment of 115 cases of amebic dysentery in which a full course of 0.065 Gm. (1 Gr.) of the drug was administered subcutaneously for 12 days, and repeated in at least half of the cases, no less than 65 (56.5 per cent) presented cysts of the ameba in the stools after the discontinuance of the treatment for varying lengths of time, while further treatment of these individuals with the drug resulted in the elimination of the infection in but 4 (6 per cent). In 40 per cent of these cases the amebae did not disappear from the stools during treatment, although the dysenteric symptoms disappeared, thus demonstrating that the disappearance of symptoms does not indicate the elimination of the infection in patients treated with emetine, and the importance of repeated stool examinations for the parasite after treatment has been completed. Emetine hydrochloride is an excellent drug for the control of the dysenteric symptoms in amebic dysentery but should not be used to eliminate the infection as other drugs are much superior to it in this respect.

The *toxicity of emetine* is much greater than that of either chiniofon or carbarsone. It is a cumulative drug and has a direct action upon the heart muscle, causing degenerative changes which may result in a myocarditis, and death may occur from sudden heart failure. Other toxic symptoms produced by this drug are severe diarrhea; excessive muscular weakness, especially of the legs; nausea; vomiting; abdominal pain; increased rapidity of the pulse; weak heart action with irregularities; muscular tremors; fainting spells and low blood pressure. In addition, Chopra (1934) states that general edema, purpuric skin eruptions, albuminuria, polyneuritis, and cerebral and pulmonary edema may occur.

It is thus evident that emetine is a dangerous drug to use unless its administration is carefully controlled and overdosage is avoided, but despite what is known regarding its toxicity, it is frequently employed in much larger doses than those which have been found to be safe, and continued over longer periods of time. The cumulative action of this drug appears to have been largely forgotten by the profession and has resulted in gross abuse in its administration and much harm to many individuals taking it. The writer has observed several cases in which death from myocarditis, or from sudden cardiac failure, was apparently caused by excessive dosage with emetine, and many more in which severe toxic symptoms were produced. Because of its toxicity and its inefficiency in eliminating infection with *Endamoeba histolytica,* this drug should be employed only to control dysentery symptoms and as little of it used for this purpose as is possible, after which the infection should be eliminated with either chiniofon, vioform or carbarsone.

Other Drugs in the Treatment of Amebiasis.—In addition to the drugs that have been considered there are a number of other drugs that have been employed as specifics in the treatment of amebiasis. The most important of these are the following:

(*a*) *Emetine Bismuth Iodide.*—This is a combination of emetine, bismuth and iodine which was first recommended by DuMez (1915) in the treatment of amebiasis. It contains approximately 29 per cent of emetine, 12 per cent of bismuth and 58 per cent of iodine. It is administered by mouth in capsules and the dose is 0.2 Gm. (3 Gr.) once a day for 12 days. It usually causes nausea and sometimes vomiting for the first day or two of treatment, and the patient must be kept in bed during the entire course of treatment. The *toxicity* of the combination is that of the drugs present, especially of emetine; and the development of excessive diarrhea, severe nausea or vomiting, or a rapid, weak or irregular pulse, with a fall in blood pressure, are indications that its administration should be stopped. Emetine bismuth iodide is an efficient amebicidal drug but possesses the great disadvantage that the patient must be in bed while it is being administered, while there is not sufficient evidence available to prove that it is any more efficient than the drugs that have already been considered. While superior to emetine alone in eliminating amebic infection, owing to its high iodine content, it is not recommended in the treatment of amebiasis for the reason that we possess other drugs that are apparently as efficient and much less unpleasant in their action. The writer believes that emetine bismuth iodide is of so little practical value in the treatment of infection with *Endamoeba histolytica* that its use for this purpose should be abandoned.

(*b*) *Treparsol.*—This drug is an arsenical which apparently acts directly upon the trophozoites of *Endamoeba histolytica* and favorable reports have been made as regards its efficiency by those who have employed it. It is furnished in tablets, each containing 0.25 Gm. (4 Gr.),

38111

and 1 tablet is administered three times a day with meals for 4 days and this course is repeated three times, with an interval of 10 days between each course of 4 days' treatment. According to Brown (1928), the tablets should be chewed with the food for the best results.

The *toxicity* of this drug is that of arsenic and care should be used in its administration. However, according to Brown (1935) of the Mayo Clinic, who has treated with it 301 patients suffering from amebiasis, the only toxic symptoms that were noted were a toxic erythema in 8 cases and nausea and vomiting in but 1 case. In view of this experience, it is evident that treparsol is not very toxic and the results that have been obtained with it in eliminating amebic infection have been excellent, according to those who have had sufficient experience with the drug.

(c) *Kurchi Bark.*—This is the bark of a small deciduous tree, *Holarrhena antidysenterica,* and decoctions of this bark have long been used in India in the treatment of dysentery. Several alkaloids have been isolated from the bark and Chopra (1933) has employed four of these alkaloids, i.e., conessine, kurchicine, kurchine and holarrhenine in combination, in the treatment of amebic dysentery by intramuscular injection. More recently, this method of treatment has been replaced by the oral administration of a preparation known as kurchi-bismuthus-iodide, a combination of the alkaloids of kurchi bark with bismuth and iodine. The dose of this preparation, in chronic amebic infections, is 0.25 Gm. (4 Gr.) orally twice a day for 10 days, while in severe amebic dysentery or diarrhea as much as 0.65 Gm. (10 Gr.) may be given orally twice a day for 10 days.

The toxicity of kurchi-bismuthus-iodide is slight and those who have employed this drug in the treatment of amebiasis have reported excellent results, with no toxic complications.

Among other drugs that have been recommended in the treatment of amebiasis may be mentioned bismuth subnitrate, dihydranol, Chaparro amargoso, emetine periodide, aburemetine, diodoquin, acetarsone, amibiarsone and gavano. None of these are as efficient as chiniofon or carbarsone and are not recommended in the treatment of this infection.

THE TREATMENT OF AMEBIASIS.—The treatment of amebiasis varies with the type of the infection. Thus the treatment of amebic dysentery is quite different from the treatment of symptomless carriers of *Endamoeba histolytica,* or of infections characterized by other intestinal symptoms. Therefore, in discussing the subject of treatment, it is necessary to divide it into the treatment of carriers, of patients presenting mild intestinal symptomatology, and of those presenting severe symptoms of the infection, as attacks of continued diarrhea or of acute amebic dysentery and amebic abscess of the liver. It is most important that carriers and patients presenting mild symptomatology be properly treated as the infection may be easily eliminated in most and thus the development of serious symptoms and complication may be avoided.

Treatment of Carriers Without Symptoms.—It has already been stated that even though definite symptoms of amebic infection may not be present, considerable ulceration may have occurred in the intestine, and amebic hepatitis and abscess of the liver sometimes develop in such cases. In view of these facts, it is most important that symptomless carriers be properly treated, not only to prevent the development of symptoms but also to prevent the transmission of the infection to others. The impression that apparently prevails among the profession that individuals infected with *Endamoeba histolytica* need not be treated unless symptoms are produced by the invasion of the intestinal walls by the parasite is most pernicious and it should be distinctly understood that **every infection with this organism should be treated even though no symptoms are present** and the individual is apparently in good health.

It is obvious that in the treatment of symptomless carriers a drug should be employed that will not necessitate the interruption of his occupation by the individual taking it, and which can be taken without discomfort or injury to health. Fortunately, we possess in chiniofon, vioform and carbarsone drugs which fulfill these requirements and which are very efficient in eliminating amebic infection in this class of cases.

In the treatment of symptomless carriers the writer has found **chiniofon** to be the most generally useful and efficient. It is administered by mouth in the form of tablets or pills, each containing 0.25 Gm. (4 Gr.), and the dose is 3 pills three times a day, after eating, for an adult weighing 150 pounds, and this dosage is continued for 8 to 10 days. If the full dose of 3 pills three times a day causes severe diarrhea, which may continue for several days, the writer usually recommends 2 pills three times a day and increase to 3 pills three times a day if possible. The diarrhea that is produced by full doses of this drug, if not excessive, increases the efficiency of the treatment, as it removes from the intestine many of the amebae and thus helps to eliminate the infection. The dosage for children should be correlated with the age and weight of the child. No precautions are necessary as regards exercise or diet while taking this drug, with the exception that rich or very sweet food should be avoided owing to the liability of gaseous distention due to fermentation and imperfect digestion.

In the vast majority of symptomless carriers one course of treatment with chiniofon has resulted in the elimination of the infection, in the writer's experience. If the infection still persists, the course of treatment may be repeated after an interval of 10 days or 2 weeks, and the second course of treatment almost invariably eliminates the infection. A careful microscopic examination should be made of the stools after the completion of the treatment, and at monthly intervals thereafter for at least three months, and if trophozoites or cysts of *Endamoeba histolytica* are found, the treatment should be repeated.

Carbarsone is sometimes effective in eliminating the infection in carriers of *Endamoeba histolytica* in those cases in which chiniofon has not been successful, but this drug is not recommended in treatment unless chiniofon has failed, for the reason that, being an arsenical, toxic symptoms of severe character may occur in individuals who are susceptible to arsenic, although carbarsone is, in the opinion of the writer, the least toxic of any of the arsenicals that have been used in the treatment of amebiasis.

Carbarsone should be administered in capsules, each containing 0.25 Gm. (4 Gr.) of the drug, the dose being one capsule twice a day for 10 days for an adult, at the end of which time the stools are examined for trophozoites or cysts of *Endamoeba histolytica*. If the stools are found to be positive the course of treatment may be repeated after an interval of 10 days without treatment, and, in most infections, a repetition of the course of treatment is necessary in order to eliminate the infection. This drug should be administered under the supervision of a physician and the dosage recommended should not be exceeded.

Vioform is useful in the treatment of carriers and is preferred by some to chiniofon, owing to the fact that a smaller number of pills may be administered. This drug is very rarely successful in cases in which chiniofon and carbarsone have failed, but should be tried in such cases. It is administered in capsules, each capsule containing 0.25 Gm. (4 Gr.), and 1 capsule is administered three times a day for 10 days, an interval of 10 days allowed to elapse without any treatment, and the same dose repeated for another 10 days.

In the treatment of symptomless carriers the writer would recommend chiniofon as the drug of choice and if this fails a course of carbarsone. If the latter is unsuccessful in eliminating the infection, vioform should be administered. He has never observed a case of a carrier in whom the infection could not be eliminated by the use of these drugs, and **emetine should never be used in the treatment of this type of amebiasis.** With none of the drugs mentioned is it necessary for the infected individual to be in bed or to interrupt his occupation while taking the drug.

Treatment of Patients with Mild Intestinal Symptoms.—In the treatment of individuals presenting mild symptoms of intestinal amebiasis, i.e., those belonging in Class II (*q.v.*), the same drugs, administered in the same manner, are recommended as in the treatment of carriers without symptoms, and emetine hydrochloride should not be administered. With either chiniofon, vioform or carbarsone, administered alone or combined in different courses of treatment, practically all individuals presenting mild symptoms can be cured. Here, again, it is not necessary for the patient to interrupt his occupation during treatment.

Treatment of Patients with Severe Symptoms of Amebiasis.—The treatment of patients presenting symptoms of severe diarrhea or dysentery, or amebic hepatitis or amebic abscess of the liver differs essentially from that already recommended for carriers and for mild amebic infections.

In *patients having severe diarrhea* **rest in bed** is essential, and if the bowel movements exceed six or eight a day, 0.065 Gm. (1 Gr.) of **emetine hydrochloride** should be injected subcutaneously once a day until the diarrheal symptoms have subsided, after which it should be discontinued and **chiniofon** administered as already advised. In from 4 to 6 days after the beginning of the administration of emetine the diarrhea will usually have ceased. If not, the emetine may be continued until 0.8 Gm. (12 Gr.) have been administered but no more.

The *treatment of acute amebic dysentery* consists in **rest in bed,** the subcutaneous administration of 0.065 Gm. (1 Gr.) of **emetine hydrochloride** daily for a period not to exceed 12 days, and a course of **chiniofon** after the emetine has been stopped. Usually in from 6 to 8 days the dysenteric stools will have disappeared under treatment with the emetine, but chiniofon should be administered if we are to be successful in eliminating the infection. If the infection is not eliminated by chiniofon administered as already recommended in treating carriers or mild amebic infections, **carbarsone** or **vioform** may be tried, administered as already directed.

In the treatment of amebic dysentery in patients in whom emetine is contraindicated, as in those suffering from myocarditis or valvular disease of the heart, one must rely upon the administration of chiniofon, vioform or carbarsone. In such cases the administration of chiniofon both by mouth and by rectal injection may be useful, the drug being administered by mouth in doses of 2 pills three times a day, each pill containing 0.25 Gm. (4 Gr.), while a daily retention enema of 200 cc. of a 2 per cent warm water solution of chiniofon should be employed, the solution to be retained as long as possible, and this treatment continued for 8 to 10 days.

If carbarsone is employed alone in the treatment of amebic dysentery and the dysenteric condition has not been improved, this drug may be given rectally as a retention enema, oral administration being stopped. If used in this manner, 200 cc. of a 2 per cent sodium bicarbonate solution in warm water to which 1 per cent of carbarsone has been added should be injected and retained as long as is possible. Such retention enemas should be employed for at least 5 days.

In the vast majority of cases of acute amebic dysentery the use of emetine hydrochloride and chiniofon, as recommended, will be followed by recovery and elimination of the infection, and rectal injections of either chiniofon or carbarsone will not be necessary.

The *treatment of chronic amebic dysentery,* during acute exacerbations, is that of acute amebic dysentery, while between the dysenteric attacks the treatment should be that recommended in carriers and mild amebic infections, i.e., the administration of **chiniofon, vioform** or **carbarsone.**

As already stated, the treatment of amebic infection, whatever the symptomatology, should be checked by a careful examination of the stools after treatment has been completed and, if possible, by a complement fixation test. If amebae are still present, or the complement fixation test is still positive a month after completion of treatment, the treatment should be repeated.

The *treatment of amebic hepatitis* consists in the subcutaneous injection of 0.065 Gm. (1 Gr.) of **emetine hydrochloride** daily for a period not to exceed 12 days. This treatment is specific in this condition and is followed by the rapid disappearance of the tenderness over the liver, of fever and of the leukocytosis which is usually present. If the symptoms are not alleviated by the treatment, the hepatitis is not of amebic origin or abscess formation has already occurred and demands operative treatment.

The *treatment of amebic abscess of the liver* is largely *surgical,* but the fact that small abscesses may be healed by the administration of emetine renders it important that in every case of amebic abscess of the liver a course of emetine should be administered unless conditions are such as to demand immediate surgical interference. Subcutaneous injection of 0.065 Gm. (1 Gr.) of **emetine hydrochloride** should be made daily for a period not to exceed 12 days, and in some cases this will be followed by a rapid disappearance of the symptoms and complete recovery. If the condition does not improve with this treatment, resort should be had to surgical measures, as puncture and aspiration of the abscess contents, or, if necessary, to more radical procedures, which are described in works upon surgery. The treatment with emetine should be employed together with aspiration as it markedly reduces the mortality in operative cases.

The *treatment of amebic abscess of the lung* consists in the administration of **emetine hydrochloride** as in amebic abscess of the liver. Ochsner and DeBakey (1936) recommend treatment with emetine and aspiration of abscesses that are not sufficiently drained through the bronchus, while open drainage should never be practiced unless secondary infection is present. They state that the incidence of recovery in collected cases treated without emetine was 43.9 per cent as compared with 91.8 per cent when treated with emetine, while in their own cases without emetine the recovery rate was only 40 per cent as compared with 100 per cent when emetine was administered.

The *treatment of patients presenting symptoms of acute or chronic appendicitis* in whom *Endamoeba histolytica* has been demonstrated in the stools is most important. It has already been stated that many individuals infected with this parasite present symptoms of appendicitis, especially of the chronic type, and it is the writer's conviction that every patient presenting such symptoms should be examined for this parasite if possible, for the reason that he has so very frequently observed cases in which a diagnosis of appendicitis was made and an operation decided upon in which an examination of the stool showed the ameba and proper treatment resulted in the disappearance of all symptoms with the elimination of the amebic infection. Such patients should be given a course of **chiniofon** or **carbarsone** administered as in the case of carriers or those suffering from mild amebic infection.

GENERAL TREATMENT.—In the treatment of carriers and of mild amebic infections with chiniofon, vioform or carbarsone, it has already been stated that confinement to bed is not necessary and that there need be no interruption in the patient's activities or occupation. In infections in which severe diarrhea occurs and in acute amebic dysentery and the acute exacerbation of chronic amebic dysentery, confinement to bed is essential. In such patients the usual precautions should be taken as regards food and during the acute diarrheal or dysenteric symptoms a liquid or very easily digested semiliquid diet should be maintained. Care should be taken during convalescence to avoid foods that are known to irritate the intestine or that are not well borne by the individual patient, and iron and arsenic are useful in many cases during convalescence. Individuals who are infected with *Endamoeba histolytica* should avoid the use of alcohol in any form, as indulgence in alcoholic drinks often results in an acute exacerbation of diarrheal or dysenteric symptoms. The use of tobacco, in moderation, is not contraindicated in infections with this parasite except when acute diarrheal or dysentery symptoms are present, but in individual cases tobacco does appear to cause intestinal symptoms and in such individuals its use should be discontinued. Marked benefit always results in patients convalescing from amebic dysentery from a change in climate, and if such patients have been living in the tropics a change to a temperate climate is most beneficial.

BIBLIOGRAPHY

Andrews, J.: Endamoeba histolytica and
other protozoa in wild rats caught in
Baltimore, J. Parasitol., 20: 334, 1934.
Atchley, F. O.: Experimental infections of
rats with Endamoeba histolytica, J. Hyg.,
23: 410, 1936.
Bartlett, G. B.: Pathology of dysentery in
the Mediterranean Expeditionary Force,
Quart. J. Med., 10: 185, 1917.
Boeck, W. C. and Drbohlav, J.: The cultivation of Endamoeba histolytica, Proc. Nat.
Acad. Sc., 2: 235, 1925; also, Am. J.
Hyg., 5: 371, 1925.
Brumpt, E.: Differentiation of the human
intestinal amoebae with four-nucleated
cysts, Tr. Roy. Soc. Trop. Med. & Hyg.,
22: 101, 1928.
Buxton, P. A.: The importance of the house
fly as a carrier of E. histolytica, Brit. M.
J., 1; 142, 1920.
Callender, G. R.: The cytological diagnosis
of dysenteric conditions and its applica-
tion in the military service, Mil. Surgeon,
56: 686, 1925.
Clark, H. G.: The distribution and com-
plications of amebic lesions found in 185
post-mortem examinations, Am. J. Trop.
Med., 5: 157, 1925.
Councilman, W. T. and Lafleur, H. A.:
Amebic dysentery, Johns Hopkins Hosp.
Rep., 2: 393, 1891.
Craig, C. F.: The occurrence of endamoebic
dysentery in the troops serving in the El
Paso District from July, 1916, to Decem-
ber, 1916, Mil. Surg., 11: 286, 423, 1917.
———: A simplified method for the cul-
tivation of Endamoeba histolytica, Am.
J. Trop. Med., 6: 333, 1926.
———: Observations upon the cultivation
of Endamoeba histolytica, Am. J. Trop.
Med., 6: 461, 1926.
———: Observations upon the hemolytic,
cytolytic and complement binding proper-
ties of extracts of Endamoeba histolytica,
Am. J. Trop. Med., 7: 225, 1927.
———: Technique and results of a com-
plement fixation test for the diagnosis of
infections with Endamoeba histolytica,
Am. J. Trop. Med., 9: 277, 1929.
———: The Parasitic Protozoa of Man,
Phila., J. B. Lippincott Co., 1926.
———: The pathology of amebiasis in car-
riers, Am. J. Trop. Med., 12: 285, 1932.
———: Complement fixation in infections
with Endamoeba histolytica, Proc. Nat.
Acad. Sc., 14: 520, 1928.
———: Further observations upon the com-
plement fixation test in the diagnosis of
amebiasis. An analysis of the results of
the test in one thousand individuals, J.
Lab. & Clin. Med., 18: 873, 1933.
———: Amebiasis and Amebic Dysentery,
Springfield, Ill., Charles C. Thomas, 1934;
also, London, Baillière, Tindall & Cox,
1934.
———: Observations upon the practical
value of the complement-fixation test in
the diagnosis of amebiasis, Am. J. Pub.
Health, 27: 639, 1937.
———: A suggested program of control of
amebiasis by health departments, Am. J.
Pub. Health, 28: 187, 1938.
——— and Faust, E. C.: Clinical Parasitology, Phila., Lea & Febiger, 1937.
——— and Kagy, E.: A study of complement fixation in experimental amebiasis in
dogs, Am. J. Hyg., 18: 203, 1933.
——— and St. John, J. H.: The value of
cultural methods in surveys for the parasitic amebae of man, Am. J. Trop. Med.,
7: 39, 1927.
——— and Swartzwelder, J. C.: Observations upon the complement fixation test
38111

in monkeys infected with Endamoeba his-
tolytica, Proc. Soc. Exper. Biol. & Med.,
37: 671, 1938.
Cutler, D. W.: A method for the cultivation
of Endamoeba histolytica, J. Path. &
Bact., 22: 22, 1918.
Dock, G.: Amebic ulceration in an individual with no symptoms of dysentery,
Centralbl. f. Bakt., 10: 227, 1891.
Elliott, J. B. Jr.: Abscess of the liver,
South. M. J., 8: 1019, 1915.
Engman, M. F., Jr. and Meleney, H. E.:
Amebiasis cutis, Arch. Dermat. & Syph.,
24: 1, 1931.
Faust, E. C.: Susceptibility, resistance and
spontaneous recovery in dogs experimentally infected with Endamoeba histolytica, Proc. Soc. Exper. Biol. & Med.,
29: 659, 1932.
——— and Kagy, E. S.: Studies on the
pathology of amebic enteritis in dogs,
Am. J. Trop. Med., 14: 221, 1934.
———, and Scott, L. C. and Swartzwelder,
J. C.: Effect of certain foodstuffs on
lesions of Endamoeba histolytica infection, Proc. Soc. Exper. Biol. & Med., 32:
540, 1934.
——— and Swartzwelder, J. C.: Effect of
continuous passage of Endamoeba histolytica through experimental dogs, Proc.
Soc. Exper. Biol. & Med., 32: 954, 1935.
Frye, W. W. and Meleney, H. E.: Endamoeba histolytica and other intestinal
protozoa in Tennessee; a study of flies,
rats, mice and some domestic animals
as possible carriers of the intestinal
protozoa of man in a rural community,
Am. J. Hyg., 16: 729, 1932.
Futcher, T. B.: A study of the cases of
amebic dysentery occurring at the Johns
Hopkins Hospital, J. Am. M. Ass., 41:
480, 1903.
Hegner, R., Johnson, C. M. and Stabler, R.
M.: Host-parasite relations in experimental amebiasis in monkeys in Panama,
Am. J. Hyg., 15: 394, 1932.
Hiyeda, K. and Suzuki, M.: Pathological
studies of human amoebic ulcers especially those of carriers, Am. J. Hyg., 15:
807, 1932.
Huber, H.: Untersuchungen über Amöben-
dysenterie, Ztschr. f. klin. Med., 67: 262,
1909.
Ikeda, K.: Roentgenological observations of
the colon in amebic dysentery, Radiology,
22: 610, 1934.
James, W. M.: Human amoebiasis, due to
infection with Endamoeba histolytica,
Ann. Trop. Med., 22: 201, 1928.
Jepps, M. W. and Dobell, C.: Diendamoeba
fragilis, n. g., n. sp., a new intestinal
amoeba from man, Parasitology, 10: 352,
1918.
Kartulis, S.: Zur Ätiologie der Dysenterie
in Aegypten, Arch. f. path. Anat., 105:
521, 1886.
Kessel, J. F.: Amoebiasis in kittens infected
with amoebae from acute and carrier
human cases and with the tetranucleate
amoebae of the monkey and pig, Am. J.
Hyg., 8: 311, 1928.
Lösch, F.: Massenhafte Entwickelung von
Amöben im Dickdarm, Arch. f. path.
Anat., 65: 196, 1875.
Lynch, K. M.: The rat as carrier of a
dysenteric amoeba, J. Am. M. Ass., 65:
2232, 1915.
Meleney, H. E. and Frye, W. W.: Studies of
Endamoeba histolytica and other intestinal protozoa in Tennessee: IX. Further
observations on the pathogenicity of certain strains of E. histolytica for kittens,
Am. J. Hyg., 21: 422, 1935.

Musgrave, W. E.: The cultivation and pathogenesis of amoebae, Philippine J. Sc., 1:
909, 1906.
———: Intestinal amoebiasis without diar-
rhoea: a study of fifty fatal cases, Philippine J. Sc., (B) 5: 229, 1910.
Nichols, H. J.: Carriers in Infectious Diseases, Baltimore, Williams & Wilkins Co.,
p. 67, 1922.
Ochsner, A. and DeBakey, M.: Diagnosis
and treatment of amebic abscess of the
liver, Am. J. Digest. Dis. & Nutrition, 2:
47, 1935.
Quincke, H. and Roos, E.: Über Amöben-
enteritis, Berl. klin. Wchnschr., 30: 1089,
1893.
Rogers, L.: Amoebic Hepatitis and Liver
Abscess, Tropical Medicine, Rogers and
Megaw, Philadelphia, P. Blakiston's Son
& Co., 1930.
———: Amoebic Hepatitis and Liver Ab-
scess, Tropical Medicine, Rogers and
Megaw, Ed. 2, London, J. & A. Churchill,
Ltd., 1935.
Root, F. M.: Experiments on the carriage of
intestinal protozoa of man by flies, Am.
J. Hyg., 1: 131, 1921.
Schaudinn, F.: Untersuchungen über die
Fortpflanzung einiger Rhizopoden, Arb. d.
kaiserl. Gesundheitsamtes, 19: 547, 1930.
Sherwood, N. P. and Heathman, L.: Further
studies on the antigenic properties of
pathogenic and free living amebas: II.
Complement fixation in amebic dysentery,
Am. J. Hyg., 16: 124, 1932.
Simic, T.: Étude expérimentale complé-
mentaire de l'Endamoeba dispar
(Brumpt), de Skoplje, sur le chat., Ann.
de parasitol., 9: 497, 1931.
Smithies, F.: Protozoiasis occurring in
temperate zone residents, Am. J. Trop.
Med., 6: 1, 1926.
———: Parasitosis of the bile passages and
gall bladder, Am. J. M. Sc., 176: 225,
1928.

Spector, B. K.: A comparative study of
cultural and immunological methods of
diagnosing infections with Endamoeba
histolytica, J. Prevent. M., 6: 117, 1932.
Strong, R. P.: Amebic Dysentery, Osler and
McCrae's Modern Medicine, Ed. 3, Phila.,
Lea & Febiger, 1925.
Swartzwelder, J. C.: Studies of the infec-
tion of dogs with trophozoites of Enda-
moeba histolytica by the oral route, Pub.
Health Rep., 52: 1447, 1937.
Thomson, J. G.: Carriers in amoebiasis, J.
State Med., 33: 563, 1925.
Tsuchiya, H.: Complement fixation in ame-
biasis, abstr., J. Parasitol., 19: 161, 1932.
———: Studies on the cultivation of Enda-
moeba histolytica and a complement fixa-
tion test for amebiasis, J. Lab. & Clin.
Med., 19: 495, 1934.
Vallarino, J. J.: Preliminary report on the
value of the roentgen ray in estimating
the extent of amebic infection of the large
intestine, Am. J. Trop. Med., 5: 149,
1925.
Walker, E. L. and Sellards, A. W.: Experimental endamoebic dysentery, Philippine
J. Sc., (B) 8: 253, 1913.
Weiss, E. and Arnold, L.: Complement fixation test for amebiasis, Am. J. Digest.
Dis. & Nutrition, 1: 231, 1934.
——— and Arnold L.: The specificity of the
complement fixation test for amebiasis,
Am. J. Digest. Dis. & Nutrition, 1: 548,
1934.
Wenyon, C. M.: Protozoology, New York,
Wm. Wood & Co., 1926.
——— and O'Connor, F. W.: The Intestinal Protozoa of Man, London, John Bale,
Sons & Danielsson, Ltd., 1921.
Yamamoto, Y.: Investigations of amoebic
dysentery. On the formation of antibodies by amoebic dysentery, J. Orient.
Med., 24: 969, 1936.
Yorke, W. and Adams, A. R. D.: Observations on Endamoeba histolytica: I. Development of cysts, excystment and development of excysted amoebae in vitro,
Ann. Trop. Med., 20: 279, 317, 1926.

CHAPTER XXXII

BALANTIDIASIS

By Charles F. Craig, M.D., M.A. (Hon.), F.A.C.P., F.A.C.S.,
Colonel, U. S. Army Medical Corps (Retired), D.S.M.

Definition.—By the term "balantidiasis" is meant the infection of
man with the ciliate protozoan, *Balantidium coli*, often called *Paramoecium coli*. This parasite belongs to the class Ciliata of the Protozoa and
the genus Balantidium. It invades the tissues of the large intestine of
man, producing ulceration and symptoms similar to those of amebic
dysentery.

History.—The first cases of infection with *Balantidium coli* were
observed by Malmsten, in 1857, who found this parasite in the feces of
two patients suffering from dysentery. Up to this time the parasite was
unknown, so that the first description of it was based upon specimens
observed in human feces, although the organism is naturally a parasite
of hogs and man is only an accidental host. Malmsten named the parasite *Paramoecium coli* but in 1862 Stein transferred the organism to the
genus Balantidium, where it belongs, and renamed it *Balantidium coli*.
Since the description of Malmsten numerous observers have confirmed
and added to his work and have described additional cases of infection
in man.

Geographic Distribution.—It is probable that *Balantidium coli* will
be found to be present wherever its natural host, the hog, is found, but
infections in man have been observed in the following countries: the
United States, Cuba, Puerto Rico, Brazil, Venezuela, Honduras, Aus-
tria, Finland, Holland, France, Germany, Italy, Serbia, Norway, Sweden,
Russia, Siberia, China, Ceylon, Java, the Philippine Islands, Egypt,
Sudan and Abyssinia. In man *Balantidium coli* is a rare parasite although very common in the hog.

Morphology.—The morphology of *Balantidium coli* is very characteristic and the parasite is easily recognized in either living or stained
preparations. It is the largest of the protozoan parasites infecting man
and is just visible to the naked eye although impossible of recognition
without the aid of the microscope. It has two distinct stages in its life
cycle, the motile or trophozoite stage, and the cystic stage, in each of
which the morphology differs.

38111

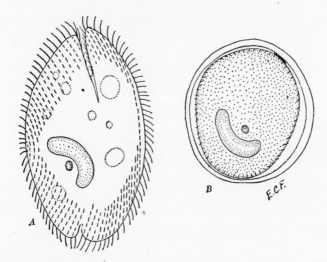

FIG. 1.—*Balantidium coli.*   *A,* Trophozoite; *B,* cyst.   (After Faust, J. Lab. & Clin. Med.)

In *unstained preparations* the motile *trophozoites* of *Balantidium coli* vary in size, measuring from 50 to 100 microns in length by 40 to 70 microns in breadth, the average measurements being from 50 to 80 microns in length by 40 to 60 microns in breadth. They are large, oval, slightly greenish bodies, covered with fine short filaments, or cilia, and possessing very active motility of a markedly progressive character, made possible by the constant swaying motion of the cilia. The anterior end is more pointed than the posterior and to one side of the median line at the anterior end there is an indentation, the peristome, which leads into a marked cleft in the body of the parasite, called the mouth or cytostome, which, in turn, leads into a short gullet, or esophagus. Within the organism may be seen two pulsating, or contractile vacuoles, one very large, situated anteriorly, while the other is much smaller and situated more posteriorly. The latter empties into a small tube connecting with the surface of the parasite through an anal opening, or cytopyge. A large kidney-shaped nucleus is present, called the macronucleus, which is usually situated near the center of the organism, and in close proximity to it, and usually lying in contact with the macronucleus, is a very small nuclear body, called the micronucleus. Food vacuoles are usually present within the endoplasm, in addition to the two contractile vacuoles that have been mentioned.

The outer surface of the body is covered with a delicate pellicle covering a small layer of hyaline ectoplasm within which is the endoplasm containing the various structures already mentioned. The outer pellicle appears longitudinally striated due to the rows of cilia, the latter arising from the ectoplasm, and becoming free after emerging through apertures in the pellicle. The movement of the trophozoites is due to the movement of the cilia and, as the body of the trophozoite is very

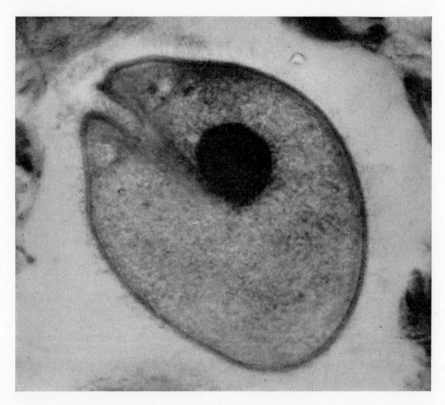

FIG. 2.—*Balantidium coli.* Trophozoite greatly enlarged. Note the cilia, especially well marked at the anterior end and within the peristome and cytostome. Stained with iron-hematoxylin. (Photomicrograph, Army Medical Museum. From preparation from collection of Drs. James and Getz, Panama.)

plastic, it is able to force its way between the epithelial cells of the mucous membrane of the intestine, perhaps aided by a cytolytic ferment, as in the case of *Endamoeba histolytica.*

In *unstained preparations* the *cysts* of *Balantidium coli* usually measure from 45 to 65 microns in longest diameter, are round or oval in shape, hyaline in appearance, and have a well-marked, double-outlined cyst wall. They contain a single parasite, which, in freshly passed feces, may be seen to revolve within the cyst, but eventually the outline of the organism becomes obscured and the cyst appears to contain a mass of granules containing the macronucleus. Such cysts are probably degenerating forms and it is probable that the only viable cysts are those containing the moving balantidium. In this species of the protozoa encystment appears to be purely protective in nature, no reproduction occurring within the cyst. Cysts containing two balantidia have been observed, but such cysts are believed to contain conjugating parasites.

38111

In *stained preparations* of the motile form, or *trophozoite,* the various structures already mentioned in the description of the unstained organism are more clearly observed and their minute details may be studied. Preparations should be wet-fixed with Schaudinn's fluid and stained with one of the hematoxylin stains to secure the best results.

In well-stained preparations the outer surface of the organism is seen to be covered with a thin pellicle which turns in at the anterior end to form the lining of the peristome, cytostome and gullet. This pellicle is marked by longitudinal striations produced by the rows of cilia which emerge through apertures in the pellicle from the ectoplasm. According to McDonald (1922), the cilia arise from hyaline-appearing bands in the ectoplasm, while between these bands are darker-appearing bands which form minute ridges upon the surface of the body of the organism. The cilia covering the body each arise from a distinct black-stained granule in the ectoplasm, pass through an aperture in the pellicle and become free, very short and delicate motile fibrils, those lining the peristome and cytostome being longer than those covering the body of the parasite. The large and small vacuoles are present as well as food vacuoles, and the macronucleus, usually kidney-shaped, has a distinct nuclear membrane, which is seldom seen except in very well stained preparations, the entire macronucleus appearing as a densely stained, black mass of chromatin with but little visible structure. The small nucleus, or micronucleus, is usually indistinguishable in stained preparations because of its small size and close contact with the macronucleus, but sometimes it may be seen as a small, spherical, black mass lying in contact with the macronucleus.

In *stained preparations* the *cysts* are usually poorly stained and show but little definite structure, although the macronucleus is usually visible as a black mass lying within the cyst. In very well stained preparations the cilia may be distinguished as well as the peristome and cytostome.

Stained preparations are not necessary for the diagnosis of *Balantidium coli* as the living trophozoites and cysts are very easily recognized.

Habitat.—The hog is apparently the natural host of *Balantidium coli,* although it may live in the intestine of man for an indefinite period. This parasite is also found in the intestine of monkeys and the orang-outang, and Brooks (1902–1903) described an epidemic of dysentery among the orang-outang in the New York Zoological Park caused by this parasite. Awakina (1937), in Moscow, found a balantidium in naturally infected rats identical in morphology with *Balantidium coli* and characteristic lesions produced by the parasite were present in the intestines of these animals and could be produced experimentally.

In man, *Balantidium coli* lives in the large intestine, being most numerous in the cecum. In the feces, trophozoites occur when the stool is fluid or semifluid in character, while the cysts occur in formed stools.

Cultivation.—This parasite has been cultivated by Barret and Yarbrough (1921), Rees (1927), Jameson (1927) and others, employing similar media to those used in the cultivation of *Endamoeba histolytica.* The morphology in cultures is similar to that observed in the intestine and conjugating pairs are sometimes observed in cultures. Trophozoites are usually observed in cultures but cysts may more rarely occur.

Life History and Methods of Reproduction.—*Balantidium coli* has a motile, or trophozoite, stage and an immotile, or cystic stage, in its life cycle, while in this species conjugation appears to play an important part in the life history. When conditions are favorable for vegetative existence the motile trophozoites live and multiply within the lumen of the bowel and in the tissues of the walls of the intestine, but when conditions become unfavorable within the lumen of the bowel, the organisms become motionless, round up and secrete a resistant cyst wall, becoming cysts. So far as known no further development occurs within the cyst, encystment in this species being purely protective in type. Two organisms are sometimes observed within a cyst, but such forms are believed to be conjugating pairs that have encysted. Encystment does not occur within the tissues.

The trophozoites multiply by binary transverse division, the micronucleus first dividing, followed by the division of the macronucleus and by the division of the body of the parasite into two organisms. As stated, multiplication does not occur within the cysts of this parasite. Conjugation of two organisms may be observed both in the feces and in cultures, and da Cunha and Muniz (1935) have described this process as regularly occurring between young trophozoites both in material obtained from the human intestine and in cultures. The writer has repeatedly observed conjugation between two trophozoites in fecal material, the conjugants uniting for variable periods of time and then separating. During union, streaming of the cytoplasm between the organisms appears to occur but whether conjugation in this parasite is sexual in nature or simply for purposes of rejuvenation has not been determined. There is no evidence that the conjugants are sexually differentiated.

Balantidium coli derives its nourishment from material present in the lumen of the intestine and from tissue cells, bacteria, starch granules, red blood corpuscles, leukocytes and other cells, and all of these substances have been observed within the food vacuoles of this organism. The food, which is captured by means of currents produced by the cilia lining the peristome, passes into the cytostome and through the gullet, or esophagus, into food vacuoles, where it is digested. The waste materials are probably excreted through the anal opening, or cytopyge, although some believe that the contractile vacuoles also rid the parasite of certain waste products.

Epidemiology.—The infection of man occurs through swallowing food or drink contaminated by hog or human feces containing the cysts of *Balantidium coli* or by direct transference of the feces of infected hogs to the mouth by the hands, which may occur in those having to do with the handling or slaughtering and dressing of hogs.

The cysts are the infective forms of this parasite and have considerable resistance to external influences. They may remain in a viable condition in hog or human feces, if the latter are kept in the shade in a moist condition for several weeks, but they are killed rapidly by direct sunlight or drying. Ohi (1924) found that cysts kept under cover in feces at temperatures varying between 50 and 70° F. (10 and 21.1° C.) remained alive for from one to one and a half months, while if the feces

38111

were kept moist the cysts were viable at the end of two months. When kept in dry feces in the shade the cysts remained alive for from one to two weeks, while if the feces were exposed to direct sunlight the cysts died within three hours. It was also found that the cysts resist an aqueous 1:1000 solution of bichloride of mercury for one hour and a 5 per cent solution of carbolic acid for six hours and they resist the action of the normal gastric juice for six hours, according to this investigator. It is evident that the cysts of *Balantidium coli* are much more resistant to drying than those of *Endamoeba histolytica* and the use of hog manure for fertilizing purposes might possibly be a source of infection under some conditions.

. The *incidence of infection* of man with this parasite is not great, for although *Balantidium coli* is a common parasite of the hog it is a rare one of man. Thus, Mathews and Smith (1919), in over 23,000 examinations of the stools of over 4000 English soldiers, did not find a single case of infection with this parasite, while Faust and the writer, in the examination of the stools of many thousands of individuals both in this country, China and the Philippine Islands, have observed about three dozen infections in all. It should be remembered, however, that individuals frequently harbor this parasite without definite symptomatology being produced, so that many infections are undoubtedly missed because there is no indication for an examination of the stool, and it is also true that only a very few of the observed infections have been recorded in the literature, but even allowing for these facts it is undoubtedly true that *Balantidium coli* is a comparatively rare human parasite. Considering its very common occurrence in the hog and the chances that exist of infection of man, it would appear that man is infected with great difficulty and that this parasite is not essentially a parasite of man but of the hog.

The infection of man sometimes occurs from direct transference of hog feces containing the cysts to the mouth by the soiled hands of individuals having to do with the handling or slaughtering of hogs. Thus, cases have been observed in hog farmers and especially in workers in slaughter houses who are employed in operations which necessitate the soiling of the hands with the feces of hogs. Young and Walker (1918) report a case of infection with this parasite in an employee in a pork-packing establishment who handled hog's intestine in his capacity of a "gut-stripper." In this case there was a very heavy infection, undoubtedly contracted through contamination by the hands of the individual infected.

Carriers of this parasite are sometimes the source of infection, as in infection with *Endamoeba histolytica,* food or drink being contaminated by such individuals if they are employed in the handling of these substances. Contamination of food or drink may also occur through a polluted water supply or through the employment of hog or human feces in the fertilization of vegetable gardens. Except in the case of workers in pork-packing establishments, or upon hog farms, it is usually impossible to trace the source of an infection, owing to the small number of cases observed due to the natural resistance of man to infection with this parasite.

The *experimental infection* of certain of the *lower animals* is possible and the cat has been infected by Casagrandi and Barbagallo (1896)

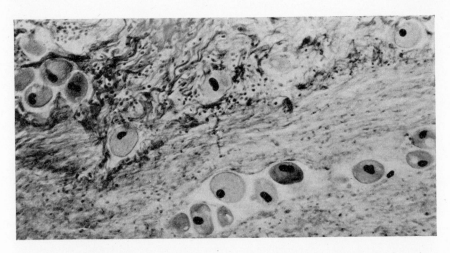

FIG. 3.—*Balantidium coli* in submucous and muscular coats of the intestine. Note areas of cytolysis around most of the balantidia. (Photomicrograph, Army Medical Museum.)

and by Behrenroth (1913); the monkey, by Brumpt (1909) and Walker (1913); while Andrews (1931) has transferred *Balantidium coli* of man from man to pigs, guinea pigs and rats.

Pathology.—That *Balantidium coli* is a pathogenic parasite of man has been abundantly proved and the lesions in the intestine which are produced by it have been studied by many observers, notably by Strong (1904) and Walker (1913). The parasite may apparently live for an unknown period of time within the lumen of the bowel without penetrating the mucous membrane, but it is believed that eventually it penetrates the epithelial lining of the large intestine, probably by reason of its motility and of a cytolytic substance which it secretes, producing noninflammatory lesions which, being quickly invaded by bacteria, become inflammatory in nature and necrosis and ulceration then occur, the result of the combined action of cytolysis and secondary inflammation. Sections of the intestine have shown that the balantidia may be found within the submucous or muscular coats of the intestine, and in the lymphatics, surrounded by an area of cytolysis, and with no small cell infiltrations characteristic of bacterial contamination.

After penetrating the mucous membrane the balantidia multiply and produce abscesses or ulcers which may penetrate to the muscular coat of the intestine. *Macroscopically* the lesions are of two types, abscesses and ulcerations. The *abscesses* lie beneath the mucous membrane in the submucous coat and may extend to the muscular coat of the gut. They consist of small cavities filled with a glairy, bloodstained exudate containing the trophozoites and frequently covered with normal-appearing mucous membrane. If a secondary bacterial infection is present the abscess contents may be purulent and the balantidia may be absent or difficult of recognition because of degenerative changes. The *ulcers* are of various size, round, oval or irregular in shape, and

38111

may be superficial or involve the mucous, submucous and muscular coats of the intestine. The edges of the ulcers are undermined and may be irregular in conformation, while the floors are covered with the glairy material mentioned or with pus. In this infection, as in infection with *Endamoeba histolytica,* the ulcers may communicate with one another by sinuses beneath or through the mucous and submucous coats of the gut. The macroscopic pathology of balantidiasis is very similar to that of amebiasis and it is impossible in most instances to make a differential diagnosis between these infections without the aid of the microscope.

Microscopically, sections of the infected intestine present a very variable pathology, depending upon the absence or presence of secondary bacterial infection. If there is no secondary bacterial infection the sections show no small round-cell infiltration or other evidence of acute inflammation, nests of the balantidia being present within the tissues or in the lymphatics, neighboring lymph glands, or even in the capillaries, evidences of the cytolysis of the invaded structures being present, the organisms being surrounded by a clear area in which all trace of structure has been lost. Hemorrhagic areas may be present and coagulation necrosis may be seen in the walls of the abscesses and ulcers. If there is a secondary bacterial infection, as is most commonly observed, there is, in addition to the picture described, marked small round-cell infiltration and the other evidences of an acute inflammatory process.

While the balantidia undoubtedly reach the portal circulation through the intestinal capillaries in the invaded areas, there is no record of this parasite being found in the liver or other organs or of the production by it of liver abscess or abscess in any of the other viscera.

Cases of infection with *Balantidium coli* have been observed in which the only lesions present were minute areas of superficial necrosis of the surface of the mucous membrane of the intestine, accompanied by slight hemorrhagic areas.

In the hog, *Balantidium coli* is most commonly a harmless parasite, although lesions have been produced by it experimentally and some authors have observed lesions in the hog similar to those observed in man. However, in the vast majority of infections studied in this animal no lesions were observed and the parasite was apparently a harmless commensal. In the monkey, *Balantidium coli* produced lesions like those observed in man.

Symptomatology.—The symptomatology of balantidiasis in man varies greatly, many individuals showing no symptoms of the infection when observed, others presenting mild gastro-intestinal symptoms, while still others present the symptoms of an acute or chronic dysentery of great severity. It is undoubtedly true that symptomless "carriers" of *Balantidium coli* exist, as in infections with *Endamoeba histolytica,* and the writer has observed cases in which the balantidia were numerous in the stools but in which there were no clinical symptoms over long periods of time. However, many patients infected with this parasite have gastro-intestinal symptoms, usually consisting of pain in the lower abdomen, gaseous eructations, slight nausea, anorexia and slight diarrhea, the stools containing much mucus. There may be tenderness over the right iliac region or low in the abdomen and sometimes the entire large intestine is sensitive to pressure. In still other patients the symptoms may be those of an acute dysentery, the stools being passed with much tenesmus and containing much blood and mucus. Attacks of diarrhea or dysentery may alternate with periods of constipation, or the stools may be fluid or semifluid in consistence over considerable periods of time without any other symptoms of intestinal irritation.

As a whole, the clinical picture closely approximates that of amebiasis and the writer believes that it is impossible to differentiate these two infections clinically. The writer has observed a few cases of combined infection with *Balantidium coli* and *Endamoeba histolytica* and the possibility of such a combination should be remembered. The mild infections with *Balantidium coli* are probably very frequently overlooked and this may account for the apparent rarity in man of a parasite so often observed in the domestic hog.

Diagnosis.—The diagnosis of infection with *Balantidium coli* must rest upon the demonstration of the parasite in the stools or in sections of the infected intestine, or in material removed from the ulcers through the proctoscope. The motile trophozoites are found in fluid or semifluid stools, while the cysts are found in semiformed or formed stools and the methods of demonstrating the parasite in the stools are similar to those employed in the demonstration of *Endamoeba histolytica* (see chapter on Amebiasis). It should be remembered that this organism is very large as compared with the various species of amebae and flagellates found in the human intestine, and the large size, combined with the very active motility of the trophozoite, enables it to be easily recognized even by one who has had little training in the study of the intestinal protozoa of man. Stained preparations are not necessary in diagnosis although invaluable for the study of the minute structure of the parasite. The simplest method of diagnosis is to place a minute portion of the liquid stool, or of the formed stool mixed with saline solution, upon a microscopic slide, cover it with a coverglass and examine with the low-power objective.

Prognosis.—Fatal results sometimes follow infection with this parasite but it is true that the prognosis in otherwise healthy individuals is good, as most infections either disappear spontaneously or may be eliminated by treatment. The prognosis is most favorable in symptomless "carriers" and least so in debilitated individuals who have suffered from attacks of severe diarrhea or dysentery. The mortality rate has been variously given by different authorities as from 5 to 30 per cent, but the writer believes that the high percentage rates that have been reported are due to the fact that only the most severe infections with this parasite are usually recognized, for where routine fecal examinations are made the percentage of fatalities has been low, owing to the fact that symptomless and mild infections have been diagnosed. In an experience covering over 40 years the writer has never observed a death which could be demonstrated to have been caused by this parasite. Though this is the personal experience of the writer, Strong (1904) found a mortality of almost 30 per cent in the Philippine Islands, and Fairley (1936) states that the mortality varies between 7 per cent in latent cases and 29 per cent in cases presenting marked dysenteric symptoms with ulceration.

Prophylaxis.—The prevention of infection with *Balantidium coli* consists in the prevention of contamination of food or drink with fecal

38111

material containing the cysts of this parasite. As the domestic hog is generally the source of infection of man, the utmost care should be taken to avoid contact with hog feces or the indiscriminate use of this material for fertilization purposes. Workers in pork-packing establishments should be warned of the danger of infection in handling the intestines of hogs and the hands should be carefully cleansed after operations requiring such handling. Those who are employed in raising pigs, and who come into intimate contact with these animals, should thoroughly cleanse their hands before eating, and hogs should not be allowed to roam freely about domestic premises if water is secured from wells or springs in the vicinity, as such water is very apt to become contaminated.

Other methods of prevention of this infection consist in the examination of food handlers in public eating places for possible infection with this parasite, the protection of food supplies from flies and other insects, and the removal of infected individuals from occupations that require the handling of food supplies. As the infection is apparently a rare one in man, its prevention is not so important as in the case of amebiasis but as much should be done in the way of prophylaxis as is possible.

Treatment.—The treatment of balantidiasis is not upon a very satisfactory basis. At the present time we have no specific treatment, but several drugs have been employed with apparently good results. Walker (1913) found that the organic silver compounds gave the best results in experimental balantidiasis in animals and **protargol enemas** have been used with success. Dutcher recommended the intravenous injection of 0.06 Gm. (1 Gr.) of **salvarsan,** while other arsenicals have been employed, notably **acetarsone** and **carbarsone,** administered as in amebiasis (*q.v.*). **High colonic irrigations with solutions containing silver nitrate, quinine** or **iodine** have been recommended by some authorities, while **methylene blue solution** (1 : 3000) has been employed with apparent success as an enema and the same drug by mouth. Other drugs recommended are thymol, oil of chenopodium, and santonin, but the remedial effect of these is very doubtful. In fact, it is most difficult to judge of the efficiency of the treatment of this infection with any drug, owing to the fact that spontaneous disappearance of the parasite from the intestine frequently occurs. Emetine is apparently useless in balantidiasis and should not be administered.

Most authorities recommend a low carbohydrate **diet** but one rich in vegetables and proteins, and **rest in bed** is essential if there are symptoms of severe diarrhea or dysentery. The **avoidance of tobacco** and **alcoholics** is important if severe intestinal symptomatology is present.

BIBLIOGRAPHY

Andrews, J.: Host-specificity in Balantidium coli, Tr. 8th Congress Far Eastern Med. Assoc., 8 : 194, 1932.

Brumpt, E.: Demonstration du rôle pathogène du Balantidium coli, Compt. rend. Soc. de biol., 67 : 103, 1909.

Craig, C. F.: The Parasitic Protozoa of Man, Phila. & Lond., 1909.

——— and Faust: Clinical Parasitology, Phila. & Lond., 1937.

Fairley, N. H.: Taylor's Practice of Medicine, Ed. 15, Lond. & Balt., 1936.

Hegner, R.: Specificity in the genus Balantidium, etc., Am. J. Hyg., 16 : 513, 1934.

McDonald, J. D.: On Balantidium coli (Malmsten) and Balantidium suis (sp. nov.), etc., Univ. California Publ. Zool., 20 : 243, 1922.

Malmsten, P. H.: Infusorien als Intestinaltiere beim Menschen, Virchows Arch. f. path. Anat., 12 : 302, 1857.

Strong, R. P.: The clinical and pathological significance of Balantidium coli, Bureau Gov't Labs. Bull., Manila, P. I., No. 26, pp. 77, 1904.

Walker, E. L.: Experimental balantidiasis, Philippine J. Sc., (B) 8 : 333, 1913.

CHAPTER XXXIII

THE INTESTINAL FLAGELLATE INFECTIONS

By Charles F. Craig, M.D., M.A. (Hon.), F.A.C.P., F.A.C.S.,
Colonel, U. S. Army Medical Corps (Retired), D.S.M.

Introduction.—There occur in the human intestine several flagellate
protozoa which, because they are believed by some to cause lesions and
symptoms, it is necessary to discuss. Many of our textbooks include a
description of the so-called "flagellate diarrheas" and some of the older
texts even describe a form of dysentery thought to be caused by one of
these flagellates, *Giardia lamblia,* under the term "giardial dysentery"
or giardiasis. As will be seen later, there is no scientific evidence of
sufficient value to demonstrate that this organism is capable of causing
lesions of itself or of initiating symptoms, and the same is true of other
intestinal flagellates, although in heavy infections their presence may
keep up a diarrhea caused by bacteria or *Endamoeba histolytica.*

Classification of the Intestinal Flagellates.—The intestinal flagellates belong to the class Mastigophora of the Protozoa, which includes
both parasitic and free-living species, all characterized by the possession
of long, threadlike flagella by means of which motility is rendered possible. The zoological position of the species of flagellates occurring in the
intestine of man, of which there are three, i.e., *Giardia lamblia, Chilomastix mesnili* and *Trichomonas hominis,* is indicated in the following
table:

Class: Mastigophora.
   Order: Protomonadida.
     Family: Octomitidae.
       Genus: Giardia.
         Species: *Giardia lamblia.*
     Family: Chilomastigidae.
       Genus: Chilomastix.
         Species: *Chilomastix mesnili.*
     Family: Trichomonadidae.
       Genus: Trichomonas.
         Species: *Trichomonas hominis.*

In addition to the three species of intestinal flagellates named above
there are two other species that are very rarely observed in the intestine

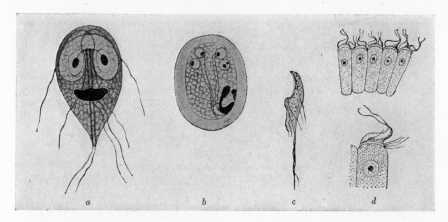

Fig. 1.—*a*, Trophozoite of *Giardia lamblia*. *b*, Cyst of *Giardia lamblia*. (After Bensen.) *c*, Lateral view of trophozoite of *Giardia lamblia*. (After Grassi and Schewiakoff.) *d*, Trophozoites of *Giardia lamblia* adherent to intestinal epithelial cells by their sucking disks. (After Jollos.)

of man. These are *Embadomonas intestinalis* and *Enteromonas hominis*, but owing to their nonpathogenic nature and rare occurrence these are of no interest to the physician and will not be described.

Infections with Giardia Lamblia.—This common flagellate of the human intestine is also known as *Giardia intestinalis* or *Lamblia intestinalis* and infection with it as *giardiasis*. It has a world-wide distribution and the incidence of infection with it varies greatly, being highest in the tropics and lowest in cold climates. Surveys for this parasite in the United States have shown that the incidence varies in different localities from 5 to 17 per cent of those examined, usually being highest in children.

This flagellate lives in the small intestine of man, the motile trophozoites being most numerous in the duodenum but occurring throughout the small intestine, while the cystic forms are found in the ileum and large intestine. The trophozoites are most numerous in liquid or semiliquid stools, while the cysts are found in formed stools. Many of the lower animals harbor giardia identical in morphology with the human species, but their species identity has not been proved.

Morphology.—The morphology of *Giardia lamblia* is very characteristic. It has two distinct stages in its life history, the motile or trophozoite stage, and the cystic stage, and the morphology is best studied in preparations stained with one of the hematoxylin stains after wet fixation.

The *trophozoite*, or motile form, differs in its morphology from other intestinal flagellates in that all of the structures of the cell are duplicated, there being two nuclei, two axonemes and four pairs of flagella. These structures stain black with the hematoxylin stains and are well differentiated in well-stained preparations.

In *unstained preparations* the *trophozoite* of *Giardia lamblia* measures from 9.5 to 21 microns in length and from 5 to 15 microns in breadth and is colorless and hyaline in appearance. It is actively motile, the motility being of a jerky, progressive character and rendered possible by the flagella.

The trophozoites are pear-shaped, the anterior end being broad and rounded while the posterior is drawn out to a sharp point, sometimes called the tail of the parasite. Dorsally the trophozoite is convex but ventrally a large ovoid concavity exists, beginning at the anterior end and occupying nearly three quarters of the ventral surface. This concavity is caused by the presence of a sucking disk, by which the organism is able to attach itself to the mucous membrane of the intestine and thus derive nourishment.

The *cyst,* in *unstained preparations,* is hyaline in appearance, ovoid in shape and measures from 8 to 12 microns in length by 7 to 10 microns in breadth. There is a well-defined, double-outlined cyst wall and the contents of the cysts appear finely granular and less refractile than the limiting membrane or wall of the cyst.

In *stained preparations* the *trophozoite* presents the following structure. Near the anterior end are two oval *nuclei,* each containing a large central karyosome. Running from near the anterior end to the posterior end are two deep black rods, the *axonemes,* which terminate at both the anterior and posterior ends in two *blepharoplasts.* There are eight *flagella* arranged in four pairs, called the anterior, middle, ventral and caudal pairs. The anterior pair originate from the blepharoplasts at the anterior end of the axonemes, cross one another, and pass along the anterior and lateral margins of the sucking disk, becoming free flagella near the junction of the anterior and middle third of the body of the parasite. The middle pair apparently arise from the same blepharoplasts, follow the course of the axonemes to the posterior border of the sucking disk, where the flagella become free. The ventral pair of flagella originate from the axonemes at the posterior edge of the sucking disk and become free flagella near the center of the body of the parasite, while the caudal pair originate from the blepharoplasts at the posterior end of the axonemes and become free at once, projecting from the posterior end of the body of the giardia. In addition to the structures mentioned there are one or two curved or rounded bodies, staining black, and situated posterior to the sucking disk, the exact nature of which is not known.

In *stained preparations* the *cysts* are very characteristic. They are oval in shape and contain from two to four nuclei, arranged in pairs, and usually situated at the anterior pole of the cyst, although there may be a pair at each end. The nuclei have a well-defined nuclear membrane and a small karyosome situated centrally or to one side of the center of the nucleus. The cyst also contains two deeply stained curved rods arranged in a V-shaped formation at the end of the cyst farthest removed from the nuclei, and curved fibrils arranged in groups of four may be present near their rods. With the iodine stain the number of nuclei may be distinguished.

LIFE HISTORY.—*Giardia lamblia,* as already stated, has two distinct stages in its life history, the "vegetative" or *trophozoite stage* and the *cystic stage.* The trophozoite multiplies by longitudinal division into two organisms as long as conditions are favorable, but when conditions become unfavorable the trophozoite loses its motility, rounds up, and develops a resistant wall about itself, becoming a cyst. The cysts are passed in the feces of the host and are the infective agents. Within the cyst the two nuclei divide, producing a four-nucleated cyst, and excystation occurs when the cysts which have been ingested reach the duodenum. According to Hegner (1927), division of the body of the giardia occurs after it leaves the cyst and some authorities believe that excystation may occur in cysts which have never left the host, owing to the fact that dividing trophozoites are very rarely encountered in the feces.

The infection of man with this parasite follows the ingestion of food or drink contaminated with fecal material containing the cysts and such contamination may occur in the various ways already described in infection with *Endamoeba histolytica*. The cysts are resistant to external conditions and may live in water for several days and in the intestinal tract of flies for at least 24 hours, while Young (1937) has found that cockroaches may pass viable cysts for as long as 12 days after feeding upon material containing the cysts.

PATHOLOGY.—Whether pathologic lesions are produced by *Giardia lamblia* is still a moot question. A few observers claim to have seen evidences of a chronic inflammatory process in the small intestine in animals infected with a giardia like that of man but, so far as the writer knows, there is no record of lesions having been observed in the intestine in human infections which were proved to be caused by this parasite.

SYMPTOMATOLOGY.—Of all of the intestinal flagellates of man *Giardia lamblia* apparently has the best claim to pathogenicity, although it has not been conclusively demonstrated that it does produce lesions or any symptoms of disease. Numerous clinicians are of the opinion that it is the cause of a chronic form of diarrhea because it is so frequently associated with this symptom, and a few claim that it is the cause of a severe type of dysentery resembling that caused by *Endamoeba histolytica*. It is true that the parasite is often found in the feces in cases presenting diarrheal symptoms, especially in children, and often in very large numbers, and it is certainly conceivable that the presence of multitudes of these organisms (which are able to attach themselves to the mucous membrane) may so irritate it, if it is already inflamed from some other cause, as to increase or prolong the diarrheal symptoms that may be present, but it may be conclusively stated that there is no evidence on record to date that demonstrates that this parasite initiates any pathologic condition within the intestine or is the initial excitant of intestinal symptomatology. In practically every case of severe diarrhea or dysentery in which it has been seen and which has been carefully investigated for the possible presence of other parasites, some other parasite has been found to be the exciting cause of the symptoms, usually either one of the varieties of the dysentery bacilli, streptococci or *Endamoeba histolytica*. Many investigators have tried to correlate the occurrence of diarrhea with the presence of *Giardia lamblia* but usually without success. Thus, Tao (1930) in Pekin studied 649 cases of infection with this parasite and could not determine any relationship between its presence and the occurrence of gastro-intestinal symptoms, 400 (61.6 per cent) having no symptoms, while 249 (38.3 per cent) presented intestinal symptomatology.

It is my opinion that *Giardia lamblia* is not a pathogenic parasite per se but that, when present in large numbers in individuals suffering from other intestinal infections resulting in diarrheal symptoms, it may increase the severity of the symptoms and prolong the diarrheal condition.

DIAGNOSIS.—The diagnosis depends upon the demonstration of *Giardia lamblia* in the feces and it should be remembered that the motile trophozoites occur only in fluid stools and the cysts in formed stools. As the motile forms are easiest recognized, a saline cathartic should be administered if the patient is passing formed stools, and a little of the material so obtained placed upon a microscopic slide, covered with a coverglass and examined with the high dry objective. The trophozoites are easily recognized by any one properly trained in fecal examinations. If the stool is formed the cysts are demonstrable by making an emulsion of a small portion of the fecal material and examining in both the unstained condition and in preparations stained with the iodine stain, as in examinations for *Endamoeba histolytica*.

PROPHYLAXIS.—As this parasite is transmitted from man to man in the same manner as is *Endamoeba histolytica* the methods of prophylaxis are the same (see Amebiasis).

TREATMENT.—It has been demonstrated beyond question that **atabrine** is a specific in the treatment of giardiasis by Galli-Valerio (1937), Brumpt (1937), Hellman (1938), Alvarez (1939) and many others. It has been found that properly administered it will eliminate infection with *Giardia lamblia* in approximately 100 per cent of the cases.

In the treatment of giardiasis, atabrine is administered by mouth in the same doses as in the treatment of malarial infections. For adults, one tablet, containing 0.1 Gm. (1½ grains), is administered three times a day for a period of five to seven days. For children from one to four years of age, one-half tablet, or 0.05 Gm. (¾ grain), twice daily for five days; from four to eight years of age, one tablet, or 0.1 Gm. (1½ grains), twice daily for five days, and for children over eight years of age the same dosage as for adults.

It is fortunate that we possess this specific as giardiasis is the only flagellate infection of man that has any real claim to importance as an infectious disease; and, even though the proof is incomplete that *Giardia* is a pathogenic parasite, it does undoubtedly aid in keeping up an intestinal irritation due to other causes and should be eliminated in all cases.

Infections with Chilomastix Mesnili.—This is a common flagellate of the intestine of man and is called, in the older texts, *Tetramitus mesnili* or *Chilomastix hominis* and infection with it is referred to as *chilomastigmiasis*. It has a world-wide geographic distribution and the incidence varies in different localities, being highest in poorly sanitated districts and in the tropics. Surveys made by different authorities in different parts of the world have shown that the incidence varies from 1.5 per cent to as high as 8 per cent and infections are more numerous in children than in adults.

The exact habitat of this parasite in man has not been definitely proved, some authorities believing that it inhabits the small intestine while others believe that it is a parasite of the large intestine. Many of the lower animals, as the rat, goat, guinea pig, etc., harbor species similar in morphology to *Chilomastix mesnili*, but the only animal which is infected with this parasite, other than man, is the monkey.

MORPHOLOGY.—This flagellate has a motile or trophozoite, and an immotile or cystic, stage of development. The exact morphologic de-

42102

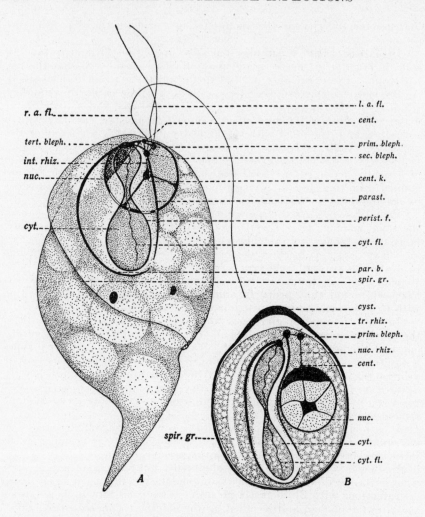

FIG. 2.—*A.   Chilomastix mesnili* (Wenyon).   Normal flagellate viewed from the ventral or oral side and showing all the structures of the body.   × 6370.

   B.   Cyst of *Chilomastix mesnili*, viewed from the ventral or oral side.   × 6370.

   Abbreviations: *cent.*, centrosome; *cent. k.*, central karysome; *cyst*, cyst wall; *cyt.*, cytostome; *cyt. fl.*, cytostomal flagellum or undulating membrane; *int. rhiz.*, intranuclear rhizoplast; *l. a. fl.*, left anterior flagella; *nuc.*, nucleus; *nuc. rhiz.*, nuclear rhizoplast; *par. b.*, parabasal body; *parast.*, parastyle; *perist. f.*, peristomal fiber; *prim. bleph.*, primary blepharoplast; *r. a fl.*, right anterior flagellum; *sec. bleph.*, secondary blepharoplast; *spir. gr.*, spiral groove; *tert. bleph.*, tertiary blepharoplast; *tr. rhiz.*, transverse rhizoplast.   (After Kofoid and Swezy.)

tails of its structure can be best observed in wet-fixed, hematoxylin-stained preparations, although both the trophozoites and cysts may be recognized in unstained preparations. The trophozoites are found in fluid or semifluid stools, while the cysts are found in formed or semi-formed stools.

In *unstained preparations* the *trophozoites* measure from 6 to 20 microns in length by from 3 to 10 microns in breadth and are usually ovoid or pear-shaped, but rarely small round forms are seen measuring from 3 to 4 microns in diameter. In freshly passed stools the trophozoites are very actively motile, the motility being of a jerky-progressive character. The organism is colorless or very slightly green in color, finely granular in appearance, and the body usually appears to be twisted upon itself. In trophozoites that are sluggishly motile the flagella and the cytostome may be visible.

In *unstained preparations* the cysts measure from 7 to 10 microns in length and from 4, 5 to 6 microns in breadth, are lemon-shaped and have a small blunt projection at the smaller end. The contents of the cysts appear granular with little or no definite structure visible. Some of the cysts may be round or irregular in shape.

In *stained preparations* the *trophozoites* present a very typical structure. The body is roughly pear-shaped but asymmetrical, and one end is broad and rounded while the other is sharply pointed. There is a *spiral groove* extending around the body from the dorsal side of the anterior end to the ventral side posteriorly and a well-marked mouth, or *cytostome*, extending backward from the anterior end ventrally for nearly one half the length of the body, having two lips within which may be seen a short free flagellum. The round or oval *nucleus* is situated near the anterior end of the body and has a well-defined nuclear membrane and a small karyosome placed to one side of the center of the nucleus. At the anterior pole of the nucleus a collection of deep black dots may be seen, the *blepharoplasts*, which are six in number. Of these, three give rise to three free flagella which project from the anterior end of the body, one to a flagellum situated within the cytostome, one to a fibril supporting the right lip of the cytostome and one to a fibril supporting the left lip of this structure. There is no posterior free flagellum as in *Giardia lamblia*.

In *stained preparations* the *cysts* present a distinct, unstained cyst wall enclosing finely granular cytoplasm in which may be seen a single round or oval nucleus lying near the anterior end, or more centrally placed in some cysts. The nucleus has a well-defined nuclear membrane, staining black with hematoxylin stains, while a deep black karyosome may be observed centrally placed or in contact with the nuclear membrane at one side of the nucleus. In some cysts the remains of the cytostome may be seen, consisting of two black lines representing the lips and a spiral black line within the lips representing the oral flagellum. The blepharoplasts may also be seen as black dots closely associated with the nucleus. Most of the cysts contain but one nucleus, but Kofoid and Swezy and Hegner have observed division of the nucleus within the cysts with the formation of two nuclei.

Life History.—Two stages occur in the life cycle of *Chilomastix mesnili*, a trophozoite and cystic stage. In the intestine when conditions are favorable, the motile trophozoites divide by binary longitudinal division, but under unfavorable conditions the trophozoites become motionless and encyst, no division occurring within the cyst, according to most authorities. The cysts are voided in the feces and are swallowed by man in food contaminated with fecal material containing them, after which excystation occurs, a single trophozoite emerging from each cyst.

38111

According to some authorities, simple, binary fission of the nucleus may occur within the cyst. Contamination of food or drink may occur in all of the ways mentioned for *Endamoeba histolytica* (see Amebiasis) and the cysts of this parasite may remain viable in the intestine of flies for as long as 80 hours after the insect has fed upon contaminated material and may contaminate food or drink for this period of time.

PATHOLOGY.—There is no evidence that *Chilomastix mesnili* is a pathogenic parasite, although it may occur in enormous numbers in the feces in both health and disease. Many individuals having this infection present diarrheal symptoms at times, but that these symptoms are caused by the parasite is not proved. No pathologic lesions that can be demonstrated to be due to this flagellate have been found in the intestine of man and it is generally regarded as a harmless commensal.

DIAGNOSIS.—The diagnosis must be based upon the demonstration of the parasite in the feces and this is accomplished by a microscopic examination of the stools of the individual suspected of harboring the parasite, unstained preparations, prepared as in the examination for *Endamoeba histolytica,* being all that are necessary in trained hands for the diagnosis.

PROPHYLAXIS.—As *Chilomastix mesnili* is not a pathogenic organism, methods of prevention are not so important as in infections with pathogenic organisms but consist in preventing the contamination of food or drink with fecal material containing the cyst by methods already discussed in the prevention of amebiasis (*q.v.*).

TREATMENT.—The treatment of infections with *Chilomastix mesnili* is not indicated as it is a harmless inhabitant of the human intestine. However, numerous drugs have been tried in endeavors to eliminate the infection but no specific for this purpose has been discovered.

Infections with Trichomonas Hominis.—This flagellate, also commonly known as *Trichomonas intestinalis,* lives in the human intestine and infection with it is sometimes called *trichomoniasis.* This flagellate has a world-wide distribution and is most commonly found in poorly sanitated regions and in the tropics and subtropics. The incidence of infection has been found to vary from less than 1 per cent to 12 per cent, but in the United States it is undoubtedly the least common of the three intestinal flagellates considered in this contribution.

Trichomonas hominis may live in the lumen of any part of the small or large intestine of man but is apparently most numerous in the ileum and the large intestine. None of the lower animals harbor this flagellate unless it be certain species of monkeys, although many of the lower animals harbor other species closely resembling it in morphology. It is claimed that monkeys and cats may be infected with *Trichomonas hominis* experimentally.

MORPHOLOGY.—Unlike *Giardia lamblia* or *Chilomastix mesnili,* this flagellate has but one stage in its life cycle, that of a motile trophozoite, for cysts have never been demonstrated in this species. The finer details of the structure are brought out in wet-fixed preparations stained with hematoxylin, but for diagnostic purposes the living, unstained parasite is sufficient.

In *unstained preparations Trichomonas hominis* is a pear-shaped, colorless, hyaline-appearing organism which is actively motile, the motility being due to the flagella and the undulating membrane. It meas-

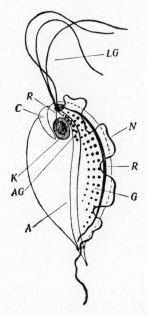

Fig. 3.—*Trichomonas hominis,* showing structural details. *LG,* Free anterior flagella; *R,* rhizoplast; *C,* cytostome; *K,* nucleus; *A,* axostyle; *AG,* axostyle granules; *N,* undulating membrane; *G,* granules. Note origin of undulating membrane and flagella from the deeply stained blepharoplasts at anterior end. (After Rodenwalt.)

ures from 7 to 15 microns in length and from 3 to 5 microns in breadth, the cytoplasm appearing granular and sometimes containing red blood corpuscles if blood is present in the feces. This organism is not usually found in formed stools, but only in fluid or semifluid stools. When motility is active the flagella and undulating membrane cannot be distinguished, but as movement becomes slower from 3 to 5 flagella may be seen to project from the anterior end and the undulating membrane may be seen as a series of minute projections along one side of the parasite, which move in a cogwheel-like manner and are very noticeable. Further structure cannot be distinguished in unstained preparations.

In *stained preparations* the cytoplasm stains a grayish-blue, while the other structures stain a deep black. Near the anterior or broad end of the parasite there is an oval *nucleus* having a central karyosome and a delicate nuclear membrane. Beginning at the anterior end there is a narrow mouth, or *cytostome,* and anterior to the nucleus is a large mass of granules, or, in well-stained preparations, a collection of separate granules, numbering from 3 to 5, the *blepharoplasts,* each of which gives rise to a flagellum. These project as free flagella from the anterior end of the organism. In addition to these blepharoplasts there are two other blepharoplasts from which arise the *undulating membrane* and the *axostyle.* The undulating membrane arises from a blepharoplast at the anterior end of the parasite and extends backward around the body, terminating at the posterior end. The free border

38111

of the membrane is formed by a flagellum which may become free at the posterior end. The *axostyle* is a rigid, spikelike structure arising from a blepharoplast near the anterior end and terminating at the posterior end where it protrudes as a sharply pointed tail.

LIFE HISTORY.—All that is known regarding the life cycle of this flagellate is that the trophozoite divides longitudinally into two organisms, division occurring first in the blepharoplasts, followed by the division of the nucleus and the body of the parasite.

The transmission of infection to man must be by swallowing material contaminated with feces containing the trophozoites, as cysts have not been observed. It has been shown by several investigators that the trophozoites of *Trichomonas hominis* are more resistant to injurious influences than the trophozoites of the parasitic amebae or other flagellates. Thus, Dobell (1934) has demonstrated that they will withstand the normal gastric juice and Hegner (1928) found they were able to remain alive in fecal material kept at room temperature for as long as eight days, so there is no reason why infection of man may not occur by swallowing the trophozoites.

PATHOLOGY.—At the present time one must regard *Trichomonas hominis* as a harmless commensal living in the intestine of man. Wenyon (1926) records finding it in the interglandular connective tissue in the intestine but states it may have reached there after death. There is no record of the experimental production of lesions with this parasite in animals with the exception of that of Kessel (1926), who claimed to have produced superficial necrosis of the mucous membrane of the intestine in kittens, but his observations have not been confirmed. As the organism is found only in semifluid or fluid stools, it naturally follows that one observes it only in the presence of diarrhea, and this fact has given rise to the supposition that it is the cause of the diarrhea. As in the case of *Giardia lamblia,* its presence in enormous numbers may aggravate or prolong any inflammatory condition in the intestine due to other causes, but that it is the cause of inflammation or intestinal symptomatology is not believed by those who have had the greatest experience in the study of infections with this parasite. When careful bacteriologic and protozoological studies have been made of cases in which this parasite was apparently producing severe diarrhea, some other organism has invariably been found to be the cause, usually one of the bacilli of dysentery or *Endamoeba histolytica.*

DIAGNOSIS.—The diagnosis of infection with *Trichomonas hominis* depends upon the demonstration of the parasite in the feces of the suspected individual, and all that is necessary for such demonstration is the microscopic examination of unstained preparations of the feces. If the patient is passing formed stools it will be necessary to administer a saline, as the parasite is not usually found in formed stools. The presence of an undulating membrane in this flagellate is characteristic and this structure can be distinguished in unstained preparations.

PROPHYLAXIS.—This is the same as for *Endamoeba histolytica* (see Amebiasis). As this parasite is apparently a harmless one, prevention is not of much importance.

TREATMENT.—The treatment of infections with *Trichomonas hominis* is not indicated, owing to the nonpathogenic nature of the parasite.

There is no known specific and the infection is difficult to eliminate. All of the drugs that have been found useful in the elimination of infection with *Endamoeba histolytica* have been tried but found unsatisfactory.

BIBLIOGRAPHY

Benson, W.: Untersuchungen über Trichomonas intestinalis und vaginalis des Menschen, Arch. f. Protistenk., 18: 115, 1910.

Craig, C. F.: The Parasitic Protozoa of Man, Phila., J. B. Lippincott & Co., pp. 1–569, 1926.

—— and Faust, E. C.: Clinical Parasitology, Phila., Lea & Febiger, pp. 1–731, 1937.

Haughwout, F. G.: The tissue invasive powers of the flagellated and ciliated protozoa, with special reference to Trichomonas intestinalis, Philippine J. Sc., (B) 13: 217, 1918.

Hegner, R.: Experimental studies on the viability and transmission of Trichomonas hominis, Am. J. Hyg., 8: 16, 1928.

Kofoid, C. A. and Swezy, O.: On the morphology and mitosis of Chilomastix mesnili (Wenyon), a common flagellate of the human intestine, Univ. California Publ. Zool., 20: 117, 1920.

Simon, C. E.: Giardia enterica, etc., Am. J. Hyg., 1: 440, 1921.

Wenyon, C. M.: A new flagellate (Macrostoma mesnili n. sp.) from the human intestine with some remarks upon the supposed cysts of "Trichomonas," Parasitology, 3: 210, 1910.

CHAPTER XXXIV

COCCIDIOSIS

By CHARLES F. CRAIG, M.D., M.A. (HON.), F.A.C.P., F.A.C.S.,
COLONEL, U. S. ARMY MEDICAL CORPS (RETIRED), D.S.M.

Definition.—Coccidiosis is the infection of the intestine of man by protozoan organisms belonging to the Sporozoa, order Coccidiida, known as coccidia. Although coccidia are common parasites of some of the lower animals they are not important as human parasites, owing to their rare occurrence and to the fact that infection with these organisms terminates spontaneously.

History.—In 1858 Gubler reported a liver infection in man with a coccidium now known as *Eimeria gubleri,* and in 1860 Kjellberg reported an intestinal infection in man with a coccidium now known as *Isospora hominis.* Both of these observations have been confirmed by more recent authorities and both species are now accepted as parasites of man by most parasitologists. Other species of coccidia have been described as parasitic in man, notably the species described by Dobell (1919) as human parasites, i.e., *Eimeria wenyoni, Eimeria oxyspora* and *Eimeria snijdersi,* but all of these were proved by Thomson and Robertson (1926) to be common coccidia of certain fish, and identical with species already described by Thelohan (1890–1892), their occurrence in man being purely accidental.

Geographic Distribution.—According to Magath (1935), about 208 cases of human infection with *Isospora hominis* have been reported to date. Geographically, these infections have occurred in the United States, Hawaii, Brazil, Uruguay, Argentina, the Philippine Islands, North and South Africa, Morocco, Portuguese East Africa, West Africa, Senegal, Nigeria, North and Central China, Indo-China, Bengal, Dutch East Indies, Persia, South Russia, Italy, Egypt, Syria, Turkey, Macedonia, Mesopotamia, Gallipoli and the Eastern Mediterranean region.

Infections with *Eimeria gubleri* are so rare that only 5 authentic cases are on record, and this species is regarded as doubtful by some parasitologists.

Etiology.—The coccidia are very frequently parasites of the lower animals and the life history of many of the species is unknown. The studies of Schaudinn and Siedlecki (1897), Schaudinn (1900) and others have resulted in the elucidation of the life history of some of the species and it is presumed that the life history of *Isospora hominis* corresponds in essentials to that of those species in which the life history is known.

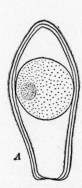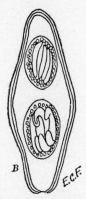

Fig. 1.—*Isospora hominis.* *A*, Oocyst from freshly passed feces; *B*, mature oocyst
from cultured feces. × 1600. (After Faust.)

The life cycle includes both an *asexual* and a *sexual* stage of development, both of which may occur in a single host.   In the *asexual cycle* the
coccidium penetrates a tissue cell of its host and is then called a *schizont.*
The schizont gradually enlarges, filling the host cell, and when fully
developed divides into several motile fusiform bodies known as *merozoites,* which are liberated by the rupture of the host cell.   The process
of division is known as *schizogony.*   The merozoites may then penetrate
other host cells and the asexual cycle is repeated.

In the *sexual cycle* some of the merozoites are differentiated into male
and female organisms, the males being known as *microgametocytes* and
the females as *macrogametocytes.*   The nucleus of the *microgametocyte*
divides and several flagellate forms develop which separate from the
parent body and are known as *microgametes.*   In the meantime, matura-
tion phenomena occur within the macrogametocytes, preparing them for
fertilization, and they are then known as *macrogametes.*   The micro-
gamete after liberation from the parent body swims about and eventually
fertilizes the macrogamete, the resulting organism being known as a
zygote or *oocyst.*   The process of fertilization may occur either within
or outside of the host cell but usually outside of the cell.   Multiplication
now occurs within the oocyst, resulting in the formation of several small
bodies known as *sporoblasts.*   Each of the sporoblasts secretes a cystic
membrane about itself and is then called a *sporocyst,* the sporoblasts now
being known as *spores.*   The nucleus of each spore divides, producing
several sickle-shaped, vermicular bodies known as *sporozoites.*   When
conditions are favorable the spores rupture, liberating the sporozoites,
which penetrate the tissue cells of the host and renew the asexual cycle,
becoming schizonts.

Two genera of coccidia are concerned in coccidiosis in man, the genus
Isospora and the genus Eimeria, as already noted.

Morphology of Isospora Hominis.—The only stage in the life cycle
of this coccidium that is known is the oocyst, the schizogonic cycle being
unknown, as well as the sexual stages of development.

In the stools of man the oocysts are found in an unsegmented condition
but develop spores after the stools have been voided.   They are elongate-

oval in shape and measure from 20 to 33 microns in length by 10 to 19 microns in breadth, one end of the oocyst being narrow and presenting a necklike appearance. They are colorless and hyaline and surrounded by a well-defined cyst wall having a double outline. Some of the oocysts are long and narrow while others are short and broad, leading Wenyon to believe that two species are involved, the larger of which he calls *Isospora hominis* and the smaller *Isospora belli*. As observed in freshly passed feces the oocysts are unsegmented, appearing as oval hyaline bodies containing a spherical mass of large granules in the midst of which the nucleus is visible as a clear, hyaline spherical area. In rare instances oocysts containing two sporoblasts may be found in freshly passed stools.

Further development within the oocysts occurs after passage from the body, the nucleus dividing into two portions, followed by the division of the granular mass in which the nuclei lie into two daughter cells, or sporoblasts. The sporoblasts become oval in shape, secrete a cyst wall and become spores. Within these spores the nucleus divides, eventually producing four sporozoites within each spore, or eight sporozoites in all. The sporozoites are long, slender, roughly crescent-shaped bodies, each having a nucleus at one extremity and lying within a mass of granules, the sporocystic residue.

It is believed that in man schizogony and the formation of the gametes occurs within the epithelial cells of the mucous membrane of the intestine, and that fertilization and the formation of the oocysts occurs in the lumen of the bowel. However, the entire cycle of development may possibly occur within the epithelial cells of the intestine.

The morphology of *Eimeria gubleri* is almost unknown. Only the oocysts have been observed and the contents of these cysts have not been described by any observer. The oocysts measure about 20 microns in length, are colorless, and have a hyaline, double-outlined surrounding membrane.

Epidemiology.—Infection with *Isospora hominis* results from ingesting food or drink contaminated with fecal material containing the fully developed oocysts. It is a parasite of the small intestine and occurs so rarely in man that one must conclude that it is normally a parasite of some lower animal. According to Magath (1935), this parasite was found but once in the examination of the stools of 60,000 patients at the Mayo clinic, and as the infection in man is self-limited, spontaneous recovery occurring in every case, it is reasonable to suppose that this coccidium is not normally a parasite of man but of some lower animal. It has not been cultivated nor has it been transmitted to any of the lower animals with the exception of the unconfirmed experiments of Fantham (1917), who claimed to have infected kittens, and of Porter (1918) who claimed to have infected cats and white rats. Nothing is known regarding the epidemiology of *Eimeria gubleri*.

Pathology.—While lesions must be produced in the intestinal epithelial cells by *Isospora hominis,* as it develops within these cells, we know nothing of the pathology of the infection, the parasite having never been observed at autopsy. In the five cases of infection with *Eimeria gubleri* observed in man, the organism produced enlargement of the liver, the coccidia being found within the epithelial cells of the liver and the bile ducts.

38111

Symptomatology.—*Isospora hominis* has been found in individuals presenting no disease symptoms and in those presenting intestinal symptomatology of varying severity. In most instances other parasites were present in cases presenting intestinal symptomatology, as one of the dysentery bacilli or *Endamoeba histolytica,* and the symptoms may have been caused by these parasites. However, in some of the reported cases the coccidium apparently was responsible for a mild diarrhea of short duration and such symptoms may have been overlooked in some cases because of the fact that the oocysts are not to be found in the stools until after the disappearance of the diarrheal symptoms. At any rate, this parasite is not considered of much importance in human pathology, as infections with it do not usually last for more than a few days, although in rare instances more persistent infections have been noted, perhaps due to reinfection rather than to continued infection.

The symptomatology of infections with *Eimeria gubleri,* owing to the extreme rarity of this parasite, is unknown.

Diagnosis.—The diagnosis of infection with *Isospora hominis* depends upon the finding of the oocysts in the stools of the infected individual. A small portion of the fecal material should be emulsified with normal saline, a drop of the mixture placed upon a microscopic slide and examined with a low dry objective. The oocysts are very characteristic bodies and should be easily recognized. No staining methods have been found of value in diagnosis. Repeated examinations are often necessary in order to demonstrate them and it should also be remembered that they may be present for a very short time, i.e., from one to four days, and that they will not be found in the stools during the diarrheal attack in most cases but only several days after the disappearance of the diarrhea. For this reason, we are very ignorant regarding the real incidence of this parasite as stool examinations are not apt to be made when intestinal symptoms are absent, and it may be more common than is commonly believed.

Prognosis.—The prognosis in *Isospora hominis* infections is always excellent as the infection is self-limited and spontaneous recovery always occurs. In infections with *Eimeria gubleri* the prognosis is unknown.

Prophylaxis.—The prophylaxis of infection with coccidia is similar to that of infections with *Endamoeba histolytica,* already described, and consists in the prevention of the contamination of food or drink with fecal material containing the oocysts.

Treatment.—Treatment is of little importance, owing to the short duration of the infection and its self-limited character. No drug has been found of specific value in coccidiosis although many of the drugs employed in the treatment of amebiasis and helminthiasis have been tried. It is obvious that, in an infection of such short duration, it would be practically impossible to evaluate the results of any drug.

BIBLIOGRAPHY

Andrews, J.: Excystation of coccidial oocysts in vivo, Science, 71 : 37, 1930.

Craig, C. F. and Faust, E. C.: Clinical Parasitology, Phila., Lea & Febiger, pp. 1–731, 1937.

Dobell, C.: A revision of the coccidia parasitic in man, Parasitology, 11 : 147, 1919.

Magath, T. B.: The coccidia of man, Am. J. Trop. Med., 15 : 91, 1935.

Thomson, J. G. and Robertson, A.: Fish as the source of certain coccidia recently described as intestinal parasites of man, Brit. M. J., 1 : 282, 1926.

Wenyon, C. M.: Coccidiosis of cats and dogs and the status of the Isospora of man, Ann. Trop. Med., 17 : 231, 1923.

CHAPTER XXXV

BACILLARY DYSENTERY

By Frederick F. Russell, M.D.

Synonyms.—Diarrhea (acute and chronic), enteritis, cholera nostras, winter cholera, intestinal grip, intestinal influenza, gastric fever, intestinal disorder, summer complaint; German, *Baccillenruhr;* French, *dysentérie bacillaire;* Italian, *dissenteria bacterica.*

Definition.—It is an infectious disease of the intestinal tract, caused by one of the bacilli of the dysentery group, occurring in both acute and chronic forms, sporadically and in small epidemics. It is characterized by frequent stools containing blood and mucus and accompanied by pain. It attacks all ages and in its severe forms has a high mortality.

Etiology.—Causative Factors.—The diarrheas of children and adults may be roughly divided into three classes: (1) those due to the dysentery bacilli, which are described here; (2) those due to protozoa, principally amebae, which are described elsewhere; and (3) those of unknown etiology. The last group is a large one, and of course cannot be accurately described. There are a certain number of cases which have all the earmarks of an infectious disease, yet neither bacilli nor amebae can be found, and it is not improbable that some of these unknowns may be due to virus infections. Another large group is that in which the diarrhea is not itself the disease but merely a symptom of some other acute infection, and lastly there is the group in which the symptoms are due to some nutritional disturbance. With improved sanitation and better nursing and medical care, the bacillary dysentery tends to diminish, leaving a higher and higher percentage of cases of nutritional diarrheas.

The disease occurs in all countries and in all climates, but is commoner in the tropics and in the warmer parts of the Temperate Zones than in colder regions; it is more frequent in the hot weather of summer than at other seasons. Both sexes and all ages are attacked. There does not seem to be any racial immunity; nor does one attack apparently give much, if any, immunity against a second attack, although we have no exact studies on this point, in which the causative organism in two successive attacks is known. It is quite possible that second attacks are relapses of latent infections rather than new infections.

3841

In well-developed communities where there is good water, adequate sewage system and efficient sanitary inspection of food and drink, particularly of the milk, the disease tends to disappear; where these safeguards do not exist, as among troops in campaign, in contractors' camps, in unsanitary settlements unprovided with sewer systems, pure water and milk, and in the backward tropics, it is still a serious problem, causing a high morbidity and mortality.

It also occurs not infrequently in institutions, particularly those for mental cases, where the personal hygiene of the patients is difficult to control, and where a common kitchen, in which the patients perform part of the work, is in use. In such institutions it is easy to understand how a patient with an acute attack, in the earliest stage of the disease, or a chronic carrier, who is perhaps temporarily on duty in the kitchen or dining room, may infect many in the institution. In addition, it is quite possible that the patients themselves may be more easily infected than normal healthy individuals.

Cross-infections among children and infants entering hospital wards for other diseases have been reported by Reed,[1] and it is, therefore, necessary to surround these patients with the same precautions used in typhoid fever wards; and in any event the stools, the bed and body linen must be disinfected and separate nurses and utensils must be furnished.

The disease is not infrequently a terminal infection in the case of cachectic patients and of those suffering from chronic disease.

The part played by flies in the distribution of the infectious material is probably quite important, as in some localities the dysentery season runs nearly parallel with the fly season. Under such circumstances both in hospitals and at home, even breast-fed children may develop the disease, although in such an event the infection may be mild in character.

Water-borne epidemics, more especially in the smaller communities where the water supply system is not continually under good supervision, are not infrequent.

C. J. Hunt[2] studied nine epidemics of dysentery occurring in cities and towns of Pennsylvania. Out of a total population of 152,000 involved, 55,000 cases (about 36 per cent of the population) were reported. In each case the disease might have been prevented by proper supervision of the water supply, as it was found that the infectious material had been distributed through that channel. In five out of the nine epidemics studied, a second outbreak, this time due to the typhoid bacillus, followed the dysentery in from ten to twenty days.

Bacillary dysentery is the cause of an enormous morbidity and mortality in the tropics and subtropical regions. Both natives and foreigners suffer from it; the foreigners, because of the better conditions under which they live, being perhaps less subject than the natives. Expeditions from northern countries to the tropics have always suffered severely and will no doubt continue to suffer, as it is hardly to be expected that there will be proper and adequate sanitary conditions in tropical ports for many years to come. The great prevalence of the disease among natives requires further study and differentiation into its various types.

That there is a considerable amount of latent dysentery in the southern and tropical regions has long been known, and J. Cunningham[3] has found that under proper and suitable conditions a survey of a community will give a total enteric index (of course, including all forms) comparable to the malarial index arrived at by spleen and blood examinations. Cunningham's studies were made in a jail in India, in a locality where dysentery was endemic. The macroscopic examination of the stools of the prisoners for mucus, and for blood and mucus, showed latent dysentery in prisoners who were, to all intents and purposes, in good health. The writer concluded that a series of ten successive examinations is sufficient to reveal all latent dysenteries in a given population. From Cunningham's data, MacKendrick found that 23 per cent of the population were abnormal in this respect, and that the chance of detecting an abnormal person at one examination was about one in three; that with five examinations one could expect to detect about 90 per cent; and with eight examinations about 97 per cent. The importance of latent dysentery with reference to the spread of the disease is obvious. Individuals in this condition are ordinarily classed as healthy carriers.

Acute and chronic carriers play the same role as in typhoid fever. The dividing line between the two classes is arbitrarily drawn at the expiration of three months from the time of the first symptoms. Healthy acute carriers are almost unknown. Healthy chronic carriers are not uncommon; a good example of this condition is described by Fletcher and Mackinnon.[4] The patient was a convalescent from rheumatism. He remembered having a slight attack of diarrhea soon after he first entered the hospital. Although his stools were formed and never contained mucus or blood, the Flexner bacilli were isolated "thirty-one times in forty-one examinations, frequently constituting from 50 to 80 per cent of all the colonies present on the plates." He was still a carrier eighteen months after the first symptoms appeared.

The ordinary chronic carrier, however, gives a good history of an acute attack and usually of remissions and exacerbations of his disease. With suitable employment and careful diet the carrier of the Flexner-"Y" bacillus remains free from symptoms and is able to work the greater part of the time. The Shiga carrier, however, is rare, as he seldom recovers sufficiently to be considered healthy, even for a time, and is therefore more properly considered a chronic case.

The excretion of the bacilli is intermittent, as with typhoid carriers, and none may be found for weeks or months together; they return in gradually increasing numbers until more dysentery colonies may be found on the plates than colon bacilli. Fletcher,[4] who studied the dysenteries of the Federated Malay States, attributes the carrier state, and the intermittent excretion of bacilli, to the formation and rupture of cysts and abscesses in the scar tissue of the colon. At autopsy many such cysts and abscesses may be found in chronic cases and carriers, and in the pus from them the bacilli are usually found.

Another explanation is offered by Nichols,[5] who notes the fact that blood cultures are occasionally positive in dysentery, and that bacilli of the dysentery group have at times been recovered from the gallbladder at autopsy.[6]

Reasoning from analogy with carriers of typhoid, paratyphoid and cholera organisms, Nichols believes that further work will show gallbladder infections in chronic dysentery carriers and suggests the necessity for further examination of cases, with this point in view. Cultures should be made at autopsy from the gallbladder and other viscera because of the possibility of a portal system septicemia, and during life the bile should be examined by means of Einhorn's duodenal tube, a method which has given excellent results in the study of typhoid and paratyphoid carriers.[7]

The duration of the carrier state in the apparently healthy is unknown, although instances are given in which it has lasted over two years without any indication of change in the future. Fletcher and Mackinnon found that all of their 13 Shiga carriers were persistent carriers, whereas only 13 out of 61 of the Flexner-"Y" group were persistent.

House and family epidemics constitute one of the characteristic features of the disease, and in rural communities, the greater number of a household have been known to die in the course of a few weeks. Of course, proper hygiene and good sanitation would prevent such catastrophes, but we know that the knowledge of good personal hygiene penetrates slowly among the masses of the people. As in secondary cases of typhoid fever, the history not infrequently shows that the mother of the household acts as nurse for the patient and as cook for the well, and sooner or later in some manner or other contaminates the food.

C. M. Lyon, writing from Huntington, West Virginia,[8] has contributed interesting and important epidemiological studies. He finds that, in his region, 15 to 80 per cent of children suffer from dysentery at some time before the age of five. Thirty-seven per cent of the urban children under observation, 52 per cent of the semi-urban, and 72 per cent of children coming to a baby welfare clinic were affected.

The epidemiological factors were the presence in the neighborhood of patients with dysentery; the improper disposal of excreta (the absence of sewers and the use of open and poorly constructed privies) and infestation with house flies.

He concludes with the statement that the private practitioner alone cannot succeed in lowering the morbidity very much; that he must have the help of the health department in improving environmental conditions, particularly the method of excreta disposal and fly control, and in measures for the special isolation needed for dysentery patients and convalescents. Bojlen's[9] studies have also shown the necessity of isolation for not less than two months after apparent recovery of dysentery cases occurring in institutions. Bojlen's[9] studies from Denmark, where both the Sonne and the Flexner-"Y" types are found, are the most impressive investigations of recent years. He found that each village and each ward in an institution might have a characteristic strain which would be common to all cases in that location. If, however, the patient was transferred to another ward, or place, he might acquire, in addition, an infection with the organism prevailing in the new location; in which case, two different strains might be isolated from his stools. The second or superinfection, being acute, might end in complete recovery, after which only the original strain could again be cultured, or he might become a carrier of both strains for an indefinite period.

The great importance of the disease has been well summarized by Barker,[10] who states that in the tropics it destroys more lives than cholera and has been more fatal to armies than powder and shot, and that it has been responsible for a greater amount of invalidism and deaths than has any other single disease.

BACTERIOLOGY.—The *Bacillus dysenteriae* was first described by Shiga,[11] who isolated it during a severe epidemic which occurred in Japan in 1898. The method which he employed had often been used before, but rarely with success. It consisted in agglutinating a large series of organisms isolated in pure culture from the stools of dysenterics with the serum from convalescents. In this way, he found an organism which reacted positively with convalescent serum. On the basis of his early experiments, he also believed the bacillus to be motile. On the culture media in use at that period he was unable to differentiate it from the typhoid bacillus, except by its slight motility and by the agglutination reaction. Shiga has recently stated (Harvard Tercentenary Address, 1936) that the Shiga variety of dysentery bacilli has disappeared from Japan in recent years.

Subsequent studies by Kruse,[12] Flexner,[13] Lentz,[14] and Hiss and Russell[15] made it clear that the organism was nonmotile and that it could be differentiated from typhoid by that character alone; this, together with the very clear-cut serologic differences, established the identity of the dysentery bacillus.

The same series of studies showed that there were differences among the dysentery bacilli themselves, and Kruse, by means of agglutination reactions, divided them into two classes, true and pseudodysenteries. In the first class he placed the organism discovered by Shiga in Japan and by himself in Germany, and in the second, or pseudodysentery class, the bacillus of Flexner and the organisms which he had isolated from cases of asylum dysentery in Germany. The term pseudodysentery was soon dropped because both varieties of the dysentery bacillus produce dysentery, and clinically the cases cannot be distinguished one from another, and it became customary in America to speak of the nonacid or nonmannite fermenting strain of bacilli (Shiga, which does not form acid from mannite), and of the acid or mannite fermenting strains ("Y," which ferments mannite only; Flexner, which ferments mannite, sucrose, dextrin and maltose; and Strong,[16] which ferments mannite and sucrose).

With this division into two principal classes and into three varieties of the second class, the subject rested until the outbreak of the World War, when the return of patients to England from the Eastern Mediterranean revived interest in the subject in English-speaking countries.

Another rough classification is into the toxic and nontoxic, or slightly toxic varieties. The Shiga bacillus produces a soluble exotoxin as well as an endotoxin, and as a result toxic symptoms, paralyses, and involvement of the articular and serous cavities are not infrequent. With all other varieties of the bacillus these toxic symptoms are absent, since only the Shiga produces the soluble exotoxin. The distinction is of some importance when it comes to treatment with serums.

The failures of early investigators to find a single causative organism upon which they could agree led them to accept the hypothesis that the disease was caused by the commoner and well-known bacteria of the intestine, which in some way had acquired great virulence. French and Italian authors reported the presence of a colon bacillus, called by them *Bacillus coli dysentericus*, which was pathogenic for cats and dogs, producing dysenteric lesions in the colon, including ulcers (Magiori, Levaran, Armand, Celli, Fioca [1895] and Escherich).

3841

In Japan, Ogata [17] described a gram-positive bacillus with liquefied gelatin and produced dysenteric lesions in laboratory animals. It has never been reported since except by Vivaldi, in a small epidemic in Italy.

Calmette isolated the *Bacillus pyocyaneus* from a form of dysentery common in Cochin China, where it is known as endemic enterocolitis; Lartigan in New York, Adami in Canada, and Barker in Baltimore, found the same organism in small epidemics, but no further references are found to this organism in the literature in recent years.

Many observers have noted the frequency with which streptococci (*Streptococcus intestinalis*) and other cocci are found in the stools in dysentery, and in the summer diarrheas of children, and have particularly observed their presence in enormous numbers in green stools. No one has recently attributed any pathologic importance to them, however (Zancard, Silvestri, Bertrand, Bauscher and Ascher).

In 1906 Morgan,[18] working in London, published a study of the bacteriology of the summer diarrheas of children. He noted that the clinical picture of the disease in England was somewhat different from that reported in America; for example, he found blood in the stools to be quite exceptional there, whereas in America it is not infrequent. He found none of the usual dysentery bacilli, but did isolate a series of organisms from stools and autopsy material. His method was as follows: The stools were plated on MacConkey's bile-salt, neutral red, lactose agar and all colonies unable to ferment lactose were transferred to lactose broth fermentation tubes. After three days' incubation all the lactose fermenters were discarded and transfers then made to gelatin; after three weeks' incubation all liquefying cultures were discarded and the remainder retained for study. Morgan examined 304 cultures and found an organism since known as *Morgan's bacillus No. 1*, which is a gram-negative, motile bacillus, producing acid and gas in dextrose, but not fermenting mannite, dulcite, lactose or sucrose. It turns litmus milk alkaline and produces indol. It caused death preceded by diarrhea in young laboratory animals, and was regularly isolated from the animal's spleen after death. Filtrates from young broth cultures were found to be quite toxic for rabbits. The stools of healthy children were repeatedly examined, but with uniformly negative results. Morgan's results from agglutination tests, using the patient's culture and serum, were disappointing, as only one serum out of forty examined showed agglutinins for the bacillus from the corresponding patient.

Kligler [19] has shown that while culturally these organisms appear to represent a single, definite species, serologically they are quite diversified. Among seventeen cultures examined, six different groups were found. In view of these wide antigenic differences it seems improbable that the organisms can be specifically related to any of these disease processes or to each other.

Up to the time of the publication of the papers of Kruse, 1901, and of Lentz, 1902, and of Hiss and Russell, 1903, and of Park and Dunham, 1902,[20] the various dysentery organisms had not been differentiated. These studies showed, however, that the Shiga bacillus fermented glucose only, and that the bacillus brought from Manila by Flexner in 1900 could be differentiated from the Shiga by its power of fermenting mannite, an alcohol which had not been used before that time by bacteriologists. Hiss and Russell showed, furthermore, that a third variety, which they called the "Y" bacillus, could be differentiated from the Shiga by reason of its power to ferment glucose and mannite only, whereas the Flexner cultures also fermented maltose, sucrose and dextrin.

In 1903, during a small epidemic near New York, Park and Carry [21] isolated another form which was like the Shiga in the fermentation reactions, but different from it in possessing the power to produce indol and in not being agglutinated in either Flexner or Shiga serum. It is possible, therefore, that they anticipated the discovery of what is now known as *Bacillus ambiguus* or Schmitz' bacillus.

Thus it is seen that during the first years after the discovery of the organism much work was done, particularly in Germany and the United States, which resulted in showing the widespread distribution of the bacilli of dysentery; of late years, however, until the outbreak of the World War, very little more was contributed to our knowledge of the bacteriology of the disease. The reason for this becomes evident when one considers the nature of the investigations upon intestinal organisms during the period. Drigalski and Conradi,[22] and soon after, Endo [23] and MacConkey, described new plating media for the isolation of typhoid bacilli from the stools and urine, making use of dyes as indicators. In the course of time these media, particularly the Endo, came to be used as a routine measure for the examination of stools in laboratories all over the world. Although these media are highly successful for the typhoid and paratyphoid bacilli, they are not equally suitable for the dysentery bacilli. In this country the eosin-methylene blue plates of Teague and Holt, Harris and of Levine are the most satisfactory. The plate medium consists of peptone 10 Gm., agar 15 Gm., lactose 5 Gm., saccharose 5 Gm., dipotassium phosphate 2 Gm., yellowish eosin 0.2 Gm. and methylene blue 0.05 Gm. Final pH 7.2 $\pm$.

The addition of saccharose hastens the production of acid by the slow colons, and the dipotassium phosphate acts as a buffer and stabilizes the reaction. The inhibiting action of the dyes is very slight and typhoids, paratyphoids and dysenteries all grow well. On this medium the typhoids, paratyphoids and the dysenteries are clear and transparent, and are easily differentiated from the colon bacilli which have dark, often metallic, centers. In Europe and especially in Denmark, Bojlen and others have used a modified Conradi-Drigalski, the basis of which is trypsin-digested casein (Cole and Onslow, 1916; Kristensen, Lester and Juergens, 1925).

Technic of Stool Examination.—In 1918 Kligler and Olitsky [24] reinvestigated the technic of stool examination for dysentery bacilli, and made certain definite recommendations, of which the following are the more important:

"*Selection of Stool Specimens for Examination.*—Too much emphasis cannot be laid on the importance of choosing a satisfactory sample of stool. If possible, one containing blood and mucus with little or no fecal matter should be used. It is desirable to plate the stool directly or very shortly after it is collected. Experiments with artificial mixtures of the Shiga bacillus with feces showed a 50 per cent reduction in four hours and from 85 to 90 per cent in twenty-four hours, when kept at room temperature."

While it is desirable to make plates as soon as possible from the suspected stool, it is, nevertheless, possible to preserve the stool for relatively long periods, two and even three weeks, by putting a small portion of the stool, the size of a pea, into not less than 5 cc. of 20 per cent glycerin in normal salt solution, and keeping the specimen in the refrigerator. The preservative power of the glycerin is, of course, limited and is completely destroyed if too large a particle of stool is put into the glycerin-salt mixture.

The idea that the stool must be plated immediately is widespread, and may be due to the fact that immediate examination is needed in the case of amebic dysentery; in bacillary dysentery this preservative works well and is useful when it is impossible to make plates immediately (Knud Bojlen [9]). Studies of artificial mixtures of dysentery bacilli and feces show a very rapid death rate of dysentery bacilli, but experience with clinical material does not altogether substantiate the finding with artificial mixtures. Bojlen found that Flexner-"Y" and Sonne dysentery stools could be preserved with glycerin for one or two weeks when kept at low temperature.

The two sorts of media which Kligler and Olitsky found most suitable are prepared as follows:

"(1) The modified Endo's medium is prepared as follows: To veal or beef-infusion 1.5 per cent agar, titrated (and this is important) to pH 7.6 to 7.8, is added 1 per cent lactose and 1 per cent by volume of decolorized basic fuchsin indicator. The latter is prepared by adding 1 cc. of 10 per cent basic fuchsin to 10 cc. of 10 per cent sodium bisulphite solution. Of course, the lactose and the indicator are added separately before plates are poured.

"(2) The eosin-blue medium is prepared by adding to the veal-infusing agar, titrated to pH 7.2 to 7.4, 1 per cent lactose, and 2 cc. of 2 per cent solution of yellow eosin and 2 cc. of 0.5 per cent solution of water-soluble methylene blue."

The usual technic of inoculation of fermentation and other test tubes by means of a loop of culture is not always satisfactory for this organism. Better results are sometimes obtained with a large inoculum; 0.5 to 1 cc. of a broth culture is transferred to each new tube by means of a sterile pipette, in the same manner that is customary with cultures of the pneumococci and streptococci; it insures immediate and abundant growth and clear-cut fermentation and indol reactions.

It is often timesaving, in the long run, to use the technic of Jordan; that is, to set up three parallel series of tubes, all treated in the same manner, and if the three fail to agree, the source of error can be immediately traced down. It is also advantageous to incubate with the organism being tested an uninoculated tube on each medium used as a control of the sterility of the medium itself.

In systematic studies of dysentery bacilli one cannot have too many controls.

Preservation of Dysentery Cultures.—It is the general experience that cultures disassociate rapidly under ordinary laboratory methods of care, and soon consist almost entirely of rough variants. Proper preservation, therefore, becomes essential for those cultures which are to be used in producing agglutinating serums.

The best method is to freeze, and dry the cultures while frozen, according to the method of Swift,[25] which he has used so successfully in the preservation, without loss of virulence, of streptococcus and pneumococcus cultures.

A simpler method of freezing and drying both cultures and serums is described by Mudd, Reichel, Flosdorf and Eagle,[26] and by Road.[27] It is almost essential in order to have smooth strains for the production of antiserums to use one of these methods. If, however, this is not possible, stock cultures should be stored in the coldest part of a good refrigerator.

Kligler and Olitsky's procedure for isolation of the bacillus from the stools, as briefly stated by them, is as follows:

"*Procedure.*—On the basis of these tests, and of experience in practical work and class work, we recommend the following procedure for the isolation and rapid identification of dysentery bacilli from stools:

"A fresh specimen of stool, preferably with blood and mucus, is collected and promptly cultured. A shred of bloody mucus, if present, is selected, washed three or four times with sterile saline, to remove all fecal matter, and spread successively on a veal infusion eosin-methylene-blue and a modified Endo plate. The plates are then incubated from eighteen to twenty-four hours at 37° C.

"The plates are now examined and the suspicious, colorless colonies inoculated into each of two differential tubes:

"(a) A small tube containing 1 cc. of a 0.5 per cent glucose broth.

"(b) A double sugar tube, on the principle of the Russell double sugar medium, containing 0.1 per cent glucose, 0.5 per cent mannite, and 1 per cent Andrade indicator.

"The colony is picked off with a small loop and inoculated first into the broth and then stabbed in and streaked on the double sugar tube.

"After from two to four hours the broth tubes are usually sufficiently turbid for an agglutination test with a polyvalent antidysenteric serum. A faint visible turbidity is sufficient, and when it appears, 0.1 cc. of a 1:50 dilution of a potent polyvalent antidysenteric serum is added and the tubes re-incubated for one hour. A definite clumping is a good presumptive test for the presence of dysentery bacilli.

"The double sugar tube is incubated over-night. A red butt without gas, and a colorless slant indicates a Shiga bacillus. If the entire tube is red and gas absent, it corresponds to a Flexner type. The surface growth is now washed off with saline and a confirmatory agglutination test is made with specific type and polyvalent serum. If desired, an agar slant and various agar mediums may be inoculated for further study, or an animal inoculation made.

"By the use of the two tubes, one can obtain a presumptive diagnosis about a day after the collection of the stool—a matter of great importance for epidemiologic and therapeutic purposes."

Any tube showing gas formation may be immediately discarded, since none of the dysentery bacilli form gas.

For the double-sugar tube phenol red is the most useful indicator, and has practically superseded the use of litmus and of Andrade's indicator. The phenol red turns a brilliant yellow in the presence of acid.

Alternative Medium.—A simple and satisfactory medium has been devised by Max Levine,[28] working in the author's laboratory, for the isolation of these organisms from stools:

Distilled water .... 1000 cc.
Agar .... 15 Gm.
Peptone (Difeo) .... 10 Gm.
Dipotassium phosphate .... 4 Gm.

The hydrogen ion concentration of this medium is 7.4 to 7.5. It therefore needs no adjustment, and if the agar is clean and white, need not be filtered. To each 100 cc. is added:

Lactose, 20 per cent solution .... 5 cc.
Glucose, 5 per cent solution .... 1 cc.
Rosolic acid (1 per cent in 90 per cent alcohol) .... 1 cc.
China blue (0.5 per cent in water) .... 1 cc.

The dysentery bacilli grow as luxuriantly on this as on any other medium, and the nonlactose fermenters are readily isolated. Colonies fished from these plates are first agglutinated in a polyvalent serum of high titer and transferred to double-sugar tubes in the manner recommended by Kligler and Olitsky (see under Procedure).

For a further study of the organism giving the presumptive cultural and serologic reactions, it is well to replate the cultures, since those fished from plates inoculated by streaking the surface with material from a stool are frequently contaminated; consequently further study of the organism cannot be carried out until pure cultures have been obtained by replating.

The culture is then transferred to milk, using bromcresol purple or litmus as an indicator, to peptone solution and to fermentation tubes containing 0.5 per cent solutions of the carbohydrates given below, in Levine's peptone dipotassium phosphate medium, or sugar-free broth. Levine's medium contains peptone 1 per cent, and dipotassium phosphate 0.4 per cent in distilled water. This should give a pH value of 7.6 which is a satisfactory reaction for this group. The carbohydrates for confirmation of the presumptive test already made, and for further study, are glucose, lactose, sucrose, mannite and dulcite, and to a limited extent maltose and dextrin.

It has, however, been pretty clearly shown, by numerous studies, that the greatest value of carbohydrate fermentations is in the separation of the dysentery bacilli into four characteristic groups: Shiga, Sonne, Schmitz and the Flexner-"Y" group. Further subdivision of the last must be made by agglutination with immune serums. The first three classes are serologically homogeneous.

In studying the group by means of fermentation reactions it is essential to have pure sugars, and the best test for their suitability is the use of control fermentations with pure cultures of known dysentery organisms. Impurities in the maltose are not uncommon; but even when pure some of the sugars are easily broken down during the sterilization, which must be carefully controlled. An exposure of ten minutes at ten pounds' pressure is sufficient, if the tubes are small. In either case the tubes should be packed loosely in the baskets, to permit rapid and uniform heating. Mudge [29] has shown that the temperature to which the sugar medium is submitted is less important than the time, and he finds that there is less hydrolysis of the sugar when the medium is sterilized in the autoclave than when it is sterilized in the Arnold. As a rule ten minutes' exposure to ten pounds' pressure in the autoclave gives a satisfactory medium. As an indicator of the reaction of the medium phenol red will be found superior to litmus.

Cultural Characteristics of the Dysentery Bacillus.—The dysentery bacillus is about the same size as the typhoid bacillus, the difference being that it is slightly shorter and thicker. In a stained preparation from a pure culture considerable variation in size and shape is seen, many bacilli being so short and broad that they resemble cocci. The organism stains readily with all the usual dyes and is regularly gram-negative. In hanging-drop preparations an active brownian movement is seen but no true motility. The absence of motility is readily demonstrated in cultures made in the semisolid medium of Hiss, which shows that the bacillus is unable to grow away from the line of inoculation and consequently leaves the medium clear, in contrast to the motile typhoid bacillus, which causes a diffuse cloud throughout the medium.

Gelatin is not liquefied. On agar plates the colonies resemble typhoid colonies, yet are much smaller and grow less rapidly; they are moreover much more sensitive to the reaction of the medium. Luxuriant cultures on agar plates have a characteristic odor. Dissociation into rough and smooth colonies takes place rapidly, and most old laboratory strains are rough. The dissociation is most marked in the Sonne variety in which two forms of colonies, rough and smooth, are found usually in the first plates (Thjøtta and Waaler [30]). Milk is not coagulated, but shows a primary acidity with a subsequent reversion to alkalinity.

None of the dysentery cultures produce gas in glucose fermentation tubes. The remaining cultural reactions vary so much with the different strains of the organism that each must be considered separately.

Toxin Formation.—Kraus and Doerr [31] and Todd [32] have shown that the Shiga strain, unlike the other members of the typhoid-colon-dysentery group, is able to produce a soluble toxin of great power. The soluble toxin is not only fatal to laboratory animals but reproduces in them many of the lesions of the disease, which are comparable to those found in human beings. The toxin is usually obtained by filtering young broth cultures, but a potent toxin may be obtained by emulsifying agar cultures in salt solution, shaking, for a short period, and then filtering. It will withstand a temperature of 60 or 70° C. for one hour but is destroyed at 80° C. if exposed for the same length of time.

The toxin, as will be seen from the symptoms, exerts its effect upon the mucous membranes of the colon, conjunctiva and urethra, on the nervous system, and on the synovial and pleural membranes, and it is probably, therefore, a complex body, consisting of two or more toxins.

Therapeutic Antidysenteric Serum.—This was formerly prepared by inoculating horses subcutaneously with cultures or filtrates of cultures, over long periods of time—nine months or a year. Flexner and Amoss [33] have described a rapid method which makes it possible to bring a horse to the productive stage in as short a period as ten weeks. The essential points in this method consist in giving three intravenous injections of toxins, or of killed, and finally of living, cultures on three successive days, followed by a period of seven days' rest, when the three successive doses are repeated and the animal is again allowed to rest. By alternating in the use of Shiga and Flexner-"Y" strains, a potent polyvalent antidysenteric serum which will have a high agglutination titer and which will protect laboratory animals against lethal doses of cultures can be produced in a relatively short time.

Pathogenicity for Animals.—Except perhaps in the case of monkeys it has been impossible to reproduce the disease in animals by feeding experiments. By inoculation with both living and killed cultures, however, dysenteric lesions can be produced in most laboratory animals. The toxin is particularly fatal to rabbits which develop a rapidly fatal paralysis of the hind quarters. The intestinal lesions can also be reproduced: swelling, injection, hemorrhages, necrosis, ulceration and, in occasional cases, scar formation may be seen.

Differentiation of True Dysentery Bacillus from Allied Organisms.—The rapid and exact differentiation of the true dysentery bacilli from allied organisms has been attempted in various ways, and the classification given by Andrews [34] in 1918 was a step in advance.

Cultures die out very quickly on ordinary media, but Andrews finds that it is possible to preserve them on Dorset's egg medium in sealed tubes; he has succeeded in keeping them alive on this medium for months, merely by paraffining the cotton stopper.

As a basis for his sugar media he used the ovomucin suggested by Winter. [35]

The medium consists of 45 Gr. (3 Gm.) of dried commercial white of egg, dissolved in a liter of cold water. It is steamed in the Arnold to coagulate the albumin and globulin and filtered while hot until clear. One-half per cent of sodium chloride and the same amount of the sugar to be used is added, together with a suitable indicator; Andrade serves very well. The mixture should be pink while hot, but colorless when cold. The sugars found desirable for a satisfactory differentiation were glucose, lactose, mannite and dulcite. Andrews does not consider that sucrose or maltose is necessary.

Agglutination in specific monovalent serums, when carried on properly to the full titer, must of course be used in any system of identification of these organisms. The reaction must, however, be carried out systematically, since neither a positive nor a negative agglutination test will of itself establish the diagnosis. For example, some Flexner-"Y" strains may not agglutinate in any available serum, and on the other hand, nonrelated organisms, particularly *Bacillus coli*, may agglutinate to the full titer of the serum. However, when unrelated organisms are excluded by cultures and all the conditions are properly controlled, the agglutination test will establish the identity of the culture in question.

Andrews recognized the Shiga and Flexner-"Y" types as true dysentery bacilli and separate from them three related organisms which he called *Bacillus ambiguus* (Schmitz' bacillus), *Bacillus alkalescens* and *Bacillus dispar* (the Sonne bacillus). He gives his results in the following table:

	Lactose	Glucose	Mannite	Dulcite	Indol	Alkali Formation	Acid Agglutination	Specific Serum Agglutination	Pathogenicity for Laboratory Animals
Bacillus of Shiga	−	+	−	−	−	Slow	−	To titer	Very high
Bacillus ambiguus	−	+	−	−	+	Slow	+	Negative	Negative
Bacillus of Flexner-"Y"	−	+	+	−	±	Mod.	−	To titer	Marked
Bacillus alkalescens ...	−	+	+	+	+	Rapid	+	Negative	Negative
Bacillus dispar	+	+	+	−	±	Rapid	+	Negative	Marked

Further work has been done by Murray [36] on the serologic reactions of the dysentery group, and his conclusion is briefly that the dysentery group can be divided primarily by cultural reactions into four classes:

1. *Bacillus dysenteriae* (Shiga).

2. *Bacillus ambiguus* (Schmitz' bacillus). This is like the Shiga type, except in the serum reactions and in producing indol. He accepts it as pathogenic.

3. *Flexner-"Y."* This class contains several varieties which cannot be separated by cultural reactions, but which are evident serologically.

4. The Sonne bacillus or *Bacillus dispar* of Andrews (Class E of Kruse). This organism, besides fermenting glucose and mannite, produces acid in lactose after long incubation—sometimes as long as 14 days—and there is sometimes a late clot in milk.

We see, therefore, that the dysentery group has been enlarged as the result of the investigations carried on during the war, that Class 2 of Murray (*Bacillus ambiguus* of Andrews) has been added to the Shiga or nonmannite fermenting type, and that Class 4 of Murray (*Bacillus dispar* of Andrews) has been added to the mannite fermenting type, and further, that Flexner-"Y's" and nearly related strains (Class 3 of Murray, and Flexner-"Y" of Andrews) have been consolidated into a single class. Murray's four classes can be arranged as follows:

Bacillus dysenteriae (Shiga) .... Class 1
Bacillus ambiguus (Schmitz) .... Class 2
Bacillus dysenteriae Flexner " Y " .... Class 3
Bacillus dispar (Sonne) .... Class 4

Andrews' classification as modified by Murray has been further modified with time; *Bacillus alkalescens* has been dropped out of the dysentery bacilli; *Bacillus ambiguus* is now commonly known as Schmitz' bacillus, and *Bacillus dispar* is the Sonne bacillus. All four are regarded as dysentery bacilli, and Andrews' division in true dysentery and related organisms has been dropped.

3841

Para-agglutination is an expression which has come into use to express the fact that bacteria other than those used as the antigens in producing the serums will sometimes be agglutinated. For example, *Bacillus coli* isolated from a case of dysentery may be agglutinated in Shiga serum in as high a dilution as the Shiga itself. It has been stated [37] that *Bacillus coli* and even intestinal cocci may acquire the property of being agglutinated by specific dysentery or typhoid serum, when growing in the body in association with these pathogenic organisms. The inference, on finding para-agglutinable bacteria, is that further search will reveal the causative organism, or that the patient's serum will agglutinate it. Although the direct value of these observations is probably not great, it does serve to emphasize one of the pitfalls of agglutinations in this group. It must not be overlooked that a positive agglutination of an unknown organism in dysentery serum does not identify the culture as *Bacillus dysenteriae*, and that complete cultural study is always necessary. The para-agglutinins are not group agglutinins, as can be shown by absorption reactions. Furthermore, the para-agglutinable bacilli may lose this property on repeated transfer to culture media.

Knud Bojlen [9] in Denmark has made extensive studies over a period of four or five years of the bacteriology, serology and epidemiology of dysentery and he finds that they can be divided into constant groups according to their fermentation reactions. Three of these groups—Shiga, Sonne and Schmitz—are serologically, as well as biochemically, distinct and constant; the Flexner–"Y" group can be subdivided into Flexner, which ferments saccharose, and "Y" which does not, but the serologic classification is not so simple. By agglutination tests the Flexner–"Y" group can be subdivided into about five varieties.

He found that the fermentation reactions of old laboratory cultures, which usually give rough colonies, might vary more or less, from the reactions with freshly isolated cultures, but the differences as a rule were not great. In his hands the fermentation tests were of real value and were particularly helpful in epidemiological studies, when it is advantageous to have as many different categories as possible.

PATHOGENESIS.—As with other enteric diseases, the infectious agent enters through the mouth with contaminated food, or drink, or is conveyed to the mouth on the fingers. It passes through the stomach and begins to multiply in the small intestine, where the bacilli can be found in enormous numbers. As they increase in number, one or more toxins are produced which are absorbed into the circulation. One of the toxins is excreted by the mucous membrane of the colon, and in passing through its walls, produces characteristic changes and gives rise to the dysenteric symptoms.

Flexner and Sweet [38] made extensive studies on the pathogenesis of the disease, and demonstrated quite conclusively that the endotoxins, which are elaborated in the course of the disease by autolysis of the bacilli in the small intestine, are absorbed, with the aid of the bile, from both the small and large intestines. In rabbits with or without section or ligature of the ducts, absorption of a toxin capable of producing lesions in the colon does not take place, although without the bile the neurotoxin is absorbed in sufficient quantities to produce death from paralysis.

After absorption into the blood, the toxin is excreted by the mucous membrane of the colon, which is greatly damaged in the process. The lesion, as shown in sections of the colon from early cases, begins in the submucosa around the blood and lymph vessels rather than on the surface. The lesion and the pathologic process resemble, in fact, those in mercurial poisoning, from which they differ only in intensity.

Geographic Distribution.—In the United States we have representatives of all four groups. (1) Shiga organisms are rare but can be found in certain localities such as West Virginia, and in the western part of Virginia. (2) The Sonne group is widespread throughout the United States and has been frequently reported from Massachusetts and New York since 1929. Some of the epidemics occurred in institutions for children and for adults, and some took the form of food-poisoning outbreaks.[39] (3) The Schmitz bacillus was first reported from Rumania and apparently is not widely distributed in the United States. However, an extensive epidemic was reported by Schleifstein and Coleman,[40] New York State Health Department. There were 200 cases in an institution with a total population of 5000. With a few exceptions the cases were relatively mild, although in two instances the temperature rose to 104° F. (40° C.). Apparently there were no fatalities. The onset was sudden, with abdominal pain followed by diarrhea with blood and mucus, which persisted for two or three days.

Symptomatology.—CLINICAL HISTORY.—*Period of Incubation.*—The exact period is not well established, but there is abundant reason for believing that it is short. Strong and Musgrave [41] report that it is probably less than forty-eight hours in the Philippines. Older statements giving periods as long as seven days are probably incorrect.

Mode of Onset.—The disease usually (80 per cent of the cases) begins suddenly, often with rigors, headache and vomiting, particularly in the severer forms found in the tropics and southern regions. From the beginning it is characterized by great prostration. Even on the first day of the disease the patient may appear extremely ill and exhausted. The temperature is usually only slightly elevated, although it may reach 103 or 104° F. (39.4 or 40° C.), and it does not show a characteristic curve. A continuously high temperature or marked irregularity in the curve may indicate the onset of some complication. The pulse is increased in frequency and is quite small.

Course of Disease.—The tongue is heavily coated, and as the disease progresses it becomes swollen and shows the imprint of the teeth. If the mouth is not well cared for the coating increases and becomes brown and dry; coating is less in evidence in subacute and chronic cases, and the surface may become bright red, smooth and shining like a piece of fresh beef. The swelling continues to be prominent until well into convalescence.

The characteristic symptoms are, of course, the *frequent bloody stools* and the abdominal pain, accompanied by great prostration. The number of stools is always large and may reach thirty or forty a day for short periods, except in the acutely toxic cases, when death may occur without much change in the number or character of the stools. The stool itself is quite characteristic, and at the height of the disease is quite unlike the stool in any other disease, not excluding amebic dysentery. It is small and consists exclusively of blood and mucus, without a trace

3841

of fecal matter. Under the microscope—and dysenteric stools ought always to be examined microscopically, on the chance of finding ameba, flagellates or ciliates—one sees red blood cells in enormous numbers, and epithelial cells in masses as they are thrown off by the mucous membrane. These are often to be recognized as columnar epithelial cells, arranged like closely set pickets on a fence, like a typical textbook picture. In addition, single epithelial cells in all stages of swelling, degeneration and necrosis are seen; the single swollen cells are often roundish and suggest at first quiescent amebae, but they do not possess the power of motion, or the ability to send out pseudopods, like amebae. They may also be readily distinguished from amebic cysts by the large size and different character of their nuclei. If stains are added to the stool, such as Donaldson's stain, as used by Kofoid,[42] it will be noted that the degenerated and necrotic epithelial cells take up the eosin readily, in sharp contrast to the amebae, which are stained yellow with the iodine. Everywhere through the microscopic field are enormous numbers of leukocytes. These various elements are embedded in masses of glairy and stringy mucus. As the disease progresses and increases in severity, the character of the stool changes from that described above; the epithelial masses increase in size until one sees sloughs of large ulcers, or even a pseudomembranous cast of the entire circumference of the gut. Under the microscope it is no longer possible to make out the structure of the epithelial cells, since the entire mass is coagulated and necrotic. The fluid part of the stool is no longer watery but serous, and dark from altered hemoglobin. Such stools are extremely offensive.

A single stool is often no more than a teaspoonful, yet the patient complains of an incessant desire to go to stool. Vesical tenesmus is also a frequent and troublesome symptom. As a result of the excessive loss of fluid from the body, the patient complains bitterly of thirst, and the need for liquids in treatment is apparent.

In very severe infections, and where the case does not come under treatment early, the patient becomes more and more prostrated and toxemic, and death occurs in the first few days.

Some cases have a striking resemblance to cholera. The onset is sudden, the prostration marked, the stools are frequent and very watery, and soon become of the consistency of rice water; the face and hands, because of the great loss of fluids from the body, quickly become shriveled and shrunken, and the abdomen sunken and boat-shaped. In the presence of cholera it is, of course, impossible to make a differential diagnosis on clinical grounds alone, and such cases are treated as cholera until bacteriologic examinations have shown the safety of releasing them from observation.

Milder cases, and those which come under treatment early, may begin to improve toward the end of the first week; the stools become less frequent, and change in character, becoming less bloody and more feculent, showing some staining with bile.

The *pain*, which is so important a symptom of the disease, manifests itself in two forms: tormina and tenesmus. *Tormina* or griping pains (cramps) are felt anywhere in the course of the colon, although they are usually localized in the transverse colon. They occur also during the course of the acute digestive disturbances where the colon is healthy, but in dysentery they continue to occur after the gas and offending food have been passed, and are then probably due to spasmodic contractions of the muscular coat of the inflamed and swollen colon.

Tenesmus is essentially an exaggeration of the usual sensation felt when the bowels are evacuated; due to the inflamed condition of the sigmoid and rectum the sensation becomes an intense and penetrating pain, recurring after every stool, no matter how small.

Vesical tenesmus does not depend upon the severity of the dysentery, but may appear in even the milder cases, and when marked may lead to retention of urine. In the case of children and of stuporous cases, special attention must be paid to the bladder and catheterization must be performed when needed.

The *urine* is scanty, highly colored and of increased specific gravity. It frequently shows the presence of albumin, hyaline and granular casts and, in rare cases, of red blood cells. The liver and the bile ducts may be involved, and jaundice may appear. The spleen may be enlarged and tender.

In adults the disease is usually self-limited and runs its course in from ten days to two weeks, but some cases become subacute and last for a month or more, and of these a few become chronic and last for months or years with periods of remission.

In infants the character of the stools varies greatly. Blood is usually present, although not in every stool, either in small specks or streaks on the surface of the mucous masses, or as fluid blood; the stool may consist entirely of blood and mucus. Mucus is always present, often in large quantities, either alone or mixed with curds and undigested food. As a rule the stools are green in color and may be quite numerous. Their passage is regularly accompanied by tenesmus, although careful observation is necessary to detect the symptoms in some cases.

The duration of cases of infantile dysentery which recover varies from one to four weeks; death occurs most frequently during the first or early in the second week, although the illness may end in death after as long a period as six weeks.

Relapses occur, comparable to those in typhoid fever, but they are not common or clean-cut.

L. Jacob [43] has described a series of cases in which the temperature rose on the nineteenth to the twenty-second day. The period of normal temperature preceding the relapse varied from one to three weeks. The intestinal symptoms were absent, or the stools were milky, amounting to little more than a diarrhea. Nevertheless, he isolated both Shiga and Flexner-"Y" strains from the stools during relapse. In spite of the mildness of the intestinal symptoms, the fever, malaise and anorexia were marked. Headache and joint pains were frequently present and severe. Relapse after surgical operations (for hernia) have been reported; the thorough purgation preparatory to the operations seemed to be the exciting cause.

At the beginning of the attack the abdomen is distended, but later it is sunken and boat-shaped; palpation of the colon is painful throughout the course, but particularly over the sigmoid, cecum or the flexures. Among infants and children in hospital practice about 20 per cent die in the first two days, but in private practice the mortality is lower. Seventy per cent have a normal temperature by the sixth day and their stools become normal by the fourteenth day.

Chronic Cases.—The symptoms do not differ from those of the acute form except in their severity. The patients are greatly emaciated; in fact, some become mere skeletons before they die. On the other hand, there are periods of remission during which the patient seems to have entirely recovered. Fletcher and Mackinnon [4] call attention to the difference in the symptoms between Shiga and Flexner-"Y" cases, which consists principally in the severity of the symptoms present. Without exception the patients with the Shiga type were very sick, greatly emaciated, and suffered from mental depression. They had frequent stools, usually containing blood and mucus. The Flexner-"Y" patients, on the other hand, usually looked well, and were often well nourished and had remissions during which the stools were normal. Such men were quite capable of doing ordinary work, and in civil life, where they could choose their occupation, would get along quite well.

Diagnosis.—The diagnosis of dysentery is readily made, but to differentiate this disease from amebic or balantidial dysentery is not possible on clinical symptoms and signs alone. The fresh stool, as soon as possible after it is passed, should be examined under the microscope, in order to exclude the dysenteries which are due to amebae and other animal parasites. The description of the microscopic appearance of amebae in dysenteric stools will be found under the subject of Entamebic Dysentery, and will not be referred to further here. It is true that the ameba of dysentery, in the summer in the North and all the year round in the tropics, will preserve its motility for several hours. While vacuum bottles or water-heated containers are desirable for the preservation of specimens, they are not absolutely essential.

The serum reactions are not of much practical value in diagnosis, since agglutinins, for example, do not become evident in the patient's serum until relatively late in the disease. They are rarely present before the end of the first week, and usually not until the second week, and may not appear until the third or fourth week. Bacteriologic examination of the stools is of more value, since it makes possible the determination of the main types of dysentery bacilli, and when followed by agglutination with type serums, shows finally the kind of bacillus involved. The severity and prognosis are much worse in those dysenteries due to the Shiga bacillus than in the forms due to other members of the group. Details of the laboratory methods in use will be found in the first part of this chapter.

The agglutination reaction is of inestimable value in epidemiological investigations of outbreaks in hospitals, institutions and communities, since many mild, unrecognized cases occur, which could not otherwise be diagnosed or identified. The length of time that agglutinins are present in the blood after an attack is not well established, but reports show that they may be present for six or seven weeks, and probably for a much longer period. Agglutinins may be present long after all bacilli have disappeared from the stools.

DIFFERENTIAL DIAGNOSIS.—Frequent stools with blood, mucus and tenesmus are caused not merely by the dysentery bacilli but also by organic disease of the rectum and colon, such as carcinoma, adenomatous polypi, tuberculosis and syphilis. These conditions must be excluded by physical examination and by the history of the onset.

Toward the end of a dysentery epidemic caused by a polluted public water supply, cases of typhoid fever are apt to appear, as has been shown by Hunt. The pollution of a water supply by sewage would naturally be expected to reproduce all the water-borne diseases which were present in the community from which the contaminating sewage came. Attention must therefore be directed to the possibility of a change in the type of infection. Because of the length of the illness and the higher mortality, the second or typhoid epidemic may overshadow the first or dysenteric outbreak.

Dysenteric symptoms are common in other diseases, and each of these must in turn be excluded before a presumptive diagnosis of bacillary dysentery is established. Malaria, kala-azar and infections with the ciliates, such as *Balantidium coli,* and with the flukes, *Fasciolopsis buskii,* *Schistosoma japonicum* and *Schistosoma mansoni.* These all produce dysenteric symptoms and are rather easily excluded by proper laboratory examination. The exclusion of amebic dysentery is not always so easy, although close attention to the clinical history, with its slow rather than rapid onset, the character of the stools and the presence of the ameba in the discharges should make the diagnosis clear. The problem would be easy were it not for the presence of the *Entamoeba coli,* and of other nonpathogenic species of entamebae which render careful examinations by an experienced worker quite necessary.

Intestinal disturbances due to eating spoiled food have an acute, stormy onset, and the patient shows great prostration, but the stools are large, fecal and offensive, and lack the dysenteric character.

Foreign bodies, such as fish and small bones of chickens, when lodged in the rectum may cause the evacuation of stools containing blood and mucus, and pain, but the other symptoms of dysentery are lacking in such cases.

In the case of children, intussusception causes an acute illness with great prostration, pain, rapid pulse and stools containing blood and mucus. This condition should be considered in making a diagnosis.

It should not be forgotten that acute bacillary dysentery and some one of the diseases mentioned above may exist in the same patient; for example, there are pathologic specimens in the Army Medical Museum showing the lesions of acute dysentery and chronic tuberculous ulceration side by side.

Complications.—Excoriations of the skin surrounding the anus are the rule in severe cases. Prolapsus ani is not infrequent in severe cases, and is more apt to occur in children than in adults. In rare cases a further complication, ischiorectal abscess, may appear.

The diphtheritic membrane in severe cases may extend from the colon to the bladder in men, but this is more commonly the case in women, where it may also involve the vaginal mucous membrane.

During the Civil War and again in the Spanish-American War, and in occasional cases reported in the current literature, typhoid fever and dysentery have been known to coexist in the same patient, the symptoms of dysentery being more or less obscured by those of typhoid, or vice versa. At autopsy the characteristic lesions of both diseases were seen side by side. Most frequently the dysenteric symptoms preceded those of the typhoid, but terminal infections of typhoid patients do occur and constitute a very fatal complication.

3841

JOINT AFFECTIONS (Rheumatism, Rheumatoid Affections).—In some epidemics these conditions are not uncommon. Woodward reported many cases during the Civil War occurring among northern soldiers. In the World War many cases were reported. Usually there is an interval of three or four weeks between the acute attack of dysentery and the appearance of the joint lesion, which is not infrequently preceded by mild conjunctivitis, lasting a few days only, and by acute urethritis, which is also mild.

The joint most commonly affected is the knee, often the ankle, and less frequently the toes. The upper extremities are not often involved, but the elbow and shoulder are sometimes attacked and the wrist and fingers in rare cases. As each new joint is involved there is a moderate rise of temperature. The heart shows signs of involvement in about one third of the cases[44] and greatly influences the prognosis. This group of symptoms is spoken of by French writers as the conjunctivo-urethro-synovial syndrome, and the intestinal group as the choleriform syndrome.

SEROUS MEMBRANE AFFECTIONS.—The serous membranes may also be involved and transient effusions in the pleura may appear.

NERVOUS AFFECTIONS.—The complications on the part of the nervous system are important, but they vary in their frequency in different epidemics and on the whole do not seem to be very common in cases occurring in the Temperate Zone, although they are numerous enough in the tropics. They are usually noticed in the second and third week of the disease, and may take the form of transient paraplegia or monoplegia, or of paralysis or paresis of isolated muscle groups. Laryngeal paralysis is not infrequent. The nerves of the heart may be attacked by the toxin and a variety of symptoms ensue, the commonest of which is brachycardia. Hiccup and herpes labialis have also been reported.

It is seen that the greater number of these complications are due to the absorbed neurotoxin and not to the multiplication of the bacteria at the site of the complication; the prognosis is therefore excellent. The paralyses pass off in a few months and all symptoms of joint involvement, which are slower to improve, disappear in four or five months from the beginning of the illness.

Sequelae.—In the older literature reports of scars from large ulcers in the colon are not uncommon; they contract in healing and cause a puckering, contraction and actual diminution in the size of the lumen of the intestine. Such cases are, however, quite rare. Woodward in his review of almost a thousand cases did not encounter any.

Clinical Varieties.—As Flexner pointed out in 1900, the clinical terms, catarrhal, tropical, epidemic and diphtheritic, are far from signifying sharply defined entities. Other terms are in common use, such as dysenteric diarrhea and chronic diarrhea, yet they merely describe the severity of the symptoms in a particular case. Colitis haemorrhagica, colitis necroticans, colitis pseudomembranacea, colitis ulcerosa and colitis fibrinosa are all stages in one and the same disease.

In sporadic cases one may find any of the several varieties of the dysentery bacillus as the causative agent. In small contact outbreaks, presumably starting from a carrier, only one variety is apt to be found, while in the larger outbreaks, which occasionally occur, due to polluted water, any or all varieties may be found in the same group of cases.

Treatment.—PROPHYLAXIS.—As has been pointed out under Etiology, in the presence of **good sanitation** and with average **personal hygiene,** such as we find in the larger cities, the disease tends to disappear. In the presence of a case, careful attention to all the details of personal hygiene and sanitation of the sick room will tend to prevent the infection of others in the same household.

The following measures are recommended by Lyon:

1. The feeding of whole lactic acid-evaporated milk mixtures to children under two years of age.

2. The boiling in their final containers of all sweet milk mixtures for children under two.

3. Thorough washing of the mother's hands after handling excreta of a child sick with dysentery and before she handles food for children.

4. Keeping excreta and soiled linen, from the patients, in covered buckets containing soap powder and water until they can be boiled.

5. Screening of house to keep out flies.

Special measures, such as **vaccination** and **passive immunization** with therapeutic serums, are theoretically correct, and under suitable conditions should give good results. Yet practical experience shows that these measures are rarely used and, in fact, are rarely necessary. Under special conditions, it is conceivable that vaccines might be useful, yet during the World War they do not seem to have been used systematically, at least in the fields where American troops were used, and apparently in those fields they were hardly necessary, as dysentery on the western front was not, except for a short period, a serious disease.

The vaccine itself is prepared in much the same way as the vaccine commonly used against typhoid fever, i.e., it is a suspension in salt solution of killed dysentery bacilli of various strains, representing, as far as possible, the members of the group causing the epidemic. The Shiga bacillus secretes a soluble toxin and it cannot be used in as large numbers as others of the group. The vaccines should be given in two or more doses, usually three, at intervals of a week or ten days; an idea of the worth of any particular vaccine may be obtained by testing the blood of the immunized patient for agglutinins after the course of the prophylactic treatment. If the patient has been successfully immunized, his serum will show agglutinins for all of the varieties used in the vaccine.

Sensitized vaccines are reported by Gibson [45] and by Boehncke [46] to be less toxic than the simple saline vaccine, and several favorable reports may be found in the literature. Vaccines against dysentery, no matter how prepared, have been used very little, and in practice it is evident that their field of usefulness is quite limited.

In hospitals a most important prophylactic measure is the isolation of the dysenteric cases from all others, and the institution of a ward technic which will prevent the spread of the infection to other patients or attendants.

Bojlen [9] found that in mental hospitals and institutions for children it was necessary to keep all dysentery cases in isolation for at least two months after apparent recovery. After this system was instituted, it became for the first time possible to eradicate the disease from the institution. Patients and individuals newly admitted were, of course, isolated for an observation period to ascertain if they were free from infectious

3841

diseases, including dysentery. Chronic carriers in such institutions must be kept in permanent isolation.

TREATMENT OF ACUTE CASES.—*General Treatment.*—Although many mild attacks occur, the disease should always be taken seriously, and the patient should be put to bed, on a **simple, liquid diet** and proper treatment. In this, as in the other acute infectious diseases, early treatment is of the very greatest importance, and there is good reason to believe that the earlier the patient receives proper care, the better the prognosis. The **rest in bed** should be complete, and the patient should use a bedpan and not be permitted to get up to go to stool. Because of the great prostration, special attention should be paid to keeping the patient **warm,** and he should be given enough liquid to allay thirst. **Rice** and **barley water** are satisfactory drinks, and strained **gruels, whey, albumin water** and **clear soups** may be given as bland and liquid foods.

In former times purgation was considered the first and most important part of treatment, and of course many patients did well, particularly after purgation with the salines, magnesium or sodium sulphate or sodium phosphate. Of late years, as the disease is now properly considered as an acute, self-limited infection, less stress is laid on the purgative treatment. Most pediatricians believe it is not merely unnecessary but positively harmful in infants and young children. The disease itself produces active purgation and great loss of body fluids.

In *children*, therefore, the best treatment is that for dehydration. **Water,** with saccharin if necessary, is given by mouth every hour, and **salt solution** or **glucose** intravenously. In general, the patients are given all the fluid they will take.

The feeding consists of **whole lactic acid milk,** 1 to 2 oz. at each feeding, gradually increasing to larger amounts; 2.5 per cent **cane sugar** is usually added to the milk—2.5 Gm. (½ teaspoonful) to 100 cc. of milk (3 oz.). When the stools become formed the amount of cane sugar may be doubled and tripled.

An alternative, if the stools are quite loose, is the feeding of **casec** (calcium caseinate), 7.5 per cent, in place of the 7.5 per cent of sucrose. It is not as fluid as milk alone, and nipples with large openings are used. If the child vomits he should receive nothing by mouth for twelve to twenty-four hours, and saline may be given subcutaneously.

Scraped ripe apples in a dose of two to four tablespoonfuls every two to four hours have been recommended (up to 20 apples daily have been given). Heisler, and later Moro, obtained good results in treatment by the use of apple pulp, fresh-scraped apples, to the exclusion of all other food for a two-day period. This has been found effective in this country also.[47] The scraped apple acts as an adsorbent agent, to which the toxin is attached, and is in this way rapidly eliminated from the body. The symptomatic improvement is remarkable. **Apple powder** is now available for treatment and may occasionally be more convenient than fresh apples.[48] **Kaolin** has been used extensively as a substitute for scraped apple, with excellent results; it is given in aluminium jell and it adsorbs the toxins in the same way as scraped apple. It is available in several forms.

Infants who are restless or in pain may be given small doses of **paregoric** and Davidson[49] states that no other drugs are of value. Neither serum nor bacteriophage has been of any value in the treatment of dysentery in children. The little patients recover more quickly if kept in a cool room, and in emergencies a room may be cooled by playing an electric fan over a tub of ice.

The disease is always most severe in young children and old persons.

In *adults,* purgation is still used but less regularly than in former days. **Rest in bed** is essential in the severe cases, and should be carried out in all cases. If the patient is unable to obtain any rest, because of frequent stools and severe tenesmus, **opium** (paregoric) is indicated.

Although there are in the literature many reports of the value of *treatment with serum,* the results on the whole do not seem to be encouraging.

Dehydration occurs in adults as well as in children, and every effort should be made to **replace promptly the large amount of fluid lost in the frequent stools.**

When the stool loses its dysenteric character and becomes again fecal, **bismuth subnitrate** may be given, 2 to 4 Gm. (30 to 60 Gr.) three or four times a day.

Lactic acid milk or **buttermilk** is valuable in adults as well as in children, and the same may be said of **scraped apples** and other fruit. In general they are fed the same as patients with typhoid; custards, ice cream, milk, and eggs are added early. Fruit juices, potatoes and rice are added next.

Local Treatment.—For the pain and abdominal discomfort it is well to apply **heat,** in the form of a **hot-water bag** or **hot fomentations.** The tenesmus may be so disturbing that **morphine** must be given hypodermically; or **opium suppositories** [½ Gr. (0.03 Gm.)] may be substituted. **Atropine** will often give relief when the pain is severe.

Enemas of warm normal salt solution are stimulating to the patient, and usually result in giving him a few hours' rest, undisturbed by frequent movements or tenesmus; in many cases they seem to be of distinct value. Incidentally it is worth remembering that the saline solution washings of the colon are particularly good laboratory material for the isolation of the bacillus. Enemas of **silver nitrate,** as described under the Treatment of Chronic Cases, are often effective. Brill[50] reports the treatment of a series of cases with serum in large doses, which improved under treatment. Being unable to obtain additional serum he substituted enemas of silver nitrate. The mortality of the two series of cases was the same, while a shorter period of convalescence followed the silver nitrate treatment and only one case of recurrence was noted after this treatment. If collapse is threatened, subcutaneous injections of warm saline solution must be given. They should also be given when nausea and vomiting are troublesome and when it is impossible to supply the necessary quantity of fluid to the body by mouth or by enemas of warm saline solution.

In excoriations of the skin surrounding the anus which complicate the disease in severe cases, **soft absorbent cotton** may be substituted for toilet paper to advantage. The skin itself should be **washed with soap and water,** and **alcohol,** and be protected with a **dusting powder.**

3841

In prolapsus ani, the prolapsed part should be reduced by pressure with **compresses moistened in warm saline solution.** Ischiorectal abscess, which may appear, should be treated according to the usual **surgical principles.**

TREATMENT OF CHRONIC CASES.—The first and most important point in the treatment of a case of chronic bacillary dysentery is to be quite sure of the diagnosis. This is never quite so simple as in entamebic dysentery, where finding *Entamoeba dysenteriae* clinches the diagnosis. The various diseases mentioned under Differential Diagnosis must each be excluded by appropriate examinations, and finally the dysentery bacillus concerned must be isolated in pure culture and tested against the patient's serum for the presence of agglutinins, together with a known culture of the proper strain of the dysentery bacillus as a control. Work of this character presents many technical difficulties, but it can be done by the laboratories of the better hospitals and boards of health.

General Treatment.—It is characteristic of the chronic cases to present alternating periods of remission and exacerbation. During the relapse the treatment should be the same as for the acute cases; during the subacute and chronic stages, the **diet** must be carefully **controlled** and the **patient confined to bed.** **Milk,** either plain or boiled, peptonized or fermented, full strength or diluted with Vichy water, lime water, gruels, or buttermilk, must be the mainstay of the diet. **Whey, beef juice, thin soups** and **eggs** or, in some cases where the whole eggs cannot be digested, the white only, may be added early; later, dishes made from milk and eggs, and milk toast may be added gradually.

Drugs administered by mouth are not of great value, yet **castor oil** in small doses from time to time produces good results. **Bismuth subnitrate** should be given in large doses, from 2 to 4 Gm. (30 to 60 Gr.) three times daily. **Opium** and **morphine should be avoided,** for the reasons already given and because of the danger of forming a habit by their continued use in chronic cases.

Local Treatment.—Local treatment of the colon should be carried out if a proctoscopic examination of the rectum shows ulcers, or if trial treatments are followed by appreciable benefit. The vogue of local treatment in the past may possibly have been due to the failure to differentiate between bacillary and entamebic dysentery, since in the latter disease ulcers low enough down in the rectum to be seen through the proctoscope are common and respond well to **irrigations.**

The simplest of the irrigating fluids is a cleansing one of **normal saline solution** given at body temperature in quantities of a few ounces, at first, and retained as long as possible. Later, as the colon becomes less sensitive, larger and larger quantities up to two liters may be given. **Silver nitrate solution,** beginning at a strength of 1:5000 and increasing to a dilution of 1:500, has been used ever since the Civil War and has given good results. Other astringents may be used from time to time, such as **alum** in a 2 per cent solution, **tannic acid,** 3 per cent, **salicylic acid,** 1 per cent, or **boric acid,** 2 per cent. All irrigations must be given with the fluid at the temperature of the body and should be introduced slowly through a large soft catheter or soft rectal tube. The patient should lie on the left side, with the hips slightly elevated, and the enema should be retained as long as possible.

Vaccine Therapy.—Vaccines are sometimes of value in the chronic relapsing cases and may be given in small, frequently repeated doses over a long period of time, until convalescence is established or, when no improvement is evident, until the patient is highly immunized as shown by an agglutination reaction with his blood serum.

When all other measures have been exhausted a **change of climate** or residence will sometimes bring about improvement or a cure. From the tropics and the South patients are regularly sent to some more northern latitude.

DIET DURING THE ATTACK.—This has already been referred to in a general way. It remains to be noted that **milk**, particularly in children, is generally agreed **not to be a suitable food** during the height of the disease; **broths, strained gruels, barley, rice** and **albumin water** should be substituted for a time. This is particularly necessary when there is nausea, vomiting or other gastric disturbance. In milder cases and in those past the height of the disease, milk, diluted or modified for children, is necessary to keep up a fair state of nutrition and to prevent the great loss of weight which occurs on diets of low caloric value.

When the patient is far enough convalesced to tolerate them, **fruit juices, fresh fruits** and **vegetables** are very gradually added to the diet in increasing quantities to maintain the normal intake of vitamins.

Prognosis.—The prognosis varies greatly in different epidemics and under different circumstances. In Japan and in the tropics the mortality reaches 30 per cent of the cases. In the United States it is rarely so high. The mortality among children and among the aged is high, and as a terminal infection in other diseases it is, of course, very fatal.

As regards chronic infections, the prognosis is not as good in the Shiga type of cases as in the Flexner-"Y" type. The patients with the former type are sicker, have fewer and shorter remissions, and are seldom able to carry on any occupation. Flexner-"Y" cases, on the other hand, tend to improve, and so long as the patient has good surroundings and suitable diet, he is able to carry on his work. In the Army, however, patients suffering from chronic or recurring dysentery are useless as soldiers, since they quickly break down whenever they take the field. The more robust may be given light duties under good surroundings in the home territory, but the others should be discharged from the service and sent to their homes, provided they can be given proper medical care and the health authorities will assume responsibility for them. To prevent the infection of others, they should be prohibited from handling foodstuffs and be instructed in personal hygiene and taught the measures necessary to prevent the spread of the infection.

The mortality varies much in different epidemics and in different localities. According to the statistics of Lentz, the mortality of Flexner-"Y" infections averaged 0.5 per cent, although in occasional outbreaks it ran as high as from 8 to 13 per cent; in Shiga infections the mortality was usually from 10 to 20 per cent, although in certain severe epidemics it rose to from 35 to 50 per cent. In the case of children and of elderly persons the mortality is higher than the average. Where the severe forms prevail, as in Japan, the average mortality may be as high as 30 per cent.

Pathology.—The lesions are confined to the colon and, to a lesser extent, to the lower part of the ileum. Blood cultures, except in very

3841

rare instances (Darling), are negative, and no metastatic infections are found in distant parts of the body. The lesion is most marked in the colon. In acute cases the entire extent of the mucous membrane is swollen and injected with small hemorrhagic areas scattered over the surface. The superficial epithelium is necrotic over large areas and comes off in masses, leaving a deeply injected base which may bleed easily. The lesions are most marked on the ridges or the folds of mucous membrane, but the characteristic which differentiates the bacillary from amebic dysentery is the general diffuse character of the lesion. Ulcers may be absent or extremely minute, yet the whole lining membrane may be thickened, swollen, edematous and hemorrhagic, or the lesions may be well developed only in the sigmoid, splenic and hepatic flexures and in the cecum, where fecal masses tend to accumulate and act as mechanical irritants. In some cases a well-developed diphtheritic pseudomembrane will be found. In very acute, fatal cases the colon may show large or small areas of necrosis and gangrene.

As the necrotic mucous membrane sloughs off, larger or smaller ulcers are left, which may become confluent with the extension of the process. The margin of the ulcer is irregular but is never undermined to the same degree as in amebic dysentery. The deeper ulcer may be seen at autopsy through the serous coat of the intestine, which is injected or discolored. Although occasional ulcers may be quite deep, perforation of the intestinal wall is quite unusual.

The picture at autopsy does not in the least resemble dysentery due to the entameba, where the areas involved in the infection show deep ulceration and are isolated from each other, and surrounded by apparently healthy mucous membrane.

Abscesses in the liver are almost unknown in bacillary dysentery but are common in the amebic form.

In the chronic cases many and complicated changes will be found; the glandular coat may be atrophied or it may be thickened and thrown into corrugations or into irregularly disposed polypoid masses; it may also be replaced by scar tissue. Some cases may show small cysts from the retention of mucus. From the small cysts and sinuses from which pus may be expressed, the dysentery bacilli may usually be isolated, and this explains the intermittent excretion of the bacilli in the stools. Unlike typhoid, no bacilli are ordinarily found in the gallbladder. The connective tissue and the muscular coats may be hypertrophic or atrophic, depending, perhaps, on the state of the disease at the time of death. The ulcers may penetrate the mucous coat only, or invade the submucosa, or even the muscularis. In any case, the resulting inflammation leads to swelling, edema, hemorrhage and necrosis in the surrounding tissues, and ultimately to an increase in the thickness of the wall due to the overproduction of connective tissue in the process of repair. It is the subsequent contraction of this newly formed tissue which leads to irregularities in the size of the lumen of the colon, amounting at times to obstructing bands. When the inflammation has extended to the peritoneal coat, adhesions, more or less extensive, naturally follow.

The following is a condensed protocol of one of Flexner's autopsies done in Manila on an acute case:

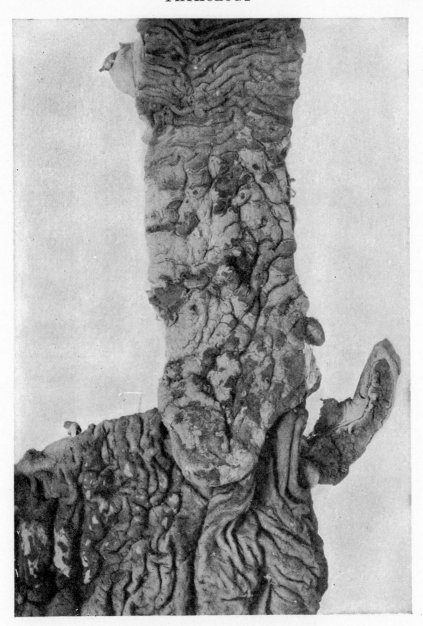

FIG. 1.—BACILLARY DYSENTERY (Shiga).

"Death ensued on the sixth day of the disease. The colon is dilated and its walls are thickened. The serous coat is injected but otherwise normal. The mucous membrane is swollen and thickened and the normal folds are thrown into coarse elevated corrugations. The general

3841

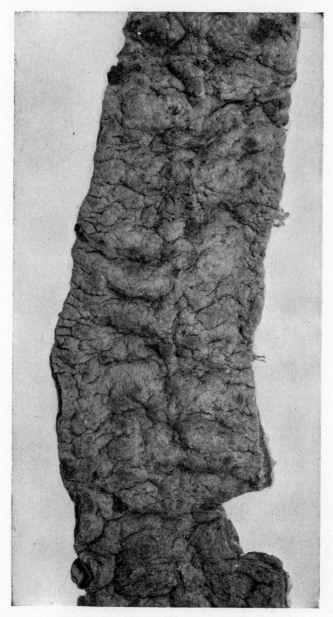

FIG. 2.—BACILLARY DYSENTERY (Shiga).

color is red, but there are seen many small hemorrhagic points. No diphtheritic membrane is seen, but there is present an exudate which is readily washed off. The normal velvety character of the mucous membrane is lost and, on close examination, a number of minute ulcers may be seen, particularly on the crests of the coarse corrugations. The lesions, as a rule, are not limited to given areas of the mucous membrane, leaving other areas normal, but the entire lining of the colon and of the lower end of the ileum is involved in the process.''

In exceptional fulminating cases the bacillus is found in the blood stream by culture (Darling, Maer). The bacteremia causes great prostration and toxemia, often with a slight temperature reaction, marked cerebral symptoms, and mild or absent abdominal signs; tenderness, pain and tenesmus may be slight or absent. At the autopsy, nevertheless, extensive dysenteric lesions will be found.

Many of the changes referred to above may be seen in Figures 1 and 2. Both specimens are from the same case of Shiga dysentery (Army Medical Museum, A. E. F., 1429). The figures show swelling, necrosis, hemorrhagic areas and a pseudomembrane, which is peeling off, leaving a lighter colored base. In this case it will be noted that the lesions extend to the vermiform appendix and to the lower portion of the ileum.

CASE I.—The clinical history of the case is briefly as follows:

" He was admitted to hospital August 10, 1918, with a diagnosis of ' under observation for appendicitis.' His illness began August 8, with a sharp, cramplike pain across the abdomen at the level of the umbilicus, followed two hours later by vomiting; he has been vomiting at irregular intervals since. Diarrhea for past four days with eight to ten stools a day. Has taken no food for past twenty-four hours; cannot retain food. Stools bloody and patient complains of burning sensation at defecation. Physical examination showed patient's abdomen to be flat. There is tenderness over ascending colon, but no rigidity. Preliminary diagnosis of intercolitis, severe, hemorrhagic. White blood-cells, at this time, 7,950. August 22, notes indicate that patient has had frequent small bloody stools with tenesmus. No leukocytosis. Reports of feces show much blood and mucus. August 26, *Bacillus dysenteriae* (Shiga) reported in culture from feces; the diagnosis was made on agglutination with specific sera and on cultural characteristics on differential media.

" *Peritoneal Cavity.*—On opening the peritoneal cavity the collapsed flat condition of the gastro-intestinal tract was found to be remarkable. The small intestine and large intestine showed some congestion of the subserous vessels. The omentum was healthy in appearance and was well down over the coils of the small intestine. It was adherent along the descending colon and sigmoid.

" *Pleural Cavities.*—The pleural cavities seemed remarkably large in comparison to the size of the lungs. After removing the breast plate, it was found that each cavity was apparently empty. There was no evidence of fluid or exudate in either cavity.

" *Pericardial Cavity.*—The pericardial cavity was thin, and even before it was opened one could see that there was excess of fluid in the cavity. This fluid was perfectly clear and of a pale straw color. There was nothing of an inflammatory character in the pericardial cavity.

" *Heart.*—The heart measured 10 x 8 x 4 cm. and weighed 163 grams. The heart was very small and flabby. This was especially marked in the right ventricle. The heart-muscle was pale and the cut surface was swollen. The left ventricle averaged only 1 cm. The valves showed nothing of special interest. The left ventricle measured 12.5 cm.

" *Lungs.*—The left lung measured 17.5 x 10.4 cm. and weighed 167 grams. The lung was remarkably small and had a curious doughy consistency, although it crepitated throughout. The cut surface showed a pale, dry, apparently partially collapsed lung tissue, remarkable chiefly for its dense, almost meaty, and at the same time, soft structure and for its dryness. The trachea and bronchi were clear. The peribronchial lymph-nodes showed caseous and calcified tuberculosis.

3841

"The right lung measured 20 x 14 x 4 cm. and weighed 160 grams. The right lung was in all respects like the left.

"*Spleen.*—The spleen measured 12 x 7 x 4 cm. and weighed 162 grams; it was fairly firm. Its outline was most irregular. On section, the malpighian bodies stood out prominently from a red, firm spleen.

"*Liver.*—The liver measured 23 x 19 x 8 cm. and weighed 1599 grams. The liver showed nothing unusual on the surface and on section showed slight congestion and cloudy swelling. The gall-bladder was negative.

"*Gastro-intestinal Tract.*—The stomach was small and contracted, with prominent rugae. It contained a quantity of gray-green material. There was a little hemorrhage beneath the mucosa on the ridges of some of the folds. There was no evidence of ulceration. The small intestine contained a quantity of bile-stained mucus, but was otherwise negative throughout the duodenum, the jejunum and the first part of the ileum. The last 40 cm. of the ileum showed a tense congestion, most marked at the crests of the mucosal folds and about 20 cm. from the ileo-cecal valve; small superficial ulcers with grayish-green necrotic membrane, covering their bases, were found. These were present in rapidly increasing numbers and the last 10 cm. of the ileum showed extensive superficial ulceration with a thick, opaque, grayish-green membrane which could be scraped away in the case of the smaller ulcers, revealing a rough red granular base. The appendix showed an intense swelling and intense congestion of the mucus and a few small ulcerations. The large intestine in the cecum showed less extensive ulceration than did the terminal portion of the ileum, but above the cecum and throughout the remaining extent of the tract there was an extremely intense ulcerative process with diffuse necrotic-looking exudate similar to that previously described. At intervals a particularly congested fold appeared, denuded of its exudate. As the descending colon and cecum were reached, the exudate became more extensive and more dense, absolutely covering every portion of the mucosal lining.

"*Pancreas.*—Negative.

"*Adrenals.*—The cortex of the adrenals had lost its usual opaque, yellow color and was swollen and translucent with here and there an occasional yellow patch. The medullary substance was decreased in amount.

"*Kidneys.*—The left kidney measured 10 x 5 x 4 cm. and weighed 135 grams. The kidney was rather small and soft. The capsule peeled easily, revealing a pale cortex on which the fetal lobulations were somewhat prominent. The cut surface showed a pale, swollen tissue with some congestion of the capillaries and a general haziness of the usual markings. The right kidney measured 9.5 x 5 x 3.5 cm. and weighed 113 grams. This kidney was like the left in all respects. In each instance, the pelvis and ureter were negative.

"*Bladder and Prostate.*—The bladder was distended with urine but was otherwise negative."

The change in the adrenals has also been noticed by Remlinger,[51] in cases from the Argonne, and by many German and Austrian writers, usually, however, in connection with Flexner-"Y" dysentery.

CASE II.—Figure 3 is from a case of mixed entamebic and bacillary (Shiga) dysentery (A.M.M., A.E.F. 1428). The clinical data and autopsy findings are as follows:

The patient was admitted August 11, 1918, with a history of having had a severe diarrhea for the preceding six days, with bloody stools, cramps and vomiting. August 13th, cramps still present. About thirty bowel movements in the last twenty-four hours. August 16th, diarrhea better, but still has very marked pain. August 20th, relapse. August 22nd, patient quite prostrated; frequent bloody stools with many clots. Temporary improvement followed administration of emetin, but the drug was continued without further beneficial

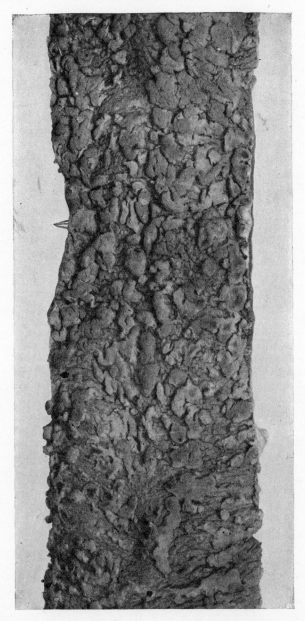

Fig. 3.—Mixed Bacillary and Entamebic Dysentery (Shiga).

results. Steady downward course, with rapid circulatory failure a few minutes before death. August 24th, 10:20 P.M., death occurred.

"*Pathological Findings in Gastro-intestinal Tract.*—The stomach was moderately distended and contained thin liquid and air. The gastric mucosa was perfectly smooth and healthy in appearance. The pyloric valve was clear.

3841

The small intestine showed duodenum and jejunum clear. The ileum was slightly distended, so that the folds flattened and the walls thinned and there was slight injection of the blood-vessels. The Peyer's patches were clear and the mucosa showed no evidence of necrosis or ulceration. The large intestine showed extensive destruction of its intestinal lining. The condition was well marked throughout the whole of the colon, sigmoid and rectum. The lesions took the form of rounded and irregular punched-out areas of necrosis of the mucosa and submucosa with frequently extension of the necrosis along the submucosa beneath still visible bridges of mucosa. Marked inflammatory reaction was not a feature of the lesions. There was a little congestion in one or two places, but for the most part the grayish necrotic-looking mucosa with the numerous coalescing punched-out areas of necrosis was characteristic of the entire large bowel. There was no evidence of perforation or hemorrhage, and there was no exudate on the surface of the mucosal lining. The abrupt line of demarcation at the ileocecal valve between the cecum and ileum was most striking.

"*Bacteriological Findings.*—(1) Cultures from stools of life; *Bacillus dysenteriae* (Shiga) by cultural characteristics and by agglutination with available serum.

"(2) Cultures from stools at autopsy; negative for *Bacillus dysenteriae.*

"(3) Feces, in life, by microscopical examination, forms typical of *Entamoeba histolytica,* but non-motile, always found.

"(4) Sections of colon showed *Entamoeba histolytica* in submucosa in moderate numbers."

Among troops during the late war, mixed infections were not uncommon, and particular care must, under such conditions, be paid to making a complete diagnosis and to keeping the diagnosis up to date, as the entamebic infection often lags behind the bacillary. If the nature of the complication is not realized, the treatment will be unsatisfactory and the disease will be prolonged.

Sections of the colon show a large amount of small round-cell infiltration, especially around Lieberkühn's glands and around and in the solitary lymph nodules. The infiltration is especially well marked around the edges and bases of the ulcers. Some of the latter are formed by the sloughing of the coagulated and necrotic mucous membrane and others, which are small and deep, by necrosis of the solitary follicles and overlying epithelium. Around the blood vessels, particularly the small ones, are seen red and white blood cells, fibrin and altered tissue cells, the whole forming a coagulated and necrotic mass. Later in the disease the coagulation necrosis is less marked and the small round-cell infiltration becomes more evident; still later, the connective tissue shows evidences of active proliferation. The ulcers heal over by the extension of the epithelium from the border, but the ulcer remains covered with scar tissue and not with normal epithelium.

Historical Summary.—The disease has been recognized throughout the ages, and the names which Hippocrates gave to the two principal forms of intestinal disturbance, diarrhea and dysentery, have been in continuous use among physicians of all schools up to the present day, although with changes in the definition of dysentery, and such qualifications and limitations as were necessary to exclude symptomatically related conditions. Of course it was impossible, on clinical grounds alone, to separate bacillary from entamebic dysentery, and the differentiation had to wait upon the development of protozoology and bacteriology. This did not reach a helpful stage until about 1900, since which time progress has been continuous and rapid. Until recent years, therefore, many diverse conditions producing frequent stools containing blood and mucus, and accompanied by tenesmus, were classified under this diagnosis. From a historical point of view the most important study is that of Woodward [52] in the Medical and Surgical History of the War of the Rebellion, and any student of the history of medicine will derive great pleasure and profit from its perusal.

REFERENCES

1. Reed: Studies from the Rockefeller Institute for Medical Research, New York, 2: 175, 1904.
2. Hunt, C. J.: Bacillary dysentery, J. Am. M. Ass., 59: 919, 1912.
3. Cunningham, J.: Latent dysentery with a mathematical note by Major A. J. MacKendrick, Indian J. M. Research, 6: 68, 1918.
4. Fletcher, Capt. William and Mackinnon, Doris, L. A.: Contribution to the study of chronicity in dysentery carriers. National Health Insurance, Special Report Series, No. 29, Med. Research Comm., London, 1919.
5. Nichols, Henry J.: Experimental observations on the pathogenesis of gallbladder infections in typhoid, cholera and dysentery, J. Exper. Med., 24: 497, 1916.
6. Ghon, A. and Roman, B.: Wien. klin. Wchnschr., 28: 579, 1915.
7. Einhorn, M.: J. Am. M. Ass., 66: 1908, 1916.
8. Lyon, G. M.: Am. J. Dis. Child., 49: 367, 1935.
9. Bojlen, Knud: Dysentery in Denmark, Copenhagen, 1934.
10. Barker, L. F.: Johns Hopkins Hosp. Bull., 11: 26, 1900.
11. Shiga: Über den Erreger der Dysenterie in Japan, Centralbl. f. Bakteriol, 24: 599, 1898; 24: 817, 870, 913, 1899. Studien über die epidemische Dysenterie in Japan, Deutsche med. Wchnschr., 26: 741, 765, 783, 1901.
12. Kruse: Etiologie der epidemischen Ruhr, Deutsche med. Wchnschr., 27: 370, 1901.
13. Flexner, Simon: Acute tropical dysentery, Johns Hopkins Hosp. Bull., 11: 231, 1900.
14. Lentz: Ztschr. f. Hyg., 39: 41, 1902.
15. Hiss, P. A. and Russell, F. F.: A study of bacillus resembling the bacillus of Shiga, from a case of fatal diarrhea in a child, with remarks on the recognition of dysentery, typhoid and allied bacilli, Med. News, 82: 289, 1903.
16. Strong, R. P. and Musgrave, W. E.: Report on the etiologies of the dysenteries of Manila. Report of the Surgeon General of the Army to the Secretary of War, Washington, 1900.
17. Ogata: The etiology of dysentery, Centralbl. f. Bakteriol. u. Parasitenk., 1ste Abt., 11: 264, 1892.
18. Morgan, H. de R.: Bacteriology of summer diarrhea in infants, Brit. M. J., 1: 908, 1906.
19. Kligler, I. J.: The agglutination reactions of the Morgan bacillus No. 1, J. Exper. Med., 29: 531, 1919.
20. Park and Dunham: New York Univ. Bull. Med. Sc., 2: 166, 1902.

21. Park, W. H. and Carry, H.: The presence of the Shiga variety of dysentery bacilli in an extreme epidemic of dysentery with notes upon serum reactions observed, J. Med. Research, 9: 180, 1903.
22. Drigalski and Conradi: Ztschr. f. Hyg., 39: 283, 1902.
23. Endo: Über ein Verfahren zum Nachweis der Typhusbacillen, Centralbl. f. Bakteriol. u. Parasitenk., 1ste Abt., 35: 109.
24. Kligler, I. J. and Olitsky, Peter K.: J. Am. M. Ass., 71: 2126, 1918.
25. Swift, Homer: J. Exper. Med., 32: 69, 1921.
26. Reichel, Flosdorf and Eagle: Am. J. Path., 10: 662, 1934.
27. Road, E. T.: J. Immunol., 29: 1, 1935.
28. Levine, Max: Studies of the group of dysentery and allied bacilli. (Not yet published.)
29. Mudge, Courtland S.: The effect of sterilization upon sugars in culture media, J. Bact., 2: 403, 1917.
30. Thjøtta, T. and Waaler, E.: J. Bact., 24: 301, 1932.
31. Kraus and Doerr: Die experimentelle Grundlage einer antitoxischen Therapie der bazillären Dysenterie, Ztschr. f. Hyg., 55: 1, 1906.
32. Todd: J. Hyg., 4: 480, 1904; 2: 16, 1907.
33. Flexner, Simon and Amoss, H. L.: The rapid production of antidysenteric serum, J. Exper. Med., 21: 515, 1915.
34. Andrews, F. W.: Differentiation of the true dysentery bacilli from allied species, Lancet, 1: 560, 1918.
35. Winter: Ztschr. f. Hyg., 70: 283.
36. Murray, E. G. D.: J. Roy. Army M. Corps, 31: 257, 353, 1918.
37. Fratzek, A.: Deutsche med. Wchnschr., 43: 200, 1917.
38. Flexner, S. and Sweet, J. E.: The pathogenesis of experimental colitis in animals and man, J. Exper. Med., 8: 514, 1906.
39. Health News, Albany, New York, February 15, 1937.
40. Schleifstein, J. and Coleman, M. B.: J. Bact., 33: 111, 1937.
41. Strong, R. P. and Musgrave, W. E.: Report on the etiologies of the dysenteries of Manila, Report of the Surgeon General of the Army to the Secretary of War, Washington, 1900.
42. Kofoid, C. A. et al.: Criterions for distinguishing the entameba of amebiasis and other organisms, Arch. Int. Med., 24: 35, 1919.
43. Jacob, L.: Klinische Beobachtungen bei Bazillenruhr, Ztschr. f. Hyg. u. Infektionskrankh., 83: 467, 1917.
44. Stettner, Ernst: München. med. Wchnschr., 64: 854, 1917.

45. Gibson, H. Graeme: Results obtained from the use of antidysenteric sero-vaccine in the field, with regard to the reduction of case incidence, J. Roy. Army M. Corps, 30 : 476, 1918.
46. Boehncke: Dysbacta-Boehncke, München. med. Wchnschr., No. 29, p. 785, 1918.
47. Dodd, K., Minot, A. S. and Casparis, H.: Am. J. Dis. Child., 43 : 1, 1932.
48. Bitter, J. E.: Northwest Med., December, 1936.
49. Davidson, W. C.: Bacteriological and clinical consideration of bacillary dysentery, Medicine, 1 : 389, 1922. Round-table discussion, J. Pediat., 7 : 568, 1935.
50. Brill, E. H.: Ruhrbehandlung mit Argentum nitricum, München. med. Wchnschr., 64 : 1643, 1917.
51. Remlinger, P. and Dumas, J.: La dysentérie de l'Argonne, étude bactériologique, Ann. Inst. Pasteur, 29 : 498, 1915.
52. Woodward, Joseph J.: Medical and Surgical History of the War of the Rebellion, Part Second, Medical Volume, Washington, 1879.

THE TYPHUS FEVERS

By Charles F. Craig, M.D., M.A. (Hon.), F.A.C.P., F.A.C.S., Colonel, U. S. Army Medical Corps (Ret.), D.S.M.

Introduction.—The typhus fever group of infections are all caused by organisms belonging to the genus *Rickettsia*, the exact biologic position of which is still undecided although they are undoubtedly more closely related to the bacteria than to the protozoa and, perhaps, are still more closely related to the filtrable viruses. Several species of rickettsiae have been described as causing disease in man and similar organisms also occur in the tissues of arthropods and other animals. Rickettsiae live in the living tissue cells where they multiply and eventually destroy the host cell, and they cannot be cultivated except upon living tissue, as the chorio-allantoic membrane of the chick embryo. Morphologically, the rickettsiae vary much in size and shape, from almost invisible organisms to others measuring as much as 2 microns in length. They occur in the form of minute granules, usually diplococcoid in appearance, within the infected tissue cell, stain well with the Giemsa stain and are gram-negative.

The Typhus Group of Fevers.—Recent investigations have demonstrated that there are a large number of acute febrile conditions caused by rickettsiae, which are closely related etiologically and clinically, and may be collectively classified as the typhus group of fevers. In this discussion, the only infections which will be considered will be epidemic and endemic typhus, though some prefer to place in this group other infections, as tsutsugamushi disease (Japanese river fever), Q fever of Australia, fièvre boutonneuse of the Mediterranean countries and even Rocky Mountain spotted fever of the United States. All of these infections are caused by rickettsiae which may be differentiated serologically or otherwise, but it is considered best to regard as true typhus infections only the epidemic and endemic forms of the disease, including the variety known as Brill's disease.

As regards the general subject of rickettsial disease it may be stated that, at present, three fairly well distinct groups of infections caused by these organisms have been separated. The *first*, or *typhus*, *group* includes epidemic and endemic typhus and Brill's disease. Etiologically, epidemic typhus is caused by *Rickettsia prowazeki* var. *prowazeki*, while endemic typhus is caused by *Rickettsia prowazeki* var. *mooseri*, Brill's disease being also caused by *Rickettsia prowazeki* var. *mooseri*. The *second group* of rickettsial infections includes Japanese river fever, or tsutsugamushi disease, and related fevers occurring in Japan, southern Asia, Formosa and the islands of the southwestern Pacific, the causative organism being called *Rickettsia tsutsugamushi*, *R. orientalis* and *R.*

42101

niponica by different authors. The *third group* includes Rocky Mountain spotted fever, the São Paulo exanthematic fever of Brazil, the fièvre boutonneuse of the Mediterranean region and South African tick fever. Etiologically, *Rickettsia rickettsii,* or variants of this organism, cause these infections. Besides the infections mentioned above other diseases have been described as caused by rickettsiae, as Q fever of Australia and a similar fever occurring in Montana, known as American Q fever, the causative organism being called *Rickettsia diaporica,* by Cox (1940), probably identical with *R. burnetti* (Derrick, 1938), the rickettsia found in Australian Q fever. All of these infections present certain clinical features which are similar but it is believed that, at present, it is best to consider only epidemic typhus, endemic typhus, and the variant known as ''Brill's disease'' as belonging to the typhus group, although all of the other infections mentioned have the common factor of being caused by species of rickettsiae.

Epidemic Typhus Fever

Synonyms.—Jail fever, famine fever, ship fever, louse typhus, tabardillo, typhus exanthematicus, typhus fever.

Definition.—Epidemic typhus fever is an acute, infectious disease, caused by *Rickettsia prowazeki* var. *prowazeki,* and characterized by a sudden onset, a continuous fever lasting usually about two weeks, of remittent type and terminating by crisis. A characteristic skin eruption occurs about the fifth day of the disease, spreading from the abdomen to the trunk and extremities. The causative organism is transmitted from man to man by lice.

Etiology.—Epidemic typhus fever is caused by a rickettsia known as *Rickettsia prowazeki* var. *prowazeki.* This organism was first noted by Ricketts (1909–1910), in the blood of patients suffering from the disease and also in the blood of monkeys and guinea pigs inoculated with blood from typhus patients. His observations were confirmed by Rocha-Lima (1916), as well as the observation by Ricketts that the same intracellular organisms occurred in lice that had bitten typhus patients. Wolbach and his colleagues, who studied typhus in Poland in 1920–1922, also demonstrated the rickettsiae in lice that had bitten typhus patients and showed that, in man, these organisms were largely situated in the cells of the blood vessels. Since these observations it has been definitely accepted that *Rickettsia prowazeki* is the cause of epidemic typhus fever.

The morphology, staining reactions, cultivation and relation of this species to other species of rickettsiae have been previously discussed and will not be repeated here.

Epidemiology.—Epidemic typhus fever is transmitted from man to man by lice, either *Pediculus humanus* var. *corporis* or *Pediculus humanus* var. *capitis,* the former species being the one almost always concerned, although the latter is capable of transmitting the infection. The role of the louse in the transmission of epidemic typhus was first described by Nicolle, Comte and Conseil (1909), who produced the disease in monkeys by means of body lice that had fed upon typhus patients. Their work was confirmed in this country by Ricketts and Wilder (1910) and by Anderson and Goldberger (1912), while Arkwright and Bacot (1923) demonstrated that the rickettsiae may remain alive in the excreta of infected lice for as long as eleven days after passage, at room temperature.

The infection of man occurs from the feces of the infected lice, which swarm with the rickettsiae, the latter being forced into the wound made by the bite of the louse during scratching. Lice become infective about the end of the fourth to the seventh day after biting a typhus patient and remain infective indefinitely. The rickettsiae are not present in the salivary glands of the louse, so that infection does not occur through the bite but is purely contaminative in nature. The relation of the transmission of this disease to lice demonstrates why it occurs most commonly where living conditions are most crowded and where cleanliness as to clothing is not observed. The old names—jail fever, famine fever, ship fever and war fever—indicate the relationship of this infection to crowded and insanitary conditions, while under such conditions deficient diets contribute to the susceptibility of those exposed to the disease. The body louse, the species generally concerned in the transmission of epidemic typhus fever, lives in the clothing, especially in the seams, and under favorable conditions, as in crowded barracks, jails and ships, the transference of lice from the clothing of one individual to another invariably occurs and hence causes rapidly spreading epidemics of typhus if the lice are infected.

Until the demonstration of the transmission of epidemic typhus by the louse, this disease was considered as one of the most contagious of all diseases, and while it is now generally accepted that contagion enters little, if any, into the picture of transmission, it cannot be said that the disease is never contagious. Instances of infection are not uncommon in which it has been impossible to incriminate the louse. The relatively great mortality from typhus among physicians, who have taken precautions against infestation by lice, indicates that perhaps contagion may play a part in the epidemiology of the disease. It has been suggested that, as inflammatory conditions of the pharynx, mouth and nose are frequently observed in typhus, droplet infection may occur, the virus being contained in the secretions that are ejected when the patient sneezes or coughs, although the virus has not been detected in such secretions. It is true that infections have occurred in laboratory workers by material from infected lice being accidentally projected into the eye. Blanc and Baltazard (1938) were successful in producing infection in human volunteers with the dried excreta of fleas infected with the endemic type of typhus by placing such excreta upon the nasal mucous membrane. Infection with this type of typhus may also occur through feeding infected material, as shown by several authorities. Certainly the high morbidity among physicians attending typhus fever cases is very suggestive of some other method of transmission than through the excreta of infected lice reaching skin abrasions, although this is certainly the most common method of transmission of the disease.

The influence of climate in the epidemiology of epidemic typhus is marked, cases being much more numerous during the late fall, winter and early spring months than in late spring, summer or autumn. The greater prevalence of the infection during the cooler seasons is readily explained by the fact that lice transmit the disease and that during these periods people are crowded together in heated houses and the conditions for the propagation of lice are most favorable, thick clothing and flannels being worn which furnish ideal breeding places for the lice. In all of the great epidemics of typhus it has been noted that most of the cases occurred in the winter, and conditions of overcrowding, lack of proper food and insanitary surroundings were present. There would appear to be no difference in susceptibility as regards age or sex if exposure to infected lice occurs; but occupations, as the practice of medicine, in which exposure to the infection is more frequent, increase the liability of contracting the disease.

Symptomatology.—The *period of incubation* varies from 4 to 16 days, the average periods varying from 10 to 12 days. During this period there are usually no symptoms but just before the onset there may be slight headache, malaise, and a feeling of depression. The onset is rather sudden with marked headache, aching in the back and extremities, and nervousness, succeeded during the next day by an increase in these symptoms and anorexia, nausea and vomiting, the last symptom being rare. Dizziness is frequently a very prominent symptom and a staggering gait is often observed during the onset, which, as in plague, has led to the arrest of the infected individual for drunkenness. Sometimes, even at this early stage of the infection, the mental condition may be one of partial stupor or slight delirium, thus adding to the picture resembling alcoholic intoxication. Distinct chills are not common but chilly sensations are frequently present. In very severe infections convulsions may occur during the onset and delirium may be intense and of a violent character.

About the end of the second day the temperature rises suddenly to 103–104° F. (39.4–40° C.) and all of the symptoms have increased in severity. The headache may be intense and located in the frontal, occipital or temporal regions, or there may be severe neuralgic pains over the entire head. The face appears greatly flushed, the conjunctivae are much congested, while the eyes have a stupid or dazed expression, the entire facial appearance resembling that of a drunken individual. As the disease progresses the temperature remains elevated, there being morning remissions of slight extent, and this remittent type of fever persists until the crisis which usually occurs in from 12 to 14 days. Constipation is usually present and the mucous membranes of the mouth, nose and throat become dry and covered with sordes, as well as the tongue, the latter being covered with a thick brown fur. The breath becomes very offensive and the patient lies in a stuporous condition much of the time. The appetite is generally completely lost and the patient has to be aroused to partake of nourishment. In some cases the onset is very rapid and most of the symptoms noted may be present by the end of 24 to 36 hours. In such cases the prognosis is exceedingly grave.

The characteristic eruption of epidemic typhus usually appears about the fifth day of the disease, although it may be noted as early as the end of the third day or as late as the seventh or eighth day. It appears first in the axillae and inner surface of the arms and upon the abdomen, extending over the trunk, flanks, back and chest and finally involving the thighs and legs. In mild infections there may be only a slight eruption, usually scattered over the inner surface of the arms, abdomen and back, but in severe infections the eruption may cover the entire body, even the palms of the hands and the soles of the feet being covered by a petechial rash.

The rash is quite characteristic in appearance and has sometimes been called a "mulberry rash" because of the resemblance of the color to that of a nearly ripe mulberry. It also resembles the rash of measles in that it occurs in the form of irregular mottling beneath the epidermis. The elements of the rash consist of roseolar macules lying within mottled areas and, when fully developed, the livid color of the eruption is striking. In severe cases it always becomes petechial and even in cases of moderate severity the eruption is usually petechial in character before it disappears, while in the mildest cases only the roseolar macules, few in number, may be observed. In the most severe cases the eruption may be hemorrhagic and in these cases melena, hematemesis and hematuria usually occur. The eruption lasts for from a few days to ten or more days and fades away very slowly without leaving a scar. In dark-skinned peoples the typhus eruption is hard to see and the most careful inspection is necessary to demonstrate its presence.

With the occurrence of the eruption the symptoms increase in severity and cardiac collapse may occur. The mental dullness increases, the movements of the hands and feet are tremulous, the tongue is heavily coated with a dark brown fur and is protruded with difficulty, constipation is present, and by the end of the first week muttering delirium is often present and the patient is aroused with difficulty and is often very irritable and hard to manage. Fatal infections usually terminate between the tenth and fourteenth days of the disease, the patient usually being unconscious at the time of death. Hemorrhages from the bowels and kidneys may occur in severe cases, and incontinence and suppression of urine are sometimes observed.

If the patient is to recover, the clinical symptoms begin to show improvement about the middle or latter portion of the second week and the fever usually falls rapidly, by crisis, or more slowly, by a comparatively rapid lysis. With the disappearance of the fever the symptoms also disappear and the patient usually has an uninterrupted convalescence, but, because of a greatly weakened condition caused by the acute symptoms, convalescence may be slow and may be complicated by cardiac weakness or nervous irritability.

In some cases the fall in the temperature is not followed by any improvement in the mental symptoms, but, instead, active delirium may develop or the patients may become unconscious. In such cases the patient usually dies in coma preceded by either suppression of the urine or incontinence of urine and feces. In still other cases the rapid decline in the fever may be accompanied by cardiac failure which may prove fatal.

The physical signs in typhus, aside from the characteristic eruption, consist of an enlarged spleen, decreased blood pressure, a weak, often irregular and rapid pulse, weak heart sounds, and a slow weak pulse during convalescence, easily excited by movement or nervous excitement, when it becomes rapid and very weak. Albuminuria is present in severe infections and hematuria is sometimes observed. A bronchitis is often present about the time of the appearance of the eruption and a cough may persist throughout the entire course of the disease. A slight leukocytosis is often present, the white cells numbering from 10,000 to 12,000 per c.mm., with a slight increase in the polymorphonuclear neutrophils.

Complications.—The complications of epidemic typhus fever are numerous and often the cause of death. In great epidemics, where medical attention and nursing are often impossible, because of the excessive number of cases, complications are almost universally the rule and probably cause as many deaths as the infection itself.

Bronchopneumonia is a frequent complication, especially under the conditions just mentioned, and often results fatally. A severe bronchitis is often observed and may be accompanied by much cough and the expectoration of large amounts of thick sputum. This cough may persist throughout convalescence. Parotitis sometimes complicates epidemic typhus, and otitis media and mastoiditis sometimes occur. Abortion is common in women who are less than three months pregnant, and in such cases puerperal septicemia is apt to occur. Dementia and mania have been noted as complications, persisting even after the patient has become convalescent, and attacks of dizziness and an ataxic gait sometimes complicate convalescence.

Gangrene of the toes is sometimes seen during an attack of epidemic typhus, and Shattuck, quoted by Strong (1942), observed symmetrical gangrene of the extremities during the great Serbian epidemic of typhus and also noted that boils and abscesses were not uncommon during convalescence from this form of the disease. Pain in the legs and feet was often noted by Shattuck during convalescence.

Sequelae.—Observers have not recorded any sequelae of permanent character following an attack of epidemic typhus, and convalescence is usually rapid and complete.

Diagnosis.—The diagnosis of typhus fever of epidemic type must be based upon clinical symptoms and the results of the Weil-Felix reaction.

CLINICAL DIAGNOSIS.—A clinical diagnosis of epidemic typhus fever cannot be made before the appearance of the characteristic eruption, as the early symptoms of this infection are similar to those of some other acute infectious diseases, especially plague.

DIFFERENTIAL DIAGNOSIS.—Epidemic typhus must be differentiated from typhoid and paratyphoid fevers, Rocky Mountain spotted fever, cerebrospinal meningitis, relapsing fever, malaria and measles.

Typhoid and Paratyphoid Fevers.—Epidemic typhus is differentiated from typhoid and paratyphoid fevers by the much more sudden onset, the much greater prostration during the first three days following the onset, the more profound mental lethargy, the occurrence of the characteristic eruption which differs greatly from the rose spots of typhoid, and the shorter course of the febrile reaction. The Widal test and the demonstration of the causative bacteria in blood cultures should enable one to quickly differentiate the typhoid group of infections from epidemic typhus. The Weil-Felix reaction is negative in both typhoid and paratyphoid fevers.

Plague.—The onset and early symptoms of typhus fever are so similar to those generally observed in plague that the two infections could be easily confused were it not that in bubonic plague the presence of the bubo is conclusive, while in pneumonic plague the character of the physical findings, the peculiar sputum which is coughed up in large amounts by the patient, and the presence of plague bacilli in the sputum differentiate it from epidemic typhus fever. In addition, no skin eruption is observed in plague and in the bubonic type the plague bacilli may be easily cultured from the buboes.

Rocky Mountain Spotted Fever.—In regions where both infections may occur, which fortunately are limited, the differentiation of Rocky Mountain spotted fever from epidemic typhus presents considerable difficulty. The symptoms of onset are similar and the skin eruption that occurs in both presents a similar morphology. The history of a tick bite in Rocky Mountain spotted fever helps and, if evidences of such a bite are present, is conclusive of the nature of the infection. The Weil-Felix reaction is positive in Rocky Mountain spotted fever as well as in epidemic typhus but cannot be obtained in as high dilutions. The blood serum of Rocky Mountain spotted fever agglutinates Proteus OXK, while that of epidemic typhus patients does not agglutinate this strain of the organism. The recent observations of Pinkerton (1940) would appear to demonstrate that Rocky Mountain spotted fever may be clearly differentiated from epidemic typhus by cross-immunity tests, the effect of the inoculation of guinea pigs, and by the fact that in tissue cultures and in the tissues of man the causative rickettsiae of this infection multiply in the cytoplasm of tissue cells but never invade the nuclei of the cells, while in epidemic typhus the rickettsiae grow in both the cytoplasm and nuclei but are few in number in the cytoplasm of the cells but exceedingly numerous in the nuclei.

Cerebrospinal Meningitis.—Cerebrospinal meningitis may resemble typhus in its early symptomatology but there should be little trouble in differentiating it when the disease is fully developed. In addition, the bacteriologic examination of the spinal fluid and the negative Weil-Felix reaction enable us easily to differentiate the two infections.

Relapsing Fever and Malaria.—These infections may be differentiated by the blood examination and the demonstration of the causative spirochetes or plasmodia in this fluid. In both of these infections the Weil-Felix reaction is negative.

The differentiation of epidemic and endemic typhus rests upon laboratory methods which will be discussed later.

LABORATORY DIAGNOSIS.—The laboratory diagnosis of epidemic typhus fever depends upon the reaction of the patient's blood serum and certain strains of *Proteus vulgaris*. It has been demonstrated that when the blood serum of patients suffering from this form of typhus fever is added to properly diluted cultures of the strain of this bacillus known as OX_{19}, the bacilli are agglutinated in high dilutions; while agglutination of another strain, known as OX_2, occurs in lower dilutions. This is not a specific reaction, as *Proteus vulgaris* is not concerned in the etiology of typhus fever, although it has been isolated from the urine, blood and organs of certain cases of typhus fever. The agglutinins appear in the blood as early as the fifth day of the disease and increase in amount until by the end of the febrile period high titers are obtained. An agglutination titer to Proteus OX_{19} of 1:25 to 1:30 may be present by the end of the fifth day of the disease and by the end of fourteen days a titer of 1:240 is generally present. By the end of three weeks agglutination titers as high as 1:2,500 have been obtained and titers between 1:320 and 1:640 are always present by the end of this period. The titers obtainable with Proteus OX_2 are much lower, but in epidemic typhus agglutination occurs with both OX_{19} and

OX_2, while no agglutination occurs with OXK, another strain of *Proteus vulgaris*. The Weil-Felix reaction is a heterologous and not a specific reaction from the standpoint of immunity, but a positive reaction with the Weil-Felix test is considered specific for both epidemic and endemic typhus for the reason that the reaction is positive in these infections and negative in other infections classed with typhus groups with the exception of Rocky Mountain spotted fever, in which disease low agglutination titers are obtained with OX_{19}, OX_2 and OXK strains of *Proteus vulgaris*.

No satisfactory explanation of the peculiar relation of *Proteus vulgaris* to typhus has yet been given, but the observations of Zinsser, Castaneda and Zia, demonstrating that there is a common antigenic factor in suspensions of the murine type of rickettsiae and Proteus OX_{19}, may explain the positive reactions obtained in typhus fevers.

The inoculation of guinea pigs with the epidemic typhus strain of *Rickettsia prowazeki* is not followed by swelling of the scrotum, thus differentiating this type of typhus from endemic typhus, in which swelling of the scrotum follows experimental inoculation; while in the rat the epidemic form of the typhus rickettsia causes an inapparent infection in contrast with the endemic, or murine, form of the rickettsia, in which a febrile infection follows inoculation, with the presence of rickettsiae in the tunica vaginalis and swelling of the scrotum.

Prognosis.—The prognosis of epidemic typhus fever has varied greatly in different epidemics and the mortality has varied from as low as 10 per cent to as high as 70 per cent. Strong (1942) states that in the great Serbian epidemic of 1915 the mortality reached 70 per cent, but that in more recent European epidemics the mortality was from 8 to 12 per cent. It is altogether probable, as suggested by Strong, that the virus in some epidemics having a low mortality was really of the endemic, or murine, type, in which the mortality is known to be very low. Bad prognostic signs are high, continuous fever; very pronounced eruption; suppression of urine, and marked mental symptoms.

The mortality of epidemic typhus is greatly influenced by all conditions depressing the natural resistance of the patient. Thus undernourishment, especially semistarvation, overcrowding, the conditions which accompany war, as mental strain, exposure to the elements, grief and fright, all contribute to a high mortality.

Other conditions being equal, age is of great importance. In the young, epidemic typhus is much milder than in the old, and in children it may be a very mild disease. Old people usually perish from a complicating bronchopneumonia, but even though this complication may not occur the prognosis of typhus in the aged is always very grave.

The mortality and morbidity of epidemic typhus among physicians are unusually high and it is generally accepted that in no other disease do so many medical attendants contract and perish from it as in this form of typhus fever. The morbidity in physicians attending epidemic typhus has averaged well over 50 per cent and the mortality has varied from 30 to as high as 50 per cent in different epidemics.

Treatment.—The treatment of epidemic typhus fever is unsatisfactory as we possess no drug that is specific, and treatment must be purely symptomatic. **Good nursing, the removal of the patient from insanitary conditions, proper nourishment,** and **treatment of serious symptoms as they arise** must be relied upon in the treatment of this disease and, fortunately, are successful in combating the infection in a majority of the cases.

The **patient should be kept in bed in a recumbent position** until the symptoms have disappeared and should not be allowed to leave the bed at any time during the active period of the disease. The **care of the skin,** in order to prevent bed sores, and **proper attention to the hygiene of the mouth,** are essential in the treatment of this infection. A mixture of equal parts of **boric acid solution, lemon juice** and **glycerin** is recommended by Strong (1942)

42101

for swabbing out the mouth several times a day, or a simple boric acid solution may be used for this purpose. The bowels should be kept open by **enemas** and excessive fever treated by **cold sponging.** The nervous symptoms may be relieved by the administration of the **bromides, veronal** or by **lumbar puncture,** according to the severity of such symptoms. The severe headache may be alleviated by **acetylsalicylic acid** (aspirin) or by **ice cap** to the head.

In epidemic typhus fever cardiac weakness is pronounced and cardiac collapse not uncommon. The use of various **stimulants** to combat the cardiac weakness is necessary. Of these, alcoholics, especially in the form of port wine, are usually administered, but care should be taken not to give large amounts. Eight ounces of port wine a day is enough and this amount should not be exceeded. For the treatment of cardiac collapse **caffeine** has been recommended, while Shattuck recommends the **intravenous administration of normal saline** in those cases in which the condition appears to be caused by lack of vascular tone. **Tincture of digitalis** or other digitalis preparations are also recommended as cardiac stimulants.

If the patient is violently delirious the administration of **hyoscine** is indicated and persistent insomnia may be relieved by the administration of **chloral, veronal** or the **barbiturates,** employing the last with great caution and only in the most severe cases of this condition.

The **sulfanilamide** drugs have been suggested as useful but there is little evidence to date that these preparations have a curative action in typhus fever. The same statement is true of the serum treatment of the infection. Several authorities have used **convalescent serum** in treatment, notably Asheshov, in Russia, who employed serum obtained from convalescent typhus patients, after the temperature had been normal for periods varying between four and fourteen days. Asheshov found that the administration of such serum did not shorten the course of the disease but did appear to render the symptoms less severe than in untreated patients. Other authorities have found that the administration of convalescent serum neither shortens the course nor mitigates the symptoms, so that, at present, the serum treatment of epidemic typhus is seldom employed.

The typhus patient should be in a very well ventilated room or, preferably, in a tent, as **fresh air** is an important adjunct to the treatment of the infection. The **diet** should be ample and nourishing and given in small amounts at frequent and regular intervals. The patient should be urged to drink water freely and iced drinks, as orangeade or lemonade, are generally gratifying and may be freely given. If anorexia is present the sipping of champagne sometimes affords relief and stimulates the appetite.

Good nursing and the proper treatment of symptoms as they arise is the secret of success in the treatment of this disease.

IMMUNE SERUM THERAPY.—The employment of immune sera in treatment of epidemic typhus has not been followed by success and has been practically discarded. The only serum treatment that has given a promise of being beneficial or curative is that of Zinsser and Castaneda, who reported favorable results in the treatment of murine typhus (endemic typhus) in Mexico, using immune serum obtained from horses immunized to the murine strain of typhus. However, the same serum used elsewhere has failed either to render the symptoms less severe or to cure the infection, so that, at present, the real value of this serum in therapeutics remains to be determined.

PROPHYLAXIS.—The prophylaxis of epidemic typhus may be divided into personal and general methods, and its success depends upon the **destruction of body lice, protection against their invasion of the clothing,** and **disinfestation of persons and habitations.**

Personal prophylaxis consists in the disinfestation of the clothing and bodies of individuals and preventing the access of lice to the person. All patients suffering from the disease should be deloused as well as those in contact with typhus patients and, if possible, the entire population of the localities in which the disease is occurring. In delousing the patients, or others, the following steps should be followed:

1. The entire body and head should be shaved, paying especial attention to the head, axillae and pubis, forearms, thighs and legs.

2. The individual should be given a bath in water containing cresol or the body may be scrubbed with a kerosene emulsion soap prepared by boiling 1 part of soap in 4 parts of water and adding 2 parts of kerosene oil. This is thoroughly mixed and the resultant jelly is mixed with 4 parts of water, and freely used in scrubbing the individual.

3. After the bath, the entire body should be rubbed with kerosene and the kerosene allowed to remain as long as it does not produce marked irritation of the skin.

The clothing which harbors the lice, must be disinfested, for the lice may remain alive on clothing for 8 to 10 days and the eggs for as long as 40 days. The clothing may be disinfected by either moist or dry heat, but to kill the lice a temperature of 55° C. (131° F.) for 30 minutes is required, while the eggs are killed at a temperature of 60° C. (140° F.) maintained for 15 minutes. Boiling the clothes for five minutes kills both the lice and their eggs, while soaking the clothes in a 5 per cent compound cresol solution for 30 minutes will also kill both lice and eggs.

To prevent access of the lice to the person—a prophylactic measure of great importance in epidemics, especially for those coming into contact with the sick, as physicians and nurses—various dusting powders have been recommended, the most used being the so-called **N.C.I. powder,** consisting of commercial naphthalene, 96 Gm.; creosote, 2 cc.; and iodoform, 2 Gm. Another powder, known as **Moore's powder,** consisting of creosote, 1 cc.; sulfur, 0.5 Gm.; and talc, 20 Gm., is recommended as more effective than the N.C.I. powder and less obnoxious and irritating.

If it is impossible, for any reason, either to boil clothing or to expose it to dry heat, as recommended above, the ironing or heating in some other way of the seams of the clothing will be found quite efficient in killing the lice and their eggs.

General prophylaxis consists in the application of all measures of known efficiency to the population as a whole in times of epidemic prevalence of the disease. Such measures consist in the mass disinfestation of the populace by treatment of the clothing and person in a disinfestation building suitable for the purpose, the limitation of travel from affected regions to unaffected regions, the disinfestation of dwellings in which typhus cases have occurred, the establishment of typhus hospitals or the segregation of typhus patients in separate wards in already established hospitals, disinfestation of railroad cars and public conveyances, proper sanitary inspections and all other methods that may be employed for the protection of the public. The application of all these general methods of prophylaxis is a function of the public health authorities and the rules governing such application are prepared and enforced by such authorities.

PROPHYLACTIC VACCINATION.—Within recent times much research has been devoted to the preparation of a vaccine that will give an immunity to typhus fever. Spencer and Parker (1925) were the first to demonstrate that it was possible to confer immunity to a disease of the typhus group by vaccination. They found that with a phenolized vaccine prepared by grinding the viscera of ticks infected with the rickettsiae of Rocky Mountain spotted fever it was possible to protect monkeys and guinea pigs against infection. Previously, Weigl (1924) had prepared a vaccine from the intestine of lice infected with typhus, but the results were not conclusive and the great difficulty of preparing this vaccine precluded its use except in a limited manner. Other authorities, as Laigret, have recommended a living vaccine, but vaccination with such a vaccine is dangerous both to the individual and the community, for obvious reasons. Zinsser, Fitzpatrick and Wei (1939) have developed a vaccine prepared from killed rickettsiae cultivated in living tissue upon a special agar medium and this vaccine has apparently given good protection in the hands of those who have employed it in the prophylaxis of epidemic typhus.

The vaccine that is being used for protection against epidemic typhus at the present time in the United States Army is the one developed by Cox (1938), consisting of a suspension of killed, louse-borne, epidemic typhus rickettsiae which have been cultivated in the yolk sac of fertile hen's eggs. The initial vaccination with this vaccine consists of three injections of 1 cc. each, given subcutaneously, with intervals of from seven to ten days between the injections. Subsequently, a dose of 1 cc. of the vaccine may be administered every four to six months as long as there is danger of infection, and further doses of the vaccine may be administered, either before the period mentioned, or afterward, if it is believed that great danger exists of contracting the disease.

While the Cox vaccine, so far as the protection of experimental animals is concerned, is efficient, it has not been tried in epidemics of the disease in man, and the whole question of the protection of man by typhus vaccines must be said to be still in the experimental stage.

Pathology.—The patient dying of epidemic typhus does not present any *macroscopic* lesions that are peculiar to the infection, with the exception of the eruption which may still be present after death. The skin may show areas of hemorrhage and gangrene may be present in areas of varying size in fulminant cases. The spleen is usually moderately enlarged during the acute disease and at necropsy it is much decreased in consistence and greatly congested. The heart, liver and kidneys show cloudy swelling. The mesenteric glands are not enlarged and the intestinal tract appears normal. The lungs frequently present the usual signs of a bronchopneumonia. The blood is darker in color than usual but otherwise appears normal.

Microscopically, the viscera show great congestion, the spleen especially being engorged with blood, while there is a reduction in the lymphoid cells and marked phagocytosis of red blood corpuscles. In the brain and viscera, and in sections made through the skin showing the eruption, the characteristic "typhus nodules" that are diagnostic of the infection occur. In the brain these nodules resemble miliary tubercles in size and may be situated in the cortex, basal ganglion, and medulla, and rarely in the white matter and the cerebellum. These nodules are formed by localized collections of plasma cells and lymphocytes, together with cells derived from the multiplication of mononuclear phagocytes and neuroglia, the process resulting in collections of cells which are characteristic of the disease. The eruption itself is caused by a localized necrosis of the walls of the smaller blood vessels, in which collections of plasma cells and lymphocytes in the adventitia occur. Similar characteristic miliary nodules occur in the viscera.

History.—The history of epidemic typhus dates back to ancient times and it is probable that it has been one of the great plagues of armies since the dawn of history. While this is true, it was first described by Fracastoro in the sixteenth century. In the seventeenth century, during the Thirty Years' War, it spread throughout Europe. Since that time, epidemic typhus has continued to cause severe epidemics in various parts of the world and has prevailed wherever wars have occurred or conditions of overcrowding, poverty and insanitary surroundings have reduced the natural resistance of large numbers of people to infection. Every war in modern history has been accompanied by epidemics of typhus and during the first World War one of the greatest epidemics of the disease occurred among the Serbians in 1915. Strong (1942) states that this epidemic "was characterized not only by its magnitude but its high virulence and high mortality." He states that as many as 2,500 cases were admitted daily to the military hospitals during the height of the epidemic and that the mortality varied from 30 to 60 per cent, and in complicated cases as high as 70 per cent. Over 150,000 people died of the disease during this epidemic.

The last great epidemic of the disease of which we have record is that occurring in Russia between 1919 and 1922, during which it is estimated over 5,000,000 people suffered from the infection.

Prior to 1909, epidemic typhus fever was considered as very contagious, but in that year Nicolle demonstrated that it is transmitted from man to man by lice and it has since been amply proved that, in the absence of lice, epidemic typhus is not transmitted by contact, although the possibility of droplet infection deserves further study.

Geographic Distribution.—As already stated, epidemics of typhus have occurred throughout the world in the past, almost always beginning in Europe, where two endemic foci exist at the present time, one in Russia and one in Poland. Since 1933, epidemic typhus has caused epidemics in most of the eastern European countries, South Africa, Egypt, in equatorial Africa, North Africa, Asia Minor, Syria, Palestine, Iran, Afghanistan, India, Indo-China and China. In the United States no epidemic of this disease has occurred since 1883, when cases were described as occurring in Philadelphia. In this city an epidemic occurred in 1836, and it was during this epidemic that Gerhard first differentiated typhus fever from typhoid fever, with which it had been previously confused. However, it should be noted that the Mexican type of typhus, known as tabardillo, which is transmitted by lice, has caused localized outbreaks of typhus in Iowa, California and New Mexico since 1917. The endemic type of typhus and Brill's disease exist in the United States, the former in our Southern States and the latter especially in the Eastern and Middle Atlantic States.

ENDEMIC TYPHUS FEVER

Synonyms.—Brill's disease, flea typhus, murine typhus.

Definition.—An acute infectious disease caused by *Rickettsia prowazeki* var. *mooseri* and transmitted to man by the rat fleas, *Xenopsylla astia* and *Xenopsylla cheopis*. It is characterized clinically by symptoms resembling those of epidemic typhus but of much less severity, and by a much lower mortality rate.

Etiology.—The endemic type of typhus fever is caused by an organism belonging to the genus *Rickettsia* and known as *Rickettsia prowazeki* var. *mooseri*. Morphologically it is identical with *Rickettsia prowazeki* var. *prowazeki*, and serologically it gives a positive Weil-Felix reaction with Proteus OX_{19} and OX_2, and a negative reaction with Proteus OXK, as does *Rickettsia prowazeki* var. *prowazeki*, the cause of epidemic typhus fever. There is also some cross-immunity between these two forms of typhus, but the method of transmission of the two infections is entirely different and the clinical pictures produced by the inoculation of susceptible animals, as the guinea pig and rat, also are distinct, as will be noted later.

What has already been stated as regards the morphology and biology of the rickettsiae of the epidemic type of typhus is equally true of the rickettsiae of the endemic type, both consisting of coccoid bodies or very minute bacilliforms living within certain cells of the infected animal or individual and capable of cultivation in living cells, as those of the chick embryo. Certain tissue reactions in susceptible animals serve to distinguish the two strains of rickettsiae. Thus, when the variety producing the epidemic form of typhus is inoculated into male guinea pigs the inoculation is followed by only a very slight rise in temperature at most and, in many cases, by no evidences of infection whatever; but if the guinea pig is inoculated with the endemic variety of the rickettsiae, a marked fever follows and a swelling of the scrotum with an exudate into the tunica vaginalis which swarms with the rickettsiae. Exactly similar reactions occur in rats after inoculation with the two varieties of rickettsiae and it is thus possible to differentiate them by these characteristic reactions.

Epidemiology.—Unlike epidemic typhus, transmitted from man to man directly by lice, endemic typhus is transmitted to man by the rat fleas, *Xenopsylla astia* and *Xenopsylla cheopis*, the rat acting as a reservoir of infection for man. The infection is transmitted from rat to rat by the same fleas and also by the rat louse, *Polyplax spinulosa*, but the rat louse plays no part in the transmission of the rickettsiae to man as this species of louse does not bite human beings. There is some evidence that the rat mite, *Liponyssus bacoti*, may transmit the infection, as claimed by Dove and Shelmire (1931). The infection is not transmitted to man by the bite of the fleas but by rubbing the feces of these arthropods into the wound made by biting or into abrasions near the site of the bite, when scratching. The infection in the fleas produces no observable injuries and infected fleas may harbor the infection for months and remain infective during that time. The rickettsiae multiply rapidly in the fleas although no apparent disease is produced. In the rat louse, however, which transmits the infection from rat to rat, the rickettsiae cause the death of the arthropod within from two to three weeks.

Until 1931 the method of transmission of endemic typhus was unknown, although in 1926 Maxcy had called attention to the association of this form of typhus with rats and grain stores. In 1931 Dyer, Rumreich and Badger demonstrated the presence of the rickettsiae of endemic typhus in rats and experimentally proved that the rat fleas transmitted the disease. Their observations were soon confirmed by others, and the typhus fever of Mexico, or tabardillo, was shown to be etiologically identical with the endemic typhus of the Southern States of this country by Mooser, Castaneda and Zinsser (1931), who demonstrated the rickettsiae in the brain of rats caught in Mexico.

There is some evidence that the endemic type of typhus may be transmitted to animals through the alimentary tract, as shown by Wolbach (1940) and others. Nicolle has demonstrated that the rickettsiae of endemic typhus are present in the urine of infected rats and suggests that the contamination of food with such urine may be a method of transmission of the infection to man. The endemic, or murine, strain of rickettsia is much more virulent for the rat than the louse, or epidemic, strain, and may exist in the brain of rats for many weeks, during which time these animals may act as reservoirs of infection for man.

The virus of the Mexican form of typhus, or tabardillo, is identical with that of the endemic, or murine, strain although it produces an epidemic type of the infection and is transmitted by lice. This again illustrates how closely these two strains of rickettsiae are related and speaks eloquently of the possible identity of both the epidemic and endemic strains, the clinical and epidemiologic differences that undoubtedly exist having been brought about by unknown biologic conditions. Be this as it may, it is true that today we must recognize the existence of the epidemic and endemic types of typhus, etiologically, epidemiologically and clinically. In the United States, for instance, the endemic, or murine, type of typhus is increasing in distribution and is the only type which is prevalent in this country.

Season has much to do with the epidemiology of endemic typhus, the great majority of the cases occurring in the summer and fall. *Sex* is also of importance, males being more frequently attacked than females, while *race* is also of importance, as it has been noted that the Negro suffers less from the disease than the whites. *Occupation* has some influence in that individuals pursuing occupations that bring them into possible contact with rats, as working in storehouses, groceries and similar occupations, are more apt to become infected than office workers or those employed in labor that will not bring them into contact with these animals.

Symptomatology.—The symptoms of endemic typhus, while similar to those of the epidemic type, are much less severe and the mortality is very low, not exceeding 1 per cent. The *onset* may be gradual or sudden. If sudden, chilly sensations or a chill usually ushers in the attack and the temperature rises to 38–39° C. (100.4–102.2° F.) by the end of twenty-four hours. If gradual, there may be several days of malaise, aching in the muscles, headache and mental depression, the temperature rising gradually to 39–40° C. (102.2–104° F.) or higher. After reaching its fastigium the temperature remains more or less constant, with slight remission, for a period of from ten to twelve days, the entire attack usually covering about two weeks. During the febrile period the symptoms are like those occurring in the epidemic form of typhus but are much less severe, especially the mental symptoms.

As in epidemic typhus, a characteristic rash is present in this infection, appearing between the fourth and fifth days of the disease upon the chest, abdomen and arms. This rash may be rather discrete or it may cover the whole body with the exception of the feet and the palms of the hands. It consists of rather dark red macules and is not apt to be petechial, as in the epidemic type of typhus. It usually does not have the dusky purplish hue of the epidemic type of eruption, although in the most severe cases the rash may very closely resemble the latter. It may last for less than two days or persist for as long as eleven days and disappears without leaving a scar or desquamation.

Convalescence is usually rapid and uneventful in endemic typhus and the more severe symptoms so common in the epidemic type, already described, are very rarely encountered in this type of the disease.

Complications.—These are practically unknown except in the fatal cases when they are similar to those of the epidemic type of typhus already described.

Sequelae.—No sequelae of importance have been described.

Diagnosis.—The diagnosis of endemic typhus fever rests upon the clinical picture, the response to the Weil-Felix test and to animal inoculation. The course of the infection and the characteristic eruption should cause one to employ the Weil-Felix test. If the blood serum of the patient gives an agglutination reaction with Proteus OX_{19} and OX_2 and a negative reaction with OXK, the diagnosis will rest between epidemic and endemic typhus, and the latter can be distinguished by its reaction with comparatively low titers of the serum, the epidemic form reacting with much higher dilutions of the serum than the endemic form.

The inoculation of guinea pigs will serve to distinguish the epidemic and endemic strains of rickettsiae as the inoculation of these animals with the epidemic strain results in no scrotal swelling, while inoculation with the endemic strain results in swelling of the scrotum. In rats the inoculation of the epidemic strain causes no apparent symptoms, while the inoculation of the endemic strain results in fever and pronounced swelling of the scrotum.

The differential diagnosis of endemic typhus from other conditions does not differ from that of epidemic typhus already described.

Treatment.—The treatment of this form of typhus is similar to that of the epidemic form already described.

PROPHYLAXIS.—The prevention of endemic typhus depends upon the eradication of rats and protection of man from contact with these animals. Rat-proofing of buildings is the most efficient preventive method, while poisoning and trapping these animals are also very valuable preventive measures. *Prophylactic vaccination* is not warranted, as this type of typhus is not a serious infection from the standpoint of public health, the cases are comparatively few and are sporadic in occurrence, and the vaccination of the general populace is not necessary.

Prognosis.—The prognosis of endemic typhus is excellent and, as already stated, the mortality rate is not above 1 per cent at most and is probably a small fraction of 1 per cent.

Pathology.—The pathology is similar to that of epidemic typhus already described.

History.—Maxcy, of the United States Public Health Service, was the first to call attention to the occurrence of the endemic type of typhus fever in Georgia.

In 1926 he suggested that this infection might be transmitted to man from infected rats and mice by fleas, ticks or mites. In 1931 Dyer, Rumreich and Badger found the rickettsiae in rat fleas and demonstrated that the fleas transmitted the infection. These observations were soon confirmed by others and prophylactic vaccines have been prepared by Weigl, Zinsser and Castaneda, Cox and other investigators.

Geographic Distribution.—Endemic, or murine, typhus is distributed in the United States, Chile, Peru, Africa, Manchuria, Malay States, Indo-China, China, Manchuria, Greece, Syria and possibly in the Philippine Islands. It has also been described as occurring in Australia, Russia, North and South Africa, and Palestine. In the United States it is especially prevalent in Georgia, but numerous cases have also been reported in Tennessee, Alabama, Louisiana and Texas. A few cases have been reported recently from New York, New Jersey, Delaware, Maryland and Virginia, but the chief endemic areas in this country are in the Southeastern and Southern States.

BRILL'S DISEASE

Most authorities regard Brill's disease as synonymous with endemic, or murine, typhus but some authorities, notably Zinsser, regard it as a recrudescence of epidemic typhus in infections acquired in Europe. Brill in 1898 first described a mild form of typhus fever occurring in New York City but it was not until 1910 that he compared the symptomatology with that of epidemic typhus and concluded that the disease described by him was a mild form of typhus fever. In 1912 Anderson and Goldberger demonstrated by animal experiments that Brill's disease was a form of typhus fever, and the later observations of Maxcy (1926) and others upon the murine type of typhus occurring in the Southern States, which is symptomatically identical with Brill's disease, has led most authorities to regard the latter as identical with endemic, or murine, typhus. Zinsser's interpretation of Brill's disease as a recrudescence of epidemic, or European, typhus was based upon his study of over 500 cases observed in New York and Boston, over 94 per cent occurring in Russians who had probably suffered from epidemic typhus before arriving in this country. While this evidence would appear to be quite conclusive, it is not accepted by the majority of authorities as establishing Brill's disease as differing from endemic typhus, and most authorities quote the name as a synonym of endemic, or murine, typhus.

BIBLIOGRAPHY

Anderson, J. F. and Goldberger, J.: Pub. Health Rep., 27 : 149, 1912.

Arkwright, J. A. and Bacot, A. W.: Parasitology, 15 : 43, 1923.

—— and ——: Brit. J. Exper. Path., 4 : 70, 1923.

Blanc, G. and Baltazard, M.: Compt. rend. Acad. d. sc., 209 : 419, 1939.

Brill, N. E.: N. York M. J., 67 : 48, 77, 1898.

——: Am. J. M. Sc., 139 : 484, 1910.

Cox, H. R.: Am. J. Trop. Med., 20 : 463, 1940.

Craig, C. F.: Brennemann's Practice of Pediatrics, Hagerstown, Md., W. F. Prior Company, Inc., Vol. 2, Chap. 32, 1942.

Dove, W. E. and Shelmire, B.: J. A. M. A., 97 : 1506, 1931.

Dyer, R. E.: Am. J. Trop. Med., 21 : 163, 1941.

——, Rumreich, A. and Badger, L. F.: Pub. Health Rep., 46 : 334, 1931.

Liu, W. T. and Zia, S. H.: Proc. Soc. Exper. Biol. & Med., 45 : 823, 1940.

Maxcy, K. F.: Pub. Health Rep., 41 : 1213, 2967, 1926; 43 : 3084, 1928; 44 : 589, 1735, 1935, 1929.

Mooser, H., Ruiz Castaneda, M. and Zinsser, H.: J. Exper. Med., 54 : 567, 1931.

Nicolle, C.: Compt. rend. Acad. d. sc., 149 : 157, 1909.

Nicolle, C., Comte, C. and Conseil, E.: Compt. rend. Acad. d. sc., 149 : 486, 1909.

—— and Laigret, J.: Arch. Inst. Pasteur de Tunis, 21 : 357, 1933.

Ricketts, H. T. and Wilder, R. M.: J. A. M. A., 54 : 463, 1304, 1373, 1910.

da Rocha-Lima, H.: Arch. f. Schiffs- u. Tropen-Hyg., 20 : 17, 1916.

Shattuck, G. C., Sellards, A. W., Zinsser, H., Hopkins, J. S. and Strong, R. P.: Rep. Amer. Red Cross, p. 29, 1920.

Spencer, R. R. and Parker, R. R.: Pub. Health Rep., 41 : 35, 1926.

Strong, R. P.: Stitt's Diagnosis, Prevention and Treatment of Tropical Diseases, Ed. 6, Revised by Strong, Philadelphia, 2 : 923, 1942.

Weigl, R.: Med. Klin., 20 : 1046, 1924.

Weil, E. and Felix, A.: Wien. klin. Wchnschr., 29 : 33, 1916.

Wolbach, S. B.: J. M. Research, 41 : 1, 1919.

Zinsser, H.: Am. J. Hyg., 20 : 513, 1934.

——: Am. J. Hyg., 25 : 430, 1937.

—— and Ruiz Castaneda, M.: J. Exper. Med., 52 : 649, 1930.

—— and ——: Proc. Soc. Exper. Biol. & Med., 29 : 840, 1932.

—— and ——: New England J. Med., 209 : 815, 1933.

——, Fitzpatrick, F. K. and Wei, H.: J. Exper. Med., 69 : 179, 1939.

There is an intentional break in the continuity of these page numbers. This space will be utilized by future revisions of the text in this volume.

TYPHOID FEVER

By Alpheus F. Jennings, M.D., and Don R. Mathieson, M.D.

The present authors in the rewriting of this chapter have retained much from the splendid clinical description of ''Typhoid Fever'' contributed by the late Dr. C. G. Jennings and Dr. P. F. Morse to this Practice of Medicine.

Definition.—Typhoid fever is an acute general infection caused by the invasion of the body tissues by the *Eberthella typhosa*. It is characterized, clinically, by a continued fever of peculiar type, a cutaneous eruption of small maculopapules, a specific enteritis, splenic enlargement

The authors wish to express their thanks to Drs. Silas Willard Wallace and Ralph A. Johnson for their valuable assistance in the preparation of this chapter.
40101

and a toxemia with distinctive nervous phenomena; anatomically, by hyperplasia and ulceration of the intestinal lymph follicles, hyperplasia of the mesenteric glands and spleen and by parenchymatous changes in the various organs of the body. Multiplicity of symptoms and complications and variability in the clinical history are marked features of the disease.

ETIOLOGY

Prevalence.—Typhoid fever is widely distributed throughout all the countries of the world. There is a marked variation in the prevalence of the disease and it may be fairly stated that the typhoid rate of any country is an index of the efficiency and observance of the laws of sanitation.

The reported cases of typhoid fever in 1935 in various countries, taken from the Annual Epidemiological Report of the League of Nations, are shown in Table I. The number of inhabitants of each country are those published in the Rand McNally World Atlas 1936.

In the United States there has been a steady decline in the disease since 1910. Table II shows the mortality from typhoid and paratyphoid fevers in the United States Registration Area. Table III shows the mortality and death rate per 100,000 population for 1937 of typhoid fever in seventy-eight cities. The rate is still higher than the rates of the countries of Western Europe.

TABLE I

LEAGUE OF NATIONS HEALTH ORGANIZATION ANNUAL EPIDEMIOLOGICAL REPORT *

Locality	Typhoid Fever Cases	Approximate Number of Inhabitants	Locality	Typhoid Fever Cases	Approximate Number of Inhabitants
Egypt	4,334	15,377,000	Bulgaria	5,217	5,956,200
Morocco, French	353	5,063,271	Denmark	78	3,623,000
Anglo-Egyptian			Scotland	584	4,916,000
Sudan	246	5,728,551	Spain	16,364	23,564,000
Union of South			Irish Free State	404	2,992,000
Africa	4,377	8,488,300	Finland	321	3,720,752
Bahamas	17	62,679	France	4,203	41,834,923
Bermudas	14	27,789	Greece	4,090	6,620,000
Canada	1,809	10,376,786	Hungary	12,085	8,837,349
(Quebec)	(1,709)		Northern Ireland	288	1,280,000
Chile	711	4,442,462	Italy	33,842	41,177,000
Cuba	1,742	3,962,344	Netherlands	359	8,290,108
United States	18,324	125,701,634	Poland	13,590	33,024,000
Jamaica	1,117	1,773,500	Portugal	3,428	6,826,000
Mexico	4,532	16,552,722	Rumania	6,780	18,176,757
Puerto Rico	559	1,543,913	Sweden	439	6,190,364
Persia	4,479	15,055,115	Switzerland	103	4,066,400
Japan	38,357	67,238,600	Czechoslovakia	5,118	15,017,347
Palestine	2,060	1,035,154	Turkey	3,813	13,660,275
Philippines	2,245	12,082,366	U.S.S.R. in Europe	51,661	122,114,545
Germany	3,064	66,020,000	Ukraine	25,301	31,901,400
England and Wales	956	40,350,000	Jugoslavia	5,142	13,934,038
Austria	620	6,748,826	Australia	487	6,438,999
Belgium	361	8,247,950			

* Corrected Statistics of Notifiable Diseases for the Year 1935. Published by the Health Section, Geneva, 1937.

TABLE II

MORTALITY FROM TYPHOID AND PARATYPHOID FEVERS IN THE
UNITED STATES REGISTRATION AREA, 1920–1937

Year	Number of Deaths	Rate per 10,000
1920	6,805	7.8
1923	6,635	6.8
1926	6,826	6.5
1929	4,854	4.2
1932	4,441	3.7
1935	3,531	2.8
1937	2,695	2.1

TABLE III

TOTAL TYPHOID RATE FOR SEVENTY-EIGHT CITIES, 1910–1937 *

Year	Population	Typhoid Deaths	Typhoid Death Rate per 100,000
1910	22,573,435	4,637	20.54
1913	24,457,989	3,285	13.43
1916	26,257,550	2,191	8.34
1919	27,735,083	1,151	4.15
1922	29,473,246	963	3.26
1925	31,315,598	1,079	3.44
1928	33,158,150	628	1.89
1931	35,137,915	563	1.60
1934	35,401,715	413	1.17
1937	35,771,787	280	0.76

* Condensed from the Twenty-sixth Annual Report of Typhoid in the Large Cities of the United States in 1937. (J. Am. M. Ass., 111: 414, 1938.)

TABLE IV

DEATH RATE PER 100,000 POPULATION FROM TYPHOID AND PARATYPHOID FEVER BY
GEOGRAPHIC DIVISIONS OF THE UNITED STATES BY COLOR, AND URBAN AND RURAL
AREAS FOR THE 3-YEAR PERIOD 1930–1932 *

Geographic Division	White			Colored		
	Cities 10,000 and over	Cities 2,500 to 10,000	Rural	Cities 10,000 and over	Cities 2,500 to 10,000	Rural
United States	1.9	4.2	3.6	6.3	17.5	13.6
New England States	0.9	0.7	0.7	0.8	0	2.5
Middle Atlantic States	1.3	2.0	1.6	2.5	5.6	3.1
East-North Central States	1.5	2.4	2.6	2.4	6.5	9.4
West-North Central States	2.4	5.1	2.8	2.8	8.3	13.5
South Atlantic States	4.6	10.3	5.8	9.9	18.7	14.6
East-South Central States	5.1	3.0	5.7	9.1	11.2	8.7
West-South Central States	10.6	14.2	9.6	22.1	33.6	19.5
Mountain States	3.4	8.4	2.3	14.8	25.0	8.0
Pacific States	1.2	2.9	1.5	3.7	6.5	4.6

* Condensed from the Statistical Bulletin, Metropolitan Life Insurance Company, November, 1935.

40101

TABLE V

INCIDENCE OF TYPHOID FEVER IN THE CIVIL WAR, THE SPANISH-AMERICAN WAR AND THE SOUTH AFRICAN WAR *

War	Average Annual Strength	Admissions	Deaths	Admission Rate per 1,000
Civil Union Army 1861–1866	532,198	79,462	29,336	29.86
Spanish-American U. S. Army 1898	147,795	20,926	2,192	141.59
South African War British Army 2.5 years	209,404	59,750	8,227	114.13

* Compiled by Lieutenant Colonel Siler and Major Lambie in the Medical Department of the United States Army in the World War, Volume IX.   (Communicable and Other Diseases.)
Note.—Considering the recorded number of deaths in the Civil War, the recorded number of admissions is probably considerably less than the actual number of cases.

TABLE VI

INCIDENCE OF TYPHOID FEVER IN THE FIRST WORLD WAR *

Army	Total Mean Annual Strength	Admissions	Deaths	Admission Rate per 1,000
United States 2.75 years	4,128,479	1,529	227	0.37
Great Britain 4.25 years	4,970,902	6,807	260	1.02
France	8,410,000	124,991	15,211	14.86
Italy	5,615,000	58,451		6.24
Belgium	267,000	3,217	523	3.59
Germany	11,000,000	112,364	11,405	
Austria	7,800,000	171,601	17,399	

* Compiled by Lieutenant Colonel Siler and Major Lambie.

Table IV, compiled by Dublin, indicates the incidence in the various sections of this country. The disease is more prevalent in the Southern States. The rate in the colored races is higher throughout the country than in the white races, reaching endemic proportions in some areas. The rate is lowest in the large cities, highest in the small cities and villages, and intermediate in the rural areas. Outside of the endemic areas the majority of the cases follow the infection of food by a carrier.

Typhoid Fever in Armies.—Until the first World War typhoid fever was the greatest scourge of armies in the field. The alarm and indignation that followed the high rates that prevailed in the Spanish-American and South African wars, together with the realization that means existed for the control of the disease, resulted in determined efforts to eliminate it. Sanitary measures were first applied by the Japanese Army in the Russo-Japanese War in 1904–1905. The opposing forces were approximately equal, but the typhoid incidence of the Japanese Army was only one-fourth that of the Russian. In the United States Army, typhoid

TABLE VII

INCIDENCE OF THE PARATYPHOID FEVERS IN THE UNITED STATES ARMY DURING THE FIRST WORLD WAR *

Area	Total Mean Annual Strength	Paratyphoid A		Paratyphoid B	
		Admissions	Deaths	Admissions	Deaths
U.S.A.	2,235,389	32	0	11	1
Europe	1,665,796	95	6	56	4
Other Countries	22,294	7	0	11	0
Total	3,923,479	134	6	78	5

* Compiled by Lieutenant Colonel Siler and Major Lambie.

TABLE VIII

ANNUAL RATES OF CASES PER 100,000 STRENGTH IN THE CIVILIAN CONSERVATION CORPS

1933—24 1934—25	1935—26 1936— 8	1937—5 1938—3.4

fever prevailed in unduly high rates despite sanitary discipline until antityphoid immunization was made compulsory, following which it decreased to its present low incidence.

The incidence of typhoid fever in the armies of the first World War is shown in the tables compiled by Lieutenant Colonel Joseph F. Siler and Major John S. Lambie (Tables V–VII). They state: "Typhoid and paratyphoid fevers were of minor importance as causes of sickness in the United States Army during the World War. This negative condition is of all the more present interest in view of the fact that in previous wars our experience with typhoid fevers was quite different." Their report bespeaks mainly the benefits of antityphoid vaccination.

In the United States Army the typhoid rate in the cantonments was less than one-half that of the Expeditionary Force in France, and the same proportion prevailed in comparison to a similar age group in civil life.

In Europe there was ample opportunity to acquire the disease. The water supplies were unsafe, there was typhoid in the civilian population, and our troops occupied sections where typhoid had been prevalent. Four hundred and thirty-five cases resulted from grossly contaminated water and improper sanitation. One fourth of the cases developed after the cessation of hostilities. Siler and Lambie state that not over one hundred cases would have occurred in the American Expeditionary Force in France had the rules of sanitation been rigidly followed.

The low incidence of typhoid fever in the Italian Expeditionary Force in Ethiopia is equally remarkable. The troops numbered 500,000 and there were 458 cases with 161 deaths over a period of eight months. Immunization by Castellani's tetravaccine, containing the typhoid, paratyphoid A and B, and cholera organisms, was made universal both for the troops and for the civilians of occupied territory, pure water was supplied, and sanitation was rigidly enforced.

The tables show that the incidence of typhoid fever in the European armies in the first World War was greatly below that of previous wars, yet in comparison with the incidence in the American Army it was quite high. The incidence was much higher in the first two than in the last two years. Siler and Lambie attribute it to the rapid mobilization of the forces with neglect of vaccination. The desperate nature of the fighting must have made observance of sanitation extremely difficult. One of us (A.F.J.) has previously experienced the stubborn determination of the enlisted man to deposit his excreta where he wishes and not where he is told. The total recorded cases for all the European armies were 477,431 and the deaths were 44,798. It would seem advisable that all persons of military age in countries anticipating war should be vaccinated.

Predisposing Causes.—SEASON.—Typhoid fever exhibits a seasonal variation, hence the synonym "autumnal fever." The seasonal curve of prevalence in the United States, as plotted by the Census Bureau in 1900, shows a wave with its lowest point about the middle of June. The line rises slowly in the latter half of June, rapidly in July and August, more slowly in September, reaching its crest in October. It then falls with about equal rapidity, reaching a low point in February. In March there is a secondary low wave and another in May.

PERSONAL CONDITIONS.—Individual susceptibility to typhoid fever varies. Of a number of persons exposed, a certain number will escape infection. A group of about 200 workmen drank water from a supply accidentally taken from the Detroit River at a point where it is highly polluted with sewage. Of the number, 156 developed gastro-enteritis within a few days after the incident. Typhoid fever developed in 56 of this group.

Group studies of agglutination reaction in persons who have not been vaccinated show an appreciable number who have significant titers. This number is higher in areas where the disease is prevalent than in areas where it is not. These individuals presumably have suffered infection without symptoms of active disease. Active robust health is no protection; those debilitated by chronic disease or other acute infection may show relative immunity.

AGE.—Approximately 70 to 75 per cent of the cases occur between the ages of fifteen and thirty years; about 12 per cent before the fifteenth, and about 18 per cent after the thirtieth, year. Infants are relatively immune. Intra-uterine infection may occur. After the age of forty the disease is exceptional. In children mild cases may be confused with other febrile disorders and hence do not appear in hospital statistics.

That childhood is a period of high susceptibility was demonstrated in a school epidemic reported by Bowdoin. The same potential exposure from infected water was present for all pupils. There were 158 in the age group six to twelve, of whom 24 acquired the disease, 13 cases being aged six and seven. There were 120 in the age group thirteen to sixteen with 3 cases and 45 in the age group seventeen to twenty-three with no cases. The percentage of those vaccinated increased with age, yet the tables demonstrated that this was not the sole cause for the difference of age incidence.

OCCUPATION AND SOCIAL CONDITIONS.—Occupation and social conditions predispose to typhoid fever only when they increase the chances of exposure to infection in the usual manner. Race, heredity, sex and altitude have no influence upon the incidence. The record of the Italian forces in Ethiopia shows that typhoid can be prevented under the worst climatic influences.

SOIL.—Soil polluted with human excrement is a common medium of infection.

Exciting Cause.—NOMENCLATURE AND CLASSIFICATION.—Our knowledge of the biology of the organisms causing typhoid and related continued fevers and the biology of closely related nonpathogenic organisms has been materially increased during the past two decades. In many instances our newer knowledge has confused rather than clarified many issues. Nomenclature and classification have become particularly difficult and complex. This is in part due to the existence of three different systems of microbic taxonomy. In the Bergey classification the typhoid bacillus is called *Eberthella typhosa*, in the British classification the name *Bacterium typhosum* is given, and in the Kauffmann-White scheme the organism is designated *Salmonella typhosa*. Although each classification has its own merits, it is certain that a general adoption of some one scheme would lead to greater uniformity of terminology in medical literature and to a clearer understanding of the bacteriology of enteric infections. All things considered, it seems that the Bergey classification in its present 1939 form is the most practical from the clinician's point of view.

The following *key* taken from Bergey presents the essential features of this classification insofar as it pertains to the coliform-typhoid-dysentery group of micro-organisms. It is followed by a general description of the classification used in England and a brief description of the Kauffmann-White scheme.

Before presenting the key it should be recalled that bacteria are generally considered as being plants belonging to the group known as the fungi. There are four large classes of fungi. The bacteria constitute one of these classes.

Class *Schizomycetes*
Order *Eubacteriales*
This order includes the true bacteria—the rods and cocci.
Family *Enterobacteriaceae*
This family includes gram-negative rods which are widely distributed in nature. Many are animal parasites and some are plant parasites causing blights and soft rots. They all grow well on artificial media. All species secrete enzymes which break down carbohydrates to acids or acids and visible gas. All produce nitrites from nitrates. When motile the flagella are peritrichous.
Tribe: *Eschericheae*
The organisms in this tribe are distinguished from all other tribes by their ability to ferment dextrose and lactose with the formation of acid and visible gas. Most members of this tribe do not liquefy gelatin.
In this tribe there are three important genera. Each of these genera

contains important species.   The genera and species with their principal differential characters are given below.

Genera:

Escherichia

Methyl red test positive. Voges-Proskauer test negative. Citric acid may or may not be used as a sole source of carbon.

The most important species of the genus and one of the most important species of the entire enteric group of micro-organisms is: *Escherichia coli* (" colon bacillus ")

Its importance will be stressed under the heading of " The Isolation of the Organism from the Stool." It is frequently the cause of genito-urinary diseases and may also be the cause of peritonitis, cholecystitis and acute appendicitis. It is said that it frequently invades the blood stream in the agonal stages of many diseases.

Aerobacter

Methyl red test negative. Voges-Proskauer test positive. Citric acid may be used as a sole source of carbon. The most important species in this genus is:

Aerobacter aerogenes

It is nonpathogenic. It is a common fecal-contaminating organism.

Klebsiella

Methyl red test usually positive. Voges-Proskauer test usually negative. Organisms are encapsulated. Of the six described species of this genus only one

Klebsiella pneumoniae (Friedländer's bacillus) is important. This organism, according to Bullowa, causes about 1 per cent of the lobar pneumonias. It is probably a frequent inhabitant of the upper respiratory system.

It should be noted that the key so far has included organisms that attack lactose and are classified in the tribe *Eschericheae*. The following organisms belong to the tribe *Salmonelleae*. The organisms in this tribe rarely ferment lactose. If fermentation occurs, it produces only acid, never visible gas. This is an important differential point.

In the tribe *Salmonelleae* there are three genera. The names of these genera, their chief differential characters and the important species are given below.

Salmonella:

All members of this genus are gram-negative, motile bacteria which produce both acid and gas in dextrose and do not ferment lactose. In this classification (Bergey) 37 species are listed. Only those of major importance and those that can be more or less readily identified by usual laboratory methods will be considered.

Salmonella paratyphi (paratyphoid bacillus A)

This organism is very closely related to the typhoid bacillus both in pathogenicity and in natural distribution. Like *Eberthella typhosa* and *Salmonella schottmülleri*, it is strictly pathogenic for man; it is not known to cause disease in any other species. Paratyphoid fever is clinically so similar to typhoid fever that a bacteriologic diagnosis must often be made to differentiate the two.

Salmonella schottmülleri (paratyphoid bacillus B)

As a rule, infection with this organism is indistinguishable from the infection caused by *S. paratyphi* and *E. typhosa*. Occasionally, however, cases of acute gastro-enteritis have been reported as being due to this organism. Its differential cultural characters are: ability to ferment inosite and to produce acid and gas from rhamnose.

Salmonella typhi murium: (Salmonella aertrycke)

The clinical picture caused by infection with this organism is strikingly different from that caused by infection with the two previously considered organisms. The onset is very sudden and the duration of the disease short. Although it resembles an acute toxemia in this and other respects, the organism can usually be isolated from fatal cases, indicating a true infection. Broth filtrates are nontoxic for laboratory animals and man. The organism's most distinguishing cultural character is its ability to produce acid from tartrate. This character distinguishes it from *S. schott-mülleri.*

Salmonella cholerae suis

Swine are the natural hosts of this organism. As the name implies, it is associated with hog cholera. It is associated with the disease in the sense that it is an important secondary invader. The primary cause is believed to be a filterable virus. This organism has occasionally been isolated from cases of acute gastroenteritis in man.

Salmonella cholerae suis, Variety from Kunzendorf

This organism is a more important human pathogen than *S. cholerae suis.* It differs from the latter by its ability to form hydrogen sulfide. It differs antigenically in lacking the specific flagellar phase.

Salmonella enteritidis (Gärtner's bacillus)

Clinically, this organism and its varieties cause symptoms of food poisoning which are indistinguishable from those caused by *S. typhi murium.* It was first isolated from the intestine of a fatal case of epidemic meat poisoning. It is widely distributed in lower animals. Numerous varieties have been described: Danysz, Variety from Chaco, Essen, Dublin, Moscow, Blegdam and from Bostock.

The second genus of the tribe *Salmonelleae* is *Eberthella.* Organisms in this genus ferment dextrose with the formation of acid but no gas. They are motile. The most important species is the typhoid bacillus itself, *Eberthella typhosa.* A discussion of the general and special bacteriology of this organism is given in subsequent sections.

The third and last genus of the tribe *Salmonelleae* is *Shigella.* This genus includes organisms which are nonmotile and which are the causes of bacillary dysenteries. Fifteen species are listed by Bergey. The most commonly encountered species are:

Shigella dysenteriae (Shiga)
Shigella ambigua (Schmitz bacillus)

These two organisms do not ferment mannite and for that reason are separated from

Shigella paradysenteriae (Flexner)
Shigella sonnei
Shigella alkalescens

These three organisms ferment mannite.

S. ambigua is serologically homogeneous. Differentiation can be made on this basis from *S. dysenteriae.* The Schmitz bacillus also produces indole when grown in tryptophan broth while the Shiga bacillus does not.

The mannite fermenting group can be quickly differentiated by their action on milk (Havens). *S. paradysenteriae* produces little change. *S. sonnei* produces a strong acidity with coagulation. *S. alkalescens* produces a strong and permanent alkalinity in milk. Other differential characters are given by Havens, to whom the interested reader is referred.

Alcaligenes faecalis is a nonpathogenic normal inhabitant of the intestinal tract. It is, therefore, encountered in all stool examinations, and must be differentiated from the other flora. This is readily done owing to its capacity to alkalinize litmus milk. It is not included in the family *Enterobacteriaceae.*

40101

In the classification used by the British bacteriologists all the organisms in the family *Enterobacteriaceae* are placed in the genus *Bacterium*. The genus is then divided into two main groups—a group including all the organisms that ferment lactose and a group including those that do not ferment lactose. The lactose fermenters are further divided into subgroups: the colon-aerogenes, Friedländer and paracolon groups. The colon-aerogenes and Friedländer groups correspond to the tribe *Eschericheae*. The paracolon group consists of lactose-fermenting organisms that, for one reason or another, cannot be included in the other groups. The non-lactose fermenters are similarly divided into subgroups: the dysentery group and the Salmonella group. Up to this point it may be argued that the British system is simpler and more readily understandable than the American system. From this point on, however, many species differentiations in the British system are based on fine serologic differences. Serologic classification is, indeed, "fraught with too many practical and theoretical difficulties."

The Kauffmann-White formula is a classification of the genus Salmonella that is based on fine differences in the antigenic structure of bacteria. The method is that of agglutination of H and O suspensions of each organism with antiserums which, by previous absorption with appropriate antigenic types, have been rendered specific for one or the other antigenic component, or a small group of such components. The theoretical concepts of this classification will be discussed below in the paragraph devoted to the antigenic structure of *E. typhosa*.

GENERAL BACTERIOLOGY OF EBERTHELLA TYPHOSA.—*Historical.*— Eberth in 1880 and 1881 examined 40 individuals who had died of typhoid fever. In 18, he found bacilli in the spleen and in the mesenteric lymph nodes. As a control, he examined 26 individuals who had died of diseases other than typhoid and found no bacilli. Thus the credit for the discovery of the typhoid bacillus has been given to Eberth and the organism has been named *Eberthella typhosa* in accordance with present-day rules of bacterial nomenclature.

Gaffky in 1884 applied the cultural methods of Robert Koch to the problem of typhoid fever and obtained pure cultures from about 25 cases. Gaffky considered that the organisms he isolated were the cause of typhoid fever. On the basis of his work, he was able to throw considerable light on the possible modes of infection and on the prophylaxis against the infection.

The discovery of the agglutinating action of serum from patients having typhoid fever was made in 1896 by Durham, Gruber, Widal and Grünbaum.

The active immunization of man against typhoid fever was first described by Sir Almroth Wright in 1896.

Morphology.—The typhoid bacillus has certain accepted morphologic, cultural and serologic characteristics. These characteristics for the most part are rigidly applicable to the freshly isolated organism. Our newer knowledge of the typhoid bacillus concerns the variations observed and studied in organisms that have been cultivated on artificial media under a wide variety of physical and chemical conditions. In the following discussion the accepted characteristics are given first and these are followed by the variations. The importance of the variations insofar as they apply to the clinical problem of typhoid fever will be given in detail.

Form.—The typhoid bacillus is a rod-shaped organism whose accepted size is 0.5 to 0.8 of a micron in thickness and 1 to 3 microns in length. Many variations in form and size occur in cultures but it is probable that these are impressed variations due to unfavorable conditions. In urine of carriers, however, typhoid bacilli have been found which are extremely long, attaining a length of 30 microns and a thickness of 1 micron.

Motility.—Typhoid bacilli are actively motile. This character provides an important differential point between typhoid bacilli and the organisms causing dysentery (Shigella) which are nonmotile. Using appropriate stains, peritrichous flagella may be demonstrated. Nonmotile strains have been isolated. Because the loss of flagella is associated with a loss of an essential antigenic substance, a great deal of work has been done by bacteriologists and immunologists on this particular type of variation.

Spores.—The typhoid bacillus is a non-sporulating organism and for this reason is not resistant to great variations in temperature. It is killed in 10 to 20 minutes at 60° C., and under experimental conditions it probably does not remain viable in ice for longer than two weeks.

Capsules.—Capsules have never been demonstrated in organisms which have been recently isolated. Under special conditions heavily encapsulated forms have been grown and photographed.

Cultivation and Growth Characteristics.—(a) *Physical and Chemical Requirements.*—The optimum *temperature* for the growth of *Eberthella typhosa* is 38° C. Only slight growth occurs at ordinary refrigerator temperatures. This fact is of some epidemiologic importance, for it has been shown that certain epidemics have resulted from the consumption of unrefrigerated food which had been contaminated by carriers. The epidemics occurred during the summer months and the food (Jello) was prepared 12 to 18 hours before eating. The combination of near-optimum temperature and a suitable medium greatly favored the growth of the contaminating organisms. It is conceivable that the epidemics would not have occurred if the food had been refrigerated.

Typhoid bacilli grow best in a neutral to a slightly alkaline solution. Growth, however, has been shown to take place anywhere between the pH range of 5 to 8.6.

Typhoid bacilli grow best in the presence of oxygen. While growth occurs under reduced oxygen tensions it is usually of a pleomorphic nature and restricted in amount.

Moisture is necessary for growth.

(b) *Growth on Routine Media.*—On *gelatin* typhoid bacilli grow readily, but the growth is not so profuse as on agar. Liquefaction does not occur. In gelatin stab cultures there is marked growth on the surface which becomes less and less as the bottom is approached. This illustrates the need for oxygen. Slight acidity is produced in *litmus milk*, due to the fermentation of the small amount of dextrose present. After 24 hours this medium becomes alkaline; clotting does not take place. In *potato* the typhoid bacillus usually develops as a transparent almost invisible streak. On *agar plates* recently isolated typhoid bacilli form characteristic colonies; they are round with very smooth edges,

40101

dome-shaped, and their surface is *smooth* and glistening. Older cultures produce colonies that are flatter and which have an irregular edge and a slightly wrinkled or *rough* surface. The first type of colony is considered to be the normal form; the latter is considered to be a variant. Associated with these differences in colony form are other important differences. The smooth form is more antigenic and more virulent. Intermediate forms have been described and will be discussed later in connection with the selection of cultures for vaccine preparation. In nutrient *broth* freshly isolated or smooth forms produce an even diffuse turbidity. Rough forms produce a more granular growth. The differences in the growth of the smooth and rough forms in broth are, however, not as a rule very marked. In *carbohydrate media* typhoid bacilli do not produce gas but they do produce acid from the following sugars: dextrose, levulose, galactose, xylose, maltose, dextrin, mannitol, dulcitol and sorbitol. They do not produce acid in media containing lactose, saccharose, inulin, salicin, arabinose, rhamnose and inosite. In *peptone broth* indol is not produced. In media containing lead acetate, hydrogen sulfide is formed which blackens the medium. Variations in biochemical activities have been reported. Certain strains, for example, have been "trained" to ferment lactose. It is unlikely that this variation occurs spontaneously under ordinary conditions.

Serologic Reactions.—(a) *Agglutinin Reaction.*—In 1896 Gruber and Durham showed that the blood serum of guinea pigs which had been inoculated with typhoid bacilli possessed the property of agglutinating suspensions of motile *E. typhosa.*

Widal and Grünbaum in the same year showed that blood serum from patients ill with typhoid fever agglutinated living broth cultures of typhoid bacilli.

The present state of our knowledge concerning the formation of agglutinins in patients with typhoid fever may be summarized as follows: "Agglutinins usually appear in the blood between the 3rd and 7th days, rise, first slowly, then more steeply to a maximum between the 16th and 22nd days, and then fall, at first steeply, later very slowly, so that they are detectable for weeks or months after convalescence. The rise in agglutinins is usually associated with a decreasing bacteremia. The maximum titer may coincide approximately with amelioration of the patient's symptoms."

The technic of the agglutination reaction, the agglutinin response to vaccination with typhoid vaccine, the relation of agglutinins to diagnosis and immunity, and the importance of this reaction in the identification of bacteria, will be described later.

(b) *Complement Fixation.*—Complement-fixing antibodies undoubtedly are produced in response to infection or vaccination with typhoid bacilli. The relative complexity of the test and the difficulties encountered in preparing suitable antigens have restricted its wide use in both research and diagnostic problems.

(c) *Precipitation.*—Precipitins may be demonstrated in typhoid immune serum by simply adding such a serum to a Berkefeld filtrate of a young 24-hour culture of *E. typhosa.* A fine cloud appears and, if allowed to stand overnight, a deposit forms in the bottom of the tube. Chemists, in attempts to isolate and purify the essential immunizing antigen in *E. typhosa,* have used the precipitin test advantageously in testing various fractions for antigenic activity.

(*d*) *Opsonins and Bactericidal Substances.*—Both of these antibodies have been demonstrated in typhoid immune serums. Their appearance and disappearance in the blood following infection or vaccination probably parallel the appearance of agglutinins, precipitins and complement-fixing antibodies.

(*e*) *Antigenic Structure of Eberthella Typhosa.*—The early work of Gruber and Durham showed that typhoid-immune serum agglutinated bacteria other than the typhoid bacillus but to a measurably lesser degree. This work implied that the typhoid bacillus was composed of not one but probably many antigens and that at least some of the antigens in each cell were *species specific* and others *group specific*. During recent years considerable work has been done to determine for each species of bacteria "the number and kind of different antigens present, their relative proportions and their position in the cell or cell appendages." It is now believed that naturally occurring smooth, motile cultures of *Eberthella typhosa* contain a heat-labile, specific flagellar or "H" antigen, two heat-stable somatic or "O" antigens and a heat-labile somatic antigen, the "Vi" antigen of Felix and Pitt. The methods used in eliciting this information have been diverse, indirect, and in many instances very complicated. In general, however, three approaches have been made: First, the method of *agglutinin absorption* introduced by Castellani in 1902; second, the study of bacterial variants; and third, the application of chemical methods.

(*f*) *Agglutinin Absorption.*—This method of antigenic analysis consists in the addition of bacterial suspensions of various species concerned in group agglutination, to the immune serum. In this manner each species added to the serum absorbs its own agglutinins and leaves the others in solution. In actual practice each species is added separately, the mixture is shaken to facilitate complete absorption and then centrifuged. After all the species concerned in the group agglutination have been added and removed in this manner, only the species-specific agglutinins remain. In the serologic diagnosis of typhoid fever this procedure is usually not necessary because the species-specific agglutinins are present in sufficiently large amounts to give a reaction when the serum is highly diluted. The method was used to prove the existence of the specific somatic and flagellar antigens of *E. typhosa* and to classify the closely related members of the Salmonella group.

(*g*) *Bacterial Variation.*—The historical approach to this subject is necessary if a clear understanding is to be realized. The first suggestion that bacterial variants might be antigenically different from normal forms was made by Smith and Reagh in 1903. They isolated a non-motile form of the hog cholera bacillus and compared its agglutination reactions with those of the normal, motile, flagellated type of this organism. They noted that a serum prepared with the normal form agglutinated both the motile and the nonmotile strains. The titer was higher for the homologous strain and there was a distinct difference in the appearance of the agglutinated floccules. The nonmotile organisms agglutinated slowly in small granular clumps and the motile forms agglutinated rapidly in large and fluffy clumps. A serum prepared by injecting animals with the nonmotile variant agglutinated both forms to the same degree and gave in each case the slow, granular type of agglutination. The serum prepared against the motile form, when

40101

absorbed with the nonmotile strain, lost its power of agglutinating the nonmotile bacilli but retained its power of agglutinating the motile strain. The serum prepared against the nonmotile form lost its agglutinating power for both strains when absorbed with the motile strain. Smith and Reagh concluded that the normal, motile hog cholera bacillus had two kinds of antigens: one contained in the flagella, the other in the cell body. The variant had lost its *flagellar antigens* but had retained its *somatic antigens*.

In 1917 Weil and Felix reported a similar type of variation in a strain of *Proteus vulgaris*. They had observed that this strain X 19, had a nonmotile variant which produced colonies on agar which were quite different in appearance from those formed by the normal, motile type of proteus bacillus. These colonies instead of being spreading and confluent with one another were compact and isolated. They named the variants producing the abnormal colonies *Ohne Hauch* forms, meaning the *non-spreading* variety. The normal, motile forms were called *Hauch* forms to signify their *spreading* nature. *Hauch* and *Ohne Hauch* subsequently came to be abbreviated ''H'' and ''O.'' It seems unfortunate that this terminology used by Weil and Felix to describe the colony morphology of Proteus X 19 should be used extensively today to designate the flagellar and somatic antigens of the typhoid bacillus!

Another type of variation related in some way to antigenicity and virulence was observed by Arkwright in 1920–1924. He noted that there were marked differences in antigenic structure between organisms that produced smooth-surfaced and those that produced rough-surfaced colonies on agar. The smooth type colonies reacted specifically with antiserum; the rough type colonies were agglutinated by antiserums prepared against many other bacteria. Other differences between the rough and smooth forms were noted. The smooth forms produced a diffuse turbidity in broth and showed no tendency to agglutinate spontaneously in 0.85 per cent salt solution. On the other hand, the rough forms produced a granular growth in broth and were auto-agglutinable in normal saline. Arkwright's work was of fundamental practical importance, for it pointed the way to subsequent studies by others showing that variants are unsuitable for use as vaccines and as agglutinogens in diagnostic agglutination tests. In the latter procedure the organisms tend to agglutinate spontaneously and give false positives if suitable controls are not employed.

Variations in the agglutinability of recently isolated strains of *E. typhosa* have been noted by laboratory workers ever since the Widal test was first described. As a matter of fact, early workers advocated rapid passage of inagglutinable strains through broth before being used as antigens. In 1934 Felix and Pitt undertook a study to determine why freshly isolated strains were often inagglutinable when tested with known high-titered serum. In the course of their work they observed that these inagglutinable strains were more virulent for mice than agglutinable strains. They attributed the increased virulence to the presence of a heretofore undescribed somatic antigen which they named the ''virulence'' or ''Vi'' antigen. In explaining why these strains were inagglutinable they stated that the ''Vi'' antigen ''masked'' or inhibited the dominant ''O'' antigen and that in order to get normal agglutinability, strains must be devoid of ''Vi'' antigen. Although a great deal of work, some of which will be mentioned subsequently, has been done on the chemical nature of this antigen, its exact biologic significance is still obscure.

(*h*) *Chemical Studies.*—The chemical nature of the antigens of the typhoid bacillus and closely related micro-organisms has been intensively investigated in recent years. Besides the theoretical and academic aim of this work, the practical aim has been to isolate a chemical or a chemical fraction from typhoid bacilli which is soluble, specific, stable, standardizable, free from properties producing harmful reactions, and equal or superior to present whole-cell vaccine in its ability to stimulate active immunity against typhoid fever. The progress that has been made toward achieving these aims is summarized as follows: Furth and Landsteiner in 1929, Boivin and Mesrobeanu in 1936, Topley and colleagues in 1937, Henderson and Morgan in 1938, and Wakeman in 1939, isolated materials from typhoid bacilli which they believed to be the essential somatic antigen. The procedures employed were all different, but the final products were strikingly similar. Regardless of whether the typhoid bacilli were extracted with diethylene glycol, or precipitated with trichloracetic acid or killed with acetone and then digested with trypsin, the antigenic substance was found to be predominantly carbohydrate in nature and to contain only small amounts of protein and lipoid substances. In spite of the fact that these workers implied that their products were "the complete antigen" or "the essential immunizing antigen" or "the specific soluble substance" of typhoid bacilli, proof is still lacking that they can be used in place of whole intact cells in typhoid prophylaxis. Chemical studies of the H and Vi antigens have shown that they are both quite sensitive to heat and chemicals. It is likely, therefore, that their immunizing quality is reduced by treatment with moderate heat (65° C.) or preservatives such as formaldehyde or phenol. Distinct chemical differences exist between the Vi and the O antigens.

For a detailed and critical review of the work herein summarized the reader is referred to Weil's recent publication in the *Archives of Pathology.*

Classification Based on Antigenic Structure.—The knowledge of the antigenic structure of the typhoid bacillus gained by the methods above outlined has served as the basis for the very precise and detailed classification of the Salmonella group (British) (*Salmonelleae,* Bergey) proposed by Kauffmann and White. Agglutination of H and O suspensions with antiserums, previously absorbed with appropriate antigenic types, resulted in the discovery of some thirteen different somatic antigens, twenty-eight specific flagellar antigens and six group flagellar antigens. Each of these antigens is labeled or named according to a scheme proposed by Kauffmann. The somatic antigens are accorded Roman numerals, these at present ranging from I to XIII. The specific flagellar antigens are given small letters, a to z, z_1, z_2, z_3, and so on. Group antigens are given Arabic numerals, which run from 1 to 6.

It seems unlikely that this classification will meet with general acceptance by clinical bacteriologists, at least not for routine use. The technical pitfalls are many in number!

Pathogenicity and Toxicity of Eberthella Typhosa.—So far as is known, man is the only animal in which the typhoid bacillus produces

40101

true typhoid fever. Massive doses of living typhoid bacilli administered orally to chimpanzees produce a disease which is similar, but not identical, to typhoid fever in man. The intraperitoneal or intravenous injection of living typhoid bacilli under a wide variety of special conditions may with regularity produce death in mice, rats, guinea pigs and rabbits. Presumably death is due to the toxemia produced by the disintegration of the injected bacilli, as no true exotoxin has ever been found and there is no good evidence that the organisms proliferate to any great degree. Recent work indicates that the "complete antigen" of Boivin and Mesrobeanu is the same substance produced by the disruption of the typhoid cell and referred to as the "endotoxin." According to Weil, both produce similar marked changes in experimental animals, such as extreme weight loss, delayed recoveries and similar symptoms when given in lethal doses. The subject is an interesting one, for on the basis of toxins always hinge the possibilities of antitoxins and toxoids.

The pathogenicity of typhoid bacilli for mice requires especial attention because mice have been used to compare the antigenicity and "virulence" of different strains and variants of *E. typhosa;* to evaluate the antigenicity of chemical fractions of *E. typhosa;* to evaluate the effectiveness of chemotherapeutic reagents and for studies on the duration of immunity following typhoid vaccination.

Grinnell (1932) was the first to utilize in a practical manner the fact that *E. typhosa,* when injected intraperitoneally in mice, produced death. He compared the virulence of twelve Rawlins strains by determining the number of organisms of each strain necessary to kill mice. In this manner he showed that some of the strains used in vaccine production were inferior to others; that the inferior strains were "rough" strains and the superior strains were "smooth." He also showed that virulence and smoothness were correlated with mouse protective properties. Mice immunized with vaccines made from smooth strains were better protected against lethal doses of organisms than mice immunized with rough strains. To Grinnell must be given the credit for initiating the many studies which have since followed on this important subject.

Rake (1935) was the first to show the marked effect that hog gastric mucin had upon increasing the "virulence" of smooth motile strains of *E. typhosa* for mice. Rake noted that the number of organisms required to produce the death of a mouse could be reduced from 100,000 to 1,000,000 times if the organisms were suspended in 5 per cent mucin instead of saline. He further showed that, by using mucin to decrease the number of organisms necessary to kill, it was possible to measure more accurately than by the Widal test antibody changes in human serums. For example, he demonstrated that two serums which showed no agglutinins for *E. typhosa* protected mice against 1,000 killing doses. This test is called the passive mouse protection test and will be referred to later under "General Prophylaxis."

Grasset and Lewin (1936) used the passive protection test in mice to evaluate different types of antityphoid serums. They did not use mucin.

Felix and Pitt (1934) used passive protection tests in mice to help prove the existence of the Vi antigen in O inagglutinable and virulent strains of *E. typhosa.*

Colonel Siler (1937, 1939) used the same test proposed by Rake to study the virulence of different strains of typhoid bacilli; to measure the immunogenic properties of vaccines made from different strains, and in studies designed to determine the duration of immunity induced by vaccines; to determine the effect of revaccination by the intradermal route. The results of these studies are taken up in their proper place under "Prophylaxis."

Henderson (1939) used the passive protection tests in mice to study the relationship of virulence to the protective value of the Vi and O antibodies.

Henderson and Morgan (1938) used the passive protection test for the measurement of the antigenicity of extracts of *E. typhosa*.

Only time will show the extent to which information obtained by killing mice in a highly artificial manner applies to problems of human typhoid fever.

Distribution Outside the Body.—The typhoid bacillus has no normal breeding place outside the human body. When the organism is discharged from an infected person, it finds its way to sewage, water supplies, soil, fomites, fingers, milk and food. In these it remains alive from one to many weeks. It eventually tends to die out as a result of drying, sunlight, warmth and bacteriophage. A temperature of 60° C. (140° F.) kills it in a short time. It remains viable when frozen. Gay states that the organism has been found to persist in the effluent from septic tanks. It may multiply enormously under favorable conditions in food as in the Hanford epidemic cited by Gay.

Modes of Conveyance.—Every case of typhoid fever is caused by infection with *Eberthella typhosa*, conveyed directly or indirectly from a previous case of the disease. Infection may be conveyed by any route which permits the bacilli excreted by a typhoid patient or carrier to reach the mouth and gastro-enteric tract of any individual.

(*a*) *Water.*—Water is the most important medium of conveyance and in the temperate zone, at least, typhoid fever is the most important water-borne disease. Where the disease is endemic, approximately 80 per cent of the cases result from infected water. In Michigan, where sanitary conditions are excellent, 5 per cent of the cases of typhoid are water-borne. The marked general reduction in the typhoid rate in the United States and its virtual elimination in some areas has been accomplished almost solely by the purification of public water supplies.

Water supplies are infected in a number of ways. The most important mode of pollution is by sewage which, because of typhoid carriers, constantly contains typhoid bacilli. Horwood states that municipal treatment of sewage is not adequate to destroy the bacillus. Nor is distance from the source of pollution to be relied upon. In 1892 an extensive outbreak in Detroit was traced to the discharge into the St. Clair River, fifty miles above the Detroit intake, of a great volume of mud and sewage dredged from a small river. In its journey the sewage traversed a shallow lake fifteen miles across. In lakes, disturbances from winds and barometric pressure variations create strong currents which can carry sewage many miles in a few hours. Excreta may be discharged directly into the water or washed into streams, lakes or reservoirs from the surface of water sheds. Wells and springs may be contaminated by surface washings, by percolation through porous soil or through underground passages. Infection is usually through surface waters, but ground water is not at all times safe. Outbreaks have re-

40101

sulted from accidental connection of sewers to mains, because of faulty plumbing or broken drains and by siphonage. Recently the hotels of a large city were inspected for plumbing hazards, wherein polluted water might become mixed with a potable supply. Eighty-two such hazards were discovered. One epidemic in the army is believed to have resulted from the use of an open tank for drinking water into which each soldier dipped his cup.

Water-borne epidemics are explosive in character, restricted to areas supplied by the polluted water, and may occur at periods out of the regular typhoid season. The rise in the incidence of typhoid in March and May is attributed to contamination of the water supplies by surface washings.

The enormous dilution of sewage in water supplies is evidence of the small number of organisms capable of causing infection in humans.

(b) *Contact Infection.*—The risk of contracting typhoid by contact is great. Stebbins states that the incidence of typhoid fever in the households of carriers is forty-two times that of the general population and in the households of cases one thousand one hundred and ninety times that of the population at large. The percentage frequency of contact cases rises when the water-borne frequency decreases. In Detroit in the three years 1917 to 1919, when the death rate was 8.1 per hundred thousand, 13.9 per cent of the cases were traced to contact infection. Nurses, doctors and hospital employees are especially exposed to the disease. The typhoid rate among nurses in Michigan is five times that of the state as a whole. Only one of fifteen cases studied had been properly immunized. The organism is spread by unclean hands, utensils, linen, flies and direct contact.

In Michigan in 1936, 19.1 per cent of the cases resulted from contact with persons suffering from the disease.

(c) *Conveyance by Food Usually Results from Contamination by a Carrier.*—*Milk* is the most important food that may act as a vehicle for the spread of typhoid fever. This food is safe when pasteurization and carrier control are strictly enforced. It is dangerous when they are not. Wherever sanitary regulations are observed in the production and distribution of milk, milk-borne typhoid is reduced to a minimum. In Detroit, no case of conveyance by milk has been traced since the adoption, in 1915, of an ordinance requiring the pasteurization of general milk supplies. Recent surveys cited by Senftner and Coughlin and Havens indicate that the incidence of carriers in dairy farm workers is the same as in the population at large. Even now the importance of pasteurization of milk is not appreciated by distributors in the smaller towns. Milk-borne epidemics are still common in them. Eight and six-tenths per cent of the typhoid cases of the years 1932–1936 in Michigan (one hundred and eighty in number) were milk-borne.

Milk may be infected by contaminated water used in washing the containers. Foods made from milk such as ice cream, buttermilk, butter and cheese may harbor the bacillus. Outbreaks have resulted from cream puffs, custards and jellies.

Milk outbreaks develop abruptly like water-borne epidemics and subside quickly. Often two or more members of a household are taken sick at the same time. Children and women are chiefly affected. It appears that under certain conditions the typhoid bacillus multiplies in milk and becomes less virulent. Therefore, cases due to milk infection may have a short period of incubation and may be mild in type.

Oysters and other shellfish grown in sewage-polluted water have been the medium of transmission of typhoid fever in a number of outbreaks. In 1894 an outbreak of this type involving 25 cases occurred among the students of Wesleyan University at Middletown. Isolated cases of oyster-borne infection undoubtedly occur which are not traced to their common source of infection.

Vegetables which are eaten raw may carry the disease. They may be grown in infected soil, washed in infected water or handled by carriers. Any infected food consumed in an uncooked state may transmit the disease.

(d) *Contamination of the Soil.*—Contamination of the soil by typhoid excreta is frequent in rural districts, in newly built unsewered towns, in camps and in territories occupied by armies in the field. In some countries, intensive soil infection results from the use of human excrement as a fertilizer. Under ordinary conditions of heat and moisture, typhoid bacilli live in the soil from one to two months. On frozen ground, they may remain virulent for several months, as shown in the Plymouth and New Haven epidemics.

The bacilli may be conveyed from soil to mouth by way of infected surface water—by soiled boots, clothing or by flies. This was a frequent mode of indirect contact infection in the camp epidemics during the Spanish-American War.

(e) *Flies.*—Sedgewick in 1892, and Kober in the same year, suggested that flies were an important factor in the transmission of typhoid fever. In the report of the Typhoid Fever Commission of the Spanish-American War, Reed, Vaughan and Shakespeare emphasize the role of flies as the medium of indirect contact infection.

Conveyance by flies occurs whenever human excrement is exposed. Flies carry the organisms on their bodies, wings and feet and in their alimentary tracts. They have been found to retain the bacilli as long as twenty-three days after infection. As a rule, flies infect only at short range. It is possible, however, for them to transport the bacilli for long distances. On the Great Lakes the late Dr. C. G. Jennings has many times sailed through swarms of flies from ten to fifteen miles off shore.

(f) *Fomites.*—Articles of clothing and bedding soiled by typhoid excreta may transmit typhoid fever. Washerwomen may be infected from unsterilized linen. Hospital inmates may be infected from soiled towels and clothing, and soldiers from infected blankets. Such articles have been shown to harbor living bacilli for two or three months.

SYMPTOMATOLOGY

CLINICAL HISTORY

The commonly accepted division of the clinical history of typhoid fever into weekly periods, while arbitrary, is convenient and practical. In the average uncomplicated case of moderate severity the first week is the period of onset or invasion, during which there is a gradual increase in the severity of the symptoms. The second and third weeks correspond to the fastigium, the period of the height of the disease.

The fourth week is the period of decline. The fifth week marks the period of beginning convalescence. The course of the specific pathologic changes in Peyer's patches roughly follows this division into weekly periods.

Typhoid fever is a disease of remarkable variability in symptoms and course. Epidemics and outbreaks show many differences in type, and the character of the disease endemic in a certain community is apt to change from year to year. Individual cases in the same outbreak are often so erratic in onset and progress that identification from the symptom-complex alone is very difficult, often impossible. No symptom or sign is necessarily present and no symptom or combination of symptoms is impossible.

Sudden severe outbreaks may occur which show such bizarre symptomatology that health authorities and physicians are in doubt as to the identity of the epidemic until accurate laboratory methods of diagnosis reveal the true nature of the malady. In a disease of such protean manifestations it is impossible in a single continuous description to include the multitude of symptoms it may present. It will be well to give a short sketch of the clinical phenomena of the disease as it is commonly observed in communities where typhoid fever is endemic, describing in fuller detail under separate headings the various individual symptoms and their variations from type.

Period of Incubation.—This is the interval between the time of infection and the onset of the symptoms of the disease. The exact time of these two events is so difficult to determine that the duration of this period is more or less a matter of speculation.

Ingestion of the typhoid bacillus and infection of the body by the organism are not synchronous. A longer or shorter interval may elapse between the entrance of the pathogenic organisms into the intestinal tract and the actual invasion by them of the body tissues through some portal of entry. That this interval may be indefinitely prolonged is shown in the case of healthy carriers, who may harbor the bacillus for long periods. It is not improbable that cases showing an unusually long period of incubation are instances of delayed invasion of the intestinal wall.

The average time for symptoms to appear is from ten to fourteen days after exposure to infection. The period may be as short as two days or prolonged to twenty-three days. In 750 cases studied by the Spanish-American War Commission the average incubation period was ten and one-half days, the shortest six days. In an outbreak in Hanford, Cal., reported by Sawyer and cited by Gay, 93 people were infected by eating spaghetti prepared by a typhoid carrier. One half the cases showed symptoms before the eighth day, 1 on the third, 12 on the fifth, and 19 on the sixth day. In 56 cases in an outbreak among the employees of a local manufacturing plant, distinctive typhoid symptoms appeared in from ten to twenty days after the ingestion of highly polluted water. Murchison has reported a small outbreak in which the period of incubation in 20 out of 22 cases was not longer than four days.

In a number of instances of laboratory infection reported in recent literature the period of incubation has been determined with greater accuracy than is possible in ordinary clinical observation. An assistant working in Gay's laboratory received from a blocked syringe a mass of a thick suspension of recently isolated typhoid bacilli on the left cheek and conjunctiva. On the third day she felt a distinct malaise and on the fifth day she was ill with a temperature of 104° F. (40° C.). A blood culture taken at this time was positive.

Kissalt's study of 50 cases of laboratory infection gives the usual incubation of about fourteen days, although cases developing in five, six and eight days are mentioned. Voisin reported two interesting cases of laboratory infection. A girl aged nineteen years swallowed a virulent culture of typhoid bacilli with suicidal intent. On the third day headache and fever developed; on the seventh day abdominal pain, and on the eighth day rose spots. The fever ran a typical course. In the second case a young physician accidentally aspirated a small amount of a bouillon culture of typhoid bacilli into his mouth while making a Widal test. Although he promptly rinsed his mouth with bichloride solution, typhoid fever developed. The first symptoms appeared on the fifth day and splenic enlargement and rose spots on the thirteenth day.

Usually no symptoms mark the period of incubation, although careful inquiry often brings out a history of headache, lassitude and loss of appetite for a few days before the onset of the fever. These symptoms tend to increase in severity and are merged into the more well-defined illness of the onset of the disease. Often no sharp increase of symptoms marks the beginning of the period of invasion. There is an insidious aggravation of all the feelings of discomfort, and the patient finally stops work and takes to his bed. Without temperature observations and a clear history of the beginning of fever this event must be taken as indicating the first day of the stage of invasion.

Course of the Disease.—FIRST WEEK.—Chilliness followed by the flush and general aching of fever will often identify the first day of onset. A well-defined chill occurs in a small percentage of the cases. In Osler's series of 79 cases treated in one year at Johns Hopkins Hospital, 13 were ushered in by a chill. In addition, there are excessive fatigue, dizziness, anorexia and abdominal pain or discomfort. Occasionally there is vomiting. The bowels are constipated, or there may be a diarrhea, usually excited by a cathartic. Headache, severe and unyielding, is a most important and characteristic symptom. Epistaxis is common on the second or third day.

The temperature taken on the first or second day shows an evening rise to 100 or 101° F. (37.8 or 38.3° C.). The pulse is 90 to 100, full and soft, becoming dicrotic in the last days of the week. The pulse rate is slow in comparison with the height of the temperature and the severity of the general symptoms. The tongue is moist and coated, the breath heavy. A mild bronchitis with unproductive cough, and sometimes dyspnea, is a common initial manifestation.

The symptoms continue and increase in severity. The temperature rises a degree or more each day, with morning remissions and evening exacerbations, until, toward the end of the first week, it reaches from 103 to 104° F. (39.4 to 40° C.) in the evening. The daily range of the remissions is from one to two degrees. The headache continues and is complained of bitterly by the patient. Sleeplessness is frequent and a dreamy confusion makes the nights restless. The skin is hot and dry, with occasional short periods of perspiration. Thirst and anorexia increase. The abdomen is slightly distended and there is usually tender-

40101

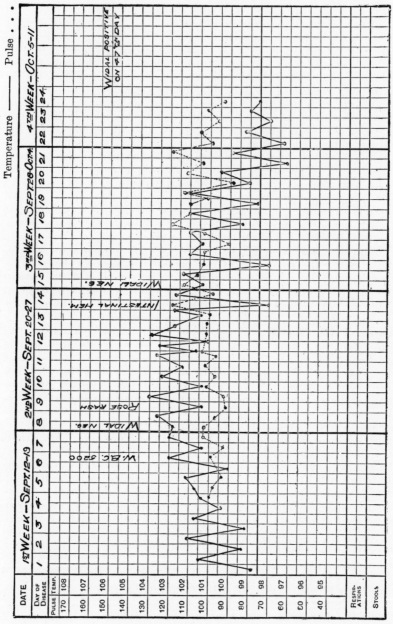

FIG. 1.—CHART IN MILD TYPHOID FEVER.
Hemorrhage on 14th day. Patient aged 36.

ness in the right lower quadrant with gurgling on pressure. Constipation persists, or there may be one or two loose stools a day. This group of symptoms, all of which are more or less common to the febrile state from any cause, continues for about seven days, the first week of the disease.

SECOND WEEK.—In the beginning of the second week, from the seventh to the twelfth day, the characteristic rose rash appears upon the skin of the abdomen or chest, and enlargement of the spleen can often be demonstrated. The symptoms of the first week continue and some of them increase in severity. The fever reaches from 103 to 105° F. (39.4 to 40.6° C.) each evening, with slight or no morning remission. The pulse becomes more rapid and is soft and dicrotic. The subjective symptoms tend to increase up to the middle of the second week. The headache then diminishes or ceases and the patient becomes dull and apathetic. In the severe cases there is delirium, especially at night. This is usually of a mild muttering type; occasionally it is more noisy. The lips are dry and crack easily. The tongue is coated and may be dry. The abdomen is distended and the gurgling and tenderness in the right lower quadrant become more pronounced. The rose rash continues, appearing in crops of a few macules each day or two. Diarrhea, if present early, is aggravated, with several pale yellow, offensive movements of characteristic pea soup consistency during the day; or it may first show itself at this time. Constipation requiring measures for its relief is equally or more frequent. The urine is scanty and often shows a febrile albuminuria with a few casts.

The second week may end the period of continuous high temperature and defervescence may begin (Fig. 1). This mild course is rarely seen except in the typhoid fever of children. Death may occur late in the second week from intense toxemia or from hemorrhage or perforation.

THIRD WEEK.—Usually the foregoing symptoms continue into the third week, the patient failing under the continued high temperature and toxemia. Toward the end of this week the temperature may begin to show more decided morning remissions. The pulse becomes weaker and faster, 100 to 130, loss of flesh is rapid and prostration is great. The face is pale with occasional flushings, the pupils are dilated and the expression is dull and heavy. The mouth and tongue are dry, and the tongue is often red and glazed. Without constant care the lips and teeth become covered with sordes. Diarrhea continues and involuntary evacuations may occur. Profuse perspirations are common; excoriations and bed sores may appear. Delirium persists, with subsultus tendinum and picking at the bedclothes in highly toxic cases. This is the condition designated as the "typhoid state." Inefficient nursing and bad feeding are often responsible for the severity of some of these symptoms. Intestinal hemorrhage, perforation, bronchopneumonia and other grave complications are most frequent at this time. Progressive asthenia or one of these complications may cause death.

FOURTH WEEK.—This is the period of decline. Defervescence is by lysis, the disease ending gradually as it began. In rare cases a crisis terminates the period of high temperature, and convalescence begins abruptly. (Fig. 2.)

The temperature curve shows characteristic oscillations or "spikings." Increasing morning remissions with sharp evening rises give a

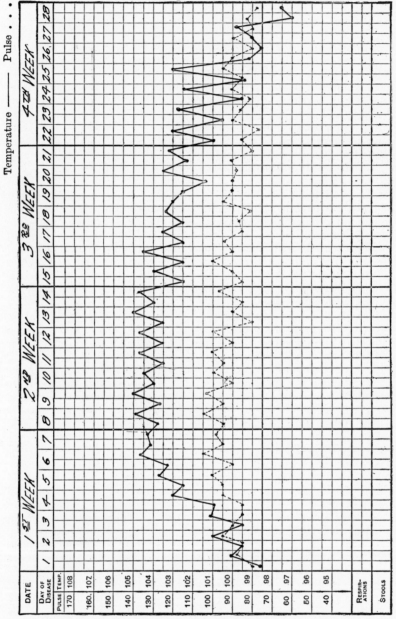

Fig. 2.—Chart in Uncomplicated, Moderately Severe Typhoid Fever. Typical Temperature Curve.

daily range from 101 to 104° F. (38.3 to 40° C.), the maximum diminishing each day by a degree or more. The pulse becomes slower, or it may increase in rapidity from myocardial weakness.

The tongue moistens and cleans off, the appetite begins to return, and the thirst lessens. The diarrhea abates, the abdomen becomes flat, and the spleen shrinks. The general symptoms improve, delirium ceases, and natural sleep replaces the wakeful and restless nights.

FIFTH WEEK.—With the fall of the temperature to normal convalescence begins. The pulse becomes slower and stronger. The appetite is keen, often ravenous. Nutrition improves and weight and strength increase. Diarrhea abates and a troublesome constipation obtains. The urine increases in amount and the albumin and casts disappear, if previously present. The temperature remains low, with fluctuations below and above the normal line. In children and nervous adults the afternoon temperature often holds at from 99 to 100° F. (37.2 to 37.8° C.) for several days. Recrudescences are common, with a rise of 101 to 102° F. (38.3 to 38.9° C.). They are excited by slight disturbances of digestion, physical exertion or nervous excitement, and last two or three days. The skin may desquamate and the hair fall out. The spleen is no longer palpable. Should it remain large the possibility of a relapse must be borne in mind. Murchison considered convalescence established when the temperature remained normal for two successive evenings.

Variations in Symptoms and Course.—Divergence from the ordinary type of typhoid fever outlined above is common. There may be variation in the mode of onset, or in either the severity or the duration of the attack. Again, the brunt of the attack may be borne by a particular system or organ. Such localization of the infection gives a special character to the symptoms and course. An intercurrent complication may hold the field during part, or throughout the whole course of the disease. The use of complex terms like pneumotyphoid, meningotyphoid, etc., to designate some of these unusual types is becoming obsolete. Although occasionally used, these terms are unnecessary and may be confusing.

Variations in Mode of Onset.—ABRUPT ONSET.—Instead of the gradual accession of the symptoms of the period of invasion the onset of typhoid fever may be abrupt. With but insignificant premonitory symptoms the fever may rise sharply to 102 or 103° F. (38.9 or 39.4° C.) on the first day, with or without a chill, and the general symptoms reach a severity that in the usual cases is not attained until the end of the first week. Sharp remissions or intermissions in the fever, during the first week, are not uncommon.

ONSET WITH PHARYNGEAL SYMPTOMS.—Severe sore throat with red pharynx, swollen tonsils and nasopharyngeal catarrh may usher in an attack. Severe facial neuralgia from invasion of the accessory sinuses of the nose may still further confuse the clinical picture and lead the practitioner astray.

ONSET WITH ABDOMINAL SYMPTOMS.—Sudden pyrexia with nausea and vomiting, abdominal pain and rigidity may mask the onset of the disease and simulate acute gastritis or peritonitis. The impetuous surgeon may be led to open the abdomen, expecting to find a diseased appendix or other variety of acute abdomen.

ONSET WITH RESPIRATORY SYMPTOMS.—Respiratory symptoms may dominate the onset. The initial bronchitis may be of unusual severity.

The high fever and sweats, rapid pulse and respiration, with the physical signs of a general bronchitis, may closely resemble acute pulmonary tuberculosis. The first symptoms may be those of pneumonia, with chill, pleuritic pain and the physical signs of lobar consolidation. The typhoid bacillus has been recovered from the lung in some of these cases; others are examples of coincident infection by the pneumococcus and the typhoid bacillus.

ONSET WITH RENAL SYMPTOMS.—In rare cases, an acute nephritis with a scant, smoky urine containing albumin, blood and casts may replace the usual symptoms of onset. The increasing and persistent fever, with abatement in the severity of the renal symptoms, should lead to the suspicion of typhoid fever.

ONSET WITH NERVOUS SYMPTOMS.—Severe, suddenly developing nervous symptoms may usher in an attack. The symptoms may be those of meningitis: headache, vomiting, delirium, photophobia, retraction of the head and positive Kernig sign. Or drowsiness, stupor or coma may develop after a day or two of the usual symptoms, and fix attention upon the nervous system.

Very rarely, in patients with a psychopathic tendency, delirium may develop with the onset of the fever, taking the form of a confusional or maniacal psychosis. In a dazed state such a patient may wander from home and end up in a hospital in some distant city, quite unable to reveal his identity; or he may be found hidden in some building where he has gone to escape fancied persecution.

Special and Characteristic Symptoms.—THE TEMPERATURE.—The ordinary form of typhoid fever shows a temperature curve which, while subject to various irregularities, is fairly characteristic and is an important diagnostic feature, which was first demonstrated and emphasized by Wunderlich and his associates. The typical chart (Fig. 2) shows a gradual rise with ascending oscillations during the first week. Normal in the morning, the temperature rises to 100 or 101° F. (37.8 or 38.3° C.) on the evening of the first day. On the following morning there is a remission of a degree or more, succeeded by an evening rise of about one degree higher than the maximum of the first day. This steplike ascent continues until about the end of the first week, when the temperature attains a height of from 103 to 105° F. (39.4 to 40.6° C.), depending upon the severity of the case.

The classical textbook ascent is perhaps exceptional, and various irregularities are the rule. Because of the insidious onset, the physician rarely sees a patient on the first day of the fever, and a temperature observation is not often made until the disease is well advanced. Patients under the late Dr. C. G. Jennings' observation who had been taken ill while in bed in the hospital, have shown the typical gradual rise of temperature. The period of ascent may be shortened to three or four days, or in severe cases the onset of the disease may be by chill followed by a persistent high fever. It is very unusual for the ascending period to be prolonged beyond the eighth day. Remissions of great amplitude or actual intermissions in the fever are occasionally observed and may be a feature of the case throughout its whole course.

During the course of the second and third weeks of typhoid fever the temperature, as a rule, tends to hold a continuous high range with small oscillations. Without apparent reason it is quite common for the

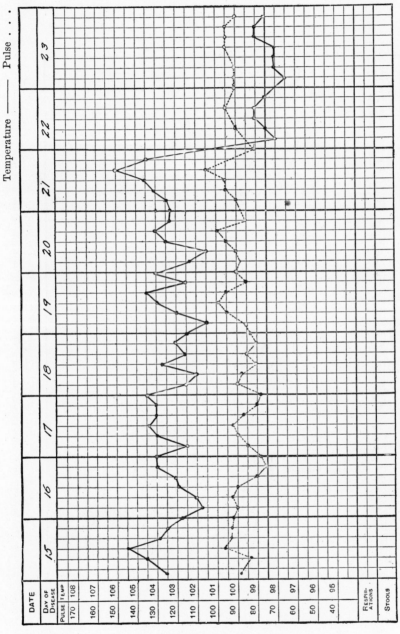

FIG. 3.—CHART IN MODERATELY SEVERE TYPHOID FEVER.
Crisis on 21st day. Four-hourly temperature. Patient aged 52.

40101

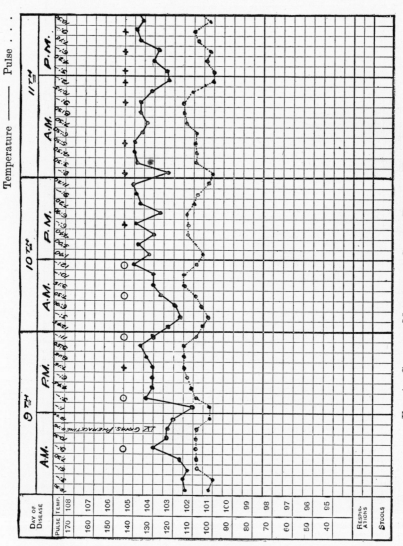

FIG. 4.—CHART IN MODERATELY SEVERE TYPHOID FEVER.

From 9th to 15th day (inclusive), showing effect of bath on temperature and pulse. O, bed bath; +, tub bath.

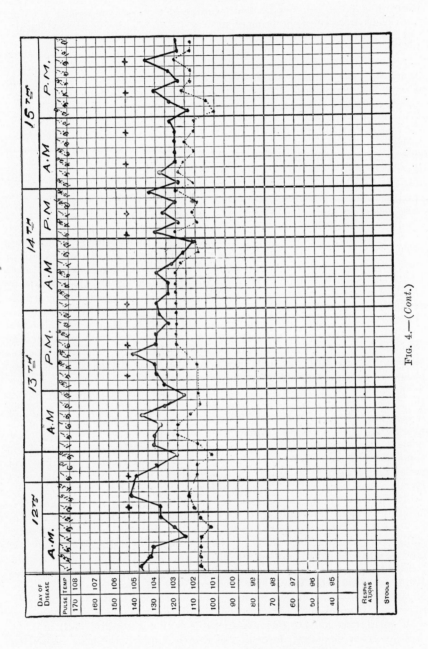

FIG. 4.—(*Cont.*)

40101

temperature to rise sharply above or fall below the average line. The study of a large number of temperature charts will emphasize the fact that every variety of curve may be met. During the height of the disease in cases of moderate severity a daily maximum of from 104 to 105° F. (40 to 40.6° C.) is the rule. The two-hour temperature chart will show two or more distinct elevations during the twenty-four hours. A midday maximum is often observed. Occasionally a reversal of type is seen, the remissions coming in the evening instead of in the morning. This is more apt to occur in children, in the aged and in persons occupied with night work.

The end of the third week or the beginning of the fourth brings an increase in the amplitude of the daily remissions. Each day the remission is greater and the maximum and minimum points lower. As the fever comes to an end the remissions decrease in range from day to day until the normal is reached. This *period of descending oscillations* is a fairly constant phenomenon of both mild and severe cases. In very rare cases convalescence begins at the end of the third week, with a sudden critical fall of the temperature to normal (Fig. 3).

The therapeutic cold bath disturbs the normal curve, and causes transient falls (Fig. 4). This is particularly the case toward the end of the fastigium. Sudden, unexpected temperature changes should always excite suspicion of the onset of some complication. Hemorrhage usually causes a drop of several degrees (Figs. 1, 5). After perforation it may either rise or fall. The complicating pus infections so frequent in typhoid disturb the fever curve, giving rise to many irregularities. Thrombophlebitis is a not uncommon cause of disturbances in the normal curve of the third and fourth weeks. The rise often begins several days before the local signs of the phlebitis show themselves. Osler has noted wide oscillations of temperature following a severe hemorrhage. Hyperpyrexia is not common. In only 4 or 5 per cent of the cases is the temperature above 106° F. (41.1° C.) and very rarely does it rise above 107° F. (41.7° C.). Hypothermia may be observed in protracted cases with great emaciation, the temperature persisting below normal for a week or more. Fever with irregular oscillations from complications and causes not always demonstrable may continue for weeks and indefinitely delay convalescence. The temperature curves of recrudescence and relapse are considered elsewhere.

CHILLS.—A chill, sometimes repeated, not infrequently marks the onset of typhoid fever and at this period has no special significance. In rare cases a relapse is ushered in by the same phenomenon. Occasionally chills occur during the course of the disease, and at this time they are always startling and may be of grave import. Osler has made a detailed study of the cases with chills under his observation at Johns Hopkins Hospital. They may occur under a variety of conditions. Most common is the chill resulting from the use of drugs, notably antipyretics. During the early experience of the late Dr. C. G. Jennings with antipyrine he saw two instances of rather alarming chill and depression from moderate doses of the drug. Chills have been caused by hypodermic or intravenous injection of typhoid vaccine, a legitimate result of the direct entrance of a foreign protein into the circulation. Two of Osler's cases resulted from the application of guaiacol to the skin.

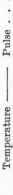
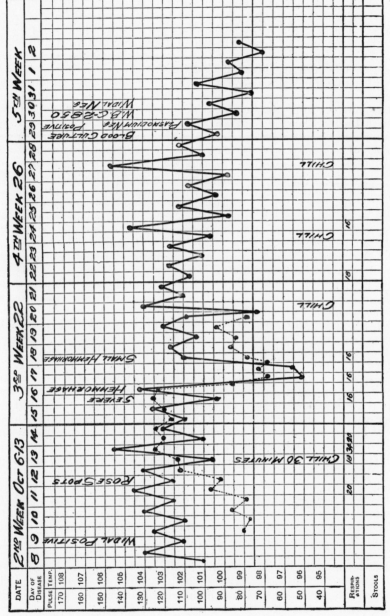

FIG. 5.—CHART IN CASE OF MODERATELY SEVERE TYPHOID FEVER.

Repeated chills during course; hemorrhage on 16th day, followed by subnormal temperature and slow pulse. Patient aged 37.

40101

A chill may serve to announce a complication. Pneumonia, perforation, appendicitis, thrombophlebitis or other complicating infections may begin in this way, although temperature variations without chills are more frequent. Occasionally a chill may precede a rapidly fatal hyperpyrexia. In a few cases a concurrent malarial infection has been proved to be the cause by the demonstration of the plasmodium. Chills may occur throughout the course of the fever and the most searching investigation may fail to reveal a local infection, a complication or any cause other than the typhoid septicemia itself. Conner asserts that chills in many of these obscure cases are due to a latent thrombophlebitis. The late author (Dr. C. G. Jennings) saw a case of this kind in consultation with Doctor Bruce of Saginaw. The patient, aged 37, was taken ill with typhoid on September 26 (Fig. 5). The disease ran the usual course of a case of moderate severity; the maximum temperature was 104° F. (40° C.). The Widal reaction was negative on the sixth day, positive on the twelfth day. On the seventeenth day the patient had a severe chill lasting half an hour, followed by a temperature of 105.5° F. (40.8° C.). The pulse was 120. After a profuse sweat the temperature returned to its former height—103° F. (39.4° C.). The phenomenon recurred on the twentieth day and again on the twenty-first day, and then throughout the subsequent course of the disease at varying intervals. After the chill of the twenty-first day there was a hemorrhage of moderate amount, followed by a period of subnormal temperature and slow pulse lasting nearly twenty-four hours. Repeated complete physical examinations and laboratory investigations failed to reveal any complication, except the hemorrhage. The Widal reaction at this time was negative. The white blood count was 2,850. The plasmodium was absent. Blood culture was positive. Although the repetition of the chills was very alarming, the other symptoms were not unusual and the patient went on to recovery.

PULSE.—The pulse characteristics in typhoid fever are the slow rate in relation to the temperature and the early appearance of dicrotism.

At the first examination of a typhoid patient the physician's attention is usually arrested by the full, soft pulse, which may be elevated slightly or not at all above the normal rate. With a temperature of 103° F. (39.4° C.) and higher, a pulse rate of 90 to 100 is not unusual. The disproportion between temperature and pulse is most marked after the first few days and continues into the second or third week. Then the rule is for it to become more rapid and variable, and to follow more closely the irregularities of the temperature curve. In many cases of moderate severity the low rate holds throughout the entire course of the disease. In 500 cases studied by McCrae, there were 176 cases in which the pulse rate did not rise above 100.

The pulse may be rapid at the onset or become so at any period during the course of the disease. In a general way the rapidity is an index of the gravity of the case. Above 120 it is always looked upon with apprehension. It may be 140 or higher in the seriously ill. In adult patients with a pulse of 150 or more the mortality is very high. An intercurrent complication is often announced by an unexpected rise. Hemorrhage of any amount quite uniformly causes a sudden jump to 120 or higher. A rapid running pulse accompanies perforation. As noted elsewhere typhoid fever of infancy and early childhood usually shows a rapid pulse, which is not necessarily of grave import. In the period of decline and during convalescence the pulse is extremely susceptible to nervous and other disturbing influences and may show wide diurnal oscillations.

At the end of the febrile period, when the temperature is subnormal, a very slow pulse, as low as 50 or 60, is not uncommon and a true bradycardia may be seen with a rate of 40 or lower. No serious import is attached to this slow pulse. Irregularity and intermittence sometimes attend the slow rate.

The dicrotic pulse is more frequent in typhoid fever than in any of the acute infections. It appears early in the first week and may continue throughout the disease. It often disappears in the second or third week, gradually becoming less pronounced as the pulse becomes more rapid.

Therapeutic measures, particularly the cold bath, change the quality and rapidity of the pulse. A reduction of ten beats or more is usual after the bath, the pulse losing its full compressible character and becoming smaller and firmer.

BLOOD PRESSURE.—The blood pressure in typhoid is almost invariably below the normal range for the individual infected. In 115 cases studied by Crile the highest systolic pressure was 138 mm., the lowest 74 mm. and the mean 104 mm. The hypotension increases as the disease advances. Crile's cases showed a mean pressure in the first week of 115 mm.; second week, 106 mm.; third week, 102 mm.; fourth week, 96 mm. To be of practical value readings must be taken at frequent intervals and continued during the course of the disease. For this reason blood pressure studies have not been popular.

BLOOD.—*The Red Cells.*—During the first week the number of red blood cells remains about normal. In the second week a reduction in the count is evident and this gradually increases and becomes greatest about the end of the febrile period. Thayer found the fall frequently accentuated in the fourth week. Regeneration of the blood begins with convalescence, or even before, should a mild fever prolong the period of decline into the fifth or sixth week. The average maximum loss is 20 per cent of the red cells. Sudden loss of body fluids from diarrhea, vomiting and profuse sweats may cause a transient, apparent increase. A sudden fall is the usual result of any considerable hemorrhage. The reduction of the hemoglobin percentage is about the same as the percentage loss of red cells.

Leukocytes.—Uncomplicated typhoid fever shows a characteristic reduction in the number of leukocytes in the peripheral circulation. In the first few days of the fever the number is normal, or there may be a slight increase. The number then progressively diminishes during the period of pyrexia, the extent of the fall depending upon the severity of the toxemia. A fall to 2,000 or even lower is not uncommon, and may indicate a feeble defense and be of grave significance. The average number at the height of the disease is from 4,000 to 5,000. In exceptional instances, from 8,000 to 10,000 may be found in uncomplicated cases. The differential count shows: (1) a progressive reduction in the percentage of polymorphonuclear cells; (2) a progressive increase in the percentage of the mononuclear cells, especially of the large forms; and (3) a constant reduction in the percentage of the eosinophils. With the establishment of convalescence the number of white cells returns to the normal, although the characteristic differential count may continue for some time. A moderate leukocytosis is not unusual during the convalescent period, often caused by some mild or hidden secondary infection.

Cold baths cause a sudden but transient increase in the number of leukocytes. The number may be increased to three or four times what it was before the bath. The relative percentage in the differential count remains unchanged. This transient increase is not a true leukocytosis. It is dependent upon the changed surface circulation. For this reason a white cell count for diagnostic purposes should not be taken for three or four hours after a cold bath.

Inflammatory complications and secondary infections by pyogenic organisms quite uniformly cause leukocytosis. The leukocytic count, therefore, is a most valuable aid in the differentiation of typhoid fever from septic conditions and in the recognition of the onset of septic and inflammatory complications. In very severe and malignant infections no increase in the number of leukocytes may take place. A high white cell count often immediately follows hemorrhage from the bowels, reaching a maximum inside of twenty-four hours and returning to the former number within a week.

Perforation of the bowel also is marked by a leukocytosis which may precede the perforation by several hours. Usually it begins a few hours after the accident and rises rapidly to 10,000, 15,000 or higher. With the onset of general peritonitis there is often a rapid fall. The rapid changes in the number of leukocytes following perforation render an hourly leukocyte count essential to the proper determination of the significance of this symptom. In perforation complicating profoundly toxic cases there is either no change or, frequently, an actual reduction in the number of cells.

THE TYPHOID RASH.—The characteristic cutaneous symptom of typhoid fever is the rose rash, a maculopapular eruption appearing chiefly upon the abdomen, chest and back. The rash can be demonstrated in from 80 to 90 per cent of cases. McCrae's white patients showed it in 93.2 per cent. It is distinctive of typhoid fever and is eagerly looked for by the physician as the earliest conclusive clinical diagnostic feature.

The rash consists of a number of discrete, circular, rose-colored spots from $\frac{1}{12}$ to $\frac{1}{8}$ inch in diameter. They are slightly elevated above the skin surface, perceptible to gentle palpation, and disappear with pressure. A minute vesicle sometimes forms at the apex of the lesion, and in severe cases some of the spots may become hemorrhagic. The eruption usually first appears at the end of the first week or the beginning of the second week—from the sixth to the tenth day. It may appear as early as the second or third day or as late as the fifteenth. In exceptional cases it is delayed until late in the attack, even after the end of the febrile period. The spots come in successive crops, a few at a time, and the individual lesion lasts from two to five days. The spots fade away, leaving a faint discoloration covered with a fine desquamation.

The duration of the rash as a whole is from one to two weeks; or it may persist during the whole febrile period. The average number of lesions present at one time is not large—from five to twenty. Only three or four may be found, or they may be very numerous: one hundred or more. The site of the rash is usually the abdomen and lower thorax, often the back and more rarely the neck, arms and legs. In quite rare cases spots have been found on the face. The typhoid bacillus can often be recovered from the blood taken from the rose rash.

TONGUE AND MOUTH.—In the early days of the disease the tongue is moist and covered with a white fur. As the disease progresses the coating becomes thicker and discolored. The oral secretions are diminished and thick and the tongue tends to become dry and cracked, often red and glazed. It is tremulous and protruded with difficulty. The red, dry, baked tongue is particularly noted in cases with severe diarrhea and great prostration. The condition of the mouth and tongue is often an index of the quality of the nursing. With modern hospital care the dry tongue and foul mouth are much more rarely seen than formerly. Any great collection of sordes on the gums or teeth is certainly an indication of neglect.

COUGH.—Bronchitis is quite a constant feature of typhoid and shows itself by an infrequent cough in the early days of the disease. It is usually restricted to the upper bronchi and causes no other symptoms. A few coarse râles are heard over the front and back of the chest. It may be more severe and attended by a frequent, distressing cough and by dyspnea. Abundant coarse and fine râles fill the entire chest.

CONSTIPATION AND DIARRHEA.—Either of these conditions may be present throughout the whole course of the disease, or there may be alternating periods of constipation and loose movements. In general, diarrhea is present in some stage of the disease in from 20 to 30 per cent of the cases. It occurs as a prodromal symptom in a small number of cases. It may appear in the latter part of the first week, or not until the second or third week. The administration of cathartics may precipitate the onset of the condition. The influence of bad feeding is very great, and the onset of loose movements after a period of constipation usually calls for a careful revision of the diet. When diarrhea is present the number of movements varies from one to two in the twenty-four hours to as many as six or eight or more. The movements are large, thin and of a dull yellow color. The reaction is alkaline and the odor offensive. The characteristic typhoid stool has the consistency and appearance of pea soup. After it has stood, a thin turbid fluid overlies a thicker, flocculent opaque stratum. Severe diarrhea is an unfavorable symptom. It drains the tissue fluids, dries up the tongue, seriously interferes with nutrition, and aggravates the exhaustion and wasting of the late period of the disease. Acute diarrhea is characteristic of infection by *S. typhi murium, S. cholerae suis, S. enteritidis* and the *Shigella* group. Any of these organisms may be ingested at the same time as the typhoid bacillus and may account for diarrhea in some cases.

ABDOMINAL TENDERNESS AND PAIN.—Abdominal tenderness accompanied by or without pain is one of the group of symptoms that help to make up the commonly recognized clinical picture of typhoid fever. The tenderness may be general over the whole abdomen or, more frequently, it is restricted to the right lower quadrant. It can often be elicited early in the period of invasion and, in that case, may be an important suggestive symptom; or it may be found at any time during the course of the fever. The specific bowel lesion is of itself an adequate cause for the symptom. Neither the tenderness nor the pain due to this cause alone is usually severe. In diarrheal cases the tenderness is

40101

greater and more widely spread over the abdomen. In these cases pain of a colicky character may precede the bowel movements or may be continuous and harassing to the patient. In certain cases severe abdominal pain may be present, with tenderness, distention and rigidity, but with no complication that can be demonstrated. Many conditions incident to the course of a prolonged fever may cause periods of pain of longer or shorter duration. Attacks of indigestion, vomiting, colic, diarrhea or constipation, and distended bladder belong to this group. Pain over the enlarged spleen is quite common. Various thoracic and abdominal complications are manifested by abdominal pain and tenderness; these symptoms, if at all severe or persistent, demand critical search for their cause. In the presence of unusual abdominal pain, perforation and hemorrhage should always be uppermost in the mind of the attendant, because of the urgent necessity of prompt diagnosis. McCrae found pain and tenderness from various causes and complications in three fifths of 500 carefully studied cases.

TYMPANITES.—Intestinal paresis, the result of inflammatory exudate in the musculature of the bowel wall, favors the development of tympanites, which is present at some time in the course of the disease in most cases of typhoid. Gurgling from intermittent pressure over the right iliac fossa may be elicited in the first week of the disease. It is found so frequently in other acute abdominal conditions that it cannot be considered a distinctive typhoid symptom, but it may complete the symptom-complex of the first week of the disease, and thus aid in arousing suspicion of the onset of typhoid fever. Mild and moderately severe cases, if properly nursed and carefully fed, rarely show tympanites of any severity. The development of the condition in these cases, as in diarrhea, calls for a revision of the dietary and attention to the alimentary tract. A clean colon is an efficient preventive.

Severe meteorism is an indication of toxemia and may be of grave import. It seriously interferes with the digestion and absorption of food, and it may precipitate hemorrhage or perforation. It may also seriously embarrass respiration and the action of the heart. A single deep ulcer has been thought to be the cause of severe intestinal distention.

SPLEEN.—The spleen is invariably enlarged. Swelling begins with the onset of the disease but can rarely be demonstrated by palpation until the end of the first week or the beginning of the second week. The spleen may not become palpable until late in the disease, or not at all. The enlargement can be determined with certainty only by palpation. Percussion is notoriously unreliable. In Osler's studies the organ was palpable in 71 per cent of all cases. It is, therefore, an important member of the group of clinical findings that permit a presumptive diagnosis of typhoid fever.

HEADACHE.—This is a constant early symptom, occurring in from 70 to 75 per cent of the cases. It may be a dull, heavy ache or an intense stabbing or boring pain. It may be frontal or occipital, more rarely parietal. It comes early, and by fixing the attention of the patient it is very useful in directing investigation to possible typhoid infection. It continues throughout the first week and lessens in severity in the beginning of the second week, when increasing mental hebetude tends to blunt the sensibilities of the patient. Headache continuing or increasing later than the end of the second week should excite suspicion of meningitis or other intracranial complication.

THE TYPHOID STATE.—This term is used to designate the symptom-complex expressing the profound asthenia that may result from severe infections or intoxications. It is not distinctive of typhoid fever. It may be met in the course of any severe and prolonged infectious disease, in abdominal inflammations, in urinary tract infections, intracranial diseases and in some intoxications like acute phosphorus poisoning. In the second week of severe cases of typhoid fever, earlier in the worst forms, the patient passes into a state of extreme physical and nervous prostration. He lies in bed relaxed and in a more or less profound stupor. Consciousness is obliterated and the special senses are dulled. He responds sluggishly to mental and physical impressions. He is aroused with difficulty and takes food and drink only when urged. The temperature is usually high, although in the aged and in alcoholic, diabetic and other debilitated patients the pyrexia may be of a low type. The pulse is rapid and weak. The respiration is quickened because of passive congestion of the base of the lungs. The tongue is brown and dry, the lips are cracked, and there is abundant dry secretion on the teeth and gums. There is a low muttering delirium, twitching of the tendons, picking at the bedclothes and grasping after imaginary objects. Involuntary discharge of the excretions may occur. This condition, when pronounced, is always a very grave one.

Relapse.—RECRUDESCENCE OR SPURIOUS RELAPSE.—The convalescent period is not infrequently interrupted by short periods of pyrexia. The typhoid convalescent is peculiarly sensitive to fever-producing influences. No adequate cause may be found, but usually the disturbance can be traced to an indiscretion in diet, constipation, a return of the diarrhea, physical exertion, or nervous excitement. An indiscreet visitor will often excite a transient rise of the patient's temperature. A careful search should always be made for a complication.

The important feature of the recrudescence is the rise of temperature. Malaise, headache and a return of the lassitude are the usual accompaniments. The temperature reaches the maximum in from one to three days and quickly begins to decline. The duration of the febrile period is from one to five or six days. Apprehension that the apparent recrudescence may be the onset of a true relapse is always in the mind of the attendant.

TRUE RELAPSE.—The true relapse is a reinfection of the patient with the typhoid bacillus, after convalescence is apparently established. It occurs after a few days of normal temperature, usually before the end of the second week after the termination of the original period of fever. It may begin as early as the second day after the temperature has fallen to normal, or its appearance may be delayed until the fourth week or longer. The longest interval in McCrae's series was 43 days. In Curschmann's experience it was 53 days.

The frequency of relapse varies in different epidemics and it is stated by writers to occur in from 3 to 16 per cent of the cases. In a collection of 28,057 cases by McCrae from European and American sources, relapse occurred in 8.8 per cent.

Liability to relapse is as great or greater in mild as in severe primary attacks. Often the mild and abortive cases are followed by severe

40101

relapses from which the diagnosis of the original attack may first be made in retrospect.

The cause of relapse is not settled. The authors are in accord with Gay, who believes that they ''are undoubtedly due to the overflowing of typhoid bacilli from their localized metastatic or ultimate foci in the body.'' Among these foci, those which have been considered to be particularly concerned in the etiology of relapse are the gallbladder, spleen and bone marrow. These tissues serve as reservoirs for the reinfection of the circulation.

Except when it follows a very mild or abortive attack, the relapse runs a shorter course than the first infection. The relapse may be multiple, two or more attacks succeeding each other at varying intervals. Osler records a case with six relapses. The onset of a relapse is usually gradual, with the steplike ascent of the temperature as in the primary attack; or it may be sudden, with chill and rapidly rising fever. The symptoms are practically the same as in ordinary typhoid. The pulse is usually more rapid and dicrotism is less frequent. The rose spots may reappear, and the spleen enlarge. It has frequently been noted that relapse is very apt to follow if splenic enlargement persists after convalescence from the original attack. A new crop of intestinal lesions may occur, and the typhoid bacillus may again be recovered from the blood.

The duration of the relapse is from one to three weeks. In exceptional cases a moderate irregular pyrexia persists for several weeks without evidence of a pus focus or other complication.

The mortality of true relapse is low, from 2 to 5 per cent. Shattuck met with one death in 21 cases. McCrae, in 172 cases of relapse, observed 5 deaths, or 2.9 per cent. In the Hamburg epidemic cited by Curschmann the death rate in 496 relapses was 4.9 per cent.

INTERCURRENT RELAPSE.—This is a term applied in this country to an exacerbation of the disease that begins during the period of decline, before the temperature has become normal. Curschmann, Sidney Phillips and other European writers speak of this form of relapse as a recrudescence. After the period of high temperature has passed and the patient appears to be well on the way to recovery the temperature again rises to a high point and all the symptoms of the fastigium reappear, continue for a week or more, and then gradually fade away. The course of this form of reinfection may be very severe and protracted. The frequent occurrence of relapse seems to indicate that immunity to typhoid infection is acquired slowly and is not fully established until some weeks after the end of the febrile period.

SECOND ATTACK.—One attack of typhoid fever usually gives immunity that continues through life. Immunity may, however, be abridged, and a second attack occasionally occurs at an interval of months or years after the first.

Some years ago the late author (C. G. Jennings) observed a boy of fifteen in the height of a typhoid attack who had passed through an equally typical attack under the same attending physician eight months before. As the diagnosis in both attacks was made by clinical findings alone, one of the infections may have been a paratyphoid. Infection by different strains of the typhoid group of bacilli may explain many if not all cases of second attacks.

DIAGNOSIS

The modern diagnosis of typhoid fever rests upon (1) the analysis of the clinical history and symptoms presented by the patient, and (2) the demonstration by laboratory methods of the typhoid bacillus in the body and the specific reactions that it produces.

Because of the high morbidity from typhoid fever in rural communities, remote from hospital and laboratory facilities, the diagnosis of the disease at the present time, in a large proportion of the cases, is based upon clinical data alone. The establishment in the last few years of public and private clinical laboratories extensively throughout the country has brought laboratory facilities for diagnosis within the reach of all.

Bedside diagnosis by experienced clinicians can usually be made with precision, and few cases running anything like the average course escape detection, although the diagnosis is often delayed until late in the course of the disease when a retrospective analysis of the symptom-complex can be made and other pathologic conditions excluded by the course of events. However, the disease presents such a variability in symptomatology, it simulates so closely other febrile diseases, and so many mild and atypical cases occur in which distinctive symptoms are missing, that diagnosis without laboratory aid may be very difficult; indeed, it is often impossible.

The laboratory is the short cut to a positive diagnosis. Its aid when available should always be sought, but it should not take the place of careful clinical observation and study. A presumptive clinical diagnosis should first be made and then checked up by laboratory examinations. Too great dependence upon the laboratory conduces to carelessness in bedside observation and tends to develop a feeble faith in clinical deductions.

In the final analysis, however, it must be admitted that no positive diagnosis of typhoid fever can be asserted without the confirmation of laboratory tests. As Gay correctly says, "If repeated and complete laboratory tests for typhoid fever, properly performed, result negatively, no definite positive diagnosis of typhoid fever should be made on the basis of the clinical examination alone."

Depending upon the period in the clinical history in which a case first comes under observation, or in which the question of typhoid infection first arises, the problem of the diagnosis of typhoid fever presents itself practically at the bedside in three phases:

First, the diagnosis in the first week of the disease.

Second, the diagnosis in the period of continuous high temperature, from the second to the fourth week.

Third, the diagnosis in cases of prolonged pyrexia in which typhoid infection is suspected.

DIAGNOSIS IN THE FIRST WEEK

Typhoid fever should be considered as a possibility in the diagnosis of every acute febrile illness, regardless of the mode of onset or the age of the patient. A provisional or positive diagnosis at the earliest possible time is important both to the welfare of the patient and for the protection of the community. With this disease in mind the physician will

40101

so direct his clinical and laboratory investigations that an early solution of the problem is made possible. The differential diagnosis of typhoid fever in the first week from the many diseases that resemble it is peculiarly the problem for the family practitioner. The symptoms are rarely so urgent as to suggest consultation or hospital care. The family practitioner should be an expert in this field of differential diagnosis.

General Diagnosis.—CLINICAL DATA.—From the clinical data alone only a provisional diagnosis of typhoid fever is possible in the first week. There are no characteristic individual symptoms of onset, but a careful study of the group of phenomena present will usually lead to a suspicion strong enough to be a guide to personal and preventive therapeutics.

The clinical data of the first week that determine the provisional diagnosis are:

Mode of Onset.—This is usually gradual, and is often preceded by a few days of vague symptoms that are ascribed to a cold, digestive disturbances, or to some other minor ailment. Chilliness, or less frequently a distinct chill, may usher in the invasion period.

Temperature.—The gradual steplike ascent of the temperature is a symptom of significance when observation begins on the first or second day. Opportunity for this early observation comes frequently to the family practitioner. Unfortunately the habit of the routine administration of an antipyretic in the early days of acute febrile diseases too often hides the suggestive curve. Such treatment is unwise when the diagnosis of a developing infection is in doubt. No variety of temperature curve, however, should exclude typhoid; exceptions to the rule of gradual rise are very frequent.

Pulse Rate.—The pulse rate, which is remarkably slow in relation to the height of temperature, quickly arrests the attention of the careful clinician. With a temperature of 102 or 103° F. (38.9 or 39.4° C.) a pulse rate below 100 is often noted. This lack of harmony is quite peculiar to typhoid fever and is a valuable suggestive symptom. The character of the pulse is full, soft, and shows dicrotism quite early. Associated with the slow rate, the dicrotism has much significance.

Headache.—Headache is often the most emphatic symptom of invasion, and while common to other acute diseases it should always direct attention to typhoid fever. It may be severe and persistent. It is quite significant in patients previously free from headaches.

Tenderness and Gurgling.—These symptoms can be demonstrated in the right lower quadrant of the abdomen during the first week, in quite a percentage of the cases. Abdominal pain, general or localized, is also frequent.

Diarrhea.—Diarrhea at the onset is very unusual in other acute febrile diseases. It is present early in from 20 to 30 per cent of typhoid cases.

Epistaxis.—Epistaxis from the second to the fourth day occurs often enough to be an important suggestive symptom.

Prostration and Mental Dullness.—In early typhoid these symptoms are quite out of proportion to the other manifestations, and should direct attention to this disease.

Cough.—Cough is present in a large percentage of cases. Associated with a rising temperature and with other symptoms disproportionate to the findings in the chest, it should suggest further examination for the presence of typhoid infection.

The foregoing group of symptoms, more or less complete, persisting over a period of a week and not manifestly due to some other infection, justifies a provisional diagnosis of typhoid fever. The prevalence of typhoid fever in the locality, the history of a recent visit to an infected community, or the possibility of personal contact with a typhoid patient, may be incidents of distinct aid in establishing the diagnosis.

LABORATORY DATA.—A positive diagnosis of typhoid fever by laboratory tests can be made in the first week of the disease in from 70 to 80 per cent of the cases. This certainty, as compared with the vagueness of clinical deductions, emphasizes the importance of resorting to laboratory methods of diagnosis in every case of acute febrile disease which is ushered in by symptoms suggestive of typhoid fever. Laboratory methods are considered in detail under a separate heading.

Blood Culture.—A positive blood culture is the most convincing evidence of typhoid fever. It is the most important single factor in the early diagnosis of the disease. Fortunately the percentage of positive cultures is highest in the first week. Any physician should be able to master the simple technic necessary to withdraw blood aseptically from a vein and to inoculate a flask of sterile bouillon. The culture can then be sent to a bacteriologic laboratory for incubation and study. This simple procedure will usually cut short the many days of embarrassing doubt that must intervene if one waits for the development of convincing clinical data.

Agglutination Test or Widal Reaction.—A positive agglutination reaction can be obtained in about 90 per cent of all cases of typhoid fever, at some period of the disease. It is a late symptom, rarely appearing before the eighth day. It is, therefore, of comparatively little assistance in making a diagnosis in the first week. While a positive result is highly presumptive of typhoid, a negative finding has no significance. As noted elsewhere, subjects vaccinated against typhoid fever give a positive agglutination test for several months following vaccination.

Leukocyte Count.—Uncomplicated typhoid fever gives a low white cell count, manifested early and continuing throughout the disease. At the onset the count is often normal or slightly increased. By the middle of the first week the number of white cells falls to from 2,000 to 5,000 per c.mm. The differential count shows the polymorphonuclear cells and eosinophils to be decreased, and the mononuclear cells increased. Increased leukocyte count is common to most diseases that may simulate typhoid fever in the first week. This simple laboratory procedure, therefore, is of great value in early diagnosis. A leukocytosis rules out uncomplicated typhoid, while a leukopenia is strongly suggestive of it.

Differential Diagnosis.—All of the acute febrile diseases must be passed in review in the differentiation of typhoid fever in the first week. In most of these diseases the appearance of distinctive clinical symptoms within two or three days eliminates the possibility of typhoid; in a certain number of cases careful matching of symptoms for several days and an early resort to laboratory aid are necessary to reach a conclusion.

THE ACUTE EXANTHEMATA.—The symptoms of the eruptive fevers before the appearance of the rash may give rise to the suspicion of the

40101

onset of typhoid fever. Sudden onset with vomiting, rapidly rising temperature, quick pulse, peculiar tongue and red, sore throat are characteristic of *scarlatina*. The eruption, appearing in from twenty-four to thirty-six hours, quickly determines the diagnosis. In rare cases a scarlatiniform erythema in the first week of typhoid may be confusing. In *variola* the longer period of invasion and the severe headache may suggest typhoid. In variola vomiting is common and the intense backache is very characteristic. The eruption comes on the third day. *Measles* may be more confusing. The invasion is more gradual and the distinctive catarrhal symptoms are frequently delayed for three or four days. The cough may resemble the early cough of typhoid, and the drowsiness may suggest the typhoid stupor. The conjunctivitis and coryza are almost never seen in typhoid. Koplik's spots are positively diagnostic of measles. The rash comes on the fourth day. In the exceptional cases in which the eruption is delayed until the fifth or sixth day, typhoid fever may be strongly suspected.

IN INFLUENZA the onset is usually sudden. In a recent epidemic, however, many cases developed gradually, with steplike rise of temperature, abdominal tenderness and relaxed bowel movements. This was followed by mild catarrhal symptoms, relatively slow pulse, low white blood cell count, headache and nosebleed—a symptom-complex impossible to distinguish from typhoid fever. The critical drop in temperature about the end of the week would determine the diagnosis of influenza, except that it might mark the end of an abortive attack of typhoid fever. A positive diagnosis is possible only by blood culture. Persistence of the continued fever through the second week renders typhoid probable, although the pyrexia of influenza may persist for two weeks or longer. A hospital patient of the late author (C. G. J.), convalescent from typhoid, surrounded by influenza, developed fever two weeks after defervescence. The question arose: was the fever due to influenza or to a typhoid relapse? A positive blood culture on the fifth day made typhoid relapse fairly certain, as the typhoid bacillus is rarely found in the circulating blood so long after the end of the fever. The subsequent typical course of the relapse confirmed the laboratory diagnosis.

PNEUMONIA may simulate typhoid fever in the invasion period. The physical signs of pneumonia in children and in the aged are often masked and the disease will run along for several days with only the symptoms of fever, a slight cough and almost no physical signs. Central pneumonia at any age may give the same confusing clinical history. In contradistinction to typhoid fever the onset of pneumonia is abrupt, usually with a chill. The temperature quickly rises to a moderate height and persists. Increased frequency of respiration is almost always present from the beginning, and is a symptom of such great significance that it should call attention immediately to pulmonary disease. Pleuritic pain may be absent or, what is more confusing, if present it may be referred to the abdomen. The expected rusty sputum may not appear for several days. Herpes, practically never seen in the first week of typhoid, is a frequent pneumonia symptom. Repeated physical examination of the chest, carefully made, searching for signs at the apex, the base and in the axillary region, will rarely fail to unmask a pneumonia after two or three days. The leukocyte count, high in pneumonia, low in typhoid, is a great diagnostic aid. Blood culture with a positive finding is conclusive. Typhoid fever with pneumonia-like onset, pneumotyphoid, giving the symptoms and the physical signs of pneumonia, is a rare condition and was never observed by the late author (C. G. J.). It would deceive the elect. Only the late history of the case will suggest the possibility of typhoid fever, and a positive diagnosis can be made only by laboratory methods.

SEPTICEMIAS AND LOCAL INFECTIONS.—The septicemias and local infections by the streptococcus, staphylococcus, gonococcus, colon bacillus and other organisms, often present the problem of differentiation from typhoid fever. The *septicemias* develop rapidly and without premonitory symptoms. The first days are marked by chills and by an erratic temperature, irregularly remittent or intermittent in type. After the initial chill the temperature may rise to a high point and persist as a continued fever. Profuse sweats are common. The pulse is rapid, quite distinct from the slow, dicrotic pulse of typhoid. The spleen enlarges early and may be a confusing symptom, although early enlargement is but rarely seen in typhoid. A portal of entry of the infection can often be demonstrated. With its usual symptoms of onset, typhoid fever would rarely be confused with a septicemia, but the early clinical history of both conditions is so variable and may be so similar that in many cases certainty in diagnosis in the first week may be obtained only by laboratory methods. A high leukocyte count with a high percentage of polymorphonuclears is characteristic of septicemia. A blood culture with positive findings would certainly differentiate the two diseases.

The fever attending hidden *local infections* by the various pyogenic organisms may be mistaken for typhoid fever before local symptoms of pus infection are pronounced. Infections of the throat, middle ears and of the accessory sinuses of the nose, particularly in the case of children, may pursue their course for several days, with fever as the only symptom, and would suggest the onset of typhoid fever. Subdiaphragmatic abscess, cholecystitis, pylephlebitis, hepatic abscess and perinephritis in the upper abdomen; salpingitis, prostatic or perirectal abscess in the lower abdomen, may begin with fever and indefinite or no localizing symptoms. The urinary septicemia of old men with prostatic disease, manifested by fever, dry, brown tongue, nervous symptoms and prostration, may arouse the suspicion of typhoid. Pyelitis in children and pregnant women causes a fever with no distinctive subjective or objective symptoms, and if a routine urinary analysis be neglected the disease may easily be mistaken for typhoid. Osteomyelitis in children has been mistaken for typhoid fever. General infection by the gonococcus may cause confusion when the local infection is concealed.

The distinction of these various infections from typhoid fever depends, *first,* upon a searching and complete physical examination—every region and organ should be examined for localizing signs—*second,* upon the results of the white blood cell count and blood culture. A high leukocyte count fixes the attention upon a pus infection and stimulates further search for the focus. It may in itself be conclusive. A blood culture is of decisive assistance.

Puerperal Septicemia.—The obstetrician occasionally is reluctant to acknowledge puerperal infection and seeks to explain a postpartum fever by the presence of an intercurrent infection like typhoid fever or malaria. The problem of differential diagnosis is the same here as in septicemia of other etiology. The fact of the puerperal state, however, is of the highest significance. It is strong presumptive evidence of a septicemia, and only the positive results of laboratory tests should be taken as proof of an intercurrent typhoid. Typhoid fever may occur in the pregnant woman and cause abortion or premature delivery. The fever persists after delivery and a differential diagnosis from septic infection may be impossible without laboratory assistance.

APPENDICITIS.—Appendicitis begins suddenly with sharp abdominal pain, circumscribed tenderness in the right lower quadrant, and muscular rigidity. Irregular fever, slight or of moderate degree, is present; the pulse is rapid; nausea or vomiting and constipation are usual. The abdominal symptoms of typhoid fever are very rarely as pronounced as in appendicitis, and an error in diagnosis should not occur. Although there may be pain and tenderness, rigidity is not present in typhoid. The leukocyte count is of great value. It is quite uniformly high in appendicitis. We have known eager young surgeons impressed with the necessity of immediate operation in appendicitis to open the abdomen in typhoid, expecting to find a diseased appendix. Typhoid fever with an early complicating appendicitis would present unusual difficulties. In army experience, antityphoid vaccination has occasionally been followed by fever, acute abdominal pain and vomiting. Such cases have been mistaken for and treated as appendicitis.

ACUTE ENTERITIS.—Acute enteritis with fever, abdominal pain, distention and tenderness, and diarrhea suggests the onset of typhoid fever. The severe forms of enteritis begin with stormy symptoms. The fever rises abruptly and all the symptoms reach their height in from twenty-four to forty-eight hours and then as a rule begin to subside. Should the fever persist longer, distinction by clinical evidence alone is impossible until the presence of the rash, the enlarged spleen, and the steady temperature curve of the second week of typhoid fever clears the diagnosis. Milder forms of gastro-enteritis are frequently met with, particularly in children, and are more difficult to differentiate. The fever is moderate; distention, gurgling, pain and tenderness in the right lower quadrant are frequently seen. Anorexia, coated tongue and headache may be added and complete a clinical picture identical with that of the first few days of typhoid fever. Such symptoms usually respond promptly to low diet and cathartic medication, but when rebellious to such treatment laboratory aid to exclude typhoid fever may be required.

EPHEMERAL FEVER, FEBRICULA, SIMPLE CONTINUED FEVER.—These terms are used to designate short, febrile attacks of undetermined etiology. Such fevers may resemble typhoid fever during the period of onset. Complete laboratory study of these cases shows that many of them are examples of mild typhoid or paratyphoid infection. Others are symptomatic of hidden local infections or due to toxic causes. A final diagnosis of febricula, which is a confession of ignorance, is justified only when thorough investigation by clinical and laboratory methods fails to reveal a definite etiology.

PARATYPHOID FEVER, A AND B—Paratyphoid fever cannot certainly be distinguished by clinical methods from typhoid fever. Either variety of paratyphoid may pursue a course identical with that of typhoid fever and present all the symptoms and complications of this disease. Practically a positive differential diagnosis is of minor importance. The therapeutics of the two diseases is identical and the measures to be adopted for the prevention of their extension in the community are the same.

Studies of groups of paratyphoid infections by observers with the armies in France have shown, however, that there are certain clinical differences between the paratyphoid and typhoid fevers which, while they are not sufficiently marked to distinguish with any certainty individual cases, may be adequate in group observation for provisional differential diagnosis. Wiltshire states that as his experience increased he found that it was possible to give a fairly sound opinion on the differential diagnosis of the two diseases, "though never with such certainty that bacteriologic examination could be excluded."

In general, the paratyphoid fevers pursue a milder and shorter course than does typhoid. The onset of paratyphoid is more frequently abrupt, and the duration of the period of invasion is shorter—from three to four days. The initial symptoms are very similar to those of typhoid. Anorexia, nausea, headache, epistaxis and insomnia are usual. Vomiting and chills are much more frequently noted than in typhoid. The temperature rises more sharply and reaches the usual maximum of about 103° F. (39.4° C.) in three or four days. The fastigium and the period of decline are both shorter than in typhoid, and the total duration of the pyrexial period is usually not more than two weeks. Early and marked remissions of the fever are the rule. The pulse is slow, as in typhoid, but dicrotism is less frequent. The tongue is more apt to be moist and is not so heavily coated as in typhoid. Gastro-intestinal symptoms are often more severe but of shorter duration. The stools are darker in color. The liver is frequently palpable below the rib line, and jaundice, very unusual in typhoid, is a frequent symptom. The spleen, although enlarged, is rarely palpable. The rose rash is present in about 60 per cent of the cases and appears rather later in the disease than in typhoid. Wiltshire gives the average date of appearance as the thirteenth day. The spots may not be distinguishable from the typhoid roseola. In about 50 per cent of the cases the rash is of the "paratyphoid type" (Wiltshire). Each individual spot is larger than the rose spot of typhoid fever, much more raised, and frequently lenticular in outline. The spots are darker in color and do not completely disappear on pressure. Pigmentation and desquamation are usual. This peculiar type of eruption is quite striking in appearance and is of considerable importance in differential diagnosis. Herpes, very rare in typhoid fever, is quite frequent in paratyphoid and when present should always suggest this disease. Perspiration is frequent, both at the onset and during the course of the disease, and is often profuse. Nervous symptoms are less frequent and less severe than in typhoid, and the typhoid state is unusual. Meningeal involvement is stated to be more frequent than in typhoid. Severe occipital pain is common.

While the foregoing group of differential symptoms may be sufficient for a presumptive diagnosis, especially when viewed in retrospect, or observed in a group of cases, positive differentiation of paratyphoid from typhoid fever can be made only by the isolation of the paratyphoid bacillus from the blood, urine or feces and its identification by cultural methods, or by the Widal agglutination reaction.

MALARIA.—The intermittent types of malarial fever bear no resemblance to typhoid fever. The onset of the remittent and the estivo-autumnal types, however, may closely resemble the onset of typhoid fever. Chills may be absent and a fever with slight remissions and increasing in severity may mark the first few days. Malaise, prostration, headache, coated tongue and diarrhea are common. There is a low leukocyte count and an early enlargement of the spleen. Differentiation can be made only by blood culture to isolate the typhoid bacillus and by the examination of the stained smear for the plasmodium. The estivo-autumnal parasite may not be found in the circulating blood for several days.

There is no such clinical entity as typhomalarial fever. The careful studies of Osler in Baltimore, where both diseases prevail, have conclusively proved that such a mixed infection does not occur. In very rare cases the two infections may be concurrent and produce a confused clinical picture.

If laboratory aid is not available for diagnosis, **quinine** in full doses may be given as a therapeutic test. Quinine has practically no effect upon the course of typhoid fever. It promptly arrests the fever of malaria.

TYPHUS FEVER—BRILL'S DISEASE.—The confusion of typhoid with typhus fever until the middle of the last century shows how closely these two diseases may resemble each other. Typhus fever is very rare in this country and occurs only under conditions which arouse suspicion of its possible presence. Typhus begins suddenly with chills, high fever, rapid pulse, great prostration, vomiting, severe headache and pain in the back and legs. The temperature rises rapidly and reaches its maximum in four or five days. Delirium and severe nervous symptoms begin early. The eruption appears from the third to the fifth day, is very abundant, darker in color than the rose spots of typhoid, and quickly becomes hemorrhagic. Mild cases, such as those described by Brill, may show a clinical course much less distinctive than the above. Differentiation from typhoid by clinical data alone may be impossible. In typhus the Weil-Felix agglutination reaction is positive.

RELAPSING FEVER.—Relapsing fever is a tropical disease, rare in the United States. It is distinguished from typhoid fever by the sudden onset with chill, high fever, nausea and vomiting, pain in the back and frequently jaundice. In from five to six days the temperature falls to normal with profuse perspiration. After an intermission of from a week to ten days there is a sudden relapse with a repetition of the symptoms of the first paroxysm. Positive diagnosis is made by the demonstration of the spirochetes in the blood.

CEREBROSPINAL FEVER.—Some cases of this disease with gradual onset may be mistaken for typhoid fever. The temperature rises slowly but irregularly. Headache is severe, vomiting is frequent and constipation marked. By the third or fifth day distinctively meningeal symptoms—rigidity of the neck, a positive Kernig's sign, and hyperesthesia—appear. A rash, appearing first on the abdomen, occurs in some cases on the third or fourth day. It is petechial in character, and quite distinct from the rose rash of typhoid. On the other hand, certain cases of typhoid fever with meningeal symptoms, *meningotyphoid,* may be mistaken for one of the forms of meningitis. Cases of true typhoid meningitis with invasion of the meninges by the typhoid bacillus have been reported. In doubtful cases the diagnosis must be made by laboratory tests. In cerebrospinal fever there is always a high polymorphonuclear leukocytosis, from 15,000 to 30,000 per c.mm. In the presence of symptoms indicating the possible onset of cerebrospinal fever, an early lumbar puncture is imperative for curative serum treatment, as well as for diagnosis. In cerebrospinal fever the spinal fluid is cloudy with polymorphonuclear cells containing the *Diplococcus intracellularis*. In typhoid fever the fluid is clear. In the rare cases of typhoid meningitis Eberth's bacillus may be demonstrated in the fluid. In unusually doubtful cases a blood culture may be decisive.

TUBERCULOUS MENINGITIS.—Tuberculous meningitis, with its premonitory stage of vague symptoms and its slow onset, may present a still more difficult problem. The white cell count is low as in typhoid. The spinal fluid in both diseases is clear and the tubercle bacillus is difficult to demonstrate. If a blood culture is available an early positive diagnosis may be made. In certain cases with a negative blood culture and with other confusing laboratory data, a differential diagnosis must be made from the clinical findings. In tuberculous meningitis the fever is very irregular in its course and not high. The pulse is often slow and arrhythmic. Vomiting, repeated several times during the first few days of the illness, is present in practically every case. It is often of the explosive type and comes at irregular intervals without adequate exciting cause. It is one of the most significant symptoms of the onset of the disease. There are present obstinate constipation and retraction of the abdomen, alternate flushing and paling of the face or extremities, rigidity of the neck, positive Kernig and Babinski signs, irregular pupils and local palsies. Stupor and coma develop comparatively early, without high fever or toxemia. As these distinctive symptoms are often of tardy development a diagnosis may not be possible in the first week.

Meningitis due to the pneumococcus, streptococcus, etc., is recognized by the demonstration of these organisms in the spinal fluid.

TRICHINIASIS.—Outbreaks of trichiniasis have been considered at first to be outbreaks of typhoid fever. In isolated cases mistakes are even more likely to occur. Trichiniasis is rather rare in this country and the possibility of the disease does not at once come to the mind of the average practitioner in the diagnosis of an acute febrile malady. Cases may readily be mistaken for typhoid fever. The onset, however, is sudden in trichiniasis. The fever is irregular in type. Usually it is remittent or intermittent; occasionally it is continuous. There are severe muscular and joint pains. The muscles are very tender, swollen and indurated, and the skin over them is often edematous. Edema of the face, particularly of the eyelids, appears early. Abdominal pain and diarrhea are common. A white blood cell count will determine the diagnosis. As first shown by Thomas K. Brown, of Baltimore, there is in trichiniasis a leukocytosis, 10,000 to 25,000 white blood cells per cubic millimeter, with the remarkable finding of from 20 to 30 per cent eosinophils. A history of the ingestion of uncooked pork can usually be obtained.

DIAGNOSIS IN THE SECOND AND THIRD WEEKS

This problem is most frequently presented to the hospital attendant and the consultant. The hospital attendant rarely sees typhoid fever in the first week. The disease is usually well under way before the pa-

40101

tient is admitted. The consultant also is not often called until the serious symptoms of the fastigium cause anxiety, or the absence of distinctive clinical signs has raised a doubt as to the diagnosis of typhoid fever.

In the second week the characteristic clinical signs of typhoid fever appear. The rose rash develops from the sixth to the tenth day, and the enlarged spleen can be demonstrated about the same time. These two phenomena, with the history of gradual onset, continued fever with slow pulse, right iliac tenderness, diarrhea and nervous symptoms, are, with rarely an exception, conclusive.

Cases entering the hospital seriously ill, unable to give a history of the previous course of the disease, with symptoms atypical in character or masked by complications, are often very puzzling and require complete clinical and laboratory investigation for their differential diagnosis.

The Widal reaction, the leukocyte count and the blood culture all are available at this period and a positive diagnosis by these methods can quickly be made, with only an occasional exception.

Differential Diagnosis.—Most of the diseases that must be considered in the early diagnosis of typhoid are eliminated by the second week of the fever. Diseases which earlier presented symptoms suggestive of typhoid either end or become distinctly differentiated before this time. The diseases most frequently confused with typhoid fever at this period are the septicemias and hidden localized pus infections; malarial, typhus and relapsing fevers; miliary tuberculosis and tuberculous peritonitis; malignant endocarditis; undulant fever and syphilis.

Acute Miliary Tuberculosis.—The differentiation of this disease from typhoid fever may be very difficult. Either disease may continue for an indefinite time with high fever, a general toxemia, and no well-defined localizing symptoms. Tuberculosis is rarely recognized or even suspected in the first week. Cases usually come up for differentiation in the second or third week of the disease, or even later, with a presumptive diagnosis of typhoid fever made from clinical data. Some irregularity in the course of the disease or some delay in the appearance of the expected characteristic signs of typhoid fever raises a doubt in the mind of the attending physician as to the correctness of the diagnosis and calls for a review of the diagnostic data.

Acute tuberculosis may show the same gradual onset as typhoid fever, with chilliness, malaise, general muscular pains, headache, nosebleed, cough, occasional vomiting and diarrhea. In miliary tuberculosis the temperature is more often irregular and shows wide oscillations. The pulse is rapid, not dicrotic, and follows the temperature curve closely. The respiration is rapid—a symptom of great significance that should always direct attention to the respiratory organs.

Anorexia is not so marked as in typhoid fever and the tongue remains moist for a longer time. The abdomen is flat, and gurgling and tenderness are absent. Diarrhea is not frequent and the peculiar typhoid stools are wanting. There is no rose rash. The spleen may be palpable as in typhoid. Pulmonary hemorrhage is distinctive of tuberculosis; intestinal hemorrhage is distinctive of typhoid.

Repeated and careful physical examination of the chest may reveal the signs of early pulmonary disease. An x-ray may be of value. Complete laboratory tests should settle the diagnosis. A low white blood cell count is found in both diseases. Tubercle bacilli in the sputum clinch the diagnosis of tuberculosis. A positive Widal reaction and a positive blood culture distinguish typhoid fever.

TUBERCULOUS PERITONITIS.—This disease pursues a long, febrile course with abdominal symptoms, and may closely resemble typhoid fever. The fever is usually not high and is remittent or intermittent in character. The pulse is rapid. Abdominal pain and tenderness, distention and diarrhea may be present in tuberculous peritonitis. The severe toxemia and the nervous symptoms distinctive of typhoid fever are not seen in peritonitis, except possibly very late in the disease. Sooner or later masses in the abdomen, or ascites, reveal the nature of the disease. The Widal reaction and blood culture are positive methods of differentiation; the tuberculin test may be of additional value.

MALIGNANT ENDOCARDITIS.—The typhoidal type of malignant endocarditis is a close counterfeit of typhoid fever. It is characterized by high fever of a remittent or continuous type with few or no definite localizing symptoms. The toxemia is severe and the patient soon falls into the typhoid state with dry tongue, delirium and picking of the bedclothes. Confusion with typhoid fever is increased by the frequent enlargement of the spleen, by the presence of petechiae, and of a mild bronchitis. The abdominal symptoms of typhoid may be simulated by a complicating colitis with distention.

The cardiac signs in endocarditis may be vague, or a systolic murmur may be attributed to an old valvular lesion. A systolic apex murmur is not infrequently found in the late stage of typhoid. A tachycardia is always found in endocarditis but is only suggestive, as it is not uncommon in the late period of typhoid fever.

A diagnosis without laboratory data is usually impossible. Leukocytosis is suggestive but does not rule out typhoid. A positive Widal is strongly presumptive of typhoid. Blood culture gives the only decisive evidence. Either the typhoid bacillus or the organism of the endocarditis may be found.

UNDULANT FEVER.—The symptoms and signs of undulant fever are in many ways similar to those of typhoid fever. It differs from typhoid in that rose spots are absent, the fever tends to fall quickly after it has reached its peak, and sacral neuritis or joint pains are common. The laboratory diagnosis of undulant fever is made by the agglutination test, the skin test for sensitivity to brucellergin and Huddleson's opsonocytophagic index test. Blood culture may be positive but special technic is necessary.

SYPHILIS.—The pyrexia of syphilis may be mistaken for typhoid fever. A period of continued fever, mild or severe, without localizing symptoms, may occur in any stage of syphilis and in the absence of a history of luetic infection may prove very puzzling. Two cases were observed by the late author (C. G. J.) before the Widal and Wassermann reactions were known, which were thought to be typhoid, until the distinctive signs of syphilis appeared. General adenopathy is very suggestive of syphilis. Involvement of the postcervical and epitrochlear glands is of particular significance. The history of nosebleed, diarrhea with abdominal symptoms, the scattered rose spots on the chest and abdomen, and enlarged spleen, point to typhoid. The laboratory findings will positively differentiate the two diseases. The positive findings in syphilis are leukocytosis and a positive Wassermann reaction. In typhoid the leukopenia, the positive Widal and the recovery of the typhoid bacillus by blood culture are decisive.

DIAGNOSIS IN CASES OF PROLONGED PYREXIA IN WHICH TYPHOID FEVER IS SUSPECTED

Occasionally the practitioner is confronted with the problem of the differential diagnosis of a prolonged pyrexia that has been classified as typhoid fever from clinical findings; or, during the course of such a pyrexia otherwise classified, the question arises: Is this a case of typhoid fever? The problem may be very difficult of solution, especially in the absence of a clear history of the onset and course of the disease. Late in typhoid distinctive clinical signs may disappear, or may be overshadowed by the symptoms of complications. The rose spots, so important in bedside diagnosis, usually fade in the third week. The enlargement of the spleen often subsides, and the diarrhea and abdominal symptoms may disappear. A rapid, small pulse takes the place of the slow dicrotic pulse of the first and second weeks. The temperature curve loses its continued type, and sharp rises or intermissions occur. The nervous symptoms and the great prostration and wasting are common to all pyrexias of long duration. The laboratory findings, also, may be uncertain. Late in typhoid a leukocytosis due to various complications is quite frequent. The percentage of positive blood cultures is reduced. The agglutination reaction, on the other hand, is usually positive, but the frequency of antityphoid vaccination at the present time takes away some of the value of this sign. The isolation of the typhoid bacillus from the urine and feces is of distinct practical value if the possibility of a chronic carrier can be excluded.

Influenza, tuberculosis, malignant endocarditis, septicemia from hidden foci of suppuration, malaria and syphilis are the common infections which may cause a prolonged pyrexia mistakable for typhoid fever. The differential diagnosis of these conditions from typhoid has been fully considered.

Pernicious anemia, leukemia and Hodgkin's disease, carcinoma and sarcoma of different organs, and cirrhosis of the liver may be marked during their progress by periods of pyrexia that may bring to mind the possibility of typhoid fever. The prolonged pyrexia of indefinite etiology that is not infrequent in children may bring up the same question. The mere mention of these causes of pyrexia will suggest the lines of investigation to be followed. A painstaking review of the history of the onset and course of the disease, a searching physical examination and a careful analysis of laboratory findings will rarely fail to lead to a definite conclusion.

In all of these conditions the isolation of the typhoid bacillus from the blood, urine or feces may be the only deciding evidence.

DIAGNOSIS OF TYPHOID FEVER IN INFANCY

Typhoid fever is so rare in infancy that it is usually the last disease considered in the diagnosis of an acute febrile disease. It should be borne in mind that infants often have elevated temperature of a few days' duration without the distinctive or localizing symptoms that make a diagnosis possible. Under such circumstances the possibility of typhoid fever should always be considered. Only by careful analysis and exclusion and the early resort to laboratory aids can the cause of such a fever be determined.

The diseases of infancy which typhoid fever may simulate are the eruptive fevers, particularly measles or smallpox; acute indigestion with fever; pneumonia; meningitis; otitis media; pyelitis; acute tuberculosis; malaria and influenza.

The usual problem presented by an infant with typhoid is to explain a persistent high fever with no distinctive or localizing associated symptoms.

In the *eruptive fevers* the appearance of the rash serves to clear up the diagnosis. The first few days of the onset of typhoid fever may closely simulate the fever of an acute digestive disturbance. The moderate fever, loss of appetite, occasional vomiting and one or two abnormal stools a day with abdominal pain and tenderness make a close counterfeit of an attack of *indigestion*. This condition is so common, particularly in artificially fed infants, that it is usually the explanation first considered. Typhoid fever should be suspected if the symptoms persist after the administration of an efficient cathartic and reduction in the food intake. An actual increase in the fever and other symptoms is is not infrequently noted in typhoid fever after a brisk cathartic. A blood culture is the only method of making a positive diagnosis in the first week. In the case illustrated in Figure 6, a positive diagnosis was made on the fifth day by blood culture. A white blood cell count of 5,000 or 6,000 would strongly indicate typhoid. The characteristic rash on the seventh and eighth day should be carefully sought. When present it clinches the diagnosis. A positive Widal is equally distinctive, but unfortunately is rarely present before the second week of the disease. In the absence of these positive findings the persistence of the fever and other symptoms beyond a week render the diagnosis of typhoid almost a certainty.

Primary pneumococcus *pneumonia* may closely resemble typhoid. Pneumonia in the infant is usually preceded by an upper respiratory tract infection with trifling or no rise of temperature. The invasion of the lung is marked by a sharp rise of temperature, rapid respiration, short, suppressed, painful cough, prostration and somnolence. The leukocyte count is uniformly high—15,000 to 25,000. The physical signs of impending or actual consolidation should be manifest in two or three days. The referred abdominal pain and tenderness often noted in pneumonia in the young patient may be a very confusing symptom. With the respiratory type of typhoid only a blood culture would make an early differential diagnosis possible.

Malarial infection is common in infants in malarial districts and will be distinguished from typhoid fever by the temperature curve. The persistent high temperature of typhoid is rarely seen in malaria. Marked daily remissions or an irregular curve with the temperature reaching normal at some time during the twenty-four hours is distinctive of malaria. The demonstration of the plasmodium in the blood is final. In the absence of this positive laboratory finding the administration of full doses of quinine is a therapeutic test of great value. The course of typhoid is uninfluenced by the drug; malarial fever promptly yields to it.

40101

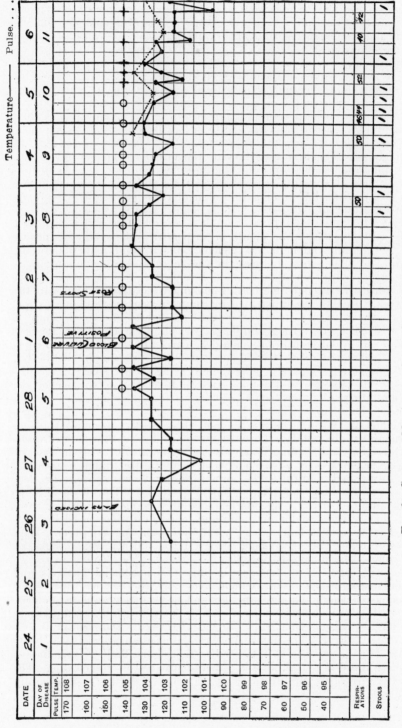

Fig. 6.—Chart in Moderately Severe Infantile Typhoid Fever.

Temperature curve modified by baths. O, sponge baths; +, tub baths. Patient aged 9 months.

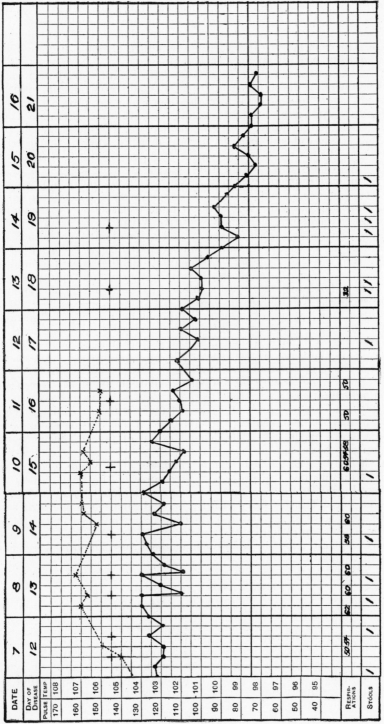

FIG. 6.—(Cont.)

40101

Otitis media is a frequent complication of typhoid fever in infants, even in the first week, and when the drums are found injected in the routine examination for diagnosis this may be thought to be the primary disease. Incision may be followed by temporary abatement of the fever, but it quickly regains its former height.

As in the adult, general *tuberculosis* of the infant may show a course which renders a differentiation from typhoid fever on the basis of symptoms alone impossible before the appearance of physical signs in the lungs, peritoneum or other organs. Only the demonstration of typhoid bacilli in the blood or excreta, or a positive Widal, will clear up the doubt. The tubercle bacillus may be demonstrated in the secretion from low in the pharynx, and is conclusive. A positive von Pirquet skin reaction is strongly suggestive of tuberculosis.

The onset of typhoid fever may be marked by nervous symptoms suggesting meningism or *meningitis*. These symptoms are usually atypical, and a close analysis will show only an imperfect picture of meningitis. The retracted abdomen, rigid neck, positive Kernig's sign, slow arrhythmic pulse, irregular respiration and coma of meningitis are practically never seen in typhoid. An early lumbar puncture is essential to the definite diagnosis and proper treatment of meningitis and should be made on the appearance of the first symptom suggesting meningeal infection. This, with the routine laboratory tests for typhoid fever, should settle the question of diagnosis.

During an epidemic of *influenza*, typhoid fever might be mistaken for this disease. Persistence of symptoms beyond the usual time for defervescence of influenza should arouse suspicion and suggest laboratory aid. Leukopenia is a characteristic of both diseases. Blood culture and the agglutination test may be the only certain means of differentiation in the absence of rose spots, enlargement of the spleen and abdominal symptoms.

Pyelitis in infancy causes a continued fever with no localizing symptoms and may be mistaken for typhoid fever if the routine examination of the urine is neglected. The demonstration of pus in the urine will clear up the diagnosis.

It should be emphasized that a diagnosis of typhoid fever in the infant is not justified, regardless of the course of the fever, unless the positive clinical signs of rose spots, splenic enlargement and abdominal symptoms, or a positive blood culture or agglutination test are present. On the other hand, it is believed by many pediatricians that many febrile attacks of short duration in the young would be proved to be mild or abortive typhoid fever if laboratory methods of diagnosis were more frequently employed.

LABORATORY DIAGNOSIS

"The only certain means of establishing the nature of an infection is the isolation and identification of the causative organism."—HAVENS

Typhoid fever may be diagnosed by laboratory means in all but the exceptionally rare case. When we consider the great variation in symptoms and signs which typhoid fever produces and when we realize the danger that results to others from an unrecognized case, the laboratory diagnosis assumes a matter of supreme importance. The diagnostic laboratory methods in typhoid fever may be grouped in the order of their importance and usefulness and under five heads, as follows:

1. The blood culture.
2. The Widal reaction.
3. The isolation of the organism from the stool.
4. The isolation of the organism from the urine and bile.
5. The blood examination.

Blood Culture.—In the early phases of typhoid and paratyphoid fever the infection is a bacteremia and the causative organism can be isolated from the blood in a high percentage of cases (60 to 90 per cent). It is, however, not uncommon in fevers of doubtful origin to obtain negative blood cultures, especially if they are made after the patient has been ill for over a week. The most favorable period, therefore, to make a blood culture is within the first few days of the onset. Blood cultures have been reported positive in apparently healthy persons even before they showed clinical signs and symptoms of the disease. Persistently positive blood cultures after the first week may be interpreted as a bad prognostic sign.

Of the various possible methods, culture in nutrient broth containing sodium tetrathionate and bile is perhaps the one which will yield the greatest number of positive cultures. Five to 10 cc. of blood drawn under rigid aseptic precautions from a superficial vein is sufficient for the inoculum. It should be carefully added to at least 100 cc. of medium, incubated at 37° C. and examined daily for at least six days. Smears which show gram-negative bacilli and hanging drop preparations which show motile bacilli should be transferred to differential media and identified as outlined for stool cultures.

In cases where blood is sent to the laboratory from an outside source for Widal test, particularly when the stage of the disease is uncertain or unknown, it is a worth-while procedure to comminute the blood clot after removal of the serum for the Widal, and transfer it to nutrient broth containing sodium tetrathionate alone or in combination with brilliant green and bile.

Often these blood clot cultures will be positive, enabling the laboratory to make a positive diagnosis of typhoid fever when the Widal test is negative or questionably positive.

Serial transfers of such cultures over a period of several days are advisable because the media support the growth of the typhoid bacillus while inhibiting the development of contaminants.

The Widal Reaction.—The laboratory diagnosis of typhoid fever by the agglutination test has become complicated by a number of factors, some of which were formerly nonexistent and some not recognized. A clear understanding, however, of these limiting factors should enable any clinician to use this diagnostic test as effectively today as fifteen years ago.

It has become increasingly clear that a diagnosis based on a *single* test is *valueless* except under unusual circumstances. These are: A very high titer (1 : 1,000) of H agglutinins in an *uninoculated* person or an O titer (1 : 250) well above the normal in an uninoculated or not recently inoculated individual. If *repeated* tests are made, preferably at 4-day

40101

intervals between the third and fourth weeks of the illness, there will be an *increase* in O titer in nearly, if not, all positive cases. Any definite *increase* (1:20 to 1:40, 60, 80, etc.) constitutes a positive laboratory diagnosis. No other laboratory evidence, with the exception of isolation of the organisms, is more valid.

The reasons that repeated tests showing an increase in specific agglutinins are so important in making serologic diagnosis are:

1. Twenty per cent of all persons in an area where typhoid fever is endemic will show a positive Widal reaction in a dilution of 1:20 or greater (Havens).

2. Individuals vaccinated with typhoid or typhoid-paratyphoid (T.A.B.) vaccine either recently or remotely may have specific agglutinins in high titers in their serums for both O and H antigens.

3. An unknown number of individuals may have had unrecognized clinical or subclinical typhoid fever and as a result have agglutinins in their serums in significant amounts.

4. Specific agglutinins for typhoid bacilli may be stimulated in individuals by nonspecific stimuli (anamnesic reaction).

Fundamentally, the agglutination test is very simple. Dilutions of the unknown serum are added to suspensions of the organism in the presence of 0.85 per cent salt solution, incubated, and observed for agglutination or clumping of the bacteria into visible aggregates which may or may not settle to the bottom of the tube.

From such a crude technic to those used today the test has run the usual gauntlet of modification and remodification, suiting, as a rule, individual circumstances and fancies. The following graduated pipette method is one recommended by the Standards Laboratory, School of Pathology, University of Oxford, England. The essential features of the test are shown in the following protocol:

Protocol

Tube No.	Unknown Serum	0.85 Per Cent Salt Solution	Suspension	Final Dilution		Results
1	0.4 cc. (1 : 10 dil.)	0.0 cc.	0.6 cc.	1 : 25	Incubate 52°C. {2 hrs. H susp. 18 hrs. O susp.	
2	0.2 cc. "	0.2 cc.	"	1 : 50		
3	0.1 cc. "	0.3 cc.	"	1 : 100		
4	0.4 cc. (1 : 100 dil.)	0.0 cc.	"	1 : 250		
5	0.2 cc. "	0.2 cc.	"	1 : 500		
6	0.1 cc. "	0.3 cc.	"	1 : 1,000		
7	0.4 cc. (1 : 1,000 dil.)	0.0 cc.	"	1 : 2,500		
8	0.2 cc. "	0.2 cc.	"	1 : 5,000		
9	0.1 cc. "	0.3 cc.	"	1 : 10,000		
10	0	0.4 cc.	"			

Glassware:

All glassware should be chemically clean and dry. Agglutination tubes should be uniform in size (0.7 by 9 cm.) and shape. One-cc. and 10-cc. pipettes should be available.

Salt Solution:

Neutral (pH 7.0 to 7.2) 0.85 per cent salt solution is used to make the serum dilutions.

Serum Dilutions:

Three serum dilutions (1:10, 1:100 and 1:1,000) are made in separate test tubes using individual 10-cc. pipettes. The 1:10 dilution is made by adding 1 part of serum to 9 parts of 0.85 per cent salt solution. The 1:100 dilution is made in a similar manner using 1 part of the 1:10 dilution to 9 parts of salt solution. The 1:1,000 dilution is made from the 1:100 dilution. These dilutions are pipetted into agglutination tubes, as indicated in the preceding protocol.

Suspensions:

Suspensions which have been standardized for agglutinability and for turbidity are recommended. These may be obtained from the Standards Laboratory, Oxford, England, or from domestic commercial drug concerns.

Temperature of Incubation:

50 to 52° C. in a water bath is recommended. The level of the water should be maintained so that not more than a third of the contents of the tubes is immersed in water. Convection currents are set up in the tubes which facilitates agglutination.

Duration of Incubation:

H suspensions should be incubated two hours, and O suspensions 16 to 24 hours, before the results are read.

Readings:

Readings are made by comparing each tube in succession with the control tube, and should *always* be made by artificial light against a black background. The highest dilution in which well-marked agglutination (without sedimentation) can be detected by the naked eye is *Standard Agglutination*. This is recorded as $+ +$ agglutination. Agglutination which leaves the supernatant almost completely clear is recorded as $+ + + +$ agglutination.

The Isolation of the Organism from the Stool.—The successful isolation of the organism from stools is dependent on the efficiency of the technic employed. There is little doubt, however, that the type of infection is a factor of some importance. In mild cases of typhoid or paratyphoid fever, such as are frequently seen in individuals well protected by inoculation, the elimination of the bacilli in the stools may be very transient. Typhoid bacilli are difficult to culture from the feces during the first week of disease. They multiply slowly, if at all, in the intestinal tract, and occur there in large numbers only after they have found their way to the gallbladder through the blood stream. In the gallbladder they proliferate freely and from there are discharged into the bowel in large numbers.

Positive cultures in 25 per cent of cases during the first week are high. During the second and third weeks the percentage of positive cultures rapidly rises and after the fourth week slowly diminishes.

Stool specimens should invariably be submitted to the laboratory at the earliest possible moment after they have been passed. The delay of even a few hours reduces the possibility of the successful recovery of the organism. This precaution is particularly necessary in warm climates and its neglect may result in a negative finding when the specimen originally contained large numbers of typhoid or paratyphoid bacilli. Unless the freshly passed specimen can be received immediately in the laboratory, it is imperative that some method of preservation be em-

40101

ployed which prevents the overgrowth of the delicate pathogenic bacteria by the hardy *Escherichia coli* and other saprophytic organisms. The simplest and cheapest method is to emulsify the fresh specimen (1 to to 3 Gm.) in double the volume of sterile 30 per cent glycerin in normal saline solution. The addition of 0.5 per cent lithium chloride will greatly enhance the preservative action of the glycerin because of its marked inhibitory effect on nonpathogenic lactose fermenters. Lithium chloride and bile, and brilliant green bile, are effective preservatives but they require very careful preparation and standardization. The difference in results under most circumstances does not justify the work entailed. Recently it has been shown that ordinary broth containing sodium tetrathionate alone or in combination with brilliant green and bile is a very good preservative medium. Specimens so treated should be subcultured for several days as it is claimed that subcultures may often be positive when the original is negative. This is due to the fact that the medium progressively favors the growth of the pathogens while restricting the saprophytes.

Fresh specimens and preserved specimens are treated alike in the laboratory. They are plated on differential media. The underlying principle of the many differential media designed for the isolation of these *E. typhosae* depends upon the fact that they do not ferment lactose, whereas the coliform bacteria split this sugar to an acid and a gas. In all of these media, therefore, lactose is incorporated with an indicator so that the organisms producing acid form colonies that can be readily distinguished by their color from colonies of nonlactose fermenters.

A large variety of such differential media are available for choice. Endo's agar, MacConkey's bile salt agar, and Wilson and Blair's bismuth sulfite agar stand out as being the most serviceable. All have some disadvantages; the careful worker uses two or even three in order to minimize the chances of missing a positive culture.

Endo's agar (peptone 10 Gm., lactose 10 Gm., dipotassium phosphate 3.5 Gm., agar 15 Gm., sodium sulfite 2.5 Gm., basic fuchsin 0.5 Gm. in 1,000 cc. distilled water) is probably the most widely used. On it colonies of *E. typhosa* appear as clear, colorless, glistening drops against the faint pink background of the medium, while colonies of *E. coli* become red and also color the surrounding medium.

MacConkey's agar (bile salts 5 Gm., lactose 10 Gm., agar 15 Gm., peptone 20 Gm., neutral red 0.05 Gm., water 1,000 cc.) supports the growth of all members of the typhoid-paratyphoid-dysentery groups, differentiating them from the lactose-fermenting organisms. Gram-positive bacteria are inhibited. The non-lactose-fermenting types do not greatly alter the appearance of the medium. Colonies of *E. typhosa*, giving a mild alkaline reaction, are uncolored and transparent, and change the color of the medium to yellow, while colonies of *E. coli* appear red and opaque.

Wilson and Blair's bismuth sulfite agar inhibits growth of the lactose fermenters, while *E. typhosa* grows well. The typical colony is black surrounded by a brownish-black zone, and exhibits a metallic sheen when viewed by reflected light. *S. schottmülleri* (paratyphoid bacillus B) has colonial characteristics essentially the same as *E. typhosa*. *S. paratyphi* (paratyphoid bacillus A) colonies appear as small, light green colonies. Occasional colonies of the coli-aerogenes group may grow. *Escherichia coli* will appear as small black, brown or greenish glistening colonies, and *Aerobacter aerogenes* produces raised mucoid colonies exhibiting a grayish-brown sheen, appreciably lighter in color than that produced by typhoid bacilli. Cultures on Wilson and Blair's medium should be incubated at least forty-eight hours, although satisfactory growth may appear in twenty-four hours.

Other Differential Media: Drigalski-Conradi agar (peptone 10 Gm., iso-electric casein 10 Gm., lactose 10 Gm., agar 15 Gm., NaCl 5 Gm., bromcresol purple 0.3 Gm., crystal violet 0.004 Gm. to a liter) is another differential medium used for the isolation of gram-negative bacteria from contaminated material such as feces, water, etc.

Crystal violet in a dilution of 1 to 250,000 inhibits quite generally development of gram-positive organisms, while having no appreciable effect on gram-negative bacteria. Bromcresol purple is an indicator sensitive to slight changes in reaction, serving to separate the lactose-fermenting from the non-lactose-fermenting organisms.

On this medium *E. typhosa* colonies are transparent, blue-white, while colonies of lactose-fermenting organisms are red and opaque and the immediately surrounding medium is turned red or bluish.

Holt, Harris and Teague's eosin-methylene blue agar (Witte's peptone 10 Gm., dibasic sodium phosphate 2 Gm., agar 15 Gm., 2 per cent eosin 2 cc., 2 per cent methylene blue 0.5 cc. to make 1 liter), used in differentiating lactose-fermenting from non-lactose-fermenting organisms, gives a sharp color change upon fermentation of lactose. Typhoid colonies are colorless, while *E. coli* colonies are opaque, black and iridescent.

All colonies which give the slightest indication of not promptly fermenting lactose, regardless of the medium used, should be regarded with suspicion. They are picked and transplanted to media designed for identification. Russell's double-sugar slants are most frequently used. Russell's double-sugar agar slants (beef extract 3 Gm., peptone 10 Gm., lactose 10 Gm., dextrose 10 Gm., sodium chloride 0.5 Gm., agar 15 Gm., phenol red 0.025 Gm. per 1,000 cc.) serve to differentiate typhoid bacilli from paratyphoid A and B bacilli and other members of the enteric fever group because of their failure to ferment dextrose. *E. typhosa* produces a pink coloration of the butt and is colorless on the slant, producing no gas. *S. paratyphi* and *S. schottmülleri* and *S. enteritidis* all produce gas.

Lead acetate agar (tryptone 20 Gm., dextrose 1 Gm., lead acetate 12 Gm., agar 15 Gm. per 1,000 cc. distilled water) serves to differentiate *S. schottmülleri* from *S. paratyphi* and *S. enteritidis*. *S. schottmülleri* turns the medium brown, while the other two do not. The separation of *S. paratyphi* and *S. enteritidis* is based on agglutination tests.

Serologic Identification.—With the exception of certain strains, to which reference is given below, the serologic confirmation by the agglutination test of *E. typhosa* and *S. paratyphi* usually presents no difculty. It is necessary only to determine that the suspension of one or the other of these organisms is agglutinated to approximately the titer of their respective antiserums. (Such serums are available commercially.) In the case of *S. schottmülleri* and *S. hirschfeldi* (paratyphoid bacillus C), however, complexity is introduced by the fact that the serum prepared against these organisms also agglutinates the allied members of the Salmonella group of bacilli. In this connection confusion is most likely to arise between these strains of paratyphoid bacilli and *S. typhi murium* (*S. aertrycke*). Differentiation can, however, be effected by means of the agglutinin absorption test. Certain fallacies, such as inagglutinability, spontaneous agglutination, coagglutination, and paraagglutination must be borne in mind when investigating the identity of these bacteria by the agglutination test.

The identification of other non-lactose-fermenting bacteria causing continued fevers and dysenteries is very difficult and requires the knowledge and ability of a trained and disciplined bacteriologist. It involves cultivation on various carbohydrate broths, peptone water, tartrate and citrate agar and, in most instances, very careful agglutinin absorption tests with individually prepared H and O suspensions of each unknown organism.

The Isolation of the Organism from the Urine and Bile.—If the patient is in a hospital and the urine may be obtained under aseptic conditions, it may be planted directly to the differential media without first inoculating it into one of the nutrient selective media.

In making the inoculations it is wise to use dilutions from 1:10,000 to 1:1,000,000 on several plates. This enables one to get isolated colonies so that typical differentiating characteristics may develop. If the urine is brought to the laboratory in a nonsterile container, inoculation first into nutrient broth, with sodium tetrathionate alone or in combination with bile or brilliant green added, and incubated overnight should be the procedure.

The cultivation of the *B. typhosus* from the gallbladder offers no difficulty. If there, it is usually present in pure culture, and inoculation of differential media may be done without preliminaries. Forsbeck and Hollon have shown that *E. typhosa* dies rapidly in a mixture of acid gastric juice and bile.

The Blood Examination.—Typhoid fever produces a rapid and rather marked anemia. There is evidence, ascertained at autopsy, of red cell destruction. Usually the hemoglobin and the red cell count fall, but often a severe diarrhea causes the apparent cell count to remain constant on account of loss of fluid. There is not a profound hemolysis as in streptococcus infections, with the development of hemolytic icterus, but a more gradually progressive anemia throughout the disease. Added to the red cell destruction, as evidenced by the intense pigmentation of the spleen found at autopsy, there is undoubtedly a defective formation of blood cells due to the bone marrow injury.

The most characteristic findings are the leukopenia and absence of eosinophils manifested as soon as the disease is well established. For the first few days we may have a mild leukocytosis up to 12,000 per c.mm., but very soon the total white cell count drops to 5,000 or less, with a relatively great diminution of the polymorphonuclears and a relative increase in the number of large lymphocytes. This sudden marked diminution of leukocytes in a febrile affection is restricted to typhoid, miliary tuberculosis, tuberculous peritonitis, malaria, colon bacillus pyelitis and influenza; but it is more regularly of value as a diagnostic aid in typhoid than in any of the other diseases. This phenomenon is very valuable in differential diagnosis. Cases of typhoid fever often have an onset strongly suggestive of acute inflammatory conditions in the abdomen, such as cholecystitis and appendicitis, and the blood count here is of great assistance. The condition which resembles typhoid fever more closely than any other, perhaps, is miliary tuberculosis with beginning meningeal involvement. In this disease a moderate leukocytosis is the rule. Army experience has shown that typhoid vaccination gives rise at times to acute abdominal pain and vomiting, closely simulating appendicitis, clinically, and here again the blood count prevents many unnecessary operations. On the other hand, the tendency of typhoid vaccination to light up slumbering infections is well known, and some of these cases following typhoid vaccination are true appendicitis and need prompt surgical intervention. The blood count usually decides this point, but it should be remembered that a sharp rise in the number of leukocytes may appear as a result of the vaccine injection. J. Wheeler Smith, Jr., showed that an average leukocytosis of from 11,000 to 12,000 per c.mm. was the rule within twenty-four hours of an antityphoid vaccination.

The blood count may also be valuable in giving warning of intercurrent pneumonia due to other organisms than the typhoid bacillus, although the response is usually not so decisive as in primary pneumonia. Perforation usually does not stimulate a leukocytosis in typhoid fever proportionate to the severity of the peritonitis, and the leukocyte increase following hemorrhage is feeble.

The depression of the leukocyte count in typhoid fever is probably due to the involvement of the bone marrow with multiple focal necroses first described by Longcope.

Examination of the Stool.—The stool in typhoid fever is usually of the thin, watery variety. Sometimes considerable free fat is recognizable, due to the diarrhea accompanying a diet containing a large proportion of milk. After the diagnosis of typhoid fever has been made, the stools should be examined daily for the presence of occult blood. A strong occult blood reaction gives warning of bleeding from the bases of the intestinal ulcerations, and measures may be instituted to ward off more serious hemorrhage. The daily occult blood test of typhoid stools should be routine, at least in hospital practice. There are several good methods of procedure. One of the simplest of the reliable methods is the modification of the benzidine test as described by Warren Vaughan.

A quantity of stool equal to about 0.5 Gm. is placed on a white card, as, for instance, a calling card, and to this a few drops of equal parts of freshly prepared glacial acetic acid solution of benzidine and hydrogen peroxide are added. A strong reaction shows a brilliant blue, fading off to pale green shades for smaller traces of blood. This method is quick of execution, and there is no glassware to be cleaned up afterward, because the white card is thrown away and incinerated. If one is not certain of a fresh, active hydrogen peroxide reagent a more certain test is the benzidine perborate test of Dudley Roberts, furnished in tablet form ready for use by Squibb & Sons. The tablets contain benzidine and sodium perborate. The tablet is moistened with the specimen to be examined and a drop of glacial acetic acid is added. The tablet turns blue or green in the presence of blood.

The bacteriologic examination of the stool in typhoid may have either of two purposes. First, it may be used as a method of finally clinching the diagnosis in a case where attempts at blood culture have been made too late in the course of the fever. Second, and most important, is the application of the bacteriologic examination of the stool in convalescent cases, to determine when it is safe to discharge patients and to allow them to mingle freely with the population at large. Nothing is plainer from the point of view of public health than that negative stools should be required before discharging a typhoid patient, just as negative throat cultures are required in diphtheria. If this practice were efficiently carried out the importance of protecting the water supplies would be correspondingly lessened.

40101

The methods for the detection of *Eberthella typhosa* in stools are fully detailed above. They are not difficult, with a little experience, but require a fairly well equipped laboratory. In private practice the stool samples may be collected in screw-capped sputum bottles, such as are used for mailing sputum samples, and sent to distant laboratories for examination. Teague and Clurman have pointed out that while the typhoid bacillus tends to be overgrown and to disappear from old samples of stool which are not examined promptly after being passed, the addition of 30 per cent glycerin to the sample preserves the typhoid bacillus and allows the examination of the specimen after several days. One part of stool is thoroughly mixed with 2 parts of 30 per cent glycerin, prepared by adding glycerin to sterile 0.6 per cent sodium chloride solution. As already mentioned, the chance of isolating the *Bacillus typhosus* from the stool is greatest in the third week of the disease, except that Krumwiede reports that in paratyphoid A infections the successes are greatest during the first week. It should be remembered that paratyphoid A has a greater resistance to brilliant green than the other members of the series, and Krumwiede reports the examination of a regiment for paratyphoid carriers where the brilliant green agar was directly standardized against the known offending strain, thus greatly lessening the labor of several hundred examinations.

Urinary Findings.—The characteristic urinary finding of typhoid fever is typhoid bacilluria. Havens found it positive on one culture in 33 per cent of the cases. It is, therefore, important diagnostic evidence though a negative finding does not rule out typhoid.

COMPLICATIONS AND SEQUELAE

Typhoid fever is remarkable for the number, variety and gravity of its complications. Practically every organ and tissue in the body may be the seat of secondary pathologic processes that tend to increase the severity of the illness, prolong its course and add to its danger. Complications, mild or severe, occur in from 25 to 30 per cent of all cases, and are responsible for from 60 to 75 per cent of all fatalities from the disease. Many of the conditions described as complications may develop late in the convalescent period or at varying times after recovery from the primary infection appears to be complete. When developing in this way these conditions may properly be classed as sequelae. To save repetition, complications and sequelae have been considered together.

Among the important diseases which may develop as sequelae to typhoid fever are thrombophlebitis, arterial thrombosis, chronic myocarditis, arterial sclerosis and arterial hypertension; pulmonary tuberculosis and pulmonary gangrene; perichondritis, osteoperiostitis and osteomyelitis; peripheral neuritis, hemiplegia and the posttyphoid psychoses; chronic derangements of digestion, prolonged or permanent impairment of nutrition, and anemia.

THE SKIN

The specific eruption of typhoid fever has been described under "Symptomatology." A number of cutaneous lesions may complicate the disease.

Erythema.—A scarlatiniform erythema is occasionally seen in the first week, preceding the eruption of the rose rash. It is of special interest at this stage, because of the possibility of mistaking it for the rash of scarlatina. It appears as a delicate scarlet rash limited to the flexor surfaces, or spread over the entire skin. The eruption fades in a day or two and may be followed by a fine desquamation. In severe toxic cases a diffuse erythema may appear in the third week and, as Phillips has shown, a large number of the reported cases showing this symptom have terminated fatally. Phillips saw one case of erythema multiforme, and Osler has reported a case of erythema nodosum appearing on the fifteenth day. A case with a morbilliform rash without the catarrhal symptoms was seen by Beevor on the third day and another by Newman in the third week.

Desquamation.—Desquamation of the skin is rather frequent. It may follow an erythema or sudamina, or it may result from trophic changes in cases with high fever. Some remarkable cases of peeling of extensive areas of the skin without apparent cause have been reported.

Sudamina.—Retention of minute drops of perspiration in the epithelial layer of the skin is common in the third and fifth weeks in cases with profuse perspiration. The eruption is most marked over the chest and abdomen. The skin appears to be covered with a multitude of droplets of water. Desquamation follows. The experience of Phillips confirms the observation of De Lacaze that the appearance of sudamina in the third week ushers in the period of convalescence.

Herpes.—Herpes is a rare skin manifestation in typhoid, in marked contrast to the frequency of the lesion in pneumonia and malaria. Different observers have noted it in the first week in 1 or 2 per cent of cases. Herpes is characteristically present in typhoid complicated by meningitis. *Urticaria* is also a rare condition dependent in some cases upon drug administration. A pemphigoid eruption of several small or large blebs is occasionally seen.

Purpura.—In the third or fourth week, in severe cases, purpuric spots may develop over the abdomen or lower extremities, sometimes following intestinal or other hemorrhage. Superficial sloughing of the skin over the hemorrhagic area has been reported. More extensive *gangrene* may occur in the case of greatly debilitated individuals.

Erysipelas.—Erysipelas is a rare complication of the period of decline. It runs the usual course, and is not necessarily a serious complication. The typhoid bacillus has been found in the affected skin.

Pus Infections.—Pus infections of the skin are quite common in the period of decline and in early convalescence. Impetigo, furunculosis, carbuncles, onychia and superficial abscess are the usual forms. Furunculosis is the most frequent. The lesions are very painful and troublesome and are often the cause of recrudescence of the pyrexia. They develop most frequently on the back and buttocks. Edsall observed a limited outbreak in the Pennsylvania Hospital, apparently due to bed pan contagion. The streptococcus and the staphylococcus are the usual infecting organisms.

Lineae Atrophicae.—In young subjects particularly, lines of atrophy similar to those seen on the abdomen after pregnancy are occasionally seen. They occur over the abdomen, on the outer aspect of the thighs, around the ankles and above and below the patella. Phillips and others have described this condition under the term "stria patellaris." The lesions involve the true skin and leave permanent scars.

40101

Bed Sores.—Modern care of fever patients has made bed sores infrequent. They occur, however, in hospitals where good nursing is the rule in about 1 per cent of the cases. A certain number result from neglect before admission. The usual cause is unrelieved pressure upon the tissues over a bony prominence. Development of the lesion is favored by soiled skin and clothing. The enforced quiet following a severe hemorrhage may be a determining factor. The common bed sore is, therefore, usually preventable by cleanliness and proper nursing technic. Sores occur as a late complication in severe cases with great emaciation. They are most frequently seen in the sacral and gluteal regions where pressure is greatest and most continuous and where the skin is soiled by the excretions. The elbows, heels and the scapular region are less frequent sites. The sore begins with a persistent area of circumscribed redness over the most prominent points of the sacral region. Unless it is promptly arrested the epidermis is eroded, the deeper layers of the skin are exposed, and a superficial slough forms, with a line of demarcation. In the more severe cases the process continues, and extensive destruction of soft tissue and bone may result. In severely toxic cases with profound disturbance of nutrition the subcutaneous type of bed sore, as it is termed by Curschmann, may develop, even with the most scrupulous care of the patient. In this author's experience it usually occurs in the lower sacral region in the depth of the anal fold. The process is a subcutaneous necrosis with suppurative softening of the connective tissue. It may become extensive before it is revealed to the attendant by alterations in the appearance of the skin.

Perspiration.—Perspiration is unusual during the period of high fever. In the period of decline and in convalescence it is quite common. In the second or third week paroxysms of chill, fever and perspiration may occur and arouse suspicion of malaria or sepsis. Hemorrhage and other complications of this period may be attended by profuse perspiration.

The Hair.—A temporary alopecia occurs after all attacks of severity, and the nails show ridges after convalescence, due to impaired nutrition. Very rarely is the baldness permanent.

DIGESTIVE SYSTEM

Mouth.—The salivary secretion is diminished and the tongue and mouth become dry in proportion to the height of the fever and the intensity of the toxemia. Without scrupulous care the tongue, lips and gums become covered with dry, brown masses of sordes. Painful cracks and fissures may form on the tongue and lips. In neglected cases flakes of thrush or a thin pseudomembrane may form on the mucous surfaces. The septic mouth may be the center for the extension of secondary infections to the parotid glands, pharynx or middle ears. Stomatitis with superficial ulceration is not infrequent under these circumstances. A circumscribed gangrene has been observed. An acute glossitis occurred at the onset of a relapse in one of Osler's series.

Parotid Gland.—Parotitis is an occasional complication in the third or fourth week or a sequel in severe protracted cases. It is due to an ascending infection from an oral sepsis to the glands through Steno's duct. In 12,173 cases collected by McCrae, parotitis occurred in 0.7

per cent. The staphylococcus is the most common infecting organism. The typhoid bacillus in pure culture was isolated from a parotid abscess by Schudnot and Blachos. The inflammation is usually unilateral, although both parotids may be infected. The infection may be mild in character or of intense virulence. The gland rapidly becomes swollen, tense and painful. A chill with a sharp increase of fever may mark the onset. Resolution without suppuration takes place in a majority of the cases. Suppuration, when it occurs, begins at the proximal end of Steno's duct and extends peripherally. The abscess may point on the face or in the external auditory canal or it may open into the mouth by way of the duct. It may burrow to the pharynx or along the great vessels of the neck into the mediastinum. Necrosis of part of the gland may occur. If suppuration impends an early incision is necessary. Parotitis is a serious complication of typhoid chiefly because it is a complication of the severe toxic cases. Reported cases show a mortality of about 30 per cent.

Pharynx.—Occasionally pharyngitis and tonsillitis dominate the clinical picture of the onset of typhoid fever and conceal the true nature of the infection. Patches of thin pseudomembrane may appear on the mucous surface, and in rare cases small, superficial ulcers have been noted on the pillars and tonsils. The typhoid bacillus has been recovered from these lesions. Pharyngitis with the same manifestations may complicate the later stage of the disease. Ouskow, cited by Hare, found evidence of pharyngitis in a majority of 439 cases coming to autopsy. Rarely invasion of the cervical lymph nodes and connective tissue by a secondary infection may occur, with great swelling and induration of the neck. It may terminate in resolution or in suppuration.

Esophagus.—Inflammatory lesions similar to those in the pharynx may be found in the esophagus. Louis and other early writers found ulceration of the esophagus of frequent occurrence. Modern observers have found it rare. Packard reviewed 5,000 cases, none of which showed ulceration. More recent literature contains descriptions of a number of cases. Baer cites 10 cases in a collection of 83 cases of typhoid with ulceration in unusual sites. In 59 autopsies in Johns Hopkins Hospital esophageal ulceration occurred in one case. In one fatal case observed by the late author (C. G. J.), showing persistent hiccup for several days before death, an ulcer 2 cm. in diameter was found in the esophagus, 4 cm. above the cardiac orifice. Streptococci and staphylococci are the organisms found associated with the ulceration. The typhoid bacillus has not been demonstrated. It seems probable that esophageal lesions are late results of oral sepsis.

Ulceration of the esophagus causes no symptoms that make it recognizable during life. Dysphagia, hiccup, and possibly hematemesis are suggestive.

Stricture of the esophagus is a very rare complication or sequela of typhoid. James F. Mitchell describes one case in Osler's series and quotes two others; one reported by Packard and the other by Summers, of Omaha.

Stomach.—Anorexia is the rule in typhoid fever. The secretory and motor functions of the stomach are greatly reduced. The digestive ferments are present in reduced amount and free hydrochloric acid is either absent or the percentage is reduced. Vomiting is decidedly the

40101

exception, both at the onset and during the course. Severe and persistent vomiting is an occasional complication of the first week. Vomiting may take place after the period of onset from indigestion or overfeeding, but it is so unusual that it should always suggest the possibility of some complication. Nephritis, appendicitis or perforation may be announced by vomiting. Hiccup is rare. The late author (C. G. J.) has noted it in one severe case, in which it was apparently a symptom of an ulcer in the esophagus at the cardiac end. It is also a symptom of perforation. Hematemesis, usually from a gastric ulcer, is a rare complication. The stomach may be involved in cases with severe meteorism.

Intestines.—Diarrhea, one of the characteristic symptoms of typhoid fever, may attain such severity as to constitute a complication. In the local outbreaks from water infection before mentioned, all of the 56 cases were complicated during the period of incubation and onset by severe gastro-enteritis. Since the water ingested was heavily contaminated by sewage, the diarrhea may have resulted from infection by one of the members of the Salmonella group other than the typhoid bacillus. In many of the cases the diarrhea was replaced by constipation after a few days of fever. In others it persisted throughout the whole febrile period. Two, at most three, loose movements a day are the limit for the normal course of typhoid. From four to ten or even a larger number may take place in severe cases. This excessive diarrhea may be due only to the specific ulceration in the ileum. An ileocolitis is the usual condition underlying a severe diarrhea.

HEMORRHAGE.—In 829 cases of typhoid fever reported by Osler from Johns Hopkins Hospital there were 50 cases with intestinal hemorrhage, representing 6 per cent. McCrae's later report from the same hospital gives 1,500 cases in which 118 cases of hemorrhage occurred, or 7.8 per cent. In 23,271 cases collected by McCrae, hemorrhage occurred in 7 per cent. Typhoid fever developing in vaccinated subjects shows a remarkable reduction in the incidence of hemorrhage, as of other complications. In the series reported by Lieut. Col. Webb-Johnson of the British Army, hemorrhage occurred in but 10 out of 821 vaccinated cases, representing 1.21 per cent, and in 40 out of 297 unvaccinated cases, or 13.46 per cent. The percentage incidence is much lower in children and up to the thirtieth year, and reaches a maximum from the forty-fifth to the fifty-fifth year. Insignificant bleedings manifestly due to hemorrhoids or fissures should not be classed with the hemorrhage which has its origin in the specific bowel lesions of typhoid fever.

The complication occurs most frequently in the second and third weeks of the disease, rarely before the seventh day. Approximately 20 per cent occur in the fourth, and 10 per cent in the fifth week. After this time hemorrhage is very unusual. It is a rare complication of relapse. The incidence of hemorrhage bears no relation to the severity of the disease. It occurs as often in the mild as in the severe cases. In the mild ambulatory cases it may be the first symptom to warn the patient that he has a serious illness. The hemorrhage may be single or several attacks may occur at varying intervals. The amount of blood in the discharge varies from a few cubic centimeters to a liter or more. In small hemorrhages the blood is mixed with the feces and is dark red or black in color, the characteristic tarry stool of an upper intestinal hemorrhage. With a profuse hemorrhage, quickly expelled, bright red blood may be passed in the fluid state or in clots. When a considerable interval elapses between the bleeding and the expulsion of the blood from the bowel, the blood appears in dark, altered clots.

The blood in small hemorrhages and in the early stage of the disease may come from intensely congested Peyer's patches and from other areas in the intestines. In later hemorrhages the necrotic and ulcerated Peyer's patch is the source of the bleeding. Gay believes that the peculiar anatomic arrangement of the blood vessels supplying Peyer's patches, as demonstrated by Professor Evans, of Berkeley, accounts for the profuse hemorrhage that may come from an ulcerated Peyer's patch. Straight, unbranched arterioles radiate from all sides into the patch, and an erosion near the margin may open up simultaneously a large number of these vessels. Hemorrhage has been attributed to a variety of exciting causes. Injudicious feeding with solid food, tympanites, or physical exertion would quite probably precipitate an impending hemorrhage. It has sometimes followed immediately after the administration of a bath or an enema.

A small hemorrhage causes no subjective symptoms. A single large hemorrhage, or a succession of small hemorrhages quickly repeated, is indicated by the usual symptoms of a sudden large loss of blood. The patient feels faint, the face pales, the skin becomes cool and moist, the pulse rapid, small and weak, and the temperature suddenly falls. Vomiting may occur. The drop in temperature may be from two to six degrees or more. The late author (C. G. J.) has seen it fall from 105 to 96° F. (40.6 to 35.6° C.) and remain at this low point for several hours. Occasionally abdominal pain precedes the bleeding. These symptoms may be present for some little time before the blood is passed from the bowel. The systolic blood pressure falls to 80 or 90 mm. Hg or lower. McCrae observed the very low pressure of 55 mm. Hg in one case. The hemoglobin content and red cell count of the blood are low in proportion to the severity of the hemorrhage. A leukocytosis often follows the hemorrhage. From a detailed study of this condition, Thayer concludes that "intestinal hemorrhage in typhoid may exercise little or no apparent influence on the number of leukocytes in the peripheral circulation. Often, however, there is a tendency toward a leukocytosis which begins immediately after the hemorrhage, reaching its maximum in from twelve to twenty-four hours. In from one or two days to a week, the number of leukocytes generally returns to the normal number for the period of the disease."

The effect of the hemorrhage upon the course of the disease will depend upon the amount of blood lost and upon the condition of the patient at the time of the hemorrhage. Strong, robust patients endure the loss of blood well. Indeed, some observers believe that a moderate bleeding may have a beneficial influence upon the subsequent course of the disease. Gay has suggested that the hyperleukocytosis mentioned above may account for the improvement.

In patients otherwise seriously ill the effect of severe hemorrhage is bad, and is often the determining factor in a rapidly fatal issue. In cases which recover, the severe anemia predisposes to a complicated and tedious convalescence.

Hemorrhage is a serious complication and always causes apprehension. The statistics from various sources give a mortality rate varying all the way from 10 to 30 per cent. Without accurate data the cases in the late author's (C. G. J.) personal experience have shown a percentage very near the low figure.

PERFORATION.—The incidence of perforation in several series of cases reported by observers in this country and Europe varies from 2 to 6 per cent. In a total of 34,916 cases summed up by McCrae perforation occurred in 3.1 per cent. Antityphoid vaccination markedly reduces the percentage. In Webb-Johnson's series of 821 vaccinated cases perforation occurred in only 0.36 per cent, while in the 297 unvaccinated cases it occurred in 2.02 per cent. It is more frequently seen in men than in women. In 661 cases in which sex incidence was noted, 471, or 71 per cent, occurred in men. It is unusual in patients over forty years of age. The complication is generally spoken of as rare in children, although among 1,550 cases of typhoid fever in children collected by Adams there were 17 cases of perforation, representing 1.09 per cent. Of 1,028 cases compiled by Holt, 12 cases of perforation were found, or 1.1 per cent.

Cases with severe general symptoms give the highest percentage, although in mild and moderately severe cases it is almost as great. In 444 cases collected by Fitz, 200 were mild or moderately severe and 14 cases belonged to the ambulatory type.

Statistics from England, Canada and the United States show that perforation is responsible for one third of all the deaths from typhoid fever.

Perforation, like hemorrhage, is a complication of the later weeks of the disease. It is very unusual before the tenth day. Accurate figures by Fitz of 193 cases show: first week, 4 cases; second week, 32 cases; third week, 48 cases; fourth week, 42 cases; fifth week, 27 cases; sixth week, 21 cases; seventh week, 5 cases; eighth week, 3 cases; ninth week, 2 cases; tenth week, 4 cases; eleventh week, 3 cases; twelfth and sixteenth weeks, 1 case each

The immediate cause of the perforation is the ulceration and necrosis of the intestine. It cannot be foretold or prevented. The final break in the bowel wall, however, may be precipitated by excessive tympanites, an attack of indigestion, vomiting, or physical exertion. These accessory causes are more or less under control.

Symptoms of Perforation.—The possibility of perforation should be constantly in the mind of the physician during the stage of intestinal ulceration. Careful inspection of the abdomen should be a part of the daily routine examination, and the attendants should be instructed to be on the alert for symptoms suggestive of rupture.

While the onset is usually without premonitory symptoms, certain objective and subjective symptoms may be forerunners of the accident. Hemorrhage, unusual abdominal pain and tenderness, distention or vomiting may have significance, and should put the physician on his guard. In certain cases a localized peritonitis at the site of an underlying ulcer sometimes causes pain, tenderness and leukocytosis, which may continue for two or three days before the bowel perforates. This condition has been termed by Harvey Cushing the "preperforative stage of ulceration." As in a case reported by him, these symptoms may disguise a perforation when it actually occurs and lead to unfortunate delay in diagnosis.

(a) *Sudden Onset.*—Sudden, severe pain in the abdomen, tenderness, rigidity, vomiting, collapse and rapid pulse are the initial symptoms,

In a few hours general peritonitis develops. The abdomen becomes more distended, pain and tenderness become general over the abdomen, the temperature rises, the pulse becomes small and very rapid, respiration increased and thoracic in character. A cold, clammy perspiration covers the surface, the face is pale and pinched, and the patient rapidly sinks. Consciousness may be retained to the end.

(b) *Insidious Onset.*—The symptoms of perforation may develop gradually. The perforation may be small and the escape of the intestinal contents slow. There may be but little pain and the symptoms of general peritonitis may be latent or absent. In 76 cases mentioned by Fitz the onset in 15 was gradual or latent, and in 5 cases there were no signs of perforation. Dieulafoy's experience led him to state that peritonitis from perforation very rarely announces itself acutely with pain and marked constitutional symptoms. In severely toxic cases with severe diarrhea, abdominal distention and profound nervous symptoms, perforation may occur and be revealed only at autopsy.

The relative frequency of the so-called characteristic symptoms of perforation is noted by Finney in 112 operated cases. "Sudden and severe abdominal pain was present in 58 cases; collapse, more or less severe, in 15 cases; nausea and vomiting in 26 cases; a marked fall in temperature in 14. In 9 of the cases the symptoms denoting perforation were not marked and came on gradually. In 5 of the cases only, was the absence of liver-dullness noted."

The *pain* is continuous or may be intermittent or colicky in character. It is usually referred to the right lower quadrant of the abdomen as general peritonitis develops. Or, like the pain of appendicitis, it may be general at first and then localized in the right lower quadrant. A referred pain in the left lower quadrant has been noted. The pain may be most intense about the navel. During the paroxysms the pain may be referred to the pubis, and with it there may be vesical irritability.

Tenderness and rigidity are emphatic symptoms, and in the first few hours are most marked in the right lower quadrant. As general peritonitis develops, the whole abdomen becomes tense and tender. More or less abdominal distention quickly follows and the liver dullness may be obliterated. Occasionally the abdomen becomes retracted, with rigid walls. Rectal examination should always be made.

Nausea and vomiting are quite constant symptoms immediately following the perforation. Vomiting is so rare during the perforation period of typhoid fever that it should always arouse the suspicion of this accident. *Hiccup* may be present at this time, but it is more frequent and persistent later.

The *pulse* quickly changes with the onset of the pain. It becomes rapid and small, and this quality persists regardless of fluctuations in the temperature. In exceptional cases the pulse rate is unchanged until the onset of general peritonitis. A rise of *blood pressure* often follows the perforation. In obscure cases this finding may be of value in the differentiation from hemorrhage. *Respiration* is quickened, shallow and thoracic in character.

A sudden, marked drop in the *temperature* is often a striking feature of perforation. The fall in temperature may immediately follow the perforation, or it may come later after an initial rise of one or two degrees. The collapse noted at the onset, with cold, moist skin, may be

40101

associated with a rise of the central temperature. A chill is a not infrequent initial phenomenon. With the development of general peritonitis the temperature shows the usual variability observed in this condition from any cause.

The *leukocyte count* is of great interest and may be of conclusive importance in diagnosis. A knowledge of the leukocyte content of the blood previous to perforation is necessary for a proper evaluation of the findings. With this knowledge even a moderate leukocytosis is of great significance. Usually an increased count follows the perforation. The number of leukocytes rises, rapidly reaching from 10,000 to 15,000 or higher in a few hours. With the development of general peritonitis a sharp fall often takes place, due to the great outpour of leukocytes into the peritoneal cavity. This fall may take place within three or four hours after the perforation, a fact which emphasizes the necessity of hourly counts when perforation is suspected. In some cases no change in the leukocyte count takes place.

Diagnosis of Perforation.—The diagnosis of perforation in typhoid fever may be very easy or extremely difficult. With a large perforation and copious extravasation into the peritoneal cavity the signs and symptoms of an acute abdomen are emphatic and unmistakable. With small perforations, and especially in the case of patients whose sensations are blunted by profound typhoid toxemia, the symptoms may be vague and misleading. Prompt recognition of the condition is so imperative that in doubtful cases every aid to diagnosis must immediately be sought. A few hours' hesitation may remove even the moderate hope which early surgical interference offers. The two most valuable symptoms for diagnosis are pain and rigidity. The less sudden the pain is in its development and the less severe it is, the greater the difficulty in diagnosis.

A number of abdominal conditions may simulate perforation. *Hemorrhage* may resemble it very closely. The sudden fall in blood pressure and the anemia are distinctive of hemorrhage; abdominal pain, tenderness and rigidity are not so marked as in perforation. The coincident occurrence of hemorrhage and perforation presents a most difficult situation.

Iliac phlebitis may be recognized by tenderness along the course of the veins extending down the thigh and accompanied by swelling.

Appendicitis gives the same clinical picture as perforation and cannot be certainly differentiated. Practically this is of little importance as the surgical indication is the same in both conditions. *Acute intestinal obstruction* from any cause may be very difficult to differentiate.

The various conditions previously mentioned which excite abdominal pain may arouse the suspicion of perforation. A small localized peritonitis may be especially puzzling. These conditions demand careful study. The absence of pulse and temperature changes and grave general symptoms of perforation are of diagnostic importance. Except in the cases of local peritonitis a low white blood cell count is a valuable sign. The great difficulty in diagnosis in these cases is clearly shown by the fact that in suspected perforation the abdomen has been opened in our best hospitals, after careful study by the ablest clinicians, and no adequate cause for the symptoms found. Such exploration, in doubtful cases and after full consideration, is justified.

Peritonitis not the result of perforation is a rare complication, usually occurring during the third week of the disease. It may result from the rupture of a softened mesenteric gland or of an abscess in any of the abdominal or pelvic organs. Migration of organisms through the intestinal wall without gross lesions seems to be the only explanation in a number of reported cases. Sudden onset with pain, tenderness, rigidity and distention is the rule. Differentiation from peritonitis due to intestinal perforation is impossible. Without operation the result is uniformly fatal.

Results of Perforation.—A number of cases of recovery following the characteristic symptoms of perforation have been reported. In how many of these cases perforation actually took place must remain in doubt. The question is well answered by Fitz. ''Since perforation of the intestine in typhoid fever may take place without any suggestive symptoms, and since suggestive, even so-called characteristic, symptoms may occur without any perforation having taken place, it must be admitted that recovery from such symptoms is not satisfactory evidence of recovery from perforation.'' Still, recovery from perforation without abscess formation must be admitted as possible. Several such cases have been verified by subsequent operation or autopsy findings.

In rare cases the peritonitis is localized and an abscess forms similar to the localized abscess which follows perforative appendicitis. Recovery may follow surgical drainage, or the abscess may discharge externally or into one of the hollow viscera. This is most likely to occur if the perforation involves a relatively quiet sector of the abdomen like the appendix region.

In the great majority of cases, general peritonitis follows perforation and, unless relieved by laparotomy, proves rapidly fatal. Death occurs, according to Fitz, in over 37 per cent on the first day following perforation, in over 29 per cent on the second day and in over 83 per cent of all cases during the first week. Even with prompt surgical interference the outlook is grave. Only about 20 per cent recover. This is a high mortality, but with the prospect of an almost certain fatal result without laparotomy, operation is not only justified but imperative.

Liver and Gallbladder.—The typhoid bacillus has a peculiar affinity for the liver and gallbladder. The organism is present in the gallbladder from the onset of the infection in practically every case of typhoid fever and, as in the case of certain healthy carriers, it may be found in the gallbladder of individuals who give no history of clinical typhoid infection. It is, therefore, remarkable that hepatic and gallbladder complications do not occur with greater frequency.

JAUNDICE.—Jaundice is extremely rare. Liebermeister found 26 cases in 1,420 cases of typhoid. German statistics, however, give a higher incidence. Posselt found icterus reported as present in from 0.14 to 7.14 per cent of the individual cases in various groups. It appears to be rarer in this country. Apart from abscess and cholecystitis it was noted in only 8 of McCrae's series of 1,500 cases. Of 52 cases of jaundice analyzed by Da Costa, 4 were catarrhal and 24 toxic. The jaundice was a symptom of pylephlebitis in 3 cases, of cholangitis in 5 cases, of abscess in 5 cases and of acute yellow atrophy in 5 cases.

Catarrhal jaundice is usually a late complication, although it has been noted in the period of onset. Coleman reports a case in the prodromal period. This complication may be mild and transient and cause no aggravation of the symptoms of the primary disease. In the more severe form the jaundice may be quite intense and accompanied by nausea and vomiting, chill and an increase in the pyrexia. Enlargement of the liver, pain and tenderness in the hepatic region are not usually present. Bile is usually absent from the stools. *Toxic jaundice* is a late complication of severe typhoid. It may be distinguished from the catarrhal form by the gravity of the symptoms and by the continued presence of bile in the feces.

HEPATIC ABSCESS.—Hepatic abscess, solitary or multiple, is a very rare complication or sequel of typhoid fever. Da Costa collected 22 cases. The solitary abscess may be the result of an infection ascending from the ulcerative lesions in the bowel, or it may be part of a pyemia with abscesses in other parts of the body. Cases following parotid abscess and necrosis of bone have been reported. Multiple abscesses may be due to a septic pylephlebitis having its origin in suppuration or gangrene in the intestine or in the mesenteric glands, or to suppurative cholangitis. The colon bacillus, the staphylococcus, the streptococcus and the typhoid bacillus have been recovered from the pus. The prognosis is very grave. Cases of solitary abscess have been successfully drained.

CHOLECYSTITIS.—In typhoid fever, as stated above, the gallbladder is a constant metastatic focus of lodgment and multiplication of the typhoid bacillus. It is generally believed and has been experimentally demonstrated that the organism reaches the gallbladder through the circulating blood by a descending infection. As a rule the presence of the organism in the gallbladder and its passage through the biliary tract to the intestine causes no inflammatory reaction. It is quite probable, however, that a mild cholecystitis not infrequently occurs and runs its course without symptoms severe enough to attract attention. In a small percentage of the cases the inflammation is of sufficient severity to cause definite symptoms. Gallstones of ancient or recent formation may be a predisposing etiologic factor. In Webb-Johnson's series of 2,500 cases of typhoid and paratyphoid fever, there were 15 cases with more or less definite symptoms of cholecystitis. The diagnosis was made in 19 of McCrae's 1,500 cases, representing 1.2 per cent. The complication is announced by chill, rise of temperature, pain in the right upper quadrant, and usually by vomiting. The pulse and respiration rate are increased. Tenderness and rigidity are present over the gallbladder area, and occasionally the enlarged gallbladder may be palpated. Jaundice may develop. There is a moderate leukocytosis, from 10,000 to 15,000. The disease usually terminates by resolution in a few days; or, in rare cases, ulceration and perforation of the gallbladder, followed by general peritonitis, may result. In only one of the 15 cases reported by Webb-Johnson was surgical interference necessary. A mild, chronic cholecystitis may result from the acute attack and be the immediate cause of the development of gallstones. In 30.9 per cent of Curschmann's cases followed over long periods, symptoms of gallstone disease were found. The infection may persist in the gallbladder without causing inflammatory reaction and may produce a temporary or permanent carrier state.

Spleen.—Perisplenitis, infarct and spontaneous rupture are rare complications of typhoid fever. One of these conditions may be suspected if pain, tenderness and rigidity in the left upper quadrant develop in the second or third week of the disease. A positive diagnosis is impossible. Abscess of the spleen may result from a failure to eliminate the typhoid bacilli from the spleen to the liver. The Mayos operated on several cases of single or multiple abscess containing pure cultures of the typhoid bacillus. In 800 cases of typhoid fever with surgical complications collected by Keen there were 9 cases of splenic abscess.

CIRCULATORY SYSTEM

Blood.—The anemia following typhoid fever is very moderate in degree, rarely exceeding a 20 per cent loss of red cells and hemoglobin. Very exceptionally posttyphoid anemia may be severe and constitute a serious complication. In 2,000 fatal cases reported by Hölscher from the Gaieme Hospital in Munich, 54 cases, or 2.7 per cent, showed severe anemia. Thayer carefully studied two cases. In one the number of red cells fell to 1,352,000 and the hemoglobin to 27.5 per cent on the thirty-fifth day of the disease. In the other the red cells numbered 1,996,000 on the thirty-second day. Both patients made very slow recoveries.

Heart.—The symptoms of *myocardial insufficiency* may appear as a complication in the latter weeks of the pyrexial period of typhoid fever or as a sequel early or late in the convalescent period. From the studies of Romberg, Hayem, and more recently of Hamman, it has been shown that the anatomic basis of the symptoms may be an interstitial myocarditis or granular or fatty degeneration of the muscle fibers. Grave and fatal cardiac insufficiency appearing in the height of the disease may depend primarily upon vasomotor paralysis, the changes in the myocardium being of secondary importance. Romberg asserted that circulatory failure during the height of an infection depends entirely upon vasomotor paralysis.

Symptoms of cardiac weakness of more or less severity usually begin in the third week of the pyrexia, sometimes earlier, without a corresponding rise in temperature. The pulse increases in frequency, loses its dicrotic character and becomes small, soft and compressible. In the average case of typhoid this pulse frequently continues into convalescence and gradually subsides, with no further evidence of myocardial weakness. In cases with more serious myocardial degeneration the symptoms increase in severity. The pulse may be intermittent or irregular in rhythm and force. Instead of a tachycardia, a bradycardia may be the first symptom of a failing myocardium. General prostration may be profound, with paleness of the skin and perspiration. Vomiting is not infrequent. Physical examination shows a feeble or diffuse apex impulse with the left border of the heart displaced to the nipple line or still further to the left. The heart sounds are feeble, or the first sound may be feeble and the pulmonary second accentuated; gallop rhythm or embryocardia may be present. A soft systolic murmur may be heard at the apex or in the third interspace, due to a relative mitral insufficiency. Dilatation is usually confined to the left side of the heart.

Although often a cause of much anxiety, myocardial degeneration in typhoid fever is rarely a direct cause of death. The symptoms usually subside gradually and the physical signs of dilatation disappear with the decline of the pyrexia. Sudden collapse, more or less severe, may occur

40101

from exertion or emotion, and some cases of sudden death during the period of decline and in convalescence are unquestionably due to acute myocardial degeneration. The above symptoms may first appear during convalescence, when the patient is beginning to be about. Instability and irritability of the heart, with subjective symptoms, may persist for several weeks or months after recovery.

Endocarditis and *pericarditis* are very rare complications of typhoid. Occasionally at autopsy recent vegetations are found on the valves. Considering the frequency of secondary infections in the declining period of typhoid fever, the immunity of the endocardium and pericardium from invasion is rather remarkable. It is only rarely that a chronic valvular lesion can be traced to an attack of typhoid fever.

Arteries.—Arteritis is rare, but it occurs more frequently as a complication of typhoid fever than of the other acute infections. The disease is apparently due to the direct invasion of the arterial wall by the typhoid bacillus. Vincent and Muratet found the arteries of the right leg to be most frequently affected. The posterior tibial, femoral, popliteal, anterior tibial and dorsalis pedis were affected in the order named. More rarely the arteries of the upper extremities or of the brain were involved. In 4 cases in Osler's series 2 were in the femoral artery, 1 in the middle cerebral and 1 in the brachial. Thrombosis of the cerebral arteries may cause the sudden development of convulsions, coma or hemiplegia. Typhoid arteritis occurs as early as the third week and as late as the eighth week, when convalescence has apparently been fully established. It appears to be as frequent in mild as in severe cases.

The onset of the complication is sudden, with pain along the course of the affected vessel, or involving more extensive areas or even the entire limb. The pain is increased by movement and pressure. Paresthesias over the affected areas are common, and tenderness is marked over the inflamed artery. Thrombus formation brings out the vessel as a hard, painful cord. Below the obstructed vessel the limb is pale or blue, swollen and cool. Pulsation in the artery is diminished or lost. The circulation may be slowly restored by the development of an adequate collateral circulation or by the formation of channels through the thrombus; or the obstruction may be complete and the process terminate in dry gangrene of the extremity.

Thayer studied the late cardiovascular condition of 183 typhoid patients treated in the wards of Johns Hopkins Hospital. From one month to thirteen years had elapsed between the attack of fever and the examination. The date of the examination was less than one year after the attack in 48 cases, between one and five years in 93 cases, and between five and thirteen years in 42 cases. The results show that arterial hypertension, palpable radial arteries, cardiac enlargement and chronic valvular disease were found with much greater frequency than in individuals who gave no history of typhoid fever. He concludes that typhoid fever is an important factor in the etiology of arteriosclerosis and cardiovascular disease.

Veins.—THROMBOPHLEBITIS.—The studies of Conner have brought forward phlebitis as one of the common and very important complications of typhoid fever, responsible for many of the irregularities in the course of the pyrexia and the underlying cause of many complicating conditions hitherto not satisfactorily explained. In general literature phlebitis is stated to occur in about 2 per cent of the cases of typhoid. Thayer found venous thrombosis in 39, or 2.6 per cent, of 1,463 cases. Da Costa reports 16 cases of milk leg in 135 soldiers treated for typhoid in the Pennsylvania Hospital, representing 12 per cent. In Webb-Johnson's series of 297 cases of typhoid fever in British soldiers not protected by antityphoid vaccination, 3.36 per cent were complicated by phlebitis. Conner analyzed 1,540 cases treated in the New York Hospital, in which there were 78 cases, or 5 per cent, of undoubted thrombosis. He believes that with more accurate diagnosis an incidence of from 10 to 15 per cent in all cases of typhoid will be shown.

Phlebitis is a late complication, rarely appearing before the third week of the disease. Nearly half of the cases develop in the third or fourth week, and about an equal number during the convalescent period.

The veins of the left leg are most frequently affected. The left femoral is the favorite site. The iliac, popliteal, internal saphenous veins, and those of the calf of the leg may be affected primarily or by extension from the femoral. The veins of both legs are affected in about 30 per cent of the cases. Quite rarely the process is confined to the pulmonary vein or to the veins of one arm, usually the left.

Autopsy findings often show thrombosis extending far beyond the site of the local symptoms as observed during life.

The onset of thrombophlebitis is often latent and insidious, and the early localizing symptoms may be absent or so mild as to escape recognition. As Aschoff has shown in his studies on thrombosis, the primary white thrombus is built up gradually, layer upon layer, from the blood platelets while the blood is still circulating. The local symptoms by which the condition is recognized develop only when complete occlusion of the vein has taken place. During this latent period, which may last for a number of days, as Conner has shown, thrombophlebitis may be manifested only by symptoms remote from the seat of thrombus formation. Small fragments may be detached from the growing, friable clot and cause pulmonary embolism and infarction. In the absence of the local symptoms of phlebitis the real nature of these small infarcts may not be suspected. Conner believes that most of the late pulmonary and pleural complications of typhoid fever have this etiology. The puzzling chills and the unaccountable irregularities in the course of the pyrexia so frequently seen in the declining period of the fever are very often due to a thrombophlebitis which has not yet shown itself by local symptoms.

The characteristic symptoms of fully developed thrombophlebitis are fever, pain, tenderness, swelling, edema and induration along the course of the thrombosed vein. Fever is present in approximately 90 per cent of the cases. Should the complication occur before defervescence the regular typhoid temperature curve is interrupted by a rise, which may be sustained for a number of days, or may persist with various irregularities, and indefinitely prolong the pyrexial period. The increase of fever usually begins with the local signs of thrombosis of a large vein. In exceptional cases the rise may precede or follow the local symptoms by several days. During the convalescent period the onset of phlebitis may cause either a sharp transient rise of temperature or a longer period of pyrexia, showing violent remissions and exacerbations; or it may cause a prolonged, mild febrile movement. In the absence of coincident,

40101

frank, local symptoms these periods of fever may be confused with recrudescence from various other causes, or with true relapse.

The evidence advanced by Conner is very strong that many post-typhoid disturbances of temperature without other apparent cause are due to a latent phlebitis. Chills, either at the onset or during the course of the complication, were noted by Thayer in 28 per cent of his cases. The relation of phlebitis to the multiple chills of the later period of typhoid has previously been considered.

Leukocytosis with moderate increase of the polymorphonuclear cells usually accompanies the complication. In all of Thayer's cases the count was above 6,000; in 54.5 per cent it was from 10,000 to 20,000. In exceptional cases the typhoid leukopenia may persist for some time after the appearance of the phlebitis.

Thrombophlebitis is a distressing and sometimes a dangerous complication of typhoid fever. Death may result directly from pulmonary embolism, or from extensive thrombosis into the abdominal veins, or indirectly, from exhaustion or complications following and dependent upon the phlebitis. It may cause much suffering and greatly prolong the period of convalescence. Some permanent disability may be left from occlusion of the large vein. Persistent swelling of the leg after exercise, varicose veins below the occlusion, and ulceration may result. Cramps in the calves of the legs are common. Gangrene is very rare.

RESPIRATORY SYSTEM

Larynx.—Routine laryngoscopic examinations during the course of typhoid show that laryngeal inflammation of greater or less severity occurs as a complication in a majority of the cases running a severe course. Jackson carefully studied the condition of the larynx in 360 hospital cases. He classified the lesions under (1) subacute laryngitis, (2) ulcerative laryngitis and (3) perichondritis. He found subacute laryngitis in 227 cases, or 63 per cent; ulcerative laryngitis in 68 cases, or 18.9 per cent; and perichondritis with or without necrosis in 17 cases, or 4.7 per cent.

No satisfactory records of the frequency of laryngeal complications in private practice are available. They are probably much less frequent than in hospital experience. However, laryngoscopic examination of the larynx is rarely made during the course of typhoid fever, and it seems quite certain that mild laryngeal complications are rarely recognized and that only the severe lesions with emphatic symptoms have received consideration in medical literature.

CATARRHAL LARYNGITIS.—The mucous membrane of the larynx participates in the catarrhal state common to the various mucous surfaces. The symptoms do not differ from those of the disease occurring as a primary affection. Jackson noted that the mucous membrane was continuously covered with a secretion, which appeared to come from the trachea and bronchi. Catarrhal laryngitis is important because of the possibility of its influence in the development of ulceration, edema or other serious conditions. Laryngeal symptoms, however mild, occurring during the course of typhoid fever, should put the physician on his guard and lead to careful laryngoscopic exploration for the presence of the more severe forms of laryngeal disease.

ULCERATION OF THE LARYNX.—Autopsy findings show that ulceration of the larynx occurs in about 10 per cent of all fatal cases. Only a small percentage of this number is recognized during life. Jackson's studies indicate that systematic examination of the larynx would reveal a much higher incidence. The high mortality rate of the cases collected by Keen and others as compared with the mortality rate of Jackson's series seems to prove that only those cases presenting serious symptoms of laryngeal obstruction are included in these reports.

The nutritional changes in the mucous membrane of the larynx, the result of the typhoid toxemia, are the important predisposing factors in the etiology of ulceration. A large majority of the cases occur in severe typhoid with high fever and intense toxemia. Immediate exciting causes are:

1. Traumatism by friction and irritation in phonation, coughing and deglutition.

2. Injudicious exposure to cold and drafts.

3. Arterial or venous thrombosis. Suddenness of onset in certain cases points to vascular occlusion as the determining factor in the ulceration. Arterial thrombosis is possible, but from Conner's studies it appears more probable that thrombosis of the small veins is the condition present.

4. Infection. The typhoid bacillus has been recovered from the ulceration in a few cases. Infection by this organism is by the blood stream. Secondary infection by pyogenic cocci is the principal factor in the immediate etiology of the complication. Drainage into the larynx of infected secretions, and food remnants from a septic mouth and pharynx, and retention through lessened cough reflex keep the mucous membrane bathed with infected material. Loss of tissue immunity determines the invasion of the mucous membrane by the organisms. A few cases have followed suppuration in the ears, or abscesses in the parotid gland and other contiguous structures. The Klebs-Löffler bacillus is rarely the infecting organism.

Laryngeal ulceration is a late complication. Sixty-seven of Jackson's cases and over 70 per cent of the cases collected by Keen and Rieser occurred after the third week. The site of the ulceration in about 60 per cent of the cases was the posterior laryngeal wall at the insertion of the vocal cords. The location in the remaining cases was the arytenoid cartilages and interspace, the aryteno-epiglottidean folds, the epiglottis and the thyroid cartilage, in the order named.

The onset of the complication is insidious, and the well-known symptoms of laryngeal inflammation may be absent, or so mild as to escape notice. Apathy, diminished sensibility or delirium may conceal the symptoms until a paroxysm of laryngeal dyspnea announces the formidable complication that is present. In Jackson's carefully observed cases, the average day of onset of the ulceration was the twenty-second; the average day of onset of symptoms was the thirty-first day.

Hoarseness, croupy cough and aphonia are the symptoms usually first noted. Pain, tenderness, dysphagia and dysphonia are present in patients whose sensibility is not too blunted. The symptoms of an apparently mild laryngitis may suddenly be followed by an alarming attack of dyspnea, or the dyspnea may be the first symptom to announce the laryngeal complication. The obstruction may be from acute edema, from an abscess in the laryngeal wall, from occlusion of the glottis by a sloughing mass, or from abductor paralysis of the vocal cords. When obstruction occurs after the period of profound toxemia the well-known violent symptoms of asphyxia are present. In the profoundly toxic patient the symptoms may be masked by the stupor, and death may take place without the attendant suspecting the gravity of the situation. A bronchopneumonia from aspiration of the laryngeal secretions may occur. The diagnosis of laryngeal ulceration is easy if the possibility of the condition is suspected and a laryngoscopic examination made. Unless particularly looked for, the complication may progress to a fatal termination without recognition.

Perichondritis and chondritis result from the extension of the ulceration into the deeper structures of the larynx. More or less extensive necrosis of the cartilages of the larynx frequently takes place. Keen, basing his opinion upon his study of the reported cases of laryngeal disease complicating typhoid, states that necrosis of the cartilages is the most common lesion. It seems quite certain, however, that Jackson's personal experience represents more accurately the relative incidence of the various lesions. The milder forms of infection are not usually recognized and do not seriously affect the ordinary course of the primary disease.

Abscess of the larynx, ulceration of the trachea and perforation with subcutaneous emphysema are occasional results of ulcerative laryngitis.

The prognosis of the severe forms of laryngeal disease complicating typhoid fever is very grave. Of the 243 cases collected, 158, or 65 per cent, died.

The influence of the early recognition and treatment upon prognosis is shown by Jackson's experience. Of his 68 cases of ulceration, which included all the cases of the serious form of laryngeal invasion, only 4 died, representing 5.8 per cent, all of them from causes remote from the larynx. Of the 8 patients upon whom tracheotomy was performed for the relief of asphyxia, 1 died from toxemia. Jackson believes that with proper local treatment the prognosis depends upon the severity of the typhoid toxemia rather than upon the local condition. Permanent deformity, impairment or loss of voice, or stenosis requiring prolonged treatment may result from the destructive lesions.

Bronchi.—BRONCHITIS.—A mild bronchitis with cough, scant expectoration and a few râles scattered over the chest is an occasional manifestation of typhoid, beginning in the first and continuing into the second week or throughout the febrile period. It usually causes but little discomfort. A severe bronchitis may complicate the onset and mask the primary disease, or it may develop at any time in the course. Occasionally the cough is severe and distressing. Like the bronchitis of measles it is a local manifestation of the general infection. The typhoid bacillus may be demonstrated in the sputum. Secondary infection by the pneumococcus, streptococcus or other organism may occur in severe septic cases. Bronchitis is rarely an important factor in a fatal issue. Osler cites one fatal case. Collapse of the lung with bronchopneumonia may result.

Lungs.—BRONCHOPNEUMONIA.—Extension of the infection from the bronchi to the lung occurs in a small percentage of cases. It is often a late event in serious cases. The lesions of bronchopneumonia are found in about one third of the fatal cases at autopsy. The typhoid bacillus, the pneumococcus, or more commonly the pyogenic cocci, are the infecting organisms. The onset is usually insidious, and is masked by the toxic state. Occasionally the complication begins with a chill. Rapid respiration, increased pulse rate and cyanosis are significant symptoms. Areas of partial or complete consolidation can be demonstrated in the interscapular and subscapular regions. The complication adds greatly to the gravity of a case. Rarely, in grave cases with myocardial weakness, edema of the lungs may result.

HYPOSTATIC CONGESTION.—Hypostatic congestion of the lower lobes of the lungs is a frequent complication of the latter half of the febrile period. In debilitated patients with severe toxemia it may occur in the first or second week. The development of the condition is favored by myocardial weakness and by the influence of prolonged dorsal decubitus. The condition causes no distinctive symptoms. There is no pain and no increase in the fever, cough or respiratory rate. The complication can be recognized only by a physical examination of the chest and will be overlooked in the absence of routine auscultation of the lungs in the back. Slightly tympanitic or impaired resonance over one or both lower lobes, absent or diminished respiration, prolonged expiration and bronchial voice and many fine râles are the physical signs which distinguish the condition.

Secondary infection of the congested area determines the development of *hypostatic pneumonia,* with the signs of complete consolidation. Elevation of temperature, rapid pulse and increased respiration are then present. With the decline of the fever and the improvement in the general condition of the patient, the consolidated area slowly undergoes resolution. The complication is grave. It was present in 121 of 1,830 cases observed by Curschmann, with 65 deaths. Careful nursing, with frequent change of the patient from side to side, tends to prevent stasis. The **bath treatment** is the most important preventive measure.

LOBAR PNEUMONIA.—In 1,420 cases of typhoid fever Liebermeister found lobar pneumonia in 52 cases, or 3.7 per cent. In Osler's series it occurred in 15 of the 829 cases, or 1.8 per cent. It is not a frequent complication. It may occur as a complication of the period of onset, of the fastigium, or of the period of decline. Typhoid fever may begin suddenly with the symptoms of a frank pneumonia and the characteristic physical signs of this disease. This is the "pneumotyphoid" of the French writers. The disease runs a course similar to that of primary lobar pneumonia for a number of days, and there is nothing in the clinical history to indicate the presence of a complicating or associated disease. Persistence of the pyrexia beyond the usual period and the appearance of rose spots, splenic enlargement, and intestinal symptoms will uncover the underlying typhoid infection. The pulmonary lesion may be a local manifestation of the typhoid bacteremia, a typhoid bacillus pneumonia, or it may be due to a complicating infection by the pneumococcus or by one of the rarer pneumonia-producing organisms. Bacteriologic studies have, up to this time, been too meager to permit a statement as to the relative frequency of the various infections.

Lobar pneumonia, complicating the latter stages of typhoid, occurs most frequently in the second and third weeks. The usual stormy onset of pneumonia is obscured by the apathy and diminished sensibility of the patient. The symptoms at this time are few and infrequent. Cough

40101

may not be increased and rusty sputum may not appear. The white cell count may or may not be increased. Increased respiration, cyanosis, rapid pulse and sharp disturbance in the temperature curve are the most important diagnostic symptoms. Physical examination of the chest will determine the nature of the complication. Curschmann states that the height of the consolidation of the lung is reached more slowly and that resolution is more often delayed than in primary pneumonia. Many cases do not advance beyond the symptoms of congestion. Lobar pneumonia is a grave complication. Of Liebermeister's 52 cases, 29 died. Marignac, cited by Hare, reported 13 cases with 10 deaths.

PULMONARY EMBOLISM AND INFARCTION.—Pulmonary embolism presents itself in two clinical forms:

1. The severe form, with suddenly developing severe thoracic pain, dyspnea, cyanosis and collapse, usually rapidly terminating in death. This form is very rare. It is caused by a large embolus detached from a cardiac or venous thrombus occluding one of the large branches of the pulmonary artery.

2. The mild form, giving rise to obscure and atypical signs of pleurisy or pneumonia. This form is relatively common. In Conner's study of 1,540 cases of typhoid fever there were 88 of pulmonary and pleural complications exclusive of bronchitis. In 63 of this number the character of the thoracic symptoms made it probable that most of them were due to pulmonary embolism. As shown above, the embolism has its origin in a thrombophlebitis.

The pulmonary symptoms may be the first evidence of a developing phlebitis. It may appear several days before the local signs of the complication, and the etiologic relation between the two phenomena may be entirely overlooked. Thoracic pain is present in practically all of the cases; usually it is the first symptom. It is sudden, sharp, and may be very severe. It is usually referred to the lower axillary region, occasionally to the hypogastrium or shoulder. Cough is usual and may begin with the onset of pain or after two or three days. Bloody sputum is seen in about one half of the cases. It appears first in small, bright red clots or as a blood-streaked mucus, the color becoming dark later. Dyspnea and thoracic oppression occur in the severe cases. A chill is occasionally noted at the onset. Rapid breathing, increased pulse rate and fluctuation in temperature are usual. The leukocyte count is usually increased. Rigidity and tenderness are occasionally observed in the upper abdomen, just below the ribs.

Physical Signs.—Conner classified the cases according to the physical signs into three groups: (1) Those with friction rubs or crepitant râles over a small area and lasting only two or three days; (2) cases with signs of a small circumscribed pneumonia, usually in one of the lower lobes, the consolidation disappearing in three or four days; (3) cases with extensive plastic pleurisy or pleural effusion.

PLEURISY.—Pleurisy is not a frequent complication. It has been observed at the onset as a localization of the typhoid infection. The thoracic symptoms may dominate the clinical picture, and the underlying typhoid infection may not be suspected until it is unmasked by the subsequent decline of local signs and the continuance of the pyrexia, with the appearance of the characteristic rose spots and splenic enlargement. More frequently it is a late complication. In patients dull with typhoid toxemia the complication may develop with few symptoms and escape recognition.

The pleurisy may be of the dry plastic variety or show effusion. The exudate may be serous, purulent or hemorrhagic. The typhoid bacillus has been found in both the serous effusion and in the empyemas. Empyema is usually due to a secondary infection by the pneumococcus or one of the pyogenic organisms. The hemorrhagic effusions are often due to tuberculosis. Small pulmonary infarctions may present the symptoms and physical signs of pleurisy. A mild complicating pleurisy does not add much to the gravity of an attack of typhoid fever. Empyema and hemorrhagic effusion are more serious.

TUBERCULOSIS.—Typhoid fever may activate a latent pulmonary tuberculosis, and the pulmonary condition may appear as a complication either during the late period of the course of the fever or as a sequel at any time after convalescence is established. The evidence is not convincing that typhoid infection predisposes to infection by the tubercle bacillus.

ABSCESS AND GANGRENE.—Abscess and gangrene are among the rarest pulmonary complications. Either of these conditions may result from one of the pneumonias or from general sepsis. In profoundly toxic patients aspiration of septic material from the larynx during the course of ulcerative laryngitis, or of food particles from the pharynx, may be the immediate cause.

RENAL SYSTEM

Retention of Urine.—This is a common and annoying condition. In the early days of the fever it may be due to the difficulty many patients experience in voiding in the recumbent position. Later it is the result of the obtunded sensibility of the typhoid state. The patient may not make a definite complaint, but will indicate his distress by restlessness or by an increase in the delirium. Physical examination will reveal a bladder tumor in the hypogastrium. Constant dribbling of urine is a suggestive symptom. Incontinence is occasionally seen in stuporous patients.

Polyuria.—Sollmann and Hofmann have shown that the eliminating capacity of the kidney for salt and water is not impaired in typhoid fever. The therapeutic use of a large water intake proportionally increases the urinary output. The urine may be increased to 5 liters or more. One of Osler's patients passed 23 liters in one day. Polyuria without excessive intake of fluid is occasionally seen in the second or third week of typhoid, and is a common phenomenon at the beginning of convalescence. It has been spoken of as a urinary crisis. The condition passes away with convalescence.

Febrile Albuminuria.—In typhoid fever the kidneys are not, as a rule, seriously affected. The slight albuminuria which is characteristic of all acute infections with fever and due to a mild parenchymatous degeneration of the epithelial cells of the tubules is common. It occurs in about 60 per cent of the cases. This febrile albuminuria should be sharply distinguished from acute glomerulonephritis. It is not of serious import and disappears in a few days or with the decline of the fever. It does not impair the functional efficiency of the kidney. The albumin rarely amounts to more than a trace. A few casts, hyaline or finely granular are usually found. In McCrae's series casts were present in 37.8 per cent of the cases.

Nephritis.—Acute glomerulonephritis is not a common complication. Curschmann gives the incidence as about 1 per cent. Talley's series of 18,000 cases shows 3 per cent. Typhoid fever may be complicated with nephritis at the onset, constituting the nephrotyphoid or renal typhoid. More commonly the nephritis is a complication of the late febrile period; or it may appear during convalescence. It may begin suddenly with edema and uremic symptoms and a scant, highly albuminous urine, containing also blood and numerous casts. The onset may be insidious, without marked edema or uremic phenomena. The complication may be overlooked in the absence of routine urinary examinations, its symptoms being obscured by those of the typhoid fever.

Nephritis at the beginning of typhoid fever is a serious complication. Cases which develop late in the disease usually recover. The condition rarely terminates in chronic nephritis.

Infections of the Upper Urinary Tract.—Bacilluria.—From the third week on, typhoid bacilli are present in the urine in about one third of the cases. The infection is usually mild, and no symptoms are present. The urine may be turbid from the presence of the bacilli, without other evidence of infection. It is generally thought that the bacilli pass through the kidney from the circulating blood in small numbers and multiply in the bladder urine. Mild local lesions in the bladder and prostate may produce the conditions favorable to the multiplication of the organisms. Bacilluria may persist for an indefinite period after recovery from the typhoid, and the host thus become a chronic typhoid carrier. Mild cases may remain latent for a number of years and then give rise to acute and severe symptoms. The colon bacillus or other organisms may be associated with the typhoid bacillus.

Pyuria.—Pus in small amount may be found in the urine without other symptoms. It may have its source in gonorrhea or in a mild catarrh of some part of the urinary tract.

Pyelitis.—Infection of the pelvis of the kidney may take place at the height of the disease or during convalescence. The complication is ushered in by an increase of temperature or, in the convalescent period, by a recrudescence of the fever preceded, perhaps, by a chill. Pus and, in the first days, blood are found in the urine. There is often a sudden leukocytosis. Bimanual palpation of the kidney will often elicit tenderness. The typhoid bacillus may be the infecting organism. Colon bacillus infection is also frequent.

The complication usually runs a course of a few days and ends with recovery; or it may persist for considerable time and be the cause of a prolonged posttyphoid febrile state. Pyelonephritis may result. Perinephritis is quite rare and is practically always due to a secondary infection by one of the pyogenic cocci.

Cystitis.—The typhoid bacillus not infrequently causes a cystitis, mild or severe. The colon bacillus and the staphylococcus are also common infecting organisms. The usual symptoms of bladder irritation are present, with fever and leukocytosis. The typhoid infections are more amenable to treatment. Chronic cystitis may result. Hugh Young reported a case of seven years' duration.

NERVOUS SYSTEM

Meninges.—Symptoms of meningitis or meningeal irritation may develop suddenly any time during the course of typhoid fever. Cases are recorded in which the symptoms appeared in the prodromal period. In some epidemics, particularly in those coincident with the prevalence of cerebrospinal fever, the incidence may be very high. During a milk infection epidemic, Curschmann observed five hospital nurses who were attacked in quick succession by typhoid fever, in all of whom meningitis symptoms predominated in the first week. Nervous symptoms of typhoid fever occurring with the onset may dominate the clinical picture and completely conceal the underlying typhoid infection. These cases have been designated as meningotyphoid by French writers.

Cole studied the meningeal complications of typhoid fever and, from pathologic findings, divided the cases into three groups: (1) meningism, (2) serous meningitis, (3) purulent meningitis. Lumbar puncture is the only means of differentiating these conditions.

MENINGISM.—Symptoms of mild, transient, meningeal irritation may occur with negative spinal fluid and insignificant autopsy findings. Curschmann and others have called attention to the condition. Wolf published twelve cases from Curschmann's clinic. In three fatal cases coming to autopsy there were no lesions of the brain or cord, and cultures from the central nervous system were negative. Such cases may be explained as due to the action of a soluble toxin upon the cortical neurons. Schultze, however, found that in certain cases, although no gross anatomic alterations could be demonstrated, small-cell infiltration was present along the course of the vessels of the meninges, and that there were similar microscopic foci in the substance of the brain and cord. Meningism has been most frequently observed in the typhoid fever of children. When the condition occurs at the onset of an attack of typhoid fever the symptoms often fade away in a few days and give place to the usual symptoms of the primary disease. When occurring later, meningism indicates a serious toxemia and is of graver significance. From our personal experience it would appear that this mild form of meningeal complication is more frequent than the reported cases indicate.

MENINGITIS.—Both serous and purulent meningitis may be produced by the typhoid bacillus. Cole's studies show that *serous meningitis* is particularly a manifestation of the localization of the typhoid organism in the central nervous system. He considers it to be caused by toxins liberated from the typhoid bacilli localized in the spinal canal. Cole reported 13 cases, 8 from the literature and 5 from the wards of Johns Hopkins Hospital. In 1917 Bayne-Jones collected 17 cases reported subsequent to Cole's communication. Serous meningitis may subside, especially after lumbar puncture, or it may continue and prove to be the early stage of a purulent meningitis. Of 13 cases reported by Claret and Lyon-Caen, 8 recovered and 5 died.

Purulent meningitis complicating typhoid may be produced by the Eberth bacillus, or it may be a secondary infection by the meningococcus, pneumococcus or one of the common pyogenic organisms. Mixed infection with one of these organisms and the typhoid bacillus may occur. In rare cases developing in the convalescent period the tubercle bacillus is the infecting agent. The identification of the infecting organism is made by lumbar puncture and examination of the spinal

40101

fluid. Lumbar puncture should be a routine diagnostic procedure in all cases presenting meningeal symptoms. Cole reported 15 cases and Bayne-Jones collected 18 additional cases. According to these data purulent meningitis may occur at any time in the course of typhoid fever. It is an exceedingly fatal complication. All reported cases have died, usually within three days of the onset of the meningeal symptoms. McSweeney has reported recovery in one case following intrathecal administration of Felix's serum.

The symptoms of meningeal invasion by the typhoid bacillus are those of acute cerebrospinal meningitis, and they do not differ in essential particulars in the two forms of the disease, serous and purulent. The symptoms are severe headache, photophobia, vertigo, pain in the spinal region with rigidity and retraction of the head. There are also cutaneous hyperesthesia, pain and tenderness in the muscles with muscular twitching and occasionally convulsions. The deep and superficial reflexes are usually increased. Kernig's sign is generally present. The onset may be with chills and facial herpes, the latter being very rarely seen in typhoid fever without meningeal symptoms.

Meningitis, serous or purulent, whether due to the typhoid bacillus or to some other organism, is a very grave complication. Most cases die. As has been noted, mild cases of the serous form occasionally recover, particularly after repeated spinal puncture.

Hemiplegia.—Hemiplegia is one of the rare complications of typhoid. It may occur at any time from the third week until well into the period of convalescence. Age does not appear to have an important influence on the incidence. Of 42 cases collected by Smithies, 9 were in children under ten years of age. In about two thirds of the cases the paralysis is right-sided, with aphasia. The cerebral lesion may be thrombosis, hemorrhage, embolism or a meningo-encephalitis. In very rare cases the lesion is a meningeal hemorrhage. According to autopsy records thrombosis appears to be the most common lesion. The clinical history of hemiplegia complicating typhoid presents no distinctive features. Six of the 42 cases reported by Smithies were fatal. Aphasia without hemiplegia and terminating in recovery at the end of a few days has been reported a number of times. Hutenel stated that this form of aphasia always occurs in children, more frequently in boys. Among the very unusual complications that have been recorded are paraplegia, monoplegia, bulbar paralysis and myelitis.

Convulsions.—Convulsions have been observed with extreme rarity. Convulsions may occur (1) as one of the phenomena of a sudden and stormy onset, especially in the typhoid of infancy or childhood; (2) during the height of the fever and toxemia; and (3) as a symptom of a vascular cerebral accident, as thrombosis or hemorrhage. Of the 42 cases of hemiplegia collected by Smithies, 10 were preceded by convulsions. As in the other acute infections, convulsions occurring at onset are not of such grave import as when they occur late in the disease as a result of serious toxemia or organic brain lesion.

Peripheral Neuritis—Peripheral neuritis sometimes occurs as a late complication. The nerves of the lower extremities are involved more often than are those of the trunk and arms. The disease may manifest itself as a multiple neuritis involving both the lower or all four extremities, or it may be restricted to a single nerve. Pain, tenderness, paresthesia, motor and sensory paresis, and trophic disturbances may result.

Neuralgia and painful areas in the muscles and skin are often seen without other evidence of organic changes in the nerves. As Conner has shown, these painful conditions are often due to phlebitis.

TENDER TOES.—In early convalescence the plantar surfaces of the toes and sometimes more extensive areas of the feet become painful and tender. Contact with the bedclothes or with any object may be exceedingly painful. This condition has been described as a peripheral neuritis. Conner believes it is due to a thrombophlebitis. Recovery takes place in a few days.

Psychoses.—Kraepelin's classification of the typhoid psychoses, which has been quite generally adopted, is the following: (1) the initial delirium, the psychoses of the period of incubation or the period of onset; (2) the febrile psychoses, developing during the height of the fever and toxemia; and (3) the asthenic or posttyphoid psychoses.

INITIAL DELIRIUM.—In the initial stage, the mental derangement manifests itself as an acute delirium or a state of mental depression. The acute delirium is characterized by profound mental obtusion with hallucinations. The patient may wander from home and conceal himself in his effort to escape fancied persecution. There may be impulses to acts of violence. The condition may closely simulate alcoholic delirium. In two such cases seen in the wards under the late author's (C. G. J.) observation, a diagnosis of delirium tremens was made on admission.

The form in which mental depression is the leading feature is rare. As the mental state may be the only outspoken symptom of the general infection, the true nature of the malady may not be suspected and the patient may be treated for a primary mental disease.

FEBRILE PSYCHOSES.—The mental derangements of the period of high fever are exaggerations of the ordinary fever delirium or stupor so frequently present in severe cases. The delirium may be of the expansive type and the stupor may assume the character of a coma vigil. In the case of a boy of fourteen years under the late author's (C. G. J.) observation, a few days of active delirium at the end of the febrile period were followed by a state of coma vigil which continued for ten days after defervescence.

ASTHENIC PSYCHOSES.—The posttyphoid insanities may develop as a continuation of the febrile delirium, or they may appear at various times during the convalescent period. Dercum recognizes the following forms: (1) acute delirium; (2) confusional insanity, stuporous insanity; (3) cerebral asthenia, pseudodementia, pseudoparesis; (4) insanity with systematized delusions resembling paranoia; (5) true mania or true melancholia. Age is not an important factor in the etiology. Many cases are observed in children.

The prognosis of the typhoid insanities, considered as a class, may be said to be good. The severe delirium of the prodromal or initial period is of grave import. About one third of the cases terminate fatally. The delirium and stupor of the febrile period usually decline with the pyrexia, and complete recovery is the rule. The prognosis of the posttyphoid psychoses is also favorable for ultimate recovery. It is true that of the cases committed to asylums only about 50 per cent recover. These figures, however, do not represent the real situation. A large per-

40101

centage of the milder cases which recover do not come under hospital care.

General Neuroses.—Various functional diseases of the nervous system may complicate the late state of the disease. Hysteria is not uncommon, and it may assume any of the well-known counterfeit manifestations of disease. Chorea, tremor, tetany, paralysis agitans and diabetes insipidus have been observed.

ORGANS OF THE SPECIAL SENSES

The Eye.—The ocular complications of typhoid have been fully studied by Geo. E. de Schweinitz. Paresis of accommodation, as a part of the postfebrile asthenia, is frequently seen. Both catarrhal and phlyctenular conjunctivitis are among the most common ocular complications. Both ulcerative and suppurative keratitis are more rare. Affections of the uveal tract are occasionally seen in the convalescent period. Iritis was seen by Sorel once in 871 cases of typhoid. Cataract may follow inflammation of the uveal tract, or it may result from nutritional disturbances without antecedent inflammation. Retinal hemorrhage is not very rare during the height of the febrile state. Embolism of the central artery of the retina has been noted. Optic neuritis with optic nerve atrophy, either partial or complete, may occur. De Schweinitz mentions amblyopia as a possible result of excessive quinine medication. Optic nerve atrophy may be caused by severe intestinal hemorrhage or epistaxis. Transient amblyopia without ophthalmoscopic changes has been reported. Thrombosis of the orbital veins, panophthalmia and paralysis of extra-ocular muscles are very rare complications.

The Ear.—Otitis media occurs in from 2 to 3 per cent of the cases. It is particularly frequent in the typhoid of childhood and infancy. It is usually a secondary infection by one of the common pyogenic organisms originating in the nasopharynx. Mastoid disease and sinus thrombosis are far less frequent than in other acute infections. The impairment of hearing and the subjective sensations of sound so characteristic of the febrile state of typhoid are apparently due to the action of the typhoid toxin on the structures of the middle and internal ear. These symptoms usually disappear with convalescence. From 1 to 2 per cent of all cases of impairment of hearing can be traced to a previous attack of typhoid fever.

GLANDULAR SYSTEM

Derangements of the Lymphatic Glands.—In addition to the enlargement of the mesenteric glands which is uniformly present, a general enlargement of all the lymph nodes may occur. It is not of importance and subsides with the decline of the fever.

Mastitis.—Mastitis is a rare complication of typhoid fever, usually appearing in females. Osler saw 4 cases in his series. It occurs late and is usually a secondary infection. The typhoid bacillus has been isolated from the pus in a few cases. It involves one or both breasts with about equal frequency. Half of the cases terminate in suppuration.

Orchitis.—Orchitis is occasionally met with, as in other infectious diseases. The epididymis is usually implicated. The disease presents no special characteristics. Chills, and fever with severe local pain and swelling, are the symptoms. The right testicle is most frequently affected, and only rarely are both involved. It runs a course of about two weeks' duration and terminates in suppuration in a minority of the cases. Atrophy of the testicle is an occasional result.

Thyroiditis.—The thyroid gland, under normal conditions, is peculiarly resistant to bacterial invasion. Bacterial thyroiditis is therefore a rare complication of typhoid, and requires for its production a very virulent infection or a greatly diminished resistance in the gland itself. Liebermeister and Hoffman found 15 cases of thyroiditis, 6 cases resulting in abscess, among 1,700 cases of typhoid. The complication appears to be more frequent in districts where goiter is common. Infection may be by the typhoid bacillus or by one of the pyogenic organisms. The disease may pursue its course as a nonpurulent inflammation and terminate in resolution, or it may result in abscess formation. It appears late in the febrile period or in convalescence. Galli has reported a thyroid abscess with pure culture of the typhoid bacillus occurring twenty-one years after the primary typhoid infection.

The symptoms are pain, tenderness and swelling of part or of the whole gland. Dysphagia and other pressure symptoms may occur. Without abscess formation the complication is not very serious. Of 41 cases of suppurative thyroiditis from all causes collected by Richardson, 9 were fatal. Crotti remarks that good surgery should reduce this mortality. Exophthalmic goiter is a possible sequela.

LOCOMOTOR SYSTEM

Muscles.—MYOSITIS.—The changes in the muscles in typhoid fever are degenerative rather than inflammatory. In convalescence, groups of muscles may become tender and painful on manipulation or with contraction. The symptoms suggest a myositis, although there is not at present satisfactory evidence that infection is the cause. The symptoms gradually disappear. *Rupture* of groups of fibers or of whole muscles may take place when degeneration is advanced, either from severe or very slight exertion. Hemorrhage at the site of rupture takes place with the development of a hematoma. The contents of the tumor may be infected and suppuration result. The typhoid bacillus has been recovered from both the blood and the pus. The muscles of the abdominal wall and of the thigh are most frequently the site of rupture. The diaphragm may be involved, with respiratory embarrassment. Sudden acute pain is the important symptom of rupture. In profoundly stuporous patients with severely degenerated and friable muscles the accident may pass unnoticed.

Joints.—ARTHRITIS.—Webb-Johnson divides the joint affections of typhoid fever into (1) acute arthritis, serous or suppurative; (2) subacute arthritis, usually serous, but which may go on to suppuration.

Acute serous arthritis complicates the first stage of typhoid. It is polyarticular, involving the knees, elbows and other joints, and closely simulates acute rheumatic arthritis, for which it may be mistaken. As a rule the affection lasts a few days only, and ends in complete recovery. In exceptional cases some restriction of motion may result, or very rarely suppuration may take place. This form is similar in its clinical course to the more common and familiar arthritis of scarlatina. Salicylates have no effect upon it. It is a local manifestation of the typhoid bacteremia.

40101

Acute suppurative arthritis may result from an acute serous arthritis or from a subacute arthritis. More frequently it is a secondary infection of the joints by the streptococcus, staphylococcus or other pyogenic organism, absorbed from various skin and mucous membrane infections of the late period of the typhoid. When due to secondary infection it does not differ from the septic arthritis complicating other infections. The typhoid bacillus alone may produce the suppuration, or it may be due to a mixed infection. Suppurative arthritis is a highly dangerous, often fatal complication.

Subacute serous arthritis occurs about as frequently as acute arthritis. This form is a complication of the late febrile or convalescent period. It is almost always monarticular and affects by preference the large joints of the lower extremities, especially the hip joint. The onset is insidious and the symptoms are mild. In apathetic patients it is easily overlooked, particularly when it involves a deeply seated joint like the hip. The course of the disease is often mild and terminates in resolution with complete restoration of joint function. It may be more severe and persistent and end in ankylosis or, rarely, in suppuration. Spontaneous dislocation is a frequent accident, due to great distention of the joint by serous effusion into the synovial sac. Dislocation is especially frequent in the subacute arthritis of the hip joint in children. In 84 cases of this type of arthritis collected by Keen spontaneous dislocation of the hip occurred in 40 cases, dislocation of the shoulder in 2 cases, and dislocation of the knee in 1 case. Subacute arthritis is undobutedly due to invasion of the joint by the typhoid bacillus. Fluid from the joint has been found to be sterile in some instances, in others to contain the typhoid bacillus.

Bones.—The typhoid bacillus uniformly localizes and multiplies in the bone marrow, which may harbor the organism for an indefinite period after recovery. The bacillus has been recovered from bone lesions, in one case thirteen years, in another twenty-three years, after an attack of typhoid. In spite of the uniform infection of the bone marrow, bone lesions are rare, occurring in less than 1 per cent of the cases. Appearing chiefly in convalescence or long after recovery, they are sequelae rather than complications. Adults are most frequently affected. The two essential forms of bone disease are (1) *osteoperiostitis* and (2) *osteomyelitis*. Osteoperiostitis is the common lesion. *Necrosis* and *caries* may result from either of the conditions. Of Keen's 237 collected cases, 110 were periostitis, 85 necrosis and 13 caries. The bones most frequently affected are, in order, the tibia, ribs, femur, ulna and humerus. Other bones may be involved. A solitary lesion is the rule. Multiple lesions may affect a single bone.

The disease begins with a tender, localized or diffused swelling over a superficial bone. There are practically no constitutional symptoms. The nodule may persist for a short or for a long time and then subside, or it may end in suppuration. Recurrence with or without suppuration is sometimes noted. The pus almost always yields the typhoid bacillus. Secondary infections with streptococcus, staphylococcus, etc., occasionally occur.

The pure typhoid lesions do not often cause serious damage to the bone. The secondary infections are much more serious and may endanger life. The x-ray is of great value in determining the character of the lesion and the extent of bone involvement.

Spine.—SPONDYLITIS.—Gibney in 1889 described a group of four cases occurring in the convalescent period of typhoid fever under the term "Typhoid Spine" in which there were pain, tenderness and rigidity of the lower spine, which he regarded as due to a perispondylitis. Carnett, writing in 1915, states that over 100 cases have been reported since Gibney's paper was published. X-ray examinations of the more recent cases support the view that an organic lesion, usually a periostitis, is the foundation of the symptoms. "The skiagrams show periostitis with effusion under the periosteum, changes in the intervertebral discs, and new formation of bone. Commonly only two adjacent vertebrae are involved, although rarely several may be. In rare instances with septic infection there may be suppuration, when caries and necrosis may occur" (Webb-Johnson). Neuroses simulating this condition possibly occur, but they should be excluded from the list of true typhoid spine cases.

The disease as a rule involves the lumbar vertebrae, either alone or together with the immediately adjacent dorsal or sacral vertebrae. The disease occurs as a late complication or as a sequela, two or three months often intervening between defervescence and the onset of the spondylitis. One case occurred four years after recovery from the primary infection. The affection occurs in both mild and severe cases and more frequently in young men, from twenty to twenty-five years of age.

The onset of symptoms is usually gradual, but may be abrupt and severe. Pain over the lumbar spine is the most constant and positive symptom. It may be very severe. It may be restricted to the lumbar area or referred along the course of the lumbar or sacral nerves. The pain is aggravated by movement. Tenderness and rigidity are present in almost all cases, and occasionally there is swelling. Some rise of temperature is usually seen. In one of our cases developing six weeks after convalescence, the temperature ranged from 101 to 104° F. (38.3 to 40° C.) during six days at the height of the disease. Sensory disturbances, muscular paresis and atrophy and changed reflexes are occasionally observed from involvement of the spinal nerve roots.

The disease usually ends in recovery in two or three weeks. It may be prolonged for several weeks. Severe cases with necrosis and caries are of course more serious.

THE CARRIER STATE

Clinical recovery from typhoid fever may not be coincident with bacteriologic recovery. With the beginning of the stage of decline the bacilli in the circulating blood diminish in number, and as a rule they disappear from the blood stream several days before convalescence begins. The bacilli, however, persist in the gallbladder, intestine and other residual foci, for varying periods after they have left the blood stream. In favorable cases, the blood and tissues are free of bacilli within a few days after the temperature becomes normal. In a certain percentage of all cases residual foci persist for months or years, in which the bacilli live and multiply and from which they are continuously or intermittently excreted. This sequela of typhoid fever is termed the *carrier state,* and an individual thus harboring typhoid bacilli in his body is termed a *typhoid carrier.*

40101

According to the channels of elimination of the typhoid bacilli, typhoid carriers are classified as: (1) *intestinal* or *fecal carriers;* (2) *urinary carriers;* and (3) *pus carriers.*

Intestinal carriers are in large majority. The bacilli are present and multiply in the gallbladder and bile ducts and elimination is through the feces. The pelvis of the kidney is the most common focus in the urinary carriers. A chronic cystitis or a spermovesiculitis is the focus in rare instances. Pus carriers are rare and of relative unimportance as sources of infection. A chronic abscess, otitis media or periostitis may be caused by typhoid bacilli. Of three thundred and fourteen cases of the carrier state collected by Prigge, 291, or 93 per cent, were fecal and 23, or 7 per cent, were urinary carriers.

Sacquépée divided all carriers according to their relation to an attack of typhoid fever into the following groups:

Group 1. *Precocious* or *incubation carriers,* who discharge bacilli before the onset of clinical symptoms of typhoid fever.

Group 2. *Recovered carriers:* (a) *convalescent carriers,* who discharge bacilli up to three months after clinical recovery; and (b) *chronic carriers,* who discharge bacilli longer than three months after clinical recovery.

Group 3. *Healthy carriers,* giving no history of typhoid fever.

At present a person is designated a chronic carrier when bacilli continue to be discharged beyond the period of one year.

Precocious Carriers.—Conradi in 1907 recorded two cases of precocious carriers. G. Mayer had already demonstrated the presence of typhoid bacilli in the stools of a patient eight days before the onset of symptoms. Battlehner has reported four precocious carriers who discharged bacilli in the feces for from twenty-one to one hundred and seventeen days before the onset of fever. Typhoid bacilli in any great numbers are not present in the feces until general infection and gallbladder localization have taken place. "It seems necessary to assume in the case of incubation carriers that the evolution of the disease symptoms has simply been delayed beyond the usual period following general invasion of the bacillus" (Gay).

Havens observed two precocious carriers in thirty-five contacts during a hospital epidemic.

Recovered Carriers.—We are largely indebted to the German investigators working along the lines recommended by Koch in 1902 for the demonstration of the incidence of the carrier state as a sequela of typhoid fever.

In a total of 2,714 persons convalescent from typhoid fever reported by nine German, English and American writers, an average of 4.1 per cent were found to be carriers for three months or longer. One group of 86 cases studied by Semple and Greig, in India, gave the exceptionally high incidence of 11.6 per cent but these were followed for a period of three months only.

Stebbins, in New York State, finds that 2.5 per cent of typhoid cases become carriers for more than one year. Anderson, of Massachusetts, accepts the figure of 2 per cent of all recovered cases in the determination of the number of carriers in any community.

Havens found 33 carriers, or 9.8 per cent, in a study of 348 individuals who had had typhoid fever one year or more previously.

Healthy Carriers.—Among 220 cases of typhoid carriers collected by Klinger, 44 individuals, or 20 per cent, gave no history of a previous attack of typhoid fever. Stebbins and Reed state that 20 per cent of the carriers in New York State were unaware of infection in the past. Elsom reported that 9 of 22 carriers under observation in Philadelphia gave no history of typhoid fever. Other authors confirm these findings. It seems conclusively proved that many persons become typhoid carriers without having passed through clinical typhoid fever.

Carriers in the General Population.—The number of carriers in the general population is proportional to the incidence of the disease in each locality. In the northeastern section of the United States and in Western Europe the rate is low. In New York State, including New York City in 1937, there were registered about 586 carriers, with a population of approximately 13,000,000, or 1 carrier to approximately 20,000 inhabitants. One-tenth per cent of 30,000 food handlers examined in the United States Army, during the first World War, were proved to be carriers. Rosenau in 1908 found 3 carriers among 993 in Washington, D. C.

Havens concludes that typhoid carriers comprise 1 per cent of the general population in regions where the typhoid rate is low and 3 to 4 per cent where it is high. A survey of some 400 dairy workers in Louisiana revealed 16, or 4 per cent, to be carriers. Scott, in Jamaica, found typhoid bacilli in the gallbladders in 3.5 per cent of 198 persons who had died of diseases other than typhoid. Havens studied 1,076 dairy employees and found 3.6 per cent typhoid carriers, 1.2 per cent paratyphoid A carriers, and 0.3 per cent paratyphoid B carriers. In Michigan, epidemiological studies revealed 198 carriers by the end of 1936; 124 of them were discovered in the last three years of that period.

Duration of the Carrier State.—The great majority of persons harboring the typhoid bacillus rid the body of them before three months and a few persist between three months and one year. Those harboring the bacillus over one year are classified as *chronic carriers* and are subject to state control.

A certain number of these are spontaneously cured. Of 368 carriers in New York State, 22 eventually were rid of the organism. In Havens' series of 348 persons who had typhoid fever, there were 12.1 per cent carriers of those who were examined from one to five years after the attack and 7.3 per cent in those who were examined more than five years after the original infection. Groninger reports the permanent spontaneous cure of a carrier fifty-one years after an attack of typhoid fever.

Urinary Carriers.—A large proportion of typhoid fever carriers excrete the bacilli in the urine. In Havens' dairy workers survey, 23 of 55 were urinary carriers and in his survey of recovered cases, 8 of 33 were urinary carriers. Two of 22 carriers studied by Elsom, in Philadelphia, were urinary carriers.

Cases Caused by Carriers.—Typhoid bacillus carriers perpetuate typhoid fever either through contamination of water supplies or by contact infection, including the contamination of food. In Michigan in 1936, 16.6 per cent of the cases were traced to carriers.

Senftner and Coughlin, and Stebbins and Reed have analyzed carrier infection in New York State. The total number of cases known to have been caused by carriers in upstate New York to June 30, 1932, was 1,875; 1,635 were caused prior to discovery of the carrier and 240 subsequent to

40101

it. Household contacts resulted in 774 cases, contaminated milk 875 cases, and other sources of contact 226 cases. Three hundred and sixty-eight carriers had been discovered during the same period. Ninety-three carriers caused no cases either prior or subsequent to discovery, 98 carriers caused no cases prior to discovery, and 316 carriers caused no cases subsequent to discovery. Two hundred and twenty-seven carriers caused 0.33 cases per person year * subsequent to typhoid fever and prior to discovery and 0.11 subsequent to discovery.

Thirty-three carriers who were dairy farm workers caused 0.91 cases per person year prior to discovery and 0.16 cases per person year after discovery.

Carrier control measures resulted in marked reduction but not complete elimination of typhoid fever.

Bacteriology of the Carrier State.—Studies of the organisms isolated from typhoid carriers and of the antibodies present in carriers have been made by numerous investigators. The principal purpose of these studies has been to discover carriers and to determine if the organisms isolated from every carrier are equally able to produce typhoid fever. The discovery of the Vi antigen and antibody has stimulated work along these lines.

Welch and Mickle studied 44 typhoid carrier strains to determine their Vi antigen content. They found that all the strains contained this antigen and concluded that a classification of strains could not be made on this basis.

Almon, Read and Stovall made a further study of the Vi antigen content of carrier strains and the Vi antibody content of serums of individuals from whom the strains were isolated. They confirmed the findings of Welch and Mickle by showing that the great majority of carrier strains contained Vi antigen and that its amount was as high in strains isolated from mild cases as from severe cases. They found the Vi antibody only occasionally and at irregular and unpredictable times in carriers. They stated that the Vi antibody level bore no relation to the swiftness of recovery or to the development of the carrier state.

Felix tested 65 known carriers for Vi antibodies, finding 60 positive, 3 negative and 2 doubtful. He demonstrated the Vi antigen in all of 25 strains recovered from carriers. Lewin studied 13 carriers. Virulent, intermediate and avirulent forms were recovered, and the serologic form was observed to change from time to time in the same carrier.

The recent work of Bhatnagar has been more encouraging. He believes that there is a definite correlation between the carrier condition and the presence of Vi antibody in the serums. As evidence he cites the records of four individuals. One proved to be only a temporary carrier. After three months no typhoid bacilli could be recovered from the urine or stools, and no Vi antibody could be demonstrated in the serum. The three persons whose serum continued to give a positive Vi reaction proved to be true chronic carriers. The organisms isolated from their feces were invariably found to be Vi-containing bacilli. If this work is confirmed and a stable and satisfactory Vi antigen-containing suspension made generally available, a significant step will have been made.

* Person years = sum of intervals from attack of typhoid fever to discovery and from discovery to June 30, 1932.

O agglutinin titers in serums from carriers are variable and cannot be relied upon for diagnostic purposes.

The Diagnosis of the Carrier State.—Diagnosis is made by bacteriologic examination. The bacilli are found in the feces and urine, in pus from suspected foci and in the bile obtained by transduodenal drainage. It is imperative that the bile specimen be free of acid gastric juice since Forsbeck and Hollon have shown that *E. typhosa* dies rapidly in such a mixture. Elimination of the bacilli is frequently intermittent, at least 30 per cent of the cases being found negative when only one examination is made. It is recommended that from three to five examinations of both urine and feces, taken at intervals of several days, be made before a suspected individual can be declared with certainty a non-carrier. The presence of the Vi antibody in the serum of a person not suffering from typhoid fever indicates that the person is a carrier.

PREGNANCY

Typhoid fever is rare in pregnant women. Authorities differ on the question of the relative immunity of the pregnant woman. In any large collection from 1 to 3 per cent of the cases of typhoid fever complicate pregnancy. The condition is one to cause anxiety. It leads to abortion or premature labor in from 40 to 60 per cent of the cases. Of 233 cases collected by Sacquin, pregnancy was interrupted in 150 cases; 37 of the patients died.

Abortion or premature labor usually occurs at the height of the fever and toxemia. When abortion occurs in the early months severe hemorrhage is common. Delivery at term usually takes place normally, and at times a healthy child may be born. Fetal death is the result of typhoid bacteremia. The organism has been repeatedly demonstrated in the blood and tissues of the fetus.

ASSOCIATION WITH OTHER DISEASES

Acute Diseases.—Typhoid fever is pre-eminently a disease of early life. Any of the acute diseases common to this period may be accidentally associated with typhoid infection, although as a matter of fact such coincidence is not frequent. Furnier collected 75 cases of *scarlet fever* associated with typhoid fever. Usually typhoid is the first infection and the scarlatina follows, probably from exposure to a passive carrier. *Measles,* a more common infection, is not readily carried and is very rarely seen. *Smallpox, chickenpox, whooping cough* and *diphtheria* have been rarely observed. *Influenza* may be an accidental associate, but it certainly does not predispose to typhoid fever. In fact there was an exceptionally low incidence of typhoid fever in Detroit during the prevalence of an epidemic of influenza. In the late period of typhoid, when complicating pyogenic infections of the skin are frequent, *erysipelas* may develop. Water-borne infections like *cholera, dysentery* and other diarrheal disease may develop with typhoid. The ingestion of highly polluted and typhoid-infected water may cause a quickly appearing *gastro-enteritis,* and this may be followed by typhoid fever after the usual incubation period.

Before the discovery of the specific organism of typhoid fever, clinicians of this country, following the lead of Woodward, concealed their uncertainty in diagnosis and lack of definite etiologic knowledge in the term *"typhomalarial fever,"* assuming the existence of a hybrid infection. This term is less ominous than typhoid fever and was widely used to designate any continued fever of doubtful etiology. Bacteriologic study has shown that there is no such pathologic entity, and the name in this sense should disappear from medical literature. The term is also given to severe continued *malarial fever* with adynamic symptoms. In French literature it is used to designate cases infected coincidentally with the typhoid and malarial organisms. In malarial districts this combined infection is occasionally seen. McCrae met with only 3 cases in his series. Chills and distortion of the temperature curve may excite suspicion of the malarial complication. Only the demonstration of the plasmodium will identify the intruding infection.

Chronic Diseases.—The association of *tuberculosis* with typhoid fever is of interest. The evidence is not convincing that either infection predisposes to the other. Both are diseases particularly incident to early life, and it would indeed be remarkable if an occasional tuberculous subject did not contract typhoid fever. The frequency of the association is not great enough to suggest anything but an accidental relation. In our experience the association is certainly rare. McCrae found only 6 cases of active clinical tuberculosis in his series. It is a noteworthy fact that in recent years there has been about an equal rate of decline in the mortality from typhoid fever and from tuberculosis. This decline may be attributed rather to the effect of modern sanitation, which affects the incidence of both diseases about equally, than to the influence of a direct etiologic relation between the two. Typhoid, like any acute debilitating disease, may activate a latent tuberculosis. Only in this sense can typhoid predispose to tuberculosis. A high percentage of consumptives give a history of one or more attacks of fever which have been thought to be typhoid, and for this reason typhoid fever has been considered to be a predisposing cause of tuberculosis. A history of a previous attack of typhoid fever in a consumptive patient should be received with suspicion. Periods of fever in cases of latent tuberculosis are very common and may closely simulate typhoid. Only laboratory evidence should be accepted as conclusive.

Association of typhoid fever with other chronic infections and with metabolic and degenerative diseases is rarely seen. The association with *syphilis* is uncommon. Before the days of antityphoid vaccination it was a particularly frequent coincidence in military medicine. *Diabetic* patients may develop an intercurrent typhoid infection. Severe cases run their course with a low temperature, although this in itself is not of unfavorable significance.

Chronic *alcoholics* are bad subjects for typhoid. Curschmann observed a mortality of 34 per cent among drunkards in Hamburg. Although the temperature generally runs low, signs of myocardial weakness develop early. Severe intestinal and other hemorrhages are frequent. Delirium, stupor and profound adynamia are frequent and grave manifestations. *Nephritis* with renal insufficiency and uremia may hasten a fatal issue.

CLINICAL VARIETIES

Infection by the Typhoid Bacillus Without Clinical Symptoms.— Infection by the typhoid bacillus without the development of clinical symptoms has been observed several times. Dennemark found typhoid bacilli in the feces of fifty-eight individuals who ate infected salad. In a study of one group of thirty-five contacts by Havens, six had positive fecal cultures; in another group of thirty-five contacts, seven excreted the bacillus. Billet made blood cultures of thirty-nine contacts and found seven positive. He made fecal cultures of sixty-four, of which thirteen were positive. All of these persons were closely observed and remained well. These studies explain the presence of agglutinins and the finding of the carrier state in those having no history of previous infection.

Mild Typhoid Fever.—Occasionally in hospital wards, quite frequently in private practice, cases of continued fever of short duration are seen which, from clinical signs alone, are difficult or impossible to classify. They have been described under the vague terms: febricula, ephemeral fever, gastric fever, simple continued fever, etc. That a certain or large percentage of such cases are examples of mild typhoid infection is the conviction of many careful and experienced observers. Louis mentions a mild case with perforation that came to autopsy. Gresinger (1864) described a form of typhoid fever in which the symptoms were mild and the duration of the disease was from eight to fourteen days. Murchison, Liebermeister and others of this period also mention a mild form of the disease. As these observations were made before the knowledge of bacteriologic diagnosis, the question was an open one. In mild cases the more positive clinical signs, the rose rash and the splenic enlargement, may not appear at all, or at least until the case has passed from observation. In fact the diagnosis of mild and atypical cases of typhoid fever by clinical means alone was, and still remains, notoriously unreliable. Laboratory aids now give certainty, and many continued fevers classified under various names have been identified as belonging to the typhoid group. French observers obtained positive serum reactions from cases of *embarras gastrique fébrile*. In a typhoid epidemic in Saarbrücken in 1904, Koch and his coworkers determined that many mild febrile cases of indefinite clinical character were typhoid infections. J. P. Bates in 1909 studied 68 cases of typhoid fever in Panama. Of these, 21 were of the short duration variety, in all of which a positive diagnosis was made by blood culture or serum reaction. Warren Coleman studied 24 cases of short duration typhoid fever in the second medical division of Bellevue Hospital. They constituted 10 per cent of all the typhoid cases admitted to the division in five years. The diagnosis in 20 of the cases was made by blood culture or serum reaction; in the remaining 4 cases, by clinical evidence alone.

The typhoid fever commission of the Spanish-American War concluded from their studies that because of their mild character a large percentage of the cases of this disease, both in civil and military practice, were not recognized as typhoid fever.

From the foregoing it seems proved that mild cases of typhoid fever of short duration are common, and in the interest of both the patient and of the public health they should be recognized and treated as such.

40101

Bacteriologic and serologic study should be made of every continued fever of more than two or three days' duration for which an adequate cause cannot be found.

The clinical history of mild typhoid shows many variations from the typical course. The fastigium of the disease is shortened and the temperature curve may exhibit many irregularities. Only exceptionally does it rise above 103° F. (39.4° C.) (Fig. 1). The stage of decline is equally variable. It may be short, or it may continue for a full week or longer, the temperature showing sharp remissions or irregularities. The symptoms are slight throughout the whole course of the disease. Diarrhea is mild or absent. Prostration is not great, and important nervous symptoms are absent. The typhoid rash is present in a majority of the cases that continue into the second week. The spleen is palpable only in a small percentage of the cases. Complications are unusual, wasting is not marked, and convalescence is usually rapid.

Abortive Typhoid Fever.—In the abortive form of mild typhoid the disease begins sharply, and all of the symptoms of an attack of moderate severity progress in the usual sequence. At the end of a week or ten days defervescence unexpectedly begins; the temperature rapidly declines, all the symptoms abate, and convalescence is established in from ten to fourteen days from the onset.

Afebrile Typhoid Fever.—A form of mild typhoid fever running its course with characteristic typhoid symptoms and without a febrile temperature is described by various authors. Diagnosis in the reported cases has usually been made from the clinical history and has apparently been confirmed in a few cases by autopsy. As elevation of temperature is an essential fact in the clinical conception of typhoid infection, a period of vague ill-health without temperature above the normal would rarely arouse suspicion of typhoid fever and lead to its identification by laboratory methods. Only an occasional case has been reported by American writers. In the present state of our knowledge a diagnosis of afebrile typhoid fever demands verification by positive pathologic or bacteriologic evidence.

Ambulatory or Walking Typhoid.—It not infrequently happens that the subjective symptoms of the initial period of typhoid fever are not of the usual severity, and a patient may continue his ordinary activities until the disease is well advanced, when an overwhelming prostration or a serious complication like hemorrhage or perforation compels him to seek medical advice.

These cases fall into two groups. Cases of the first group are observed most frequently in men of the lower classes who are not mindful of bodily discomfort and who resist the illness to the last moment. Eventually such a patient consults the physician in his office, or walks into the hospital, where he is found to be well along in the second or third week of the disease. Intelligent devotees of the various forms of mental therapeutics are also found in this group. The subsequent course of the disease in these cases is often severe and fatal.

In the second group are included the cases of mild typhoid which escape recognition as such and are thought to be cases of influenza, cold, acute intestinal catarrh or other unimportant infection. Patients of this group may pass through the disease without taking to their beds.

Malignant Typhoid Fever.—A profound toxemia characterizes this form of the disease. The onset may be sudden, with high fever, frequent and persistent vomiting, quick and feeble pulse and a rapidly developing and fatal asthenia. In other cases, after a violent onset, early adynamic symptoms develop. There are abundant diarrhea, great prostration, feeble heart action, low delirium or profound stupor. The patient is overwhelmed by the intensity of the infection and succumbs in the second week of the disease.

Subcutaneous and internal hemorrhages are occasionally seen, and constitute what is known as *hemorrhagic typhoid fever*. This form is very rare. In Osler's studies at Johns Hopkins Hospital only 1 case was observed. This was reported in detail by Hamburger. Hamburger cites Uskow's series of 6,513 cases of typhoid fever with 4 of the hemorrhagic form. Liebermeister observed 3 cases of this form among 1,900 cases of typhoid.

Typhoid Fever in Children.—Children are just as susceptible to typhoid fever as adults. They are more resistant to the typhoid toxemia, and the general course of the disease is as a rule milder. Short duration typhoid and the abortive types are frequently seen, and the individual stages of the disease are shortened. Septic and protracted cases are infrequent.

Some of the individual symptoms show variation from the adult type. The slow pulse of adult typhoid is not observed. From the onset the pulse is rapid, especially in very young children. Vomiting more often occurs at the onset and diarrhea is more constant than in the adult. Pain and abdominal distention are more pronounced. Hemorrhage and perforation are rare accidents up to six years of age. After this the incidence of these accidents increases with the age of the patient and about equals the adult percentage by the end of childhood.

In the severe cases nervous symptoms and complications are apt to occur. Convulsions at the onset and meningeal symptoms during the course are not rare. Transitory aphasia is a complication seen more commonly in children.

Recrudescence and relapse occur with greater frequency than in adult typhoid. The mortality rate is low. The Hamburg statistics show a rate of 4 per cent between the ages of two and five years and of 6.4 per cent between five and ten years.

Typhoid Fever in Infancy.—Infants enjoy a relative immunity to typhoid fever, as they do to some of the other acute infectious fevers. The disease is comparatively rare under the age of two years, and decidedly rare under one year. The occurrence of the disease in very early life has been doubted by many clinicians, but the positive findings of modern laboratory diagnosis and the accurately recorded cases of many pediatricians have demonstrated that typhoid fever is one of the diseases that must always be given consideration in the differentiation of the acute febrile diseases of infancy.

Holt states that but 11 cases of typhoid fever in infants under two years of age were observed in the Babies' Hospital in New York during a period of thirteen years. Five were under one year of age. Griffith, of Philadelphia, who has repeatedly called attention to the occurrence of typhoid fever in the young, observed 45 cases in the Children's Hospital in infants under two years of age. Nine were in infants under

40101

one year, the youngest being three months old. Cases in the newborn have been recorded. Jacobi reports a case developing on the sixteenth day after birth.

Of 145 cases of typhoid fever in children reported by A. Hand, Jr., 2 were under two years of age. In a study of 337 cases of typhoid fever in children by Adams, of Washington, 13 were in infants two years of age and in 1 case one year of age. Of 200 cases in the experience of Abt, of Chicago, 4 patients were two years of age and 2 were under one year. In the various discussions on the subject in the American Pediatric Society it has been brought out that members who have had a large experience in the care of children have all met with a few cases of infantile typhoid. During an extended personal experience with diseases of children in a city with a large typhoid fever incidence, the late author (C. G. J.) observed only 2 cases occurring in infants under one year of age. One at nine months gave a positive blood culture on the fifth day. Statistics from European sources show about the same incidence. In 3,686 cases treated in the Hamburg general hospital in 1886 and 1887, 7 were under two years of age. In the Jacobspital of Leipzig, from 1880 to 1893, there were 1,626 cases of typhoid, including 5 under two years of age. The mortality statistics of Paris from 1880 to 1889 give 36 cases under the age of one year, out of 16,036 deaths from typhoid fever.

SYMPTOMS.—The onset of the disease in infants is more apt to be abrupt and without prodromic malaise. The infant is severely ill from the beginning. Anorexia, vomiting, diarrhea and abdominal pain are frequently noted in the first day or two. In rare cases convulsions mark the onset of the disease, or they may occur in the fastigium and are then, as in other severe infections, of grave import. The temperature curve (Fig. 5) shows variations from the usual adult type. It rises to a moderate height on the first day and attains in two or three days the high level that in adult cases is not reached until the end of the first week. The remittent character of the fever in the fastigium is less marked. During this period the range of the temperature is apt to be higher than in adult cases of the same general severity. The pulse is rapid and more in harmony with the temperature, and is not often dicrotic. Diarrhea is present in about the same general proportion of cases as in adult typhoid. The dejecta, however, have more the appearance of the ordinary diarrheal stool in infancy than of the peculiar typhoid stool of adult cases. Tympanites is not severe and gurgling and tenderness are infrequent. The grave intestinal accidents, hemorrhage and perforation, are decidedly rare.

The eruption appears somewhat earlier than in the adult, but is not so constantly seen. Hand noted it in 70 per cent of his cases, an unusually high percentage. The spots are fewer in number and not so distinctive in appearance.

The normal leukocyte count in infancy varies from 9,000 to 18,000; in childhood from 8,000 to 12,000. The low leukocyte count of adult typhoid fever, so valuable in diagnosis, is not found in the very young. Only rarely is the count below 5,000, and it varies all the way to 16,000 in uncomplicated cases. The blood count in infancy is, therefore, of comparatively little value in diagnosis; a count below 6,000, however, would be strongly suggestive of typhoid fever.

The typhoid of infancy does not show the multiplicity of complications and sequelae that are so marked a feature of adult typhoid. Some cases succumb to the toxemia in the second or third week of the disease, and the milder cases recover completely.

Typhoid Fever in the Aged.—Typhoid is decidedly rare in the latter part of life. Of 5,306 cases observed by Curschmann, 60 were in patients over fifty years of age. The course of the disease is severe and the prognosis unfavorable. The mortality is from 30 to 40 per cent.

The onset and evolution of the symptoms are gradual. Chill is very rare. Repeated chilly sensations are usual the first few days of the febrile period. Resistance to the toxemia is feeble. Prostration is manifested early and soon becomes profound. Stupor and coma are early symptoms. Tremor, subsultus and muttering delirium are almost always present. In the patients who recover these adynamic symptoms are marked throughout the entire course of the disease.

The temperature is in harmony with the sluggish reaction to the infection. The curve holds at a low maximum, rarely rising above 102° F. (38.9° C.); it is erratic, with marked remissions or intermissions. The characteristic typical curve of typhoid is almost never seen. Afebrile cases occur most frequently in the aged.

Cardiac asthenia appears early. The pulse is rapid from the beginning, and becomes irregular and feeble as prostration increases. It does not show the dicrotic character of typhoid in earlier life.

Bronchitis is apt to be severe, and the feeble right heart favors the development of hypostatic pulmonary congestion and pneumonia.

Hemorrhage and perforation are of average frequency. Hemorrhage is a severe complication, even small losses of blood adding greatly to the gravity of a case. Diagnosis by clinical means is difficult. The rose spots are few, less brilliant and disappear quickly. The spleen is seldom palpable. The general picture of the disease is misleading, and laboratory aid is essential to prompt and positive diagnosis.

The disease is often long-drawn-out, convalescence is tedious, and the former state of health is rarely regained.

TREATMENT
GENERAL PROPHYLAXIS

Typhoid fever is a preventable disease. The elimination of typhoid as an important factor in the death rate from disease in the United States Army during the first World War is convincing evidence that with equally efficient administration in civil communities, of the prophylactic measures now known to sanitary science, typhoid fever would practically disappear from mortality statistics. In the present state of society, eradication of the disease is not to be expected. Under the best civil sanitary administration now possible, living bacilli will occasionally escape the protectve barriers thrown out against them and reach the alimentary canal of unprotected individuals. Typhoid fever, like smallpox, should be only a rare visitor in any community.

The prevention of typhoid fever may be accomplished by: (1) the destruction of the bacillus at its source; (2) the prevention of the transmission of the bacillus from the excreta of the typhoid patient or carrier to healthy persons; (3) the protection of the individual by antityphoid vaccination.

40101

1. **Destruction of the Bacillus at Its Source.**—The bacillus leaves the infected patient by way of the excreta: the feces, urine, sputum and, rarely, in the pus of typhoid abscesses. Could these discharges from every typhoid patient and carrier be thoroughly disinfected immediately after discharge—or, to put it in other words, could the bacillus be killed at its source—typhoid fever would soon cease to exist. This is only theoretically possible. Unrecognized healthy carriers, mild, incipient and atypical cases, cases with delayed diagnosis or under the care of thoughtless physicians or nurses give abundant opportunity for the bacillus to escape and be at large. **Early and correct diagnosis** is an important factor in the prophylaxis of the disease. In a recognized case of typhoid fever the responsibility for the prevention of further extension of the infection rests with the attending physician. To wait for the clinical and laboratory signs necessary for a positive diagnosis is a serious error. Prophylaxis should begin with the first suspicion of the presence of typhoid.

Destruction of the bacillus at its source is accomplished by the **disinfection of all excreta** as soon as they are discharged from the patient and the **sterilization of all persons or objects contaminated by them.**

STOOLS.—Disinfection of the stools requires care and time. **Heat** is the most efficient disinfectant. Its use is not practicable in home surroundings. In hospitals, camps and during epidemics, **disinfection of feces by boiling or by the action of steam** is practical and efficient. The fever wards in hospitals should be equipped with **closed hoppers for the sterilization by steam, of excretions, bed pans and urinals. Chemical disinfection** is available in all cases and if carried out with due attention to detail, the results are satisfactory. The bathroom toilet should not be used until the patient is convalescent and the stools free from bacilli. The discharges should be received in a bed pan or commode containing a small quantity of disinfectant solution. There should be added disinfectant solution in quantity equal to at least twice or three times the volume of the mass of excreta. The mixture should then be thoroughly stirred and all solid masses of feces broken up. Bacilli embedded in hard fecal masses will resist the action of the disinfectant for hours or indefinitely. The receptacle should then be tightly covered and allowed to stand for several hours—two hours at least—before final disposal. After emptying, the receptacle should be cleaned and sterilized by boiling water, steam or disinfectant solution.

Carbolic acid in 5 per cent solution is the most satisfactory and generally useful chemical disinfectant. The quantity used should be double the volume of the feces.

Fresh milk of lime is an efficient disinfectant and has the advantage of being readily available everywhere. To 100 parts of freshly burnt lime—calcium oxide—add 60 parts of water. The resulting product is slaked lime—calcium hydroxide. To prepare the milk of lime mix 1 part of this fresh slaked lime with 8 parts of water. The slaked lime must be kept tightly sealed and the milk of lime prepared fresh every day. The quantity used should be three times the volume of the feces. **Air-slaked lime is useless as a disinfectant.**

Other chemical disinfectants that may be used are **chlorinated lime,** 5 per cent solution; **compound solution of cresol,** 2 per cent; **solution of formaldehyde,** 10 per cent. Bichloride of mercury is not effective for the disinfection of feces.

URINE.—Cole states that every specimen of urine from a typhoid patient should be regarded as a pure culture of typhoid bacilli. Each specimen should be disinfected as voided, by the addition of a 5 per cent **solution of carbolic acid,** 1 part to 2 parts of urine, or 1:1000 **bichloride of mercury solution,** 1 part to 20 parts of urine. The mixture should stand for two hours. It is often convenient to keep the urine in a covered jar containing the proper amount of disinfectant for the day's excretion and to empty the jar every twenty-four hours. **The urinal should be kept immersed in a disinfectant solution when not in use.** Disinfection of the urine at its source, by the internal administration of hexamethylenamine is considered elsewhere.

SPUTUM—NASAL SECRETIONS.—Sputum and nasal secretions should be received in **gauze or paper and burned** at frequent intervals; or in **sputum cups** which are frequently **disinfected with carbolic acid or bichloride solution.**

VOMITUS, PUS AND OTHER DISCHARGES.—Vomitus, pus and other discharges should be treated like the urine or feces.

BATH WATER.—This is too frequently discharged into the house drain, without treatment. It may be efficiently disinfected by the addition of one-half pound of **fresh chlorated lime** to each 50 gallons of water.

PERSONAL AND BED LINEN.—The patient's personal and bed linen should first be **soaked** for two or more hours **in a 5 per cent carbolic acid solution, and then boiled.** Towels and handkerchiefs should be treated in the same way. Rubber sheets may be soaked in a disinfectant solution. **Mattresses, blankets and fabrics that cannot be boiled should be sterilized with dry heat or formaldehyde.**

DISHES, UTENSILS, ETC.—Dishes and tray service should be sterilized by a disinfectant solution or by boiling before being taken from the sickroom. **Bed pans, urinals, syringes, rectal tubes and all instruments must be boiled or treated with one of the disinfectant solutions and when possible kept immersed in the solution. The sickroom should be kept scrupulously clean and, at the end of the illness, thoroughly disinfected.**

THE CHRONIC TYPHOID CARRIER.—Detection and control of the chronic carrier has reduced to a material degree the number of contact cases originating from it.

Detection of Carriers.—Carriers are discovered by:

1. Epidemiologic investigation of sporadic cases and outbreaks.
2. Bacteriologic investigation of recently recovered cases.
3. Routine examinations of food handlers.
4. Routine examinations, especially the study of the bile obtained by transduodenal drainage or at operation.

An increase in detected carriers has resulted from the practice of investigation of isolated endemic cases as well as of distinct outbreaks. Accurate bacteriologic diagnosis of all persons suffering from suspicious fevers is an important factor in eliminating the chronic carrier. The health authorities should maintain supervision over the typhoid patient until bacteriologic recovery is complete.

Supervision of the Chronic Carriers.—Each carrier should be registered and visited periodically by the local health officer. He should be prohibited from any occupation involving the handling of food. Immunization should be strongly urged to all household or industrial contacts. Milk sold from a farm on which a typhoid carrier resides should be subject to strict supervision. The carrier should be directed to dispose of his excreta in such manner that transmission of the bacillus to others will be avoided. His personal clothing and linen should not be laundered without previous disinfection. He should not make a trip or change his residence without notification of the health authorities.

A carrier should be made aware of his condition and he should be educated to co-operate with the health authorities and assist in guarding the community from contact with his excretions.

Treatment of Carriers.—(*a*) *Medical Treatment.*—Vaccine therapy, drugs and radiation have not proved of value in the cure of the typhoid carrier.

(*b*) *Surgical Treatment.*—The *chronic carrier state* may be cured by **resection of the focus of infection**. In Michigan, 22 cholecystectomies have been performed for the cure of the carrier state to the year 1937. Twenty of them, or 90.9 per cent, were cured. In New York State through 1938, 86 carriers have been subjected to cholecystectomy and 47 have been cured. Coller and Forsbeck report cholecystectomy in 18 typhoid bacillus carriers, with 16 recoveries and no deaths. All of these cases are included in the Michigan report noted above. Hanssen cites 8 cases of cholecystectomy at the New York Postgraduate Hospital, of which 7 were cured and none died. Whipple reported 12 cases of cholecystectomy, with 8 cures, 2 deaths, 1 failure to cure and 1 lost to observation. In addition, two cholecystotomies were done, one of whom was cured. These authors have reviewed the literature, with findings essentially the same as their own. Nichols, Simmons and Stimmell (1919) treated 5 fecal carriers by cholecystectomy with recovery in 3.

Cholecystectomy fails to cure a small percentage of fecal carriers. Some of these are liver or biliary duct carriers. They cannot be detected preoperatively. Others are intestinal tract carriers, and in them the bile is sterile. Biliary culture should be done when operation is considered, and if negative, surgery will not effect a cure. Hammer quotes Kehr stating that in addition to removal of the gallbladder the common duct should be drained. In a majority of the cases operation is accepted for relief of symptoms of gallbladder disease. When operation is urged for the cure of the carrier state primarily, its risk should be considered, but the benefits that accrue both to the carrier and the community justify it in the presence of any reasonable hazard. Following operation the bacilli persist in the feces up to the fourteenth day, after which they tend to disappear. In one case of Coller's series they were present for 308 days, and in one of Browning's for 14 months.

As evidence of cure of the carrier state by cholecystectomy the State of New York requires that at least three biliary specimens, taken at intervals of not less than twenty-four hours, and eight consecutive liquid fecal specimens taken on successive days, be negative. The patient is eligible for release by the Michigan Department of Health after twelve consecutive fecal specimens, obtained at monthly intervals, and two bile specimens obtained during the year after operation, have proved negative.

Senftner and Coughlin have analyzed 68 cases operated upon in upstate New York previous to 1933. Cholecystectomy was done upon

61, of whom 35 were cured, 8 died, 10 were not cured and 8 were lost to observation. In 7 cholecystotomy was performed, of whom 2 died, 3 failed to be cured and 2 were lost to observation. In 4 cases cholecystotomy was first done and then cholecystectomy. Of these, 2 died and 2 were cured. No deaths occurred in patients under fifty years of age. The total mortality for this series was 14.7 per cent. That of those operated upon for relief of the carrier condition primarily was 7.1 per cent, and excluding carriers in state institutions, it was 3.7 per cent. Of 31 operated upon above the age of fifty, 32.3 per cent died.

Urinary carriers may be due to chronic cystitis, pyelonephritis, pyelonephrosis, and perinephric abscess. A urologic investigation will determine the location of the infected area. Recovery of the typhoid bacillus from both the right and left ureters is common, even though the disease is unilateral.

Barker reports one case of typhoid cystitis cured by the technic of Schottmüller. This consists in the instillation of 100 cc. of 2 per cent silver nitrate through a catheter into the bladder. This is allowed to remain five minutes and is then washed out. The treatment may be highly irritating.

Huggins and Roome collected from the literature 20 cases of typhoid bacillus pyonephrosis treated surgically. Twelve underwent nephrectomy and 10 recovered and 2 died. Three underwent nephrotomy and 1 recovered and 2 died. Cystotomy was performed once and the patient died. Two patients died without operations and the outcome of 2 was unknown. They report 2 cases of their own treated by nephrectomy with recovery. A chronic sinus with discharge of typhoid bacilli followed the operation in both cases. One healed spontaneously in ten months and the other in eleven months.

Kahle and Beacham report one case with cure by nephrotomy followed by subcapsular nephrectomy.

Treatment of the carrier state may be undertaken solely for the cure of that condition or because of symptoms resulting directly from the infection. Such an operation is a serious one and the chances of ultimate cure should be weighed carefully before it is advised.

2. **Prevention of the Transmission of the Bacillus.**—ISOLATION.—A patient suspected to be in the incubation or developed stage of typhoid fever should immediately be isolated, and every known barrier against the transmission of the disease should be thrown around him. As a general rule, this object can best be attained in a hospital where the routine for the prevention of the transmission of disease is always ready to function. In many of the hospitals of the United States typhoid fever patients are still treated in the general wards. They should, however, be **isolated in rooms or special fever wards and nurses assigned to their care who do not come in contact with the patients in the general wards.** With the usual precautions the danger of hospital infection is not great, although careless attendants are occasionally responsible for the transmission of the disease. In children's hospitals, where patients are in closer contact, the danger is greater. *If treated at home* **the patient should be in a room separated from the other members of the family and every precaution taken to prevent them from coming in contact with the patient's excretions.**

40101

Physicians, nurses, orderlies and other attendants on the typhoid sick should observe special precautions to guard against the danger of carrying the disease to others. Hands soiled with the patients' excretions are the common guilty agents. **A disinfectant scrubbing of the hands should follow each contact with the patient.** When using the bed pan or urinal the nurse or orderly should wear **rubber gloves, and a rubber apron** should protect the clothing. **Typhoid nurses should not prepare the food for other patients or serve it.** The sickroom should be screened, and excreta, soiled clothing and food remnants carefully guarded from flies.

The proper disposal of sewage and the prevention of the transmission of typhoid fever through the medium of general water and food supplies are sanitary measures that come under the control of local and state boards of health. Sterilization of the drinking water of small groups or individuals may be accomplished by treatment with **hypochlorite of lime.** Horwood recommends that one-half pound of fresh bleach be dissolved in one gallon of water. Two drops of this solution will effectively sterilize one gallon of water after stirring for five minutes. In the United States Army, one gram of the powder, issued in a tube, is first mixed into a paste and then made into a solution by stirring in a clean ordnance cup. This is then added to 36 gallons of water and allowed to stand 30 minutes before use. Efficiency of sterilization is indicated by the appearance of a blue color when 10 drops of a solution containing 10 per cent of potassium iodide and 1 per cent of soluble starch are added to a cupful of the water. Tablets of hypochlorite of lime, each sufficient to sterilize one gallon of water, may be obtained.

Previous to the introduction of antityphoid vaccination the reduction of the typhoid rate had been slowly progressive throughout the country. This reduction was due in large measure to the **protection from sewage contamination of general water supplies or to their purification by filtration and chemical treatment.** The remarkably low typhoid rate of some European cities adequately sewered and provided with an abundance of pure water is convincing evidence of the importance of these factors in the prevention of typhoid fever. An outbreak of typhoid fever should lead immediately to the **thorough investigation of the water, milk and other foods consumed by this community. Bathing in polluted waters should be prohibited.** The rural swimming hole or the urban tank may be a prolific source of infection.

3. **Antityphoid Vaccination.**—Benmer and Peiper in 1887 and Chantemesse and Widal in 1888 showed that mice could be protected from infection by the typhoid bacillus by inoculation with sterilized cultures of the organism. In 1896 A. E. Wright developed a vaccine for the immunization of human beings and in the same year Pfeiffer and Kolle published the results of the vaccination of a few men with a vaccine prepared by a method similar to that of Wright. In the few years following this original work, a number of methods of preparation and administration of typhoid vaccine were developed by various experimenters.

ANTITYPHOID VACCINATION IN ARMIES.—Vaccination on a large scale was first practiced in the British Army in India and in South Africa during the Boer War, under the direction of Wright. Wright's statistics showed a reduction in the incidence of typhoid fever among vaccinated men of at least 50 per cent with a reduction of case mortality from 16.6 per cent in the *un*vaccinated to 8 per cent in the vaccinated. These results were obtained under the conditions of active service in the field. At the close of the war, vaccination was discontinued but in 1905 it was resumed. Leishman reported that the case incidence of typhoid among vaccinated men in the British Army in India from 1905 to 1908 was 3.8 per thousand and in the *un*vaccinated it was 28.3. Leishman's statistics showed decided improvement over the original statistics of Wright, due to improvements in the method of preparation of the vaccine and in the technic of administration. Antityphoid vaccination was quickly introduced into all the armies of the world, and always with the same remarkable reduction in the incidence and mortality of typhoid fever. In the French Army no cases occurred among the vaccinated men in the garrison at Avignon in 1912 and 1913, nor in the regiment stationed at Tours in 1914. In both units there were severe epidemics among the unvaccinated men.

Vaccination was adopted in the United States Army in 1909 on the advice of a mixed civil and military medical board and was carried out under the direction of Colonel F. F. Russell, who had studied the conditions of antityphoid vaccination in England. Voluntary vaccination was begun in March, 1909, and vaccination was made compulsory for all persons in the military service under forty-five years of age in the last quarter of 1911. The decrease of typhoid fever in the United States Army following the introduction of vaccination is shown in Table IX. Despite the introduction of rigid sanitary rules following the Spanish-American War, the rate remained high until the year that vaccination was made compulsory.

TABLE IX

DECREASE OF TYPHOID FEVER IN THE U. S. ARMY FOLLOWING INTRODUCTION OF VACCINATION

Year	Vaccination	Cases per 100,000	Army Strength
1908	None	320	74,692
1909	Voluntary	335	. . . . .
1910	"	243	81,434
1911	½ Compulsory	85	82,802
1912	Compulsory	31	88,478
1913	"	4.4	90,752
1914	"	7.5	92,872
1915	"	8.0	. . . . .
1916	"	23	. . . . .

The appearance of paratyphoid fever among the troops mobilized on the Mexican border in 1916 and among the armies in France led the Medical Department of the Army to adopt preventive inoculation against the paratyphoid fevers. Castellani and others had shown that a triple vaccine containing three organisms, the typhoid bacillus, the paratyphoid bacillus A and the paratyphoid bacillus B, developed antibodies active against each of these organisms and that the reaction was no more severe than when a single vaccine was used. After an exhaustive study by Colonel C. F. Craig, of the effects of a triple typhoid vaccine prepared by the Army Medical School, this vaccine was adopted in 1917.

The incidence of typhoid fever in the armies in the first World War was published by Siler and Lambie and their abridged tables appear in the discussion of "Typhoid Fever in Armies." Their report further analyzes the effect of antityphoid vaccination. In the United States Army vaccination was universal and the full dose was administered to each man. There resulted a remarkably low attack rate. In the European Armies the troops were, at the onset, mustered with such haste that immunization was neglected. Typhoid fever was prevalent, though far below previous wars in numbers. The incidence was highest in the first two years and diminished in the final two years when the opportunity for thorough vaccination had been provided. The earlier British troops were sent to France before immunization had been completed. Nevertheless, their typhoid rate was low and there were relatively few deaths. Data are lacking on vaccination in the French, German, Austrian and Italian forces but it is obvious that the lessons of the Spanish-American and South African wars had not been heeded by them. Their rates were needlessly high and their losses were serious. In the American Expeditionary Force one fourth of the cases occurred after the cessation of hostilities, leading Siler and Lambie to conclude that for armies in the field revaccination is necessary before the usual interval of three years has passed. The Italian Expeditionary Force in Ethiopia had been thoroughly immunized before embarkation. The typhoid admission rate was about 0.8 per 1,000, which is comparable with excellent civilian rates in temperate climates.

The paratyphoid organisms were a negligible factor as a cause of disease in the United States Army during the first World War. This was in all likelihood due to immunization against these organisms with T.A.B. vaccine.

ANTITYPHOID VACCINATION FOR THE CIVIL POPULATION.—Inoculation for the prevention of typhoid fever should be practiced in the following civil groups:

1. Contacts of carriers and cases.
2. Doctors, nurses and hospital personnel.
3. Communities where typhoid is epidemic or the endemic rate is unusually high.
4. Communities where typhoid is to be expected because of floods or devastation.
5. Construction gangs or other groups living in barracks.
6. Individuals contemplating travel in countries where typhoid is endemic.
7. Individuals living in communities where pasteurization of milk is not required by law.

The protection afforded depends upon the magnitude of the infection and the time elapsed since vaccination. Many of the cases among civilians are the result of overwhelming infection from contact or from contaminated food and water.

Stebbins, from data gathered from persons exposed to carriers in New York State, and Bowdoin, who observed an epidemic from infected water in a school, both found that the attack rate of vaccinated persons was one-fifth that of the unvaccinated. In both instances the exposure was great. Malbin's recent study confirms this.

TABLE X

MORTALITY OF WATER-BORNE EPIDEMIC IN HAWAII

	Population on Castner Water System	No. of Cases of Typhoid	Cases per 1,000	Deaths		Mortality Rate per 1,000
				No.	Per Cent	
Vaccinated....	4,087	55	13.45	4	7.4	0.97
Unvaccinated..	812	45	55.41	7	15.5	8.62

Under improved sanitary conditions and more frequent vaccination the protection afforded is better. The Department of Health of New York City has published (1916) the results of vaccination of individuals exposed to typhoid fever in various ways, chiefly in their homes. Of 8,101 exposed persons, 534 were vaccinated. All of these escaped infection. Of the 7,567 persons not vaccinated 161, over 2 per cent, developed typhoid fever. Russell gives a report (Table X) of a small water-borne epidemic which occurred in Hawaii.

Lewin states that antityphoid inoculation has eliminated typhoid fever from the mines of South Africa wherever it has been universally used. In that area Grasset's endotoxoid vaccine is preferred to the bacterial suspension and vaccination is repeated yearly. Preventive inoculation was widely practiced during the floods of the Ohio and Mississippi rivers in 1937 and no increase of typhoid for that year was reported from the flooded areas.

Galloway reports the results of extensive vaccination in a southern county. There were 11,760 persons inoculated during a period of five years and of these 8 contracted typhoid and none died. About 22,000 persons living under similar conditions were not vaccinated and of these 265 had typhoid and 37 died.

Immediately following the first World War, the typhoid rate dropped appreciably. The death rate per 100,000 population in the United States registration area in 1918 was 12.6; in 1919, 9.2; in 1920, 7.8. Horwood attributes this drop to the vaccination of about four million young men during the war. This drop was predicted by C. G. Jennings and Morse in the previous edition of this article. Experience has conclusively proved that in civil communities, typhoid fever can be materially reduced under average conditions and practically eliminated under favorable conditions, by the combination of vaccination and the application of sanitary regulations.

PROPHYLACTIC TYPHOID AND PARATYPHOID VACCINES.—Since the work of Grinnell it has been accepted that the strain of the typhoid bacillus to be used in the preparation of vaccine should be the smooth form. Both the smooth virulent and the smooth intermediate strains have been employed. The rough variants are unsuitable. The tendency of all strains of E. typhosa to undergo dissociation and serologic change of form under artificial cultivation should be anticipated. For this reason strains used for vaccine preparation are routinely tested repeatedly for growth characteristics, antigenicity and agglutinability. By the use of suitable technics for the propagation of cultures certain strains have been found to retain their original characteristics for many years.

40101

Smooth virulent strains are at present believed to be superior to intermediate strains for immunization. Such strains contain the Vi antigen and the O antigen and more nearly approximate the antigenic structure of the typhoid bacillus as it occurs in clinical infection. In laboratory animals smooth virulent strains afford a higher degree of protection than does the intermediate strain. Siler and coworkers, using the mouse protection test devised by Rake, have demonstrated that humans vaccinated with this strain have better immunity than those vaccinated with the intermediate strain. Bowdoin reports satisfactory results from the use of a smooth virulent strain in Georgia. A similar strain was employed in the vaccination of the Italian Expeditionary Force in Ethiopia. Lewin employs only the smooth virulent strains in the preparation of his vaccine. It has not been found necessary to incorporate in the vaccine more than one strain.

The prime requirements of a vaccine are that it be immunogenic and nontoxic. The strain used in vaccine production up to quite recently was the Rawlings strain isolated by Wright in 1900. That this strain has been immunogenic has been amply demonstrated by the decreased incidence of typhoid fever in the U. S. Army and Navy following its introduction as a preventive measure. In spite of its demonstrated efficacy, the work of Grinnell, and Maltauer, who showed that it was intermediate between smooth and rough, stimulated interested parties to inquire into the possibility of finding a pure "smooth" strain which might be even more immunogenic. This investigation was taken up and carried to its present status by the group at the Army Medical School working under the direction of Colonel J. F. Siler.

The problem which faced this group was to find some accurate method of measuring the antigenicity of unknown strains. In their first published study (1936) they used the mouse virulence method. This consisted in determining the average lethal dose of various strains when injected intraperitoneally into white mice, and subsequently comparing the protection offered by these strains when given prophylactically. The method is known to have its fallacies, but it would seem to have served to show that several strains appeared superior to the Rawlings strain and justified further tests.

The subsequent tests were carried out, using a different method of evaluation—that of determining the passive protection offered mice by serum from individuals immunized with vaccines made from several strains. The value of these tests was enhanced by the discovery that mucin increased the virulence of *E. typhosa* for the mouse, thereby making it possible to give much smaller inoculations, and eliminating the disadvantage of nonspecific toxemias. The results of these tests confirmed their earlier findings—that No. 58 (carrier strain) was the most immunogenic strain tested. The Surgeon General of the Army then granted permission for this strain to be used in preparing typhoid vaccine for the Government Services. It is understood that commercial laboratories engaged in the production of vaccines have incorporated this strain. As pointed out by the Army workers, field tests will only establish the validity of the results obtained by the mouse tests.

Grasset's typhoid endotoxoid vaccine is prepared from disintegrated organisms treated with formalin. Smooth virulent strains are selected for use. Lewin reports that clinically and serologically it is the equal of the bacterial suspension and that its reactions are much less severe.

Certain studies previously alluded to have been directed to the stimulation of immunity by means of the chemically purified antigens. This work has been carried out by Boivin and Mesrobeanu, Topley and associates and Henderson and Wakeman. Such antigens so far isolated evoke, in mice, antibodies of the same order as the strains from which they are derived. Large scale immunization of humans by these antigens has not yet been reported.

Paratyphoid vaccines are prepared from four strains, Rogers' and Meers' paratyphoid bacillus A and Cools' and Rowlands' paratyphoid bacillus B.

There have been no studies made upon these organisms comparable to those of the typhoid bacillus. The smooth forms are, however, selected with a great deal of care.

For general use, vaccine containing the typhoid bacillus and paratyphoid bacilli A and B is advised. The concentration of the suspension is 1,000 million of the former and 750 million each of the latter per cubic centimeter. When the protection to be achieved is known to be against typhoid fever only, as in areas where the paratyphoid fevers, are rare, vaccine containing the typhoid bacillus alone is permissible. Reactions to the single vaccine are stated to be less severe than to the triple vaccine and there is some belief that vaccination with the typhoid bacillus confers a degree of immunity to the paratyphoid fevers. The Michigan State Department of Health at present recommends immunization with the typhoid bacillus alone. When the single vaccine is administered the suspension is made to contain 1,000 million organisms per cubic centimeter. The Massachusetts Department of Health was preparing to discontinue the use of the paratyphoid vaccine in 1937, but an extensive outbreak of paratyphoid fever caused them to delay their action.

In some countries, British Guiana for instance, enteric fever due to paratyphoid bacillus C (*Salmonella enteritidis* var. von Kunzendorf) is prevalent and this organism may be included in the vaccine in such instances.

Dosage.—Both the single and triple vaccines are administered in three doses, 0.5 cc. in the first injection and 1.0 cc. in both the second and third injections. It is administered at intervals of seven days, but McCoy, Gay and others have shown that the interval may be shortened to three days or it may be given on alternate days with equal effectiveness and no more severe reaction. At the present time it is believed that no more than ten days should elapse between injections. Lewin has tested the efficiency of the injection of one large dose, using the endotoxoid, but as measured by the resulting agglutination titer, the effect was of lesser degree and shorter duration than the injection of three doses.

The vaccine is injected with aseptic precautions subcutaneously into the deltoid area of the arm, behind the spine of the scapula or in the subclavicular region. Intramuscular or intravenous injection may be followed by severe reactions.

Reactions.—The local reaction consists of induration and tenderness at the site of injection. The axillary glands on the injected side or on both sides become swollen. There are pain and stiffness. The general reaction consists in fever with malaise, chilliness and headache. Pain in

40101

the back and legs, diarrhea, nausea and vomiting, dizziness and cramps are less common. Immediately following vaccination there is a leukocytosis with a count of around 11,000 per c.mm. This declines for a period of five days, and then a secondary rise occurs lasting from seven to fourteen days. The differential count shows 60 to 63 per cent polymorphonuclears. The general reactions last twelve to twenty-four hours and are most common after the second injection and least frequent after the third.

In some cases the reaction is more severe. Thirty-five thousand five hundred and fifty-two persons in the army were hospitalized. More days of duty were lost because of vaccination than from the disease itself. At rare times there are hyperpyrexia and collapse. This probably results from the accidental injection of the vaccine into a vein. No case of disability or death resulted from vaccination in the United States Army in the war (1917–1918).

Siler and Lambie describe three syndromes resulting from vaccination. One was pain and tenderness in the right lower abdomen together with fever and leukocytosis which suggested acute appendicitis. At operation the appendix was normal or slightly inflamed. Following these experiences operation was avoided unless urgent and definitely indicated. Severe meningismus with headache and stiffness of the neck muscles was the second. On lumbar puncture, the spinal fluid was found under increased pressure but was normal upon laboratory examination. Reduction of the pressure by drainage resulted in recovery. The third syndrome consisted of purpura with epistaxis, hematuria, melena and joint hemorrhage.

Precautions and Contraindications.—The injection is best given late in the afternoon and followed by rest in bed. If the symptoms of reaction persist the following day the patient should remain at rest and sedatives may be administered. Vaccination should be postponed in the presence of any acute infection, including typhoid fever, since sharp reactions may result. Vaccination is contraindicated in many of the chronic diseases, especially advanced arteriosclerosis, aortitis, myocarditis, cardiac decompensation, valvular heart disease, active tuberculosis, chronic pleurisy, diabetes and chronic nephritis. Advanced age, infancy and pregnancy are not contraindications.

Duration of Immunity.—Duration of immunity following vaccination is still imperfectly understood. Laboratory determination of immunity is decided by the agglutinin, bacteriolytic and bactericidal properties of the blood serum and the mouse protection test in use at the Army Medical School. The exact reliability of these tests has not been fully determined, but the present knowledge of the pathogenesis of typhoid fever indicates that they are of value. There is no accepted test indicative of antibodies attached to tissue cells. It must be assumed that the person in whom no antibodies are demonstrable, is susceptible to typhoid fever.

Siler and Dunham have shown by the mouse protection test that immunity is greatest shortly after vaccination and that it progressively decreases during the following two years although not to the point of ineffectiveness. Thereafter it decreases more slowly and it is present in some persons after ten years. It is subject to marked individual variation. Experience confirms these studies.

Bowdoin found vaccination effective two years after inoculation in a group of heavily infected children.

The duration of immunity after revaccination has not been determined. Field experience alone will solve this problem. It is conceivable that there may arise instances in which the presence or absence of immunity in an individual should be ascertained. Use of the above-mentioned tests may be helpful.

Revaccination.—Persons exposed to typhoid fever should be revaccinated after three years if exposure is imminent. The need for further revaccination has not been determined. The determination to revaccinate rests upon the discretion of the physician in charge and depends largely upon the degree of exposure anticipated. No set rule has been established. Maximum protection results from the administration of the full-sized three-dose course described above.

Reactions following vaccination constitute a personal and economic objection to its frequent repetition. Although no permanent disability or fatality has followed its use by the subcutaneous route, several methods are being investigated in an effort to minimize the reactions.

Siler and Dunham have reported from the Army Medical School upon revaccination by the intradermal injection of a single dose of 0.10 cc. of the standard bacillary suspension. The resulting immunity as measured by the mouse protection test is equal to that of the original inoculation. This method of revaccination is recommended by the Michigan Department of Health.

Tuft in 1931 first reported immunization by the intradermal injection of doses of 0.05, 0.10, 0.15 and 0.20 cc. of the standard bacillary suspension. Perry later confirmed his work. Effectiveness was determined by agglutination only, which resulted in titer equal to that of the usual method. Reactions following these methods are stated to be of little consequence. It is justifiable to employ one of these methods in suitable instances.

Typhoid Fever in the Vaccinated.—Absolute immunity does not exist in man and failure of typhoid vaccination to protect in some cases is to be expected. Several causes of failure are recognized. Ingestion of massive quantities of the inoculum is probably the main reason for failure. Infection from contact, from food and from small water supplies causes a large proportion of cases where sanitary conditions are otherwise good. These exposures are often overwhelming. In the past the use of a vaccine lacking in the necessary antigens may have occurred but this is not a facor at the present time when the antigens necessary to provide protection are fully understood. Finally, certain individuals are incapable of developing adequate immunity. These failures do not detract from the brilliant results of antityphoid vaccination.

Vaughan and Coburn and others state that typhoid fever in the vaccinated is clinically similar to typhoid in the unvaccinated. The mortality rate in the vaccinated soldiers of the United States Army was 14.2 per cent, which is above the accepted normal of about 10 per cent. Complicating diseases accounted for this rate. In Vaughan's 270 cases in the American Expeditionary Force the rate was 11 per cent. Other authors report reduction of the mortality in the vaccinated. The Statistics of Beck show a mortality of 2.7 per cent; those of Bernard and Paraf 5.3 per cent; those of Webb-Johnson 3.38 per cent, and of the

Michigan State Board of Health (1936) 6.2 per cent. In Malbin's 98 cases in vaccinated persons the mortality was 4 per cent.

Oral Vaccination.—Sir Almroth Wright (1904) was the first to attempt oral vaccination against typhoid fever. Seven individuals were given a heat-killed vaccine and their serums subsequently tested for the presence of specific bactericidal substances. Three individuals showed an increased response while 4 showed a diminished response.

Besredka in 1927 reported favorable laboratory and clinical studies upon a group immunized with oral T.A.B. vaccine. A control group of 268 individuals were vaccinated subcutaneously. During a subsequent epidemic, 5 of the former group and 10 of the latter group developed typhoid fever. Besredka concluded that the results of oral vaccination were as good as subcutaneous vaccination. The use of bile vaccine was in line with his theory of local tissue immunity. He believed the bile produced a specific lesion in the intestinal mucosa which permitted the organisms in the vaccine to be absorbed into the blood stream where they were believed to exert their full antigenic effect.

Since Besredka's work numerous kinds of oral vaccines have been made and sold by commercial laboratories in this country and abroad. The use of bile in connection with vaccine has been recommended. Using such commercial oral vaccines, many studies have been carried out in an endeavor to determine their prophylactic efficiency and to make comparisons with vaccine given parenterally. Evaluations and comparisons have been made on the basis of agglutinin response, incidence of typhoid fever in the orally vaccinated, the subcutaneously vaccinated and the unvaccinated, and by the mouse passive protection test.

The results of these studies are well summarized in a statement recently made in the *Journal of the American Medical Association* (111: 1124, 1938): "Judging from the available evidence, it would seem that oral vaccination should be eliminated entirely as a method of treatment. As a means of preventive immunization, however, it may be justifiable to use it in those instances in which the subcutaneous method is not practicable. Pending more conclusive evidence for the value of oral typhoid vaccination, commercially available products have not been accepted by the Council on Pharmacy and Chemistry."

The efficiency of oral typhoid vaccine should finally be judged by the relative incidence of typhoid fever in the vaccinated and in the unvaccinated—where the exposure is somewhere near equal both in quantity and virulence.

INDIVIDUAL PROPHYLAXIS

The devious and, often, hidden routes by which the typhoid bacillus is carried make it difficult for the individual, by his own efforts, to escape infection.

Individuals should be warned against direct infection through contact with typhoid patients or, in case of unavoidable exposure, **should be instructed in measures of defense.** Physicians, nurses and others in attendance upon the sick are in especial danger of contact infection. The fingers directly, or indirectly by way of food, convey the infection. **Scrupulous cleansing of the hands should follow contact with the patient or with any objects contaminated by him. A gown should protect the clothing** of all who come in contact with the patient. Indirect infection by water, food, flies or fomites is difficult to guard against. **In times of danger only cooked foods should be eaten, and water—** unless obtained from a source above suspicion—**should be boiled.** Persons traveling or visiting infected communities should be especially on their guard against infection. Most important in individual prophylaxis, however, is the immunity given by adequate **antityphoid vaccination.** It is cheaply purchased and experience shows that it will protect against all ordinary exposure.

GENERAL MANAGEMENT

A patient presenting symptoms suggestive of the onset of typhoid fever should be sent **immediately to bed.** The frequent grave or fatal course of ambulatory typhoid shows the disastrous results of wasting the patient's energies in the early stage of the disease. Unless the home is of exceptional appointments, the hospital is the proper place for the care of the typhoid patient. In the country and in small villages a hospital may not be within reach, and the physician must make the best of inadequate facilities. In a city house of modern appointments, hospital conditions can be closely imitated. The sickroom should be large, well ventilated, quiet and sunny, with bathroom adjoining and isolated as much as possible from the rest of the house. An open fireplace for heating and ventilation, and for use as an incinerator, is a useful feature. Pictures, heavy curtains and all unnecessary furniture should be removed, hardwood floors well covered with removable carpets, windows well shaded and in summer properly screened. A hospital single bed, twenty-six or twenty-eight inches in height, should be so placed as to be accessible from all sides. A soft hair mattress protected by a rubber sheet and resting on woven wire springs will give the patient the greatest comfort. The bedclothes should be light, the pillow low, and all kept scrupulously clean. A day nurse and a night nurse are essential for the best results. If the patient is a heavy man, a male nurse for night duty and to assist with the baths and other difficult attentions is a great aid. Efficiency and accuracy in the administration of the nursing routine are such important factors in the successful treatment of typhoid fever that **nurses of the best training and highest intelligence should be selected.**

In the country and in humble city homes the nursing of necessity may have to be done by members of the family or other unskilled attendants. This puts a heavy burden on the physician who must carefully instruct the attendants in the details of feeding, baths, disinfection of excreta, etc. Explicit, written instructions for each day's routine must be given. The physician even may be called upon personally to direct the baths and other difficult procedures.

The nurse should keep a **chart of the temperature, pulse, diet and other clinical notes. Attendants should be warned of the significance of the symptoms of hemorrhage and perforation and instructed to notify the physician immediately.**

With the patient's immediate necessities provided for, attention must then be given to precautions against the spread of the disease. Every effort must be made to **destroy the bacillus at its source or to prevent its penetration beyond the confines of the sickroom.** The rules given under "Prophylaxis" for the disinfection of the excreta and all infected clothing and utensils should be strictly enforced.

40101

The patient must have **absolute physical and mental rest.** He must not rise from the bed and the bed pan and urinal should be used from the beginning. Some patients have great difficulty at first in adjusting themselves to such conveniences and the nurse may have to exercise much tact and persistence in educating them.

Gossipy visitors must be excluded from the sickroom. Members of the family should have but limited admission. All business and annoying problems should be kept from the patient. Efforts to amuse and divert him are permissible only when he is mildly ill or well advanced in convalescence.

During the period of convalescence great care is required in guarding against the infection of other members of the household. The discharge of bacilli does not always cease with the end of the febrile period. The patient may remain a temporary carrier for several weeks, and **precautions against the spread of the infection must be continued until the stools and urine are free from typhoid bacilli.** Two or three negative cultures of the excretions are necessary to insure safety. The food consumed by the members of the household should receive careful supervision. **Water should be boiled and all foods should be cooked.** Finally all persons coming in contact with the patient or living in the house should be protected by **antityphoid vaccination.**

Diet.—The febrile period of typhoid fever lasts a month or more. It is attended by grave wasting of body tissue on one hand and by dangerous intestinal lesions on the other. **The selection of a system of diet adequate to repair the waste, and of such a character as not to offend the diseased bowel,** is one of the most important problems in the management of the disease. In the past the weight of authority has been in favor of a liquid diet of low nutritive value. The fear of hemorrhage, perforation and relapse has outweighed the fear of exhaustion. The tendency of modern clinicians, however, is toward giving food of greater variety and of higher caloric value. This tendency is the result of a more accurate knowledge of the metabolism in typhoid fever and the favorable experience of many able physicians with a liberal diet of high caloric content. Under the commonly prescribed fluid diet of low caloric value, the loss of weight during the course of the fever is progressive and often extreme. A loss of 10 or 15 per cent of the body weight is usual, and it may be as great as 30 per cent or more. A study of the food intake of a number of hospital cases under a milk and beef tea diet, made several years ago by the late author (C. G. J.), showed that the food value of the diet in these cases, until well into the period of convalescence, rarely exceeded 1,000 calories and often was as low as 400 calories per day.

METABOLISM IN TYPHOID FEVER.—Von Hösslin in 1882 studied a series of typhoid patients fed with a varied diet of rather low caloric value and concluded that foods were absorbed in typhoid fever almost as well as in health. A few years later several Russian experimenters, whose work is reviewed by Dubois, obtained similar results in studies made in Chadnowsky's clinic. Von Leyden and Klemperer in 1904 also found that the absorption of foods in typhoid is nearly equal to that in health. These experimenters, by liberal feeding, could prevent wasting, although they were unable to keep their patients in nitrogen equilibrium, despite the high protein content of the diet. The conclusions of these earlier observers have been corroborated and extended and the dietetic management of typhoid fever has been placed on a scientific foundation. In 1909 Shaffer and Coleman published the results of their work on protein metabolism in typhoid fever. This very important work, which fixed the attention of the profession on the possibilities of high caloric feeding in typhoid, was followed by researches along similar lines by Dubois, Lusk, Ewing and others in this country and by Kocher in Germany. The results, in part, of these investigations, upon which are based the efforts of modern clinicians *to maintain metabolic equilibrium during the long febrile period of typhoid fever,* are embodied in the following:

1. The total body metabolism in typhoid fever increases with the rise in temperature and decreases as the temperature falls; there is an average increase over that of the normal individual of about 40 per cent.

2. Increased metabolism does not result from increased food intake as the metabolism of a typhoid patient on a liberal diet is but slightly raised above that of a fasting patient.

3. Food in large amount, at least when the protein is kept relatively low, does not increase either the heat production or the fever in the febrile stage of typhoid. Food in itself has little or no dynamic action in typhoid fever.

4. In typhoid fever there is a toxic destruction of protein, as shown by the negative nitrogen balance in the excretions.

5. It is possible to maintain nitrogen equilibrium on a diet containing an excess of protein and fat. With a diet carrying an excess of carbohydrates, and representing a daily intake of from 3,000 to 5,000 calories, nitrogen and weight equilibrium can be maintained, and even a gain in weight may be shown during the febrile period.

6. Protein and carbohydrates can be absorbed throughout the disease as well as in normal individuals. Fat in large amount can be absorbed, but the percentage of absorption is somewhat lower than the normal, especially in the first and second weeks.

From the time of Graves, who wished his epitaph to be "He fed fevers," a few bold clinicians have advocated departure from the almost universal practice of limiting food in fevers to liquids of low caloric value. Trousseau and Flint in their day, and F. C. Shattuck of Boston, Kinnicutt of New York, Barrs of Leeds and Buchuyev of Russia of the present period, have insisted that typhoid patients were underfed. In this country Shattuck's influence has been very great, and many practitioners have followed his teaching and have adopted a more liberal and varied diet in their treatment of typhoid. With the support given from the laboratory side by Coleman and his collaborators, the high caloric diet is meeting with the recognition it seems to deserve.

The value of a high caloric diet in typhoid fever must be determined by the results obtained at the bedside. Theoretically it is better for a febrile patient to be on a diet that will maintain metabolic equilibrium, provided he can digest and absorb it. Starvation is no more beneficial to a febrile patient than to a person in health. The question is, can the typhoid patient take sufficient food to hold his weight and not give rise to digestive disturbances more harmful in the end than a moderate loss of body weight? Liberal feeding is in favor with the profession at the present time, and accumulated clinical experience should soon put the question beyond controversy. The feeding of typhoid patients up to the limit of their digestive capacity requires good clinical judgment and careful individualization. *The dangers of overfeeding* are distinct and it is often very easy to overstep the limits of safety. Many patients cannot take or digest the theoretical food requirement during the early febrile period. The physician must then be content with a moderate loss of weight and hold himself on the alert immediately to take advantage of an improved digestion to raise the food intake to the quantity necessary to balance tissue waste. A loss of from five to ten pounds during the period of high fever is not of any great importance. *The bad effects of underfeeding* are due to the withholding of food in the periods of decline and convalescence when the appetite is returning and digestion has reached about its normal efficiency.

The papers of Barrs, Buchuyev and Shattuck appeared at about the same time. Buchuyev's views were extreme. He gave solid food to all typhoid patients who could take it, from the time they came under observation. Meat, bread, eggs, milk and cereals were included in the diet. He reported 398 cases with a mortality of 8.2 per cent. Only four were complicated with hemorrhage and one with perforation. The number of relapses is not given.

Barrs' diet included minced meat, bacon, eggs, milk, bread and butter, cereal puddings, custards, stewed fruits and sponge cake. These articles were given in cases with moderate fever, an evening temperature of 102° F. (38.9° C.), and solid foods were not urged upon the patient, but given if asked for.

Shattuck's dietary included a wide range of foods, all of them of easy digestibility, high nutritive value and giving a small undigested residue. He gives the following list of articles and preparations which is suggestive rather than exhaustive:

> All liquids, including broths and cocoa.
> Soups—purée of oysters, clams, potato, etc., carefully strained.
> Gruels—strained, if containing rough particles.
> Ice cream, blancmange, junket, milk toast without crust, sherbet.
> Eggs—raw, soft-boiled, lightly scrambled.
> Meat—finely minced, scraped raw beef.
> The soft part of raw oysters, macaroni, rice.
> Orange and grapefruit juice.
> The soft part of baked or stewed apples.

In the Massachusetts General Hospital, from 1902 to 1910 inclusive, 491 cases of typhoid came under Shattuck's personal care and were given a liberal diet. There were 45 deaths—a mortality of 9.1 per cent. During the same period there were 2,160 cases fed on liquids under the care of other members of the staff. Of this group 238 died—a mortality of 11 per cent.

These statistics indicate that a liberal diet which includes a few simple and easily digested solid foods is not productive of harm, at least in the hands of expert clinicians. On the other hand, it must be emphasized that thoughtless attempts to force feeding with solids in all typhoid cases, regardless of the condition of the patient, will often result seriously.

The studies of Coleman and his associates on the metabolism of typhoid fever, controlled by abundant clinical demonstration, have placed high caloric feeding upon a scientific and practical basis. A daily intake of from 60 to 80 calories per kilogram of body weight—a total of 4,000 to 5,500 calories—is necessary to obtain nitrogen and weight equilibrium. Coleman has shown that nitrogen balance can best be maintained by a diet with a moderate protein content. The optimum is from 62 to 94 grams of protein, representing 10 to 15 grams of nitrogen. Carbohydrates are the most important source of energy requirement and should constitute about one half of the daily ration, reduced to calories. Fats, with their high yield of energy, are utilized in all stages of the disease. They are better borne and more completely absorbed in the third and fourth weeks and in convalescence.

Coleman advocates a diet consisting largely of milk, cream, butter, lactose and eggs, in combinations that will yield the necessary protein requirement and represent from 3,000 to 5,000 calories a day. Milk and eggs are the chief source of protein. From four to six eggs may be given in twenty-four hours. Carbohydrates are contained in the milk and cream. Lactose added to the milk and other foods supplies the bulk of the carbohydrate content. Fat is contained in the milk, cream, butter and the yolk of eggs.

The formulas suggested by Coleman, of milk, cream and lactose, giving food values from 1,000 calories up, will be found convenient as a basis in building up the dietary of the typhoid patient.

Formula Giving 1,000 Calories a Day

Milk, 1,000 cc. (1 qt.) .... 700 calories
Cream, 20 per cent, 50 cc. (1¾ oz.) .... 100 "
Lactose, 50 grams (1¾ oz.) .... 200 "

For eight feedings, each containing 130 cc. (4⅓ oz.). Approximate composition: Protein 36 grams, carbohydrate 97 grams, fat 50 grams.

Formula Giving 1,500 Calories a Day

Milk, 1,500 cc. (1½ qt.) .... 1,000 calories
Cream, 50 cc. (1¾ oz.) .... 100 "
Lactose, 100 grams (3¼ oz.) .... 400 "

For six feedings, each containing 260 cc. (8¾ oz.). Approximate composition: Protein 50 grams, carbohydrate 175 grams, fat 70 grams.

Formula Giving 2,000 Calories a Day

Milk, 1,500 cc. (1½ qt.) .... 1,000 calories
Cream, 250 cc. (8⅓ oz.) .... 500 "
Lactose, 125 grams (4 oz.) .... 500 "

For seven feedings, each containing 250 cc. (8⅓ oz.). Approximate composition: Protein 55 grams, carbohydrate 200 grams, fat 110 grams.

Formula Giving 2,500 Calories a Day

Milk, 1,500 cc. (1½ qt.) .... 1,000 calories
Cream, 250 cc. (8⅓ oz.) .... 500 "
Lactose, 250 grams (8⅓ oz.) .... 1,000 "

For seven feedings, each containing 250 cc. (8⅓ oz.). Approximate composition: Protein 55 grams, carbohydrate 335 grams, fat 110 grams.

40101

Formula Giving 3,000 Calories a Day

Milk, 1,500 cc. (1½ qt.) .... 1,000 calories
Cream, 500 cc. (1 pt.) .... 1,000 "
Lactose, 250 grams (8⅓ oz.) .... 1,000 "

For eight feedings, each containing 250 cc. (8⅓ oz.) Approximate composition: Protein 60 grams, carbohydrate 345 grams, fat 160 grams.

The daily protein requirement may be obtained by the addition of from three to six eggs to any one of the formulas. For example, four eggs added to the first formula will increase the protein content to 62 grams, the fat to 74 grams, and the total calories to 1,320. Almost any modification of the composition and energy value of the daily diet may be made by the addition of various allowable foods to some one of the milk formulas. In this way the diet can readily be adapted to the condition of the patient at any stage of the disease.

SAMPLE DIET, CONTAINING APPROXIMATELY 90 GRAMS OF PROTEIN AND 3,000 CALORIES.—Food administered in ten feedings, every two hours during the day and every three hours during the night:

220 cc. (7 oz.) of the milk formula, giving 1,500 calories, are administered at 1, 4 and 9 A.M., and at 1, 3, 7 and 10 P.M.

7 A.M.—1 egg, 1 oz. (30 grams) bread or toast, ½ oz. (15 grams) butter, 1 cup of coffee, 2 oz. (60 cc.) cream, ⅓ oz. (10 grams) sugar.

11 A.M.—4 oz. (120 cc.) bouillon, 1 egg, 1 oz. (30 grams) mashed potato, 1 oz. (30 grams) toast or crackers, ½ oz. (15 grams) butter, 4 oz. (120 grams) custard.

5 P.M.—1 egg, 4 oz. (120 grams) boiled rice, 1 cup of tea, 3 oz. (90 cc.) cream, ½ oz. (15 grams) sugar, ⅓ oz. (10 grams) butter.

Table XI gives a number of foods available for feeding the typhoid patient during the febrile and early convalescent periods, with their approximate composition and caloric value. For convenience, the composition is expressed in the number of grams and calories contained in one ounce, approximately 30 grams. Small fractions have been omitted. The figures are necessarily only approximate, but are sufficiently accurate for practical use in the ward or sickroom.

MILK AND MILK PRODUCTS.—Clean milk produced under the conditions that obtain in the modern well-conducted dairy is the most satisfactory single article of food for the typhoid patient. Except when there is a definite contraindication to its use, it should form the basis of the diet in the febrile period of the disease. The fact that, when properly prepared and administered, it is digested by the youngest infant, seems to be conclusive evidence that it is a food adapted to the enfeebled digestion of the adult febrile patient.

Milk for the typhoid patient must be clean and of the best quality. Edsall has demonstrated, with his fever patients, the indigestibility of milk with a high bacterial count. Even clean milk, however, if given unmodified to the fever patient, may be the cause of indigestion, of tympanites and diarrhea. Undiluted milk will cause the same symptoms when given to healthy infants. This is met by the pediatrician by diluting and modifying the milk in such a manner as to adapt it to the digestive capacity and nutritive requirements of the infant. The lesson

TABLE XI

Grams of Protein, Fat and Carbohydrate, and Number of Calories Contained in 1 Ounce (30 Grams)

	Protein grams per oz.	Fat grams per oz.	Carbohydrate grams per oz.	Calories per oz.
Milk Foods:				
Whole Milk...........................	1.0	1.2	1.5	20
Cream, 20%...........................	.75	5.5	1.3	60
Buttermilk...........................	.9	.2	1.5	10
Fermilac..............................	.9	.6	1.5	14
Skimmed Milk........................	1.0	.1	1.3	10
Whey.................................	.3	.1	1.5	8
Condensed Milk, unsweetened...........	3.0	3.0	3.5	50
Malted Milk, dry.....................	4.6	2.2	19	119
Butter...............................	.9	25.5		240
Ice Cream............................	1.6	3.0	5.3	55
Cottage Cheese.......................	6.0	.3	1.3	35
Full Cream Cheese....................	8.0	10.0	.7	130
Cereal Foods, uncooked:				
Wheat Flour, Farina..................	3.3	.5	23	110
Oatmeal..............................	5.0	2.2	20	120
Cornmeal.............................	2.8	.6	22	106
Rice.................................	2.4		24	105
Pearl Barley.........................	1.5	.3	25	107
Imperial Granum......................	3.3	.2	23	105
Mellin's Food........................	2.3		23	100
Cereal Foods, cooked:				
Wheat Bread..........................	2.8	.4	16	80
Crackers.............................	3.0	2.8	22	125
Shredded Wheat.......................	3.1	.5	24	110
Oatmeal, boiled......................	1.0		3.5	18
Rice, boiled.........................	1.0		7.3	34
Macaroni, boiled.....................	1.0	.5	5	26
Cereal Gruels........................	.4		2	10
Sponge Cake..........................	2.0	3.2	20	115
Potato, baked........................	1.0		6.0	30
Sugars:				
Cane Sugar ⎫				
Lactose ⎬			30	120
Glucose ⎭				
Eggs:				
1 Whole Egg, weight, 50 grams...........	6.0	5.0		70
White, 1 Egg.........................	3.6			15
Yolk, 1 Egg..........................	2.4	5.0		55
Meat Foods:				
Scraped Meat.........................	6.3	3.2		55
Meat Juice, homemade.................	1.5	.15		7
Meat, Soup, broths, bouillon..........	1.4	.1	.4	8
Beef Juice, Valentine................	3.0			12
Meat Juice, Wyeth....................	11.4			45
Beef Extract, Armour.................	4.8			19
Panopepton, 18% alcohol..............	2.0		3.5	60
Liquid Peptonoids, 17% alcohol........	1.5		3.2	55
Oysters.................................	1.7	.3	1.0	14
Wines and Spirits:				
Rhine Wine ⎫				
Claret ⎬ 9% alcohol...............				17
Champagne ⎭				
Sherry ⎫ 18% alcohol....................				34
Port ⎭				
Whisky ⎫				
Brandy ⎬ 50% alcohol.................				105
Rum ⎭				

is plain. If raw, unmodified milk causes indigestion in the fever patient, it may be made acceptable by modifying it after the manner of infant dietetics. In our experience we have found that the formulas of Coleman make a very satisfactory foundation for a modified milk diet whether or not it is desired to push the daily intake to the full theoretical requirement.

In cases in which milk is distasteful or not well borne, or in localities where good, fresh milk is not obtainable, a diet with plain milk excluded must be given, although preparations containing milk as an important constituent may be taken and well digested. Such articles are condensed milk, fermented milk, whey, junket, ice cream, custards, cream soups, cream puddings, cream cheese, tea, coffee and cocoa.

CARBOHYDRATES.—The carbohydrates have an important place in the typhoid dietary. Lusk and Shaffer and Coleman have shown that, in addition to their direct value as food, the carbohydrates have the property of sparing body protein both in afebrile and febrile conditions. In typhoid fever there is an increased need for carbohydrates and, unless this demand is met, the body protein wastes. Carbohydrates prevent loss of body protein to a greater extent than fat and even protein itself. The demonstration of this fact is one of the most important results of studies in the metabolism of typhoid fever. There is also experimental evidence that a diet rich in carbohydrates is unfavorable to the growth in the intestinal tract of organisms of the colon-typhoid group.

Sugars are utilized to build up the caloric value of the typhoid dietary. Each ounce of any one of the sugars represents 120 calories. Milk sugar is the most important of the group. This carbohydrate is easily digested and does not easily ferment. It is not very sweet and can be given in large amounts in the milk formulas, in beverages, and as the sweetening ingredient in various food preparations like ice cream, custards, gruels, etc. From eight to sixteen ounces or more may be given daily, and Coleman has found that these large amounts are well borne and do not cause digestive disturbance or predispose to tympanites. Cane sugar is too sweet to be given in large quantity; one or two ounces a day may be given in lemonade and other beverages. Glucose and malt sugar are occasionally of use. In emergencies glucose is available for rectal and subcutaneous feeding.

CEREALS.—Cereals and other farinaceous foods carry a high carbohydrate content and a small percentage of vegetable protein. Bread, crackers, zwieback, cereal gruels and puddings, porridge and mashed potatoes are light foods which can safely be given both in the febrile stage and in early convalescence. In cases in which milk must be excluded from the diet, the cereals in the form of gruel and porridge will have a prominent place. Milk and cream may be made more digestible and often are better borne if diluted with a gruel, whereas, if given pure, these foods would disagree. In the early stage of typhoid, when digestion is greatly impaired, the gruels are of especial value. All cereals must be thoroughly boiled and strained. The proprietary farinaceous and malted infant foods may be of distinct value in cases in which digestion is seriously impaired or diarrhea is troublesome. They have about the same composition as wheat flour.

EGGS.—Eggs form an important part of the typhoid dietary. They supply protein and fat in about equal proportions. Egg albumin is completely peptonized in the stomach, and the fat is well split up before it reaches the ileum; practically no undigested residue is left. From four to six eggs may be given in a day, soft-boiled, coddled or beaten up with milk or one of the fruit juices. The white of egg is agreeably given as albumin water flavored with orange or other fruit juices and sweetened with lactose or cane sugar.

MEAT FOODS.—Meat soups, broths, beef tea and bouillon are homemade infusions of beef, mutton, veal, chicken or shellfish. They are of low nutritive value—from four to eight calories per ounce. They contain a small percentage of protein but, as usually prepared, they are simply solutions of meat salts and extractives. They are popular in the home sickroom, but should be classed rather as agreeable and stimulating beverages than as foods. They have a distinct and valuable function in stimulating appetite and digestion, and in small quantities are useful in certain stages of typhoid fever, particularly in the late febrile period and in convalescence. They often have a decided laxative effect and may excite or aggravate a diarrhea. By the addition to them of eggs, milk, cream or cereals, they may be made to carry considerable nutriment.

Beef juice contains a relatively small quantity of extractives and from 4 to 6 per cent of protein. This meat preparation is easily digested and is not apt to produce diarrhea. It is of value when milk cannot be given, and as the first step to the resumption of meat feeding. The raw meat flavor of beef juice is sometimes distasteful and can be disguised by serving the beef juice in broth, milk or sherry wine. The cream soups contain milk or cream, butter, flour and eggs and have a much higher nutritive value. They are agreeable and readily digested.

Gelatin in the form of calf's foot jelly, wine jelly or the homemade product is a useful food in febrile states. In the form of iced bouillon it is very grateful to the patient. It acts as a fuel food, like the fats and carbohydrates, but differs from them in this particular—that its oxidation products are eliminated by the kidneys. It digests quickly, being completely peptonized in the stomach in one hour. The proprietary meat preparations are in general of low food value, except for the alcohol they may contain. Peptonized meat preparations are objectionable, as they are often toxic and very apt to produce diarrhea.

American practice is against the addition of meat to the typhoid dietary during the febrile period. It may be given in mild or uncomplicated severe cases when the fever is declining or in early convalescence. One-half to one ounce of scraped meat rolled into small balls and lightly broiled should be the first venture. Should this be well digested, the tender white meat of chicken or a broiled chop may follow. Until well into convalescence the quantity should be limited to from two to four ounces a day. It is quite common to see a rise of temperature follow the resumption of meat feeding.

FRUITS AND FRUIT JUICES.—Cooked fruit, like applesauce, which can be eaten as a soft pulp, is occasionally permissible in mild cases and when convalescence is well established. In all cases of severity the fruit acids are better given in the form of the fruit juices, lemon, orange, grape and grapefruit. They are excellent vehicles for the administration of the white of egg and sugar. As lemonade, orangeade, etc., they agreeably assist the increase of the daily food intake. The fruit jellies dissolved in water and sweetened serve the same purpose. The fruit

40101

acids in excess may cause abdominal pain and diarrhea, and their effect should be carefully watched.

BEVERAGES.—Water, far above the quantity taken in health, is necessary for the nutrition of the febrile patient and for the elimination of the toxins of the disease and the end products of increased metabolism. The conscious patient may be urged to drink frequently from a water bottle placed at his bedside; the delirious or unconscious patient must be given water by the nurse every hour when awake, in as large amounts as he can be made to swallow. The quantity taken should be charted and the total twenty-four-hour intake summed up for the information of the physician at his morning visit. McCrae makes the rule that three quarts be the minimum daily intake. We are inclined to doubt the advisability of risking the possibility of cardiac overstrain by forcing water ingestion to the extent advocated by the late Dr. E. F. Cushing— two to four gallons a day.

Lemonades, orangeades and other preparations, cracked ice, iced tea and coffee may be used to tempt the patient to increase the amount of fluids taken. Gravely toxic patients who cannot be made to take sufficient water by the stomach should be given saline solution per rectum. If the rectum is irritable and the demand urgent, intravenous or subcutaneous administration is justifiable. The course of typhoid fever is often made milder in patients who take water in abundance. The tongue remains moist and clean, nutrition is better; the toxic delirium and stupor are less severe.

TEA, COFFEE AND COCOA WITH CREAM AND SUGAR.—These are grateful and stimulating nutrients. They may be given hot or iced. They are apt to interfere with sleep and are best added to the morning meals. They gently stimulate the circulation and increase the urinary output. Strong coffee is a prompt and active cardiac stimulant in the shock of hemorrhage, perforation and other accidents.

ALCOHOL.—The routine administration of alcohol in typhoid fever either as a food or as a stimulant is unnecessary and unwise. The majority of patients go through the disease as well—perhaps better—without it. If other food of adequate caloric value is taken the addition of alcohol is superfluous. Children and young adults rarely require it, while it is often of distinct benefit to elderly patients and those accustomed to its use in health.

In moderate quantity and properly diluted it may be of great value as an emergency food in conditions of profound anorexia and at times when ordinary food cannot be taken or is not well borne. It does not prevent nitrogen waste, but spares fat and for a short period replaces carbohydrates in the diet. In febrile states especially it is rapidly oxidized, each gram of alcohol yielding seven calories, and one ounce of whisky or brandy approximately one hundred calories. It is a direct stimulant to gastric secretion and motility, and hastens the absorption of the products of digestion. In the intestine it stimulates peristalsis and acts as a carminative and mild astringent.

In sudden circulatory failure alcohol acts as a stimulant, either reflexly from the stomach or, after absorption, as an equalizer of the circulation. In the profound toxemia of severe cases attended with increasing cardiac asthenia and grave nervous phenomena, it improves nutrition, supports the circulation and relieves insomnia, delirium and other exhausting nervous symptoms. In the early days of the convalescence of severe and complicated cases it may be of decided benefit as a stimulant to appetite and digestion and as a general tonic. The possibility of the formation of a habit must always be borne in mind and the remedy should be discontinued at the earliest possible moment.

The effect of the administration of alcohol should be carefully noted and unless results are favorable it should be discontinued. The beginning doses should be small—2 to 4 drams of whisky or brandy every four hours. It is rarely necessary to exceed one-half ounce every three hours, or four ounces in twenty-four hours.

During the febrile period a well-aged whisky or brandy is generally the most useful form for administration. The spirit should be diluted to an alcoholic strength of from 5 to 10 per cent, 1 part of whisky to from 2 to 5 parts of water. Claret or champagne—either clear or diluted with an effervescent water—may be better taken. Burgundy, sherry or port is more suitable for administration in the convalescent stage. Unless given to fill some special indication, alcohol is most effective when administered immediately before or with the regular feedings.

MANAGEMENT OF THE DIET.—The routine of the diet for each day should be prescribed by the physician at his morning visit. A feeding chart should be kept by the nurse and the amount of food actually taken by the patient at each meal recorded. Each morning the total intake of food and fluids for the preceding twenty-four hours, with the approximate composition and caloric content, should be determined. Food should be administered at regular stated intervals and in measured quantity. Two-hourly feedings are the rule in severe cases. The frequency of the night feedings will be governed by the condition of the patient. Sleep is rarely prolonged, and in many cases the two-hourly interval can be continued throughout the night without interfering with sleep. Drowsy and stuporous patients can be aroused without detriment. The sleep that may come after a long period of wakefulness or delirium should be interrupted only in cases of necessity. Patients mildly or moderately ill who take abundant nourishment during the day may be allowed to sleep the night through or may be given one or two early morning meals.

For the first two days after the patient comes under observation only fluid food in moderate quantity should be given. Four ounces of milk diluted with two ounces of water or cereal gruel may be given every three hours. Following this the milk formula containing 1,000 calories may be given and the intake increased as rapidly as the patient's digestion will permit. Coleman has very properly emphasized the necessity of cautiously and gradually attaining the desired maximum food intake in an individual case. In the early period of the disease it is often impossible to push the intake above 1,500 calories without exciting a digestive upset.

As soon as it is shown that the milk formula is well borne the food may be increased by from 200 to 300 calories a day, until the daily intake is 3,000 to 4,000 calories, and the interval between meals shortened to two hours. One or more eggs, a cereal with cream, soft toast, custard, broth and other appropriate foods may be added and the effect of each article carefully observed. The stools should be frequently examined for curds and other undigested particles of food.

40101

The appearance of abdominal discomfort or distention or of diarrhea is a signal for prompt revision of the diet. Relief may be obtained by a change in the proportion of the various articles in the diet, or it may be necessary for a day or two to return to diluted milk, albumin water, gruel or broth feedings at longer intervals. A complete rest of the stomach for several hours may be advisable. We have seen the fever decline and toxic delirium abate as a result of a short period of food restriction and increased elimination. By observing these precautions the optimum diet for a given case can be attained with a minimum of risk.

Vitamins.—There now exists a comprehensive understanding of the results of vitamin deficiency and one may well deduce that many of the complications and sequelae of typhoid fever formerly thought due to toxemia may in reality be due to this cause.

Possible complications due to lack of vitamin A are: furunculosis, bed sores, parotitis, bronchopneumonia, conjunctivitis, keratitis, iritis, ulceration of the larynx and lesions of the tongue and pharynx.

Polyneuritis and myocardial insufficiency may be due to lack of vitamin B_1 or thiamin. The former was first recognized by Shattuck and the latter by Weiss in disease other than beriberi. The effects of the lack of the other factors of the vitamin B complex in typhoid fever are not clearly differentiated from toxemia. Sore mouth and tongue, anemia, central nervous system degeneration and digestive disturbances are known to occur in diseases due to this cause. All of these are features of typhoid fever.

Of all complications hemorrhage and perforation would seem most likely to result from the tissue injury of typhoid fever. Hemorrhage and ineffective tissue repair are characteristic of vitamin C depletion. Hartzell and associates have found that in most cases of perforation in peptic ulcer the cevitamic acid of the blood is at prescurvy levels. It is probable that the depletion of vitamin C reserves is a contributory factor at least to these dangerous complications.

The vitamin content of the sample diet given in Table XI, taken from the tables published by McCollum, is shown below. Sixty grams of meat and one hundred grams each of orange and lemon juice have been added.

	A (Units)	B_1 (Units)	C (Mg.)
Milk 1,540 cc.	1,700–9,240	154–385	4.6–44.5
Eggs 3	2,520–8,100	45–108	
Bread 60 gms.		6	
Butter 40 gms.	340–400		
Cream 150 gms.	1,500		
Potato 30 gms.	15	2–3	
Custard 120 gms.	970–3,000	15–30	
Meat 60 gms.		25–300	
Lemon juice 100 gms.		15	26–70.9
Orange juice 100 gms.	95	30	22–89
Minimum	7,140	292	52.6
Maximum	20,740	826	204.4

The minimum values given are adequate for a person in normal health but are not sufficient to meet the increased need that accompanies infection, heightened metabolism and increased excretion by the bowel, even though the food consumption is maintained. The diet should be fortified by the administration of the vitamins in concentrated or crystalline form.

Vitamin A can be supplied best in halibut liver oil, of which 1 cc., containing 19,200 international units, can be taken daily. The **vitamin B complex** is administered as dried brewers' yeast. Thirty grams contain from 400 to 2,000 international units which supply, with the food, one day's need. If yeast cannot be taken the individual factors of the B complex can be given separately. Thiamin hydrochloride is given in doses of 2 to 10 mg. (600 to 3,000 international units) daily by mouth. In polyneuritis or myocardial insufficiency, 20 to 50 mg. can be administered intramuscularly or intravenously daily. The dose of riboflavin, for a caloric intake of 3,000 calories, is 1.8 mg. or 600 Bourquin-Sherman units.

Nicotinic acid is not advised since it increases peristaltic activity. Liver extract supplies the factors of the B complex other than thiamin and can be given intramuscularly. The B complex probably contains factors additional to those just described and every effort should be made to maintain its oral ingestion.

The daily requirement of **cevitamic acid** in typhoid fever is at least 120 mg. and it may be more. It can be taken orally in amounts of 200 to 500 mg. each twenty-four hours. A certain amount of fruit juice should be taken if at all possible. Vitamin C reserve is the only one that can be tested in the laboratory. A blood level below 0.5 mg. per cent or a 24-hour urinary excretion below 30 mg. indicates that the reserves are depleted. It should then be given parenterally in daily dose of 500 mg. until the reserves are restored.

Hydrotherapy.—The cold bath is the most efficient measure we possess to combat pyrexia, toxemia and many of the grave symptoms and complications of typhoid fever. Since the earliest times the cold bath, administered in various ways, has had periods of popularity. James Currie, of Liverpool, proposed the cold effusion treatment in 1787, and it was extensively used in England and other countries. In the great British epidemic of 1817 to 1819 the method of Currie was followed with perseverance, only to be abandoned later. The water cure had become a system of quackery and was shunned by the profession. In America, Robert Jackson employed the cold bath in the treatment of fevers as early as 1774. Nathan Smith, writing in 1824, was an earnest advocate of hydrotherapy, and he considered the cold bath the only remedy that favorably influenced the fever. E. Brand, of Stettin, in 1861 revived the cold bath treatment, and his numerous publications and favorable statistics fixed the attention of the medical profession on the value of hydrotherapy in the treatment of acute febrile and toxic states.

The cold bath given as a routine from the onset in all cases of typhoid fever, and with the exact technic advised by Brand, has not been popular outside of Germany. In America, tub baths, modified from the Brand method, have been extensively used in hospitals and to a more limited degree in private practice. Hydrotherapy in some form may be considered an essential part of the therapeutics of the disease.

THE TUB BATH.—*Brand Cold Friction Bath.*—This is administered from the onset of the disease every three hours, when the rectal temperature is above 102.5° F. (39.2° C.). The patient is first given a stimulant—one-half ounce of whisky or, what is preferred by many, four

40101

ounces of hot, strong coffee or tea. He is then undressed and covered with a sheet or a napkin around the loins. Pledgets of cotton are put in the ears, and the dry skin of the hands and feet is covered with vaseline. A rubber bathing-cap is desirable for women. The patient's face is bathed with ice water and a cold water compress applied to the head, and he is gently lifted by two attendants from the bed into the portable tub placed at the bedside. Adjustable strips of canvas clamped to the sides of the tub make a comfortable rest for the patient's body and legs. The tub is filled with fresh water, not above 70° F. (21.1° C.) or below 65° F. (18.3° C.). The entire body and extremities are submerged. The head is supported by an attendant, or on a suitable head rest. Continuous brisk friction of all the skin surface is an essential part of the bath, especial attention being given to the extremities. Repeated effusions to the head with cold water are very important in cases with predominant nervous symptoms. The duration of the bath is twenty minutes, unless untoward symptoms require it to be shortened. Complaints of chilliness and blueness of the fingers are usual and are not indications for ending the bath. Continued chattering of the teeth, cyanosis of the face and a weak pulse demand removal.

At the end of the bath the patient is lifted from the tub, gently dried, except over the abdomen, and lightly covered in bed with a sheet and blanket. Hot-water bottles are placed at the feet. Another hot drink and, a little later, food may be given. The temperature is taken one-half hour after the bath. A fall of from one to three degrees is usually noted. At the end of three hours the temperature is again taken, and if above 102.5° F. (39.2° C.), the bath is repeated.

Modified Tub Bath.—The cold bath of Brand, rigidly enforced, is heroic treatment, and most physicians prefer some modification of the method that will make the bath more acceptable to the patient. By many the bath is not given until the patient's temperature is above 103 or 103.5° F. (39.4 or 39.7° C.). It is good practice to begin the bath treatment with the water at a temperature of 80 or 90° F. (26.7 or 32.2° C.) gradually reduced during the bath to 65 or 70° F. (18.3 or 21.1° C.) by the addition of cold water. As a rule we prefer to use such a graduated tub bath until the patient's confidence is obtained and his manner of reaction to the bath is determined. The warm bath gradually chilled is a modification particularly adapted to women, children and nervous men. The bath is begun with the water at a temperature of three to four degrees below the temperature of the patient and cooled three or four degrees every five minutes until it is below 90° F. (32.2° C.). The patient is then removed.

THE BED BATH.—Properly given, the bed bath is a fairly satisfactory substitute for the tub bath. It is the preferred form of hydrotherapy in many hospitals and by many physicians in the home treatment of typhoid fever. A shallow tub is made in the bed by a large rubber sheet. The sides of the sheet are stretched over a tightly rolled blanket placed on each side of the patient and held by clamps or long tapes tied to the bedstead. The ends of the sheet are stretched in the same manner over shorter rolls. The portable bath of the medical supply houses is very convenient, if available, or the sheet may be fastened to an improvised frame. Havens stretches two parallel ropes from the head to the foot of the bed and fastens the sides of the sheet to the ropes with clothespins.

In the bed bath the patient's body is only partially immersed. The water is poured over the patient from a pail or pitcher, from large sponges or from the ordinary sprinkling pot. The trunk and extremities are continuously rubbed, as in the tub bath. The bath is continued for twenty minutes or made shorter if the condition of the patient demands. At the end of the bath the water is siphoned off with a rubber tube, the rubber sheet is removed and the patient lightly dried and covered with a linen sheet and blanket. As with the tub bath, a hot drink is given before the bath and after, if necessary, and cold compresses are applied to the head.

THE SPONGE BATH.—The patient is placed on a rubber sheet large enough to protect the bed. Cold compresses are applied to the head and chest and renewed every few minutes. They may also be placed over the large vessels under the arms and along the inner surfaces of the thighs. The sponges should be large and carry an abundance of water The trunk and each extremity are successively bathed and rubbed, the whole bath lasting twenty minutes. The patient may be dried and covered as in the other baths, or allowed to remain five or ten minutes in a wet sheet and covered with blankets.

INFLUENCE OF HYDROTHERAPY ON THE COURSE OF TYPHOID FEVER.— As a rule the best results are obtained from tub baths; bed baths with effusions rank next in efficiency; sponge baths are the least disagreeable to the patient and have the least influence on the pyrexia and toxemia.

1. The febrile period of typhoid fever is not shortened by hydrotherapy, except that the baths may prevent complications that prolong the fever beyond the normal period. The immediate effect of the bath is to reduce the temperature from one to four degrees. The reduction is transitory and the temperature returns in a short time to its former height. During the remission the patient usually feels better. In the early stage when the temperature is in the ascendant, and during the height of the febrile period, the fall of the temperature after the bath may be insignificant; exceptionally a rise of a degree or more is seen. In the period of decline a sharp remission that continues for several hours is usually noted. It must be emphasized that the extent of the drop in the temperature is not necessarily a measure of the good effect of the bath. The degree of improvement in the general condition of the patient is of more significance.

2. Toxemia is reduced by hydrotherapy. Diuresis is increased, and the general improvement in the symptoms attributed to the presence of toxins in the circulation points to their increased elimination. The typhoid state is rarely seen when systematic bathing is carried out. The good effect of the bath is best seen in severe cases with delirium, stupor, subsultus tendinum and other symptoms of profound toxemia. In these cases the bath—preferably the tub bath—with the water tempered to fit the condition of the patient is a lifesaving measure and should be given thoroughly and conscientiously.

3. The circulation is improved. The heart action is slowed, the pulse becomes smaller and firmer and the blood pressure rises 15 to 20 mm. Vasomotor paresis is lessened and the circulation is equalized. Thayer found a hyperleukocytosis immediately following the cold bath, and Gay suggests that this result may explain its beneficial effect.

40101

4. The full respirations that are stimulated by the bath relieve pulmonary stasis. Passive congestion of the lungs, bronchitis and bronchopneumonia are less frequently seen and are favorably influenced if present.

5. The skin is kept clean and healthy and the liability to bed sores is diminished. Thayer has found that the addition of alum, one-half pound to the tub, is of value in the presence of boils and other skin infections.

6. The mortality rate is lowered. Hospital statistics show a decided reduction in mortality with the introduction of routine bath treatment. Osler, from his experience at the Johns Hopkins Hospital, although deploring the disagreeable features of the bath, believed that it saved from six to eight patients out of every hundred. The general experience also in the larger hospitals of New York and Philadelphia was that the mortality under the cold tub treatment was reduced approximately 50 per cent. The figures of the Brisbane Hospital, Australia, published by F. E. Hare, give a mortality of 14.8 per cent in 1,828 cases treated by the expectant method, and 7.05 per cent in 1,902 cases treated after the introduction of hydrotherapy.

The bath in itself, however, may not be the only factor in the production of the lowered mortality. The tubbed patient is, as a rule, better fed, better nursed and more closely watched than the patient treated on the expectant plan. Shattuck's results at the Massachusetts General Hospital were equally good with liberal feeding, good nursing and hydrotherapy in the form of sponge and bed baths. The advocates of an abundant diet in typhoid fever state that the beneficial effect upon the course of the disease and the lowered death rate that result from the cold bath treatment can be obtained as well without the baths if the patient is abundantly nourished. Coleman believes that high temperature is a danger only when the patient takes insufficient food, and that tubbing is unnecessary if the patient is well fed. He believes that hydrotherapy owes its value to reduction in the total metabolism. If this can be covered by food, the cold bath loses its purpose.

With all allowance for the enthusiastic statements of the advocates both of tubbing and of feeding, it may confidently be stated that **hydrotherapy and liberal feeding are the fundamental modern improvements in the treatment of typhoid fever.** Widely used they together will carry the patient through his long illness with the least possible discomfort and danger.

Brand and his followers urged that all typhoid patients should be treated by the cold tub bath. At the present time the rigid Brand treatment is carried out only exceptionally. In many hospitals where the method was systematically used for several years after its introduction, it has given way to milder forms of hydrotherapy. Patients are individualized and the various hydrotherapeutic methods are adapted to the condition of the patient and his environment.

In mild cases tubbing is unnecessary. A cold sponge bath morning and evening are requisite for cleanliness, and should be a routine measure in all cases. Two or three additional sponge baths may be given through the day, should the afternoon temperature reach 103° F. (39.4° C.). Cold compresses to the head, chest or abdomen for an hour or two at varying intervals may replace the antipyretic cold sponge. The ice bag also is a grateful substitute.

In cases of average severity the tub or bed bath will be indicated toward the end of the first week when the temperature reaches 103° F. (39.4° C.). From one to three tubs during the afternoon and evening exacerbation of the fever usually suffice. The temperature of the first baths should be from 85 to 95° F. (29.4 to 35° C.) and reduced during the bath and at subsequent baths, according to the manner of reaction of the patient and the influence upon the temperature, pulse, respiration and nervous symptoms.

Severe cases should be tubbed from the outset, if possible. If the tub bath be not available, the bed bath thoroughly carried out should be substituted for it. The sponge bath alone is too feeble a substitute. The bath should be given every four to six hours if the temperature is above 103° F. (39.4° C.), or with a lower temperature, if stupor, delirium and other toxic symptoms are marked. It will rarely be necessary to give more than three or four baths in the twenty-four hours. If a bath is given about nine or ten o'clock in the evening the effect will often carry through to the time of the natural morning remission and further night bathing will be unnecessary. In highly toxic and stuporous cases the regular intervals should be maintained night and day.

Tub baths should be begun with great caution or withheld entirely in gravely prostrated patients coming under observation late in the disease. Such patients are probably safer if treated with diligent nursing, good feeding and a few gently given sponge baths.

Infants and children respond well to the milder forms of hydrotherapy. Lukewarm sponges, packs and bed baths are agreeable to them and are efficient.

Elderly patients are better sponged or bathed in bed. Reaction in such patients is sluggish and apt to be unsatisfactory. Usually they are better pleased and as well off if given the routine morning and evening sponge and only an occasional extra bath.

Tub baths should be given with extreme care, or discontinued toward the end of the third week when sharp remissions mark the course of the temperature. Cardiac asthenia and the danger of hemorrhage and perforation require that the patient be moved as little as possible. At this period the sponge bath is safer. Only the milder forms of hydrotherapy are permissible in the treatment of relapse.

CONTRAINDICATIONS TO THE TUB BATH.—(a) *In the Presence of Complications That Demand Absolute Rest.*—Symptoms suggestive of hemorrhage or the appearance of blood in the stools require immediate interruption of all forms of hydrotherapy. Bathing should not be renewed until several days have elapsed after the arrest of the bleeding. Abdominal pain, pointing to the onset of perforation, peritonitis, appendicitis, cholecystitis or other acute abdominal inflammation, is a contraindication. Phlebitis, pleurisy, severe bronchitis and other complicating infections, remote from the abdomen, demand temporary or permanent suspension of antipyretic baths.

(b) *In the Presence of Conditions or Complications Marked by Extreme Weakness.*—Constitutionally feeble, anemic and obese patients, and subjects of arteriosclerosis, chronic nephritis, chronic alcoholism or tuberculosis should not be treated with cold tub or bed baths.

SULFANILAMIDE AND RELATED DRUGS

Cure of typhoid fever by **sulfanilamide, prontosil** and **sulfapyridine** is undetermined. Long, Myers, Coxon and Forbes, Sturgis, and Klee and Römer report failure to modify the disease. Sturgis used sulfapyridine. All gave full dosage. Another group of authors record favorable influence upon the disease. Harries and others treated six cases with prontosil or sulfapyridine with clinical improvement in all and critical fall of temperature in two. A seventh case was treated by sulfapyridine, starting on the eighth day, and serum given on the eleventh day. The temperature started at once to fall by lysis and remained normal after the seventeenth day. Brotherhood and Harkleroad each report a case with recovery in childhood. Diefenbach and Yuskis report an atypical case, the only clue to the diagnosis being the recovery of *E. typhosa* from the blood stream. The temperature was normal after seven days of treatment by 5 grams daily. Kulesza treated 37 cases with one injection of prontosil daily, the amount not being recorded. In 20 of them, he states, the patient recovered, the average number of injections being two. Among the collected cases sulfanilamide failed to clear the urine of typhoid bacilli in two and agranulocytic angina occurred in one.

Buttle and his colleagues (1937) have studied the effect of sulfanilamide on experimental mouse infection with *E. typhosa*. Their results indicated that sulfanilamide given in single doses immediately after the intraperitoneal inoculation of $100:1,000$ minimum lethal doses of organisms, gave definite and lasting protection. Kolmer and Rule state that sulfanilamide in the dose which they used showed some therapeutic effect, although the results were not so encouraging as those of Buttle and others. Kolmer acknowledges that his dose was only one-sixth that of Buttle, which might account for the differences noted.

Long and Bliss state that growth of the typhoid bacillus in 50 per cent horse serum broth was unaffected by a $1:10,000$ concentration of sulfanilamide, such as markedly inhibited the growth of beta-hemolytic streptococci. They further noted that a concentration of 250 mg. per cent in urine in vitro will kill the typhoid bacillus.

In summary, the results of the treatment of typhoid bacillus infection, either clinical or experimental, by sulfanilamide and related compounds are not as encouraging as are those in the treatment of beta-hemolytic streptococcus infections.

SPECIFIC THERAPY

Serum Therapy.—Chantemesse, Rodet, Etienne and others treated typhoid fever with antityphoid serum previous to 1920 with some degree of success. This method failed to become generally accepted because of ensuing serum reactions.

Interest in serum therapy has been revived in England because of the work of Grasset and Gory and Felix and Petrie. The latter have prepared and standardized antityphoid horse serum. The antigens which they used to immunize the horses were a killed, smooth virulent strain of *E. typhosa* and a live avirulent rough strain. According to them, the former provided the necessary O antigen and the latter the necessary Vi antigen.

Grasset and Gory in 1928 produced an antityphoid serum by the inoculation of horses with typhoid endotoxoid. This they claimed produced a satisfactory anti- O serum.

Grasset and Lewin state that in 3,500 cases treated by Grasset's serum the mortality was reduced 50 per cent. They tested, in a small series of cases, the effect of that serum as compared with one prepared by the method of Felix and found them equal in value. Lewin used serum containing both O and Vi antibodies in 13 cases, in 7 of which it was of distinct value. Felix reported the use of his serum in 43 cases. There were 5 fatalities and in 24 the toxic symptoms appeared to be controlled. McSweeney used Felix's serum in 8 cases with benefit to toxemia. One of his cases had typhoid bacillus meningitis and was treated by the intrathecal administration of serum with recovery. Shwartzman prepared an experimental serum using as antigen a cell-free filtrate of *E. typhosa*. Shwartzman and others administered their serum to 78 patients. In 39 of them, or 50 per cent, there was distinct benefit and the mortality of the treated cases was 8.9 per cent as compared with 22 per cent in a control series.

Those who have administered serum state that its effect often is dramatic, persons desperately sick recovering in forty-eight hours. Shwartzman found serum reactions to be serious in persons already exhausted by their infection. The earlier serums were unconcentrated. In the course of their studies several investigators administered normal horse serum to control cases, but its effect was distinctly unfavorable and its use had to be abandoned. Lewin found that serum-treated cases were subject to recrudescence.

Felix and Bhatnagar state that complement enters the antigen-antibody reaction. The effect of the antityphoid horse serum might, therefore, be enhanced by the concurrent administration of human serum, since, as shown by Burbank and confirmed by us, complement is often low or absent in persons suffering from severe infection.

The serum treatment of typhoid fever is still in the experimental stage but there is more promise of its value than there was two or even one decade ago.

Immunotransfusion and Human Serum Therapy.—Treatment of typhoid fever by transfusion of blood of recovered persons was first reported by Von Yaksch and Walger and it is used by Bowen with favorable results. It is surprising that this method of treatment has not been given greater attention. Theoretically it presents interesting possibilities.

The blood serum of the normal person contains small amounts of bactericidal substances, mouse protective antibodies and in some cases O antibody. The blood serum of a recovered or immunized individual contains these in increased amounts. The blood serum of carriers contains, in addition to the above, appreciable amounts of the Vi antibody. It should, therefore, be a comparatively easy matter to obtain from them a serum containing all the necessary immune substances as well as one in which the danger of serum reactions would be lessened. Cadham has shown that in streptococcus infections immune serum is more valuable than immune whole blood because of the greater availability of complement. Such serums should be administered as soon after withdrawal from the donor as possible.

40101

Vaccine Therapy.—Treatment of typhoid fever by the injection or oral administration of bacillary suspensions has been discarded because of serious reactions and failure to demonstrate beneficial results. Lewin finds, however, that Grasset's endotoxoid can be given during the disease without reaction. Thirty-two cases so treated by him suffered a mortality of 6.2 per cent, while in 84 comparable control cases it was 22.6 per cent. The first dose was 0.10 cc. and increased to 1.0 cc. at the fifth or sixth dose. Bowen administered a bacteria-free filtrate prepared by the lysis of a recently isolated typhoid bacillus by bacteriophage. One cubic centimeter was injected intravenously. Hyperpyrexia followed the treatment but did not seriously affect the patient. After one or, at most, two injections, recovery is said to occur to within forty-eight hours in favorable cases.

TREATMENT OF SYMPTOMS AND COMPLICATIONS

Fever.—Fever is a defensive reaction to infection, and within certain limits it is—according to modern views—a conservative process. Its suppression is not always desirable and its violent reduction may be a clinical error. If the tissues are well fed and abundant excretion is maintained, a temperature of the average height usual in typhoid fever is not in itself a source of danger. The chief danger in typhoid fever is the toxemia, the intensity of which is usually—but not necessarily— indicated by the height of the temperature. A grave toxic state may be present with but little rise in temperature, while on the other hand the good effects of hydrotherapy in reducing toxemia are often manifest with practically no reduction in the temperature. Coleman finds, in the use of the high caloric diet, that the temperature may be lightly regarded if the patient can take an abundance of food.

HYDROTHERAPY.—For the control of fever and the metabolic disturbances that go with it, hydrotherapy has proved to be the most efficient remedial measure. The indications for the various forms of application of the bath treatment and the technic of administration have been considered in preceding pages.

ANTIPYRETIC DRUGS.—The synthetic antipyretic drugs reduce temperature by their action on the heat-regulating nervous mechanism, lowering the point at which the temperature is maintained. They increase the dissipation of heat, and this is brought about by dilatation of the cutaneous vessels. Collapse often follows their too rapid action. They have no beneficial influence upon the toxemia of the disease. **The coal-tar antipyretics, therefore, have no place in the treatment of typhoid fever.** They are circulatory depressants and their routine use is harmful. The administration of these drugs in the early stage of typhoid fever tends to confuse the diagnosis and divert attention from proper methods of treatment. Given later in the disease, when the myocardium is weak and violent reactions are apt to follow the use of any antipyretic measure, they are a positive danger.

An occasional single dose of one of the more slowly acting members of the group, such as **phenacetin, may not be harmful when given to relieve a painful symptom** like severe headache, but other and less objectionable remedies are usually available to meet such an indication.

Quinine in large doses is an antipyretic. It acts directly upon the tissues, diminishing nitrogen metabolism. Erb advised the administration of 20 to 30 grains (1.3 to 2 Gm.) in two doses during the evening of every second day, beginning in the latter part of the second week of the disease. The effect of the drug is prolonged, lasting from twenty-four to forty-eight hours. Like other antipyretic remedies its action is most pronounced in the declining period of the disease.

Toxemia.—Free elimination should be maintained by the **liberal administration of water.** The tactful and persistent nurse may be able to give an abundance of fluids by the mouth. If not they must be introduced in other ways. *Stuporous or comatose patients* may be given **water or nutrient fluids by the stomach tube,** 500 to 800 cc. (17 to 27 fl.oz.) every eight or twelve hours. **Small enemas,** 300 to 500 cc. (10 to 17 fl.oz.) **of normal saline,** may be given two or three times in the twenty-four hours. The solution should be of body temperature or slightly warmer and injected slowly. The continuous drop method is very satisfactory. Beginning every six to eight hours, 500 cc. (17 fl.oz.) of normal saline may be given. The solution may be given a nutrient value by the addition of 2 per cent of **glucose.** A diarrhea or an irritable bowel may interfere with this treatment.

Venoclysis is a safe method for the administration of large amounts of fluids, provided the solutions used have been properly prepared. If a laboratory equipped to make up these solutions is not at hand they may be purchased ready for injection. Up to 4,000 cc. may be given daily. Solutions used are normal saline and 5 and 10 per cent glucose in either distilled water or saline. Hartmann's solution, Ringer's solution and sodium *r*-lactate solution may be given as indicated. **Hypodermoclysis** may be resorted to if other methods fail. From 1,000 to 2,000 cc. of sterile saline solution may be injected into the loose connective tissue under the breasts, in the axillary region or into the thighs—areas not subjected to pressure. Necrosis is a positive danger and the fluids must be given slowly and with care.

Malbin found that toxemia was distinctly lessened when tympanites was relieved by prostigmin.

Gastro-intestinal Symptoms and Complications.—Severe *vomiting* is an unusual symptom in typhoid. When present, the stomach should be given rest for a few hours and no food or only the blandest fluids should be given. **An ice bag or a hot compress over the upper abdomen** is useful. **Bits of ice or a carbonated water** may be given, or frequently repeated teaspoonful doses of **peppermint or chloroform water or chalk mixture.** **A hypodermic injection of morphine** will relieve when other measures fail. Other obstinate cases will respond to **gastric lavage.**

ABDOMINAL PAIN.—Severe abdominal pain is an important diagnostic sign of perforation and other grave abdominal complications. It should not be masked by an anodyne. **It is imperative that opium be withheld at least until the cause of the pain is determined.** Mild persistent pain is a symptom of indigestion and may be relieved by attention to the diet. An excess of fruit juices or cold drinks not infrequently excites colicky pain. **External applications with correction of the diet** usually bring relief. **The hot-water bag, electric heater** and **hot stupe** are useful. A carminative, like **peppermint, chloroform water or brandy** may be given in addition.

CONSTIPATION.—Constipation is the rule in typhoid patients who are carefully and properly fed. The condition is favorable and **should not**

40101

be interfered with by laxatives or purgatives. A single cathartic dose of calomel, castor oil or a saline may be given without harm if the case is seen at the beginning of the invasion period, although it will have no beneficial influence on the course of the disease. Repeated purgation, even in the first week, may excite a diarrhea difficult to control; after this time a cathartic is distinctly contraindicated. **The daily administration of a small soap and water enema** will empty the lower bowel with the least disturbance to the inflamed and ulcerated small intestine. This routine should be kept up until convalescence is established and the bowel resumes its normal function. One ounce of a good brand of **liquid petrolatum** given each evening during the declining and convalescent periods is often a very satisfactory substitute for the enema.

DIARRHEA.—Diarrhea is not a necessary symptom of typhoid fever, and, when present, its cause should be carefully sought. An unsuitable diet is the common cause. It may be a symptom of extensive ulceration involving the colon, or of a severe infection.

The appearance of diarrhea calls for an **immediate revision of the diet.** The total daily intake of food may be too high, or there may be an excess of some one article of the diet. The symptom can usually be controlled by a rearrangement of the dietary. Meat soups and extracts are a frequent cause. Milk or, more frequently, cream is the offending article. The stools should be examined, and if curds are found the milk should be given more dilute or otherwise modified, or stopped entirely. In exceptional cases it may be necessary to cut off all food for a day and give nothing except water by the mouth. As soon as the diarrhea is checked, feeding with albumin water, cereal gruels or whey may be begun and the diet again built up to the proper caloric content, with milk, eggs, cereals and lactose.

The semisolid foods in the high caloric diets are not apt to cause the trouble. Coleman has found that patients entering the hospital with profuse diarrhea develop normal stools after a few days of high caloric feeding.

It has been shown that the putrefactive bacteria predominate in the stools of patients with persistent diarrhea, and that a favorable change to the fermentation type of intestinal flora may be brought about by increasing the carbohydrate content of the food—particularly the lactose. The administration of **pure cultures of the Bacillus acidophilus** has been suggested to hasten the transformation.

Drugs may be necessary if the diarrhea resists the changes in the diet. **Bismuth subnitrate or subcarbonate,** 10 to 20 grains (0.65 to 1.3 Gm.) **suspended in chalk mixture,** 2 to 4 drams (8 to 16 Gm.) may be given every two to four hours. In severe cases **opium should be added to the bismuth,** one to two teaspoonfuls of **paregoric** or 2 to 4 grains (0.13 to 0.26 Gm.) of **Dover's powder** in capsule or syrup after each bowel movement. Given in this way the frequency of the dose of opium will be automatically regulated by the severity of the diarrhea. **Tannigen,** 5 grains (0.3 Gm.) every four hours, is a valuable astringent. Very frequent movements with symptoms of irritation of the lower bowel may be relieved by **enemas of starch water,** 6 ounces (180 cc.), and **laudanum,** 15 minims (1 cc.). Prolonged colon irrigation with **warm saline solution** is valuable in profoundly toxic cases with diarrhea and tympanites.

Intestinal antiseptics seem to have the confidence of many practitioners for the control of diarrhea and tympanites. **Salol** is the drug most frequently prescribed. It may be given in doses of 4 grains (0.26 Gm.) alone or combined with the chalk mixture and bismuth.

TYMPANITES.—Although a common symptom and, when moderate, not a dangerous one, tympanites should always receive serious consideration. Once the bowel becomes overdistended tympanites is a grave complication and very difficult to relieve. It usually—but not necessarily—is associated with diarrhea, and the same causes may be responsible for the symptom. Faulty diet is the common immediate cause. In severe form tympanites is a manifestation of profound toxemia with paralysis of the musculature of the intestinal wall.

The first appearance of meteorism demands **immediate attention to the dietary and revision in detail along the same lines as indicated for the treatment of diarrhea.** An excess of lactose or other carbohydrate may be the error in one case or an excess of protein food in another. For the milder degrees of distention, after attention has been given to the diet, the **ice bag** may be applied intermittently to the abdomen. **A hot-water or turpentine stupe**—made by wringing a flannel compress out of hot water containing one teaspoonful of turpentine to the quart—is the most useful external application. **A hot turpentine enema**—one-half teaspoonful to two quarts of water—will often give relief. If these simple measures fail **a rectal tube** may be passed carefully into the bowel and allowed to remain until expelled.

By the mouth, the simple carminatives will aid in giving relief. **Turpentine**—5 to 10 minims (0.3 to 0.6 cc.), given in emulsion or soft capsule—is the most valuable internal remedy.

Hypodermic injection of **solution of pituitary extract**—1 cc. (15 minims)—or **physostigmine sulfate**—$\frac{1}{50}$ grain (0.0013 Gm.)—should be given in severe cases. The remedies act as stimulants to the muscular wall of the bowel. Malbin used prostigmin in small fractional doses (0.25 mg. or less repeated in one-half hour). This proved effective in the treatment of tympanites. It should be used cautiously if perforation is suspected.

Several methods used in the treatment of surgical distention may be considered. Inhalation of oxygen in concentration of 98 to 100 per cent by mask as advocated by Boothby or by tent as suggested by Burgess is one. The other is the introduction of the Levin tube attached to the Wangensteen suction apparatus. The latter, naturally, relieves distention of the stomach and upper intestine only. Intestinal intubation is a trying manipulation, hardly suitable for a desperately sick typhoid patient.

INTESTINAL HEMORRHAGE.—The nurse should be warned of the possibility of hemorrhage, and instructed to notify the physician at once at the first sign of blood in the stools, to stop the administration of all food and water, and to keep the patient absolutely at rest and wait further instructions.

Hemorrhage is arrested by the formation of a clot in the ruptured bleeding vessel. The available measures favoring coagulation are (1) the arrest of intestinal peristalsis; (2) the administration of remedies which act locally upon the bleeding surface; (3) the administration of substances which increase the coagulability of the blood.

40101

The patient should be kept on his back with **complete mental and physical rest.** Every active and passive movement must be avoided as far as possible. All forms of hydrotherapy must be stopped. The patient should not use the bed pan or urinal, but should void his excretions in pads covering a drawsheet. No food or drink should be given by the mouth. He may be allowed small pieces of ice to allay thirst. A large **ice bag** should be applied to the abdomen. **Opiates must be given with caution.** Perforation and hemorrhage are frequently associated complications. Opium masks the pain and other symptoms upon which the diagnosis of perforation depends, and this grave accident may be obscured until the favorable time for surgical treatment has passed. *When the patient is very restless* the necessary quiet may be obtained by the **hypodermic administration of morphine.**

Astringents by the mouth are probably without value and they now are little used in the treatment of internal hemorrhage. **Turpentine,** advocated by Murchison, 10 minims (0.6 cc.) given in an emulsion every four hours, may be of use in adynamic cases. **Adrenalin** has a selective action upon the splanchnic area, powerfully constricting the vessels. Its use has been strongly advocated by Forchheimer and others. It should be given by hypodermic injection, 1 cc. (15 minims) of the 1 : 1000 solution, or the same quantity diluted with 500 cc. (17 fl.oz.) of normal saline, by hypodermoclysis. The possibility of increasing the bleeding by the rise in general blood pressure which it causes, before time is given for its local constrictive action, should be borne in mind.

The salts of calcium increase the coagulability of the blood. **Calcium lactate** is the preferable salt, given in doses of 20 to 40 grains (1.3 to 2.6 Gm.) every four hours. **Injections of blood serum** are sometimes of value. A number of preparations containing **thromboplastin** are put out by manufacturing chemists. They all markedly reduce the coagulation time of the blood. Prompt action may be obtained from them by subcutaneous or intravenous administration.

In profuse hemorrhage, when the patient is in collapse and life is threatened, stimulants must be given even at the risk of further bleeding. **Brandy, champagne, camphor and strychnine** are valuable. The alcoholic stimulants are of particular value because of their food content and their feeble action on blood pressure. **Normal saline administered by the drop method or by hypodermoclysis,** in quantity just sufficient to lift the patient out of the collapse, is sound treatment. **Transfusion of blood** will save life when other measures fail. The perfection of the technic of the operation has made transfusion an easy and a safe therapeutic measure.

Food and water in small quantity should be begun on the second day after the cessation of the bleeding and gradually increased in quantity. The feeding and bath routine in operation before the hemorrhage should not be reached until four or five days after the bleeding has stopped.

PERFORATION.—There is no medical treatment for perforation except measures to relieve pain. The complication is certainly fatal without surgical interference. **Surgical counsel should be called immediately** with the onset of symptoms suggestive of perforation, and the physician and the surgeon together should decide upon the advisability of operation. If the diagnosis is reasonably certain and an expert surgeon is at hand there is no alternative to immediate operation. If the symptoms are vague and the diagnosis doubtful, decision is very difficult. Many operations have been done for suspected typhoid perforation when no perforation was found. The death rate in these cases has been high, not from the operation itself, but from the grave condition of the patients at the time of operation. Of 19 such cases reported by Mitchell from the Pennsylvania Hospital, 8 recovered and 11 died. The exact diagnosis of perforation is so difficult, the danger of delay so great and the added risk from operation so small, that **exploration is justifiable if there is a reasonable suspicion that perforation has taken place.** Most authorities will agree with the opinion of Mikulicz, the first surgeon to operate for typhoid perforation, who said, "If there is suspicion, don't wait for an exact diagnosis; explore immediately for it is free from danger."

CHOLECYSTITIS.—**Rest, an ice bag over the right upper quadrant, and anodynes to relieve pain** make up the medical treatment of cholecystitis. **Urotropin** in full doses, 75 grains (5 Gm.) or more a day, will inhibit the growth of organisms in the gallbladder and may be given a trial. *Mild cases* with moderate fullness of the gallbladder usually recover under **medical treatment.** *Severe cases* with great distention and marked local and general symptoms may require **cholecystotomy and drainage.** The operation is a dangerous one and should be advised only after full consideration. Perforation of the gallbladder is a common accident in the severe cases and is uniformly fatal. Keen is "decidedly of the opinion that in distention of the gallbladder prompt surgical interference is the best. It is far better to prevent perforation than to remedy it after it has occurred."

Nervous Symptoms and Complications.—Severe nervous symptoms are manifestations of toxemia and are much less frequently seen in patients who are well fed and systematically bathed.

HEADACHE.—Headache may be severe in the first week of the disease. It usually is softened and made endurable by a **cold compress or ice bag to the head. Sodium bromide,** 30 grains (2 Gm.), repeated after an interval of three hours may give relief. In exceptional cases an analgesic may be required. The temptation is great to administer one of the synthetic antipyretics, but for reasons already given this should be withheld if possible. Probably no harm can come from the administration of 5 grains (0.3 Gm.) of **phenacetin,** repeated in one hour if necessary. If this fails to give relief it is better to allay the pain with a **hypodermic injection of codeine,** ½ grain (0.032 Gm.), or **morphine,** ⅛ grain (0.008 Gm.).

INSOMNIA.—Insomnia is best overcome by the **bath treatment.** A cool or tepid tub bath at eight or nine o'clock in the evening will usually give a few hours of sleep. This should not be disturbed and the nurse should be instructed to time the administration of food and other attentions so as to give the patient **as many hours of sleep at night as possible.** When the wakefulness is persistent one of the hypnotics may be given: **trional,** 10 to 15 grains (0.6 to 1 Gm.); **veronal** or **medinal,** 5 to 10 grains (0.3 to 0.6 Gm.); or **morphine,** ¼ grain (0.016 Gm.), hypodermically. In the insomnia of adynamic states, one-half to one ounce of whisky or brandy often acts well.

DELIRIUM.—Delirium is controlled in the same manner as insomnia. **A tepid or cold bath and ice to the head** have a decided sedative in-

40101

fluence. **Veronal,** 2 grains (0.13 Gm.) every four hours, is useful. **Morphine** hypodermically will give these patients the rest that is absolutely necessary. Violent delirium may be quieted by **lumbar puncture** and the withdrawal of 10 to 20 cc. of spinal fluid. The delirious patient should never be left alone.

MENINGITIS.—Meningitis is a very grave complication of typhoid fever. **Lumbar puncture for diagnosis and treatment** is a most valuable measure. In meningismus and the serous form it may ward off a fatal result. The puncture may be repeated every second day.

Cole believes that in typhoid meningitis the **intraspinal administration of an antityphoid serum** is indicated, if the typhoid bacillus can be isolated from the spinal fluid, using the same technic that is employed in the serum treatment of meningococcus meningitis.

PSYCHOSES.—The delirium of the febrile stage may persist into convalescence and merge into a posttyphoid psychosis. The treatment of this condition belongs to the alienist. The mental disturbance is largely an exhaustion phenomenon and is to be treated by **supportive measures.** **High caloric feeding during the febrile period** prevents the profound exhaustion so often seen in convalescence and the well-fed patient rarely shows persistent mental disturbance. Many cases can be treated at home, but, *if the psychosis is prolonged and severe,* **institutional treatment will be better.**

Circulatory Symptoms.—MYOCARDIAL WEAKNESS.—Myocardial weakness may be evident in the latter part of the febrile stage. When the blood pressure falls and the heart becomes rapid, weak and irregular, cardiac stimulation is necessary. **An ice bag over the heart** slows and strengthens ventricular contractions without the possibility of a drug reaction. **Strychnine** may be given: $\frac{1}{40}$ to $\frac{1}{20}$ grain (0.0016 to 0.0032 Gm.) every four to six hours. *In elderly patients,* alcoholic subjects and those who have been unable to take adequate food, **whisky, brandy or wine** is a valuable stimulant. It is rarely necessary to give more than 6 ounces (180 cc.) of whisky or its equivalent in the twenty-four hours. A tablespoonful in hot sweetened water every three or four hours is usually sufficient. *If the heart becomes progressively more rapid and feeble,* **digitalis** should be given. A standardized preparation in doses equivalent to $1\frac{1}{2}$ grains (0.1 Gm.) of powdered digitalis may be given every six or eight hours for two days and then the interval between doses lengthened to twelve hours. *In urgent cases* **the drug should be given hypodermically.** **Saline infusions,** 500 to 750 cc. (17 to 25 fl.oz.), every six hours are valuable. In sudden and serious heart failure, **camphor, caffeine or ether** may be given hypodermically and **aromatic ammonia or compound spirits of ether** by the mouth—$\frac{1}{2}$ dram (2 cc.)—frequently repeated.

PHLEBITIS.—**Absolute rest of the affected limb** is necessary. It should be placed on a pillow slightly elevated, and all rubbing avoided. The leg may be **covered with cotton and lightly bandaged or kept wet with a lead and opium lotion.** An anodyne—**morphine hypodermically** —is often necessary to relieve pain. The leg must be kept quiet for at least a week after the acute symptoms have subsided, and for five or six weeks it should be little used. **An elastic fabric bandage or stocking** should be worn after the patient gets up and until the swelling subsides.

Respiratory Symptoms and Complications.—BRONCHITIS; PNEU-MONIA; PLEURISY.—The mild bronchitis which is so common in typhoid fever requires no special treatment. Severe bronchitis, pneumonia and pleurisy are treated in the same manner as when these diseases are primary. **The bath treatment** is an important prophylactic of the hypostatic congestion which so frequently leads to pulmonary infection.

LARYNGITIS.—Ulcerative laryngitis may often be prevented, or serious results from it avoided, by **careful and persistent oral antisepsis.** If aphonia or dyspnea develop, **inhalation of benzoin** should be used. **A spray of adrenalin** (1:1,000) may be used in an emergency to tide the patient over a period of danger. Whenever laryngeal obstruction is present an **early tracheotomy under local anesthesia is imperative.** Postponement of operation leads to necrosis of the cartilage with deformity, stenosis and loss of voice. "All lesions disappear as if by magic after an early tracheotomy" (Jackson).

Urinary Symptoms.—RETENTION OF URINE.—Retention of the urine is a symptom of importance and should be carefully watched for. It may occur early in the disease, before the patient has become accustomed to the use of the bed pan or urinal. At this time it is usually nervous in origin and may be overcome by **hot compresses to the hypogastrium or hot rectal irrigations.** Later it is a manifestation of profound muscular debility. Overdistention favors infection, and if not readily overcome by the above applications the patient must be **catheterized.** This must be done by the physician, or at least by an expert attendant. The **strictest asepsis** is required and **urotropin** should be given after the operation.

BACILLURIA.—Typhoid bacilli may be recovered from the urine in from 25 to 30 per cent of all cases of typhoid fever at some period of the disease. They appear in the third or fourth week or during convalescence. The organisms may pass through the urinary tract without causing any signs of inflammatory reaction, or a few pus cells in the urine may indicate the presence of a mild pyelitis. Bacilluria or pyelitis yields readily to treatment by **urinary antiseptics.** If possible, **frequent cultures** should be made of the urine toward the end of the febrile period and the **administration of urotropin should be begun at once if bacilli are found.** In the absence of means to demonstrate bacilli, the urine should be frequently **examined microscopically and the antiseptics should be given if pus cells are present.** It is good practice to anticipate the invasion of the urinary tract and give urotropin in the third and fourth weeks in all cases. **Urotropin with acid sodium phosphate,** 10 grains (0.65 Gm.) of each, may be given three times a day.

A persistent bacilluria or a pyelitis may yield to treatment by a **typhoid or colon vaccine.**

Glandular System.—Either typhoid bacilli or the pyogenic cocci may invade the various glandular organs and cause an inflammation that may go on to abscess formation. Parotitis, mastitis and orchitis are the most common. The application of **ice** is the most generally useful measure. Occasionally a **hot compress** will give more relief. *When suppuration occurs* **the treatment is surgical.**

Skin.—BED SORES.—The treatment of bed sores should be **preventive.** Both physician and nurse must assume a large part of the responsibility for the development of this complication. In certain profoundly toxic

40101

cases sloughing of dependent areas of skin may take place in spite of all precautions, but when bed sores develop in cases of moderate severity it is evidence of careless nursing. Well-fed patients and those who are systematically bathed rarely have this trouble. **Frequent change of position** must be insisted upon. **Clean linen and a careful make-up of the bed** are essential. At least twice a day the **skin of the lower back and buttocks should be inspected and rubbed with alcohol.** Any areas of redness must receive special attention, and all pressure relieved from them by **ring cushions.** The suspicious areas should be cleansed with **soap and water,** bathed first with a **weak bichloride solution,** and this followed with **alcohol,** and, finally, dusted with a **borated talcum powder.** For over-red and suspicious spots **ichthyol collodion** may be applied.

If an actual break in the skin takes place, the treatment should be that of indolent ulcers under other circumstances. **Perfect cleanliness, alcohol and zinc oxide ointment** will usually suffice to stimulate healing. When the edges of the ulcer are undermined it may be packed with **iodoform gauze, or with gauze moistened with balsam of Peru.**

MANAGEMENT OF CONVALESCENCE

The convalescent typhoid patient must be carefully watched and his activities controlled until well after the end of the fever period. Experience with high caloric feeding shows that when it is possible to keep up an abundant diet during the febrile period, convalescence is shortened and the complications of this period are made less frequent.

As a rule the patient should be **kept in bed for a week after the evening temperature becomes normal,** and he may then be allowed to sit up and gradually get on his feet. A little overexertion or excitement is very apt to bring on a recrudescence of the fever and there is always the menace of true relapse resulting from it. Patients who have been kept on a low liquid diet throughout the course of the disease are very sensitive to diet changes, and **meat and other solid foods must be added with great caution.** Abundantly fed patients have little trouble in passing to a full diet soon after the fever has abated.

The possibility of hemorrhage and perforation is present during the convalescent period, and a **diet leaving little residue** after passing through the upper digestive tract **must still be adhered to. Cathartics must be withheld,** and a daily emptying of the lower bowel obtained by a **simple enema. A well-refined liquid petrolatum,** one or two ounces a day, will often keep the bowels in good condition and replace the enema.

Other complications and sequelae must be anticipated and promptly met. Secondary infections by the pyogenic organisms are not uncommon.

The patient is still a carrier. **Rigid care of the excretions** is demanded until repeated cultures from the urine and feces demonstrate that bacteriologic recovery is complete.

Some degree of anemia is usually present and a tonic of **iron, quinine and strychnine** is of value.

The resumption of business requires caution. The patient's strength returns slowly and it may be two or three months before he is able to take up his former activities. **A period of rest away from home surroundings** will hasten his return to normal.

RECRUDESCENCE AND RELAPSE

Any return of fever after convalescence has set in must be met by an **immediate return to the rigid rest and diet regime of the febrile period.** The bowels should be thoroughly emptied by an **enema** and the food reduced to the **blandest fluids** for a day or two.

True relapse is a reinfection and demands the **same treatment in all its details as the original attack.** Tubbing is, however, rarely required, although it may be necessary in severe cases. Usually milder hydrotherapeutic methods are adequate.

TREATMENT OF TYPHOID FEVER IN INFANCY

In the infant the adjustment of the diet in typhoid fever is comparatively simple. Briefly, it is the adjustment of a milk formula to suit the impaired digestion of the sick infant.

During the first and second weeks the formula which the child was taking at the time of the onset of the infection reduced 25 or 50 per cent will be suitable. Whole milk diluted with one or two parts of a 5 per cent milk sugar solution will usually be well taken. The cereal gruels may be added later and the caloric content of the formula increased by a higher percentage of milk sugar. The protein content and caloric value of each day's feeding should be recorded and an effort made to keep the food value as near the normal requirement as possible. **Malted or dextrinized cereal foods** can often be advantageously used **as additions to the milk formulas. Fermented milk or whey** may be useful if the stomach is irritable. **Beef juice, fruit juices and broths** are not so well borne but are occasionally helpful. During the period of intestinal irritability the **milk may be sterilized** by a short exposure to the boiling temperature. **An abundance of water** should be given.

Stimulants are rarely required in typhoid fever in the young child. In the third week of the disease, when nutrition is failing and the heart action is weak, the addition to the food of from 1 to 4 drams (4 to 16 cc.) of **brandy** in the twenty-four hours may be of distinct advantage. Each dram of brandy will give an additional value of fourteen calories to the food and it may be taken and assimilated when an adequate amount of other food cannot be given. **Strychnine, digitalis and other drug stimulants are of doubtful value.**

Diarrhea is present in about one half of the cases and, when the movements exceed three a day, will require correction. **Bismuth subcarbonate**—4 grains (0.26 Gm.)—**in chalk mixture**—1 dram (4 Gm.)—will best control it. It is best administered after each bowel movement. Given in this way the frequency of dosage is automatically regulated by the varying requirements of the patient's condition. The occasional addition of 5 to 10 minims (0.3 to 0.6 cc.) of **paregoric** to this prescription may be necessary. It is particularly beneficial if the movements are frequent and accompanied by abdominal pain.

Constipation will require attention. **A routine cathartic** is usually given **before the diagnosis is made,** and further administration is unwise. The lower colon should be thoroughly emptied each day by **irrigation with a simple enema.**

40101

For the control of *high temperature*, **hydrotherapy** is the most effective. **Antipyretic drugs must be avoided.** **A bath may be given every four to six hours** if the rectal temperature is 103° F. (39.4° C.) or over. **A tepid sponge may be efficient but the best results are obtained from the full bath.** The full bath is easily given to the infant. The water should be at a temperature of 100° F. (37.8° C.), and the bath continued with **gentle friction** for eight to ten minutes. The cooling of the water that will take place during the bath is all the reduction that is necessary. When nervous symptoms are marked, even a higher temperature of the water—up to 105° F. (40.6° C.)—may give better results and be followed by quiet and a moderate reduction of temperature. Infants do not endure the cool bath well, and a bath at a temperature of 90° F. (32.2° C.) often leaves the child prostrated with a cold, blue skin and a weak pulse—a result that cannot but be harmful. *For marked nervous symptoms,* in addition to the bath as above directed, **sodium bromide,** 2 to 4 grains (0.13 to 0.26 Gm.) **in syrup,** may be given.

The treatment of the *period of convalescence* is chiefly a problem in infant feeding and requires the careful adjustment of the food to the nutritional requirements of the infant and its ability to digest and assimilate it.

PROGNOSIS

Cause of Death.—Death in typhoid fever results from (1) the intensity of the toxemia; (2) severe localization of the infection; and (3) complications and sequelae.

All of the organs and tissues suffer from the lethal effects of the typhoid toxin. The heart, the vasomotor and heat-regulating mechanisms, and the nervous system are most conspicuously influenced. The effect upon mortality of the individual localizations and complications is considered in detail in another section.

In 580 fatal cases reported by Curschmann from Hamburg and Leipzig, 46.9 per cent died of toxemia, and 53.1 per cent died of localizations and complications. Perforation, hemorrhage, pneumonia and nephritis were the causes of death in 241 of the latter group of 305 cases. In this country at the present time the disease is certainly less virulent. Elsner, from a careful study of available autopsy findings, places the mortality rate from toxemia at 24 per cent. Writers generally estimate that toxemia is responsible for about one third and complications for about two thirds of the fatalities.

Mortality.—The case mortality rate of typhoid fever generally accepted at the present time is about 10 per cent. Statistics from many sources give rather wide variations from this figure.

The death rate of typhoid fever in New York City for 1917 in 1,442 reported cases was 15.8 per cent. The average annual mortality from 1908 to 1917 in a total of 28,083 cases was 15.18 per cent. This probably fairly represents the mortality in a large number of cases of all ages and conditions, under varying epidemic influences, and treated by a variety of methods, and of sufficient severity to be recognized and reported. It is quite certain that many mild and atypical cases which recovered are not included in these figures.

The mortality of hospital-treated cases varies from 7 to 22 per cent. Of 21,371 cases admitted to the hospitals of the Metropolitan Asylum

Board of London over a period of thirty-six years, 16.3 per cent died. The mortality in Osler's wards at the Johns Hopkins Hospital was 9.1 per cent. In private practice the mortality is probably lower, from 5 to 12 per cent.

Factors which influence the mortality of the disease and are valuable guides to prognosis are: (1) the age of the patient; (2) the type of the prevailing outbreak or endemic; (3) the severity of special symptoms; (4) the presence of complications; (5) the treatment; (6) antityphoid vaccination.

AGE.—After the period of infancy and childhood there is a steady increase in the mortality percentage of the disease. In infancy it is about 20 per cent. The lowest rate, from 6 to 7 per cent, is between the ages of five and ten years. From ten to twenty-five years of age the mortality is increased slowly from 8 or 9 to 10 or 12 per cent. At forty years the rate is from 18 to 24 per cent. After the age of forty years the disease has a very grave prognosis, with a death rate of from 25 to 35 per cent.

TYPE OF PREVAILING OUTBREAK.—The mortality varies greatly in different communities and in different epidemics and endemics in the same community. The type of the disease will be virulent in one section and mild in another. Sudden outbreaks in districts previously free from typhoid often show a high mortality. The disease is also apt to be more fatal at the beginning of an outbreak. In certain years serious complications are common.

SEVERITY OF SPECIAL SYMPTOMS.—Except in infants and young children a pulse rate persistently above 120 is cause for apprehension. In exceptional cases, women and nervous men have a rapid pulse from the onset of the disease, without other symptoms of gravity. Persistent temperature above 104° F. (40° C.) indicates a severe infection, and repeated elevation above 105° F. (40.6° C.) without marked remissions adds to the gravity of a case. The outlook is serious when high fever continues through the third and fourth weeks. Severe diarrhea and meteorism are common in some outbreaks, and increase the mortality rate. Cases with marked nervous manifestations are serious. Liebermeister observed a mortality of over 50 per cent in cases with early and severe delirium and of about 70 per cent in cases with continued stupor and coma.

COMPLICATIONS AND SEQUELAE.—Any complication, however mild, affects the prognosis unfavorably. It tends to prolong the illness and favors the development of other complications.

INFLUENCE OF METHODS OF TREATMENT.—It is difficult properly to evaluate a method of treatment in typhoid fever, which varies so widely in severity from year to year and in different epidemics, without the observation of a large number of cases extending over a long period. Available evidence of this kind is strongly indicative that the **bath treatment** has very favorably influenced the mortality. The statistics of the Brisbane General Hospital, Queensland, reported by F. E. Hare, are convincing. In 1,828 consecutive cases treated by the expectant method during the years 1882 to 1886 the mortality was 14.8 per cent; 1,902 consecutive cases treated with cold and tepid baths during the years 1887 to 1896 showed a mortality of 7.5 per cent. Equally satisfactory results have been obtained in a number of the hospitals of this country and Europe. It can be confidently stated that the treatment of typhoid fever as carried out in well-equipped modern hospitals is an important factor in the reduction of the mortality.

ANTITYPHOID VACCINATION.—Typhoid fever, when it occurs in individuals who have been vaccinated, pursues a much milder average course than it does in unvaccinated patients, and complications are very much less frequent and fatal. The report of Webb-Johnson of the British Army shows the influence of vaccination on mortality and on the incidence of complications. In 297 cases of typhoid fever, unvaccinated, the mortality was 57, or 19.19 per cent. In 821 cases, vaccinated, the mortality was 27, or 3.28 per cent. In the unvaccinated group complications occurred in 35.69 per cent; in the vaccinated group in 7.55 per cent.

Mode of Death.—Sudden death takes place in from 3 to 4 per cent of the fatal cases. In Osler's series of 137 fatal cases there were 4 sudden deaths. It occurs more frequently in men than in women. It is an accident usually of the third week, more rarely of convalescence. Autopsy findings are inadequate to explain the fatal result in about one third of the cases. Cerebral anemia and reflex syncope have been given as causes. In the remaining cases with positive autopsy findings, acute myocarditis, pulmonary embolism and thrombosis and cerebral embolism are the conditions that have been found.

Incomplete Recovery.—Typhoid fever is a serious disease, aside from its high immediate mortality. The weeks of bacteremia with high fever and profound toxemia gravely impair cell function and may leave the patient in a state of prolonged or permanent ill-health with disabling pathologic conditions and a decided curtailment of longevity. Many of the complications result in permanent damage to structure and function, or initiate chronic infective or degenerative diseases which are remote causes of death. The effect of typhoid fever on the mortality of recovered cases was studied by Dublin from the data of a life insurance company. Fourteen hundred and twenty-eight cases of recovered typhoid were investigated. Of this number 54 died during the first three years following recovery. The expected mortality of this group was 26.

Among the important disabling sequelae are the following: a state of permanently deranged metabolism, the patient never regaining his former trophic level; gallstone disease and chronic intestinal catarrh; chronic laryngeal obstruction from ulceration and necrosis; pulmonary tuberculosis and pulmonary abscess; chronic myocarditis, arteriosclerosis and thrombophlebitis; chronic renal or bladder infection; hemiplegia; incurable psychoses and degenerative brain and cord lesions.

PATHOGENESIS AND TISSUE CHANGES

We have the following questions to consider:

1. The manner in which the typhoid bacillus enters the body.
2. The cause of the general reaction to the infection (fever).
3. The tissue injury and tissue reactions which result.
4. The manner of elimination and healing.

As to the first of these, the portal of entry is only approximately known. The typhoid bacillus, as shown under "Etiology," is taken into the mouth from some one of the many sources, and gains entrance to the tissues somewhere in the gastro-intestinal tract. There are no adequate data fixing any particular part of the gastro-enteric tract as the point through which the *Eberthella typhosa* gains entrance to the tissues. Indeed, there is no reason whatever for believing that some one place is to be sought for rather than several loci. Suggestive facts exist favoring the tonsils and pharynx, the intestinal epithelium, and the lymphoid tissue of the intestine as occasional portals of entry.

It is certain that the typhoid bacillus does not multiply to any extent in the intestinal tract. The few bacteria taken into the mouth at the time of infection do not increase in the gastro-enteric tract, but first gain entrance to the body proper and are later eliminated into the intestine. The general assumption that gastric juice will kill typhoid bacilli is not strictly correct, since it has been shown that moderate acidity does not kill the typhoid bacillus (Kitasato). The typhoid bacilli which we cultivate from the intestinal tract in cases of typhoid fever do not represent bacteria which have been taken into the mouth at the time of infection and which have multiplied in the gastro-enteric tract, but they are bacilli that are being eliminated from the blood and tissues by way of the intestines.

It is frequently assumed that the portal of entry is the lymphoid apparatus, particularly the Peyer's patches in the ileum, because here we usually find the most characteristic anatomic changes of the disease. The fact that the Peyer's patches are injured, points rather to the intestinal lesions as the result of the susceptibility of lymphatic tissues to injury by the typhoid bacillus. The changes in the lymphatic apparatus are probably a result of the invasion of the body as a whole by the typhoid bacilli rather than a door through which they enter the body.

Goodpasture believes that the typhoid bacillus, after gaining access to the intestine, first proliferates in plasma cells of the agminated follicles and mesenteric lymph nodes. Upon the necrosis of these cells the bacilli are liberated for dissemination or they may proliferate in necrotic tissue and become ingested by macrophage cells. Metastatic foci develop in the lymph nodes throughout the body. The organisms which he observed in the plasma cells were small gram-negative rods which he was convinced were intracellular forms of *E. typhosa*. These events take place during the incubation period and this particular pathologic change is demonstrated only in the early stages of the disease. When the bacilli are liberated from the plasma cells they are exposed to the extracellular environment and are dissolved by the bacteriolytic action of the blood serum, thus mobilizing the antigens.

The typhoid bacillus gains entrance to the gastro-intestinal tract through the mouth. Somewhere in the course of its passage toward the anus it is absorbed into the lymphatics and thence passes on to the regional lymph nodes. This may be anywhere from the tonsils or pharynx to the sigmoid, but certain considerations make it probable, if not certain, that the usual portal of entry is found in the last few feet of the ileum. The relative stasis in this part of the bowel compared to the upper portions is well known, and the richness of the lymphatic apparatus and other considerations point to this portion as that especially differentiated for absorption. The fact is that the mesenteric nodes draining this region show the earliest anatomic injury in typhoid infection. The question of broken or unbroken epithelium is purely academic. Injury to the intestinal mucosa has never been shown to be necessary, and moreover the ease with which leukocytes can pass in and out of an uninjured mucosa shows that the entrance of an active organism like the typhoid bacillus might be determined by the chemotactic conditions present, and not by the presence or absence of an actual hiatus in the tissue. There is abundant evidence in the respiratory as well as in the gastro-enteric and genito-urinary tracts that unbroken epithelium of mucous membranes is not a barrier to the entrance of bacteria, but that the ability of an organism to gain entrance into these localities depends upon the specific properties of the organism itself.

Having entered the lymphatics, the bacillus is filtered out by the regional lymph nodes. Thus the mesenteric nodes are the first tissues to be subjected to the effects of the typhoid bacillus after it has gained entrance into the body.

The most significant fact in the pathogenesis of typhoid fever is the predilection the typhoid bacillus shows for the lymphatic apparatus. The organism multiplies in the lymph nodes, spleen and bone marrow as well as in the bile. From the first three of these localities it gains entrance to the blood. There is no evidence that it multiplies in the blood stream; on the contrary, it is rapidly destroyed. Even the blood of a normal individual has considerable ability to kill typhoid bacilli, and in an infected individual during the course of the disease this bactericidal power of the blood increases markedly.

It is probable that the entrance of the bacillus through the gastrointestinal tract, the invasion and multiplication in the lymph nodes, and the "overflow" into the thoracic duct and blood stream all take place during the incubation period of the disease, before the patient is sick. In other words, the bacteria could be recovered from the mesenteric apparatus and blood stream before the appearance of the first symptoms of typhoid fever.

Typhoid fever is best designated as a bacteremia, in that the bacteria are present during the course of the disease in the characteristic foci mentioned above, and also in the blood stream.

The general reaction to the infection, that course of clinical events which we call typhoid fever, does not commence until the organism is well entrenched in its various foci. The bacteria, by their presence, set up various phenomena in the host which, taken together, constitute the clinical manifestations characteristic of the disease.

The fever and other toxic manifestations of typhoid fever may be caused by the liberation of the somatic antigens resulting from the disintegration of the bacilli. V. C. Vaughan, Sr., in 1913 postulated such a theory to explain the cause of symptoms in certain infectious diseases, but the toxic effects of the antigens were not then recognized. Spanedda has produced in animals degenerative changes by the injection of purified antigen, and Weil has noted great loss and prolonged recovery time in experimental animals in the same manner. He states that these effects can be prevented by active and passive immunization.

Tissue Changes—Morbid Anatomy.—GENERAL.—A superficial inspection of the body presents no appearances characteristic of typhoid fever. The rose spots disappear after death. There is more or less emaciation, depending upon the length of the illness. Cases autopsied after long illness may show special appearances due to complications: parotitis, arthritis or decubitus. Rigor mortis is well developed.

MUSCLES.—Zenker first described the characteristic "fish flesh" transformation of the muscles known as Zenker's necrosis. The change is found only in the more severe cases in which there has been high and prolonged fever. The rectus abdominis and muscles of the thigh are most often affected. In the gross this waxy degeneration gives a whitish, waxy appearance to the sectioned muscle, which has been compared to fish flesh. Microscopically the muscle fibers are found under these conditions to have lost their striations, and their ability to take acid stains uniformly. The muscle protoplasm is collected inside of the wrinkled sarcolemma in pale, irregular lumps. There is frequently rupture of the capillaries between the fibers, giving rise to small hemorrhages. Occasionally these hemorrhages are larger, and at autopsy diffuse suggillations of blood involving the muscles, and loose areolar tissues of the whole lower half of the abdominal wall are found. These muscle changes, Zenker's necrosis and hemorrhages, are not confined to typhoid but are found more frequently in this disease than in others.

GASTRO-ENTERIC TRACT.—The upper portions of the tract are relatively little affected. In cases of long standing, ulcerations of the pharynx and esophagus are sometimes found. These are usually small, indolent ulcers, seldom over 1 cm. in diameter, and with very little reaction around their margins. Their etiology is not clear. They are not specific lesions of typhoid, but are usually classed along with ulcers of the epiglottis and laryngeal structures as "cachectic ulcers."

No changes are found in the stomach or duodenum which can in any way be referred to typhoid fever.

The small bowel, in cases uncomplicated by perforation or hemorrhage, is usually collapsed and fairly empty. On opening the lumen of the bowel we find the upper portion fairly normal or moderately congested. As the lower jejunum and ileum are approached the agminated follicles or Peyer's patches are found to be swollen and raised above the surface of the mucosa. At first they have a pinkish color by reflected light, but a little lower down we find them more swollen and presenting a blanched appearance. These represent the early intestinal lesions of typhoid. Since the earliest systematic descriptions by Chomel and Louis the progress of the intestinal lesion of typhoid fever has been divided into four stages corresponding roughly to the four weeks of the ordinary disease course:

1. *Stage of Swelling of the Peyer's Patches.*—Our knowledge of the mechanism of production of the characteristic typhoid lesion is due to Mallory. During the first week the lymphoid tissue, solitary agminated follicles and Peyer's patches become swollen and project above the surface of the mucosa. The Peyer's patches appear as oval plaques extending lengthwise of the bowel. The solitary follicles, embedded more deeply in the mucosa, may not be apparent, or may project beyond the mucosa as pedunculated points. Examined microscopically at this stage, we find the swelling to be due not so much to lymphoid hyperplasia in the strict sense—although the lymphocytes are increased in number—as to the accumulation in the lymph follicles and in the reticulum and sinuses of large mononuclear macrophages. These cells have an abundance of light-staining protoplasm and pale reticular nuclei. In many

40101

of them are found red cells, lymphocytes and tissue debris. They are variously designated as endothelial leukocytes (Mallory) and as mononuclear wandering cells. Whether they have a specific origin from endothelium by proliferation of the lining cells of the lymph and blood spaces, or whether they represent a form of undifferentiated mesodermal wandering cell or polyblast (Maximow), has not been satisfactorily settled.

The macrophages pack themselves so tightly in the sinuses and tissue spaces that the lymphoid tissue is to a degree destroyed by them, so that in a well-developed lesion the lymphocytes only appear in patches. The normal structure of the lymph node is destroyed, and the patch consists of a dense mass of these large mononuclear cells with relatively few lymphocytes. This is the stage of greatest swelling, and the swelling is due not only to the increase in the cell content of the patch, but also to the edema which develops in the tissue, due to the local circulatory disturbance. This local circulatory disturbance arises from occlusion of the blood vessels which nourish the lymphoid tissue, and is due in part to the external pressure on the capillaries exerted by the closely packed macrophages, in part to plugging of the vessels themselves by the large mononuclears loaded with tissue debris, and in part to minute thrombi (Mallory), due to the endothelium of the capillary being lifted up by the accumulation of cells and fibrin beneath.

2. *Stage of Necrosis.*—This vascular occlusion leads to anemic necrosis of the patch, with the formation of a slough. While in the gross the lesion seems well confined to the lymphoid tissue, microscopically it is evident that the wandering cells are numerous outside the Peyer's patch. The necrosis in the severer grades often extends beyond the lymphoid tissue limits laterally into the mucosa, and deeply to the muscularis or even to the peritoneum.

At the height of the stage of swelling in a mild case resolution may occur before the slough forms, and the tissue be restored to normal by the disappearance of the wandering cells. More frequently the patch undergoes necrosis as a whole or in part, and the slough forms. At this stage we may find the pale, white, swollen and feltlike patch becoming a dirty brown color, due to the imbibition of bile, or one of various shades of mottled, dark red or slate color, due to small hemorrhages. When the patch does not undergo necrosis as a whole but only in small, pitlike areas, probably corresponding to the lymph follicles around a central vessel, we get the appearance described by Chomel as "plaques à surface réticulée." Up to this stage the microscopic appearance of the lesion is unique, in that practically no polymorphonuclear cells are involved in the process. The typhoid bacillus, and whatever poisons are liberated from it throughout the body, tend to depress the usual polymorphonuclear inflammatory reaction. This is true of the lesions elsewhere in the body as well as of those in the intestine. Even secondary infections, usually accompanied by active leukocytosis, are able in the typhoid patient to stimulate only a feeble response. As the tissue of the area dies, a moderate collection of polymorphonuclears occurs at the margin between the necrotic and the healthy tissue. These begin to liberate leukoproteases that digest the coagulated lymph and dead cells and cause the slough to begin to separate. This usually occurs around the edge when massive necrosis of the patch has occurred, so that we find the edges loosening from the healthy tissue and curling up or rolling under. The separation gradually works toward the center, and finally the dead slough separates entirely, leaving the ulcer.

3. *Stage of Ulceration.*—The fact that tissue beyond the margin of the patch has been involved in the process is most evident at this stage, when the slough separates and leaves a more or less irregular ragged area extending well beyond the limits of the original Peyer's patch. Sometimes the ulceration is very superficial, including only the upper layers of the mucosa, and leaving some lymphoid tissue and epithelial crypts. But the usual typhoid ulcer extends down to the muscularis, leaving a fairly clean floor covered with a thin gray exudate and a few shreds of fibrin. Often the whole patch does not undergo necrosis but the slough separates in several larger or smaller areas, leaving irregular ulcers connected with narrow passages and separated by bridges of still intact mucosa. The ulceration is more extensive toward the last few inches of the lumen. It is not uncommon to find the last six or twelve inches a mass of confluent ulcers with bridges of mucosa left in their midst.

4. *Stage of Healing.*—The typhoid ulcer is unique in its ability to heal without scar tissue contraction and consequent disturbance of bowel function. There is apparently a complete *restitutio ad integrum.* The lymphoid tissue regenerates, and is covered in by epithelium without increase in fibroblasts and their usual hyaline transformation to scar tissue, so that after the healing of a typhoid ulcer we find perhaps at the most an atrophy of the submucosa, causing a slight depression and some increased pigmentation.

The colon is moderately involved, according to Murchison, in one third of the cases. The solitary lymph follicles show numerous ulcerations. These are more apt to occur or to be more numerous in the cecum. Sometimes a special form of typhoid, *colotyphus,* is recognized in which the ulceration of the colon overshadows that of the ileum, or is confined to the colon. The ulcerations are said to be large, with their long diameters lying transversely of the gut. Cases with extreme gaseous distention and meteorism with multiple perforations in the bowel have been recorded by Kaufmann. Excessive growth of the lactic acid bacillus has been found in these cases, accounting for the excessive gas.

The important complications of the intestinal lesions are perforations and hemorrhages. The hemorrhages occur from erosion of the exposed vessels of the area at the time of the separation of the slough. Perforations the size of pin points are found at the base of a small, deep ulcer, or in a larger area they may be even a centimeter across, at the base of a large ulcerated area. Excessive peristalsis probably plays a role in the formation of the larger perforations. Observed from the peritoneal side, the ulcer always has a blue-black or dark red, mottled, discolored margin. This is important, in view of the fact that perforations are sometimes reported which are the result of postmortem rough handling of the intestinal coils on the part of the prosector. There is very little reaction by the peritoneum and omentum after perforation does occur. The slight exudate is thin, grayish and watery. There is no well-marked plastic exudate firmly gluing the coils of the intestine together, but only the appearance of a few fibrin flakes in the exudate. It is important to remember that although perforation usually occurs in the last twelve

40101

inches of the ileum it may appear higher, and that it may be in the appendix or large bowel and is not infrequently multiple in any location.

Hemorrhage.—After death from hemorrhage a large amount of unclotted blood may be found in the bowel. The bleeding vessel cannot be found. Sometimes clots may be detached from the base of one or several ulcers. A hemorrhagic form of typhoid is sometimes recognized in which multiple hemorrhages in the skin and mucous membranes occur.

LYMPHATIC SYSTEM.—The swelling of the mesenteric lymph nodes is probably the earliest lesion of typhoid fever. Usually the nodes draining the last few inches of the ileum are most involved; they may become very large, representing in the aggregate a mass as large as an orange. In the gross they are gray, pale pink or slate colored. On section they are moist and softened, showing small areas of liquefaction necrosis. They may break down entirely and rupture into the abdominal cavity, giving rise to the indolent low-grade peritonitis characteristic of typhoid perforation. The lymph nodes in other portions of the body usually present no appreciable gross swelling. Microscopically the lesion in the mesenteric nodes is identical with that in the lymphoid tissue of the intestine. The lymphoid structure and surrounding tissue becomes packed with mononuclear macrophages and small areas of liquefaction necrosis occur from vascular occlusion. The other lymph nodes of the body show a moderate sinus catarrh. The number of macrophages escaping from the intestinal lymphatic apparatus into the thoracic duct and thus into the venous circulation may be so great as to cause small pulmonary emboli, as in the case reported by MacCallum. Hemorrhages into the substance of the lymph nodes are common.

SPLEEN.—Acute splenic tumor in typhoid is quite constant. The organ weighs from 600 to 900 grams (20 to 30 oz.) and is so extremely soft that it seems to flow and flatten out on the table when removed at autopsy. On section the pulp oozes and flows out of the capsule in the form of a thick, reddish-brown paste, and the malpighian corpuscles are scarcely recognizable. Microscopically we find the characteristic macrophages and a pathology similar to that in the lymph nodes and intestine, with the addition that the organ is extremely engorged with red blood cells. A very large proportion of the macrophages are engorged with red cells and with crystals and amorphous masses of blood pigment. The spleen may rupture, resulting in a fatal hemorrhage. Focal necroses occur within the spleen as in the lymph nodes, and large necroses beneath the capsule (infarcts) are not uncommon. Cases autopsied late in the disease, after a long illness, may show no enlargement of the spleen. The organisms tend to disappear from the spleen as the agglutinins rise in the blood, and the spleen tends to decrease in size as the disease progresses to a favorable conclusion. It is said that there is a relation between the persistence of the splenic tumor and relapse.

BLOOD AND BONE MARROW.—The most distinctive finding in the blood is the leukopenia. The white count after the first few days, during which there may be a mild leukocytosis, seldom above 12,000, shows a decrease to 4,000 or even less. This decrease is due to a falling off of the polymorphonuclears and to the practical disappearance of the eosinophils. There is a relative increase in the lymphocytes, and especially in the large mononuclear cells. Late in the course there is usually a severe anemia. A hemorrhagic diathesis may develop, and a decrease in the number of platelets is said to occur. Typhoid bacilli are more or less constantly present throughout the course of typhoid fever. They are present in greater numbers during the first week, and their cultivation from the blood serves as the best method now known for early diagnosis. The bone marrow has been shown by Longcope to undergo characteristic changes in typhoid. In general these are analogous to those in the lymph nodes and in the spleen, with the addition that the specific marrow elements are affected. There is marked invasion of the sinuses, with the characteristic macrophages. These are found to be actively phagocytosing red cells and tissue detritus. Many focal necroses occur, containing dead cells and fibrin. According to Mallory, these focal necroses represent the end-result of the characteristic typhoid reaction, a so-called "typhoid nodule" consisting of aggregations of endothelial leukocytes (macrophages). The lymphocytes are apparently increased in number and the myelocytes are distinctly reduced. The reduction in these elements explains, of course, the decrease in number of the neutrophil and eosinophil polymorphonuclears in the circulating blood. This depression of bone marrow function is such that the intercurrent peritonitis which develops after perforation usually fails to bring out a leukocytosis, and other intercurrent infections like pneumonia may fail to raise the white count above seven or eight thousand. The aneosinophilia may be diagnostic value, as was pointed out by Thayer. As recovery is established, the leukocyte count and number of eosinophils return to normal.

GALLBLADDER.—The bacteria reach the gallbladder very early in typhoid fever, and remain for an indefinitely long period. Gay and Claypole, confirming work done by Chirolanza, showed that typhoid bacilli might be isolated from the gallbladder within half an hour after intravenous injection of typhoid bacilli, even when the cystic duct was tied. The gross pathology caused by the presence of typhoid bacilli in the gallbladder is usually not great during the course of the disease. The importance of the gallbladder in this fever is rather in relation to the carrier condition and to later attacks of cholecystitis with gallstones. There is usually a mild degree of catarrhal inflammation throughout the biliary system during the course of the disease. This may be so severe as to cause the disease picture to be ushered in by gallbladder pain and jaundice, with a chill. But usually the gallbladder inflammation leads to nothing more distinctive than occasional pains in the right upper abdomen, which tend to abate as the disease progresses. Purulent cholecystitis with leukocytosis may occur. Typhoid fever must be admitted to the first rank of those diseases which have a definite etiologic relationship to gallstones.

The liver presents characteristic changes. It is usually enlarged, swollen and cloudy on section. Microscopically the characteristic "typhoid nodules" are found, which have been differently designated as "lymphomata" and as "focal necroses." It is easy to convince oneself that both of these latter appellations apply to different stages of the same lesion.

One observes many small miliary collections of cells somewhat resembling miliary tubercles, which are found to consist of large numbers of the characteristic macrophages or endothelial leukocytes crowding the sinuses between the cell cords. These macrophages are filled with phagocytosed red cells and cell detritus, or are free of other material and actively dividing. They enclose and push aside cords of liver cells and finally become so dense that they break down themselves and are replaced by tissue detritus and fibrin. The question as to whether these areas represent mechanical plugs of macrophages swept in by the portal circulation, or whether clumps of bacteria or their poisons attract them, is not clearly settled. The authors believe that they represent local reactions to the actual presence of bacilli, as in the case of the miliary tubercle. The difficulty in demonstrating bacilli in such lesions in tissue sections is well known. Besides these nodules we find the individual liver cells to be swollen and edematous, with granular, vacuolated and fat-containing protoplasm and pale-staining nuclei. Around the portal vein in the lymphatics and diffusely throughout the connective tissue of Glisson's island, we find wandering macrophages.

HEART AND BLOOD VESSELS.—There are no specific changes in the heart. The heart failure occasionally assigned as a cause of death is to be referred to degeneration of the myocardium. Endocarditis is rare, though vegetative lesions containing typhoid bacilli have been found. Pericarditis is also rare, and when found is usually part of a complicating intercurrent infection like pneumonia or pleuritis. The myocardium presents no characteristic changes, although a great variety of lesions have been described in individual cases. The heart muscle is usually soft, flabby, and dark brown in color, and somewhat mottled, due to fatty changes. Microscopically, we find marked brown atrophy evidenced by collections of brown pigment at the extremities of the muscle nuclei, more or less accumulation of fine, fat droplets within the muscle cell, albuminous granules and increase of fluid. Frequently none of these changes can be demonstrated. Interstitial myocarditis, with marked infiltration with round cells and multiple miliary abscesses, has been found.

The blood vessels are not infrequently attacked, probably because of the general tendency of the typhoid infection to affect endothelial cells and tissues. Thayer has described early arteriosclerosis as an important concomitant of typhoid fever, but this is probably as common in other severe infections as in typhoid. The growing conviction that arteriosclerosis is in large part a result of repeated infections of various types might be pointed out in this connection. Active arteritis with autochthonous thrombus formation, especially of the smaller vessels, is an occasional accident. Most frequently these occur in the extremities, ear and parotid gland. Thrombosis is more frequent in the veins, especially in the left femoral, leading to phlegmasia alba dolens. Naturally the prognosis is much better in the cases of venous thrombosis than in those of arterial occlusion.

RESPIRATORY SYSTEM.—Ulcers of the larynx occur not uncommonly in the later stages of the disease. They are found at the base of the epiglottis, in the posterior portion of the vocal cords, and in the aryepiglottidean folds. The cartilage may be involved. It is not clear that they represent specific lesions as in the case of the ulcers of the intestine. Diphtheritic laryngitis and tracheitis are rare findings.

The lungs present several types of lesion. There is a form of lobar pneumonia which occurs in cases with pneumonic onset and the physical signs of pneumonia, which probably represents an early localization of the typhoid bacillus in the lung, the so-called "pneumotyphoid." Later in the disease, lobar pneumonia may also develop, either from the typhoid bacillus, which is rare, or due to secondary invasion by the pneumococcus. The cases due to the pneumococcus are said to show a characteristic hemorrhagic type of lesion. This is an interesting observation in view of the fact that a hemolysin has been isolated from the typhoid bacillus; but hemolysis does not play an important role in ordinary typhoid fever.

Lobular pneumonia due to terminal mixed infection is a common event.

NERVOUS SYSTEM.—All writers especially remark the fact that although this disease gets its name from a nervous system manifestation, the changes in the nervous system are not anatomically recognizable. Degenerations of the peripheral nerves have been described, but are clinically and anatomically unimportant. Occasional perivascular round-cell infiltration of the cerebral vessels is noted, but this finding always raises the question of another etiology. Typhoid meningitis is occasionally met with. It may be either serous and associated with round-cell infiltration of the meninges, or typically purulent, with a spinal fluid resembling that of the epidemic form. The typhoid bacillus should be isolated from the exudate before a diagnosis of typhoid meningitis is made. Eleven cases of "clinically diagnosed" typhoid meningitis which Dr. P. F. Morse autopsied proved to be tuberculous. The exudate in purulent typhoid meningitis is not distinctive but contains a large proportion of mononuclear wandering cells.

GENITO-URINARY SYSTEM.—The kidneys show the usual parenchymatous degeneration of acute infection. Typhoid nodules like those in the liver are said to occur occasionally. Acute hemorrhagic glomerular nephritis is a rare complication. Miliary abscesses have been described. The pelvis and ureter are usually normal, although they may show petechial hemorrhage. Colon bacillus pyelitis sometimes occurs. The bladder is rarely affected, although typhoid bacilli occasionally multiply in it and are eliminated in enormous numbers. The cases showing bacilli in the urine usually have a trace of albumin. The prostate is not known to be primarily affected by the typhoid bacillus, although abscess or fibrous atrophy of the testis or typhoid epididymitis occasionally occurs.

The typhoid bacillus has been cultivated from the uterus when typhoid occurred during pregnancy. The child dies in utero or soon after birth, from typhoid bacteremia. The placenta offers no barrier to the passage of the bacilli. It has not been proved that recognizable lesions of the placenta are present in cases of placental transmission. Mastitis is a rare complication.

OSSEOUS SYSTEM.—Bone complications are not very uncommon. They sometimes occur during the febrile attack, but most frequently they are found months or years after the typhoid attack. A thickened, elevated periosteum is found, raised from the bone cortex by a thin, stringy pus which extends down into the bone substance. Sequestra may be present. Typhoid bacilli can be cultivated from the pus. The lesions are very refractory to treatment and recur easily. It is said that an acute mixed infection, especially with Bacillus pyocyaneus, occurring accidentally, has been known to effect a cure.

40101

Typhoid spine, with the x-ray evidence of spondylitis and perispon-dylitis, is not uncommon. The joints are rarely involved, but the arthri-tis, when present, may be mono-articular or polyarticular.

HISTORICAL SUMMARY

The history of typhoid fever may be divided into three periods.

The *first period* extends from the early history of medicine to the time of the final identification, upon clinical and pathologic grounds, of typhoid fever as a disease entity, distinct from typhus and the other continued fevers.

The *second period* includes the few years between the recognition of the disease as a distinct clinical entity and the discovery of the typhoid bacillus.

The *third period* extends from the discovery of the specific organ-ism of the disease to the present time.

Each period is marked by distinctive developments in our knowledge of the disease.

Hippocrates, during two successive autumns, met many cases of con-tinued fever having the clinical features of typhoid fever. Galen cer-tainly saw the disease which he described under the name *hemitritæus*.

From the early part of the seventeenth century, when Spigelius spoke of the disease as common in Italy, typhoid fever has been described by a great number of writers under a variety of names, suggested by dis-tinctive clinical features or the author's conception of the nature of the disease.

Bretonneau in 1826 first showed the constancy of the intestinal lesions of the disease, which he considered a type of inflammation of the bowels, and named it *dothienenteritis*. He also was one of the first to suggest that the disease was due to a poison and was communicable. Louis in 1829 published his elaborate work and first named the disease *typhoid fever*. This name was adopted by Chomel in his "Clinical Lectures," 1834, and since then it has been in general use, except in England, where *enteric fever* is the accepted name.

By this time—the beginning of the nineteenth century—the clinical history and gross morbid anatomy of typhoid fever had been well studied and a clear picture of the disease developed. The French observers, however, still held to the view that typhus and typhoid fevers were identical, and this confusion was general throughout other countries.

Thomas Willis, of England, in 1659 first attempted to differentiate typhoid from typhus fever. Gilchrist in 1734, Laugrish in 1735, and Huxham in 1739, added to the distinctive features of the two diseases. In England and elsewhere typhoid fever continued, however, to be con-sidered a modified form of typhus until William Gerhard, of Philadel-phia, in 1837 finally established the differential clinical and postmortem criteria of the two diseases. Gerhard states that, up to the time of his writing, no one had clearly stated that the two diseases were always distinct, until the publication of a note in the *Dublin Journal*, in Sep-tember, 1836, by Lombard, of Geneva, after his study of the fevers of Great Britain. Gerhard's views were, however, opposed by both French and English physicians. Shattuck, of Boston (1839), who studied ty-phoid and typhus fevers in England and France, upheld Gerhard's doc-trine and was supported by Valleix and Rochoux in France and Barlow in England. Murchison and other English physicians remained unconvinced until Sir W. Jenner in 1849 confirmed and amplified the distinctions laid down by Gerhard. Since that time, the view that typhoid fever is a disease distinct from typhus fever has not been seriously questioned.

The outstanding addition to our knowledge of typhoid fever in the *second period* of its history was the remarkable demonstration by William Budd, of England, in 1856, of the communicability of typhoid fever through the excreta of the patient and the routes of conveyance of the infection. From the early part of the last century the doctrine of the contagiousness of typhoid fever had been held by a few able observers. Nathan Smith, of New England (1824), from his unique experience with typhoid fever among isolated communities, considered the contagiousness of typhoid so evident that it scarcely needed demonstration. Bretonneau a little later (1829) demonstrated that the disease was transmitted from one person to another. Chomel was inclined to the contagion theory but remarked that in France not one physician in a hundred regarded typhoid fever as contagious. Louis adopted the contagion theory in the second edition of his work (1841). Murchison adhered to the theory of the spontaneous origin of the infection.

Budd demonstrated by careful epidemiologic studies (1) that the infection is contained in the intestinal discharges of the patients; (2) that the disease is transmitted from the sick to the well through the medium of the stools; (3) that the infection is conveyed to healthy persons by water, milk, etc., contaminated by the dejecta of typhoid patients; and (4) that the infection may be thrown off by convalescents for an indefinite time after clinical recovery from the disease. Budd also laid down rules for the prevention and arrest of epidemics. It is interesting to note that the observations of Budd, like those of Nathan Smith, were made in rural districts where contagion can be more readily traced than in cities.

The *third period* of the history of typhoid fever begins with the discovery of the specific organism of the disease in 1880, by Eberth. Gay gives equal credit to Klebs and Koch who independently demonstrated the organism in typhoid-infected tissues at about the same time.

The specific bacillus was found in the stools of typhoid patients by Pfeiffer in 1885, and in the urine by Hueppe in 1886. In 1887 Vilchur isolated the bacillus from the circulating blood, laying the foundation for the conclusion that typhoid fever is primarily a bacteremia and that the intestinal lesions are usual but incidental local manifestations of the infection.

In 1894 Chiari showed that the gallbladder quite regularly harbored the bacilli during and following the disease—a fact of great importance in the understanding of relapse and the carrier state. The agglutination method of differential diagnosis was introduced by Widal in 1896. The laboratory methods for the positive diagnosis of typhoid fever were then complete.

The knowledge of the bacteriology of typhoid fever enabled the methods of infection and routes of conveyance of the organism to be studied with accuracy. The dissemination of the disease by contaminated water and food, by flies and other fomites and by human carriers, could now be positively demonstrated.

40101

In 1893 Frankel suggested the specific treatment of typhoid fever by the subcutaneous injection of killed cultures of the typhoid bacillus. Antityphoid vaccination—the crowning event in the history of typhoid fever—was introduced by Wright and by Pfeiffer and Kolle in 1896. The possibilities of prophylactic vaccination against typhoid fever have been shown by the experience of the vast armies engaged in the first World War. Could preventive vaccination be made universal throughout the world the history of typhoid fever would be ended.

BIBLIOGRAPHY

Achard, C. and Bloch, S.: Typhoid vaccination by mouth, Bull. Acad. de méd., 91: 531, 1924.

Almon, L., Read, J. and Stovall, W. D.: Study of Vi antigenic fraction of typhoid bacilli isolated from carriers and cases, and antibody content of the serum of these patients, Am. J. Pub. Health, 27: 357, 1937.

Anderson, G. W., Hamblen, A. D. and Smith, H. M.: Typhoid carriers. Study of their disease producing potentialities over series of years as indicated by a study of cases, Am. J. Pub. Health, 26: 396, 1936.

Barker, L. F.: On nature and treatment of typhoid and paratyphoid bacilluria and cystopyelitis, J. Urol., 23: 387, 1930.

Besredka, A.: Local Immunization, Baltimore, Williams and Wilkins Co., 1927.

Bhatnagar, S. S.: Vi agglutination in diagnosis of typhoid fever and typhoid carrier condition, Brit. M. J., 2: 1195, 1938.

——, Speechly, C. G. J. and Snigh, M.: A Vi variant of Salmonella typhi and its application to the serology of typhoid fever, J. Hyg., 38: 663, 1938.

Billet: Quoted by L. C. Havens.

Boivin, A. and Mesrobeanu, L.: Les antigènes somatiques et flagellaires des bacteries, Ann. Inst. Pasteur, 61: 426, 1938.

Boothby, W. M.: Oxygen administration: the value of high concentration of oxygen for therapy, Proc. Staff Meet., Mayo Clin., 13: 641, 1938.

Bowdoin, C. D.: The efficacy of immunization in an acute water-borne outbreak of typhoid fever. To be published.

Bower, A. G.: Modern treatment of typhoid fever, Mil. Surgeon, 83: 70, 1938.

Brotherhood, J. S.: Treatment of typhoid fever by sulfanilamide. Personal communication.

Browning, C. H., Coulthard, H. L., Cruickshank, R., Guthrie, K. J. and Smith, R. P: Chronic enteric carriers and their treatment, Med. Res. Counc., Spec. Rep. Ser., No. 179, H. M. S., London, 1933.

Burgess, A. M.: Clinical experience with 95 to 98 per cent oxygen in the treatment of abdominal distention and other conditions, New England J. Med., 221: 299, 1939.

Buttle, G. A. H., Parish, H. J., McLeod, M. and Stephenson, D.: Chemotherapy of typhoid and some other non-streptococcal infections in mice, Lancet, 2: 681, 1937.

Cadham, F.: Septicemia: method of treatment: report of 100 cases, Am. J. M. Sc., 188: 543, 1934.

Castellani, A.: Medical aspects of Italo-Ethiopian War, Mil. Surgeon, 81: 1, 1937.

Coburn, H. C., Jr., Ostrander, F. R. and Gillespie, J. O.: Typhoid fever in vaccinated, Mil. Surgeon, 76: 133, 1935.

Coller, F. A. and Forsbeck, F. C.: The surgical treatment of chronic biliary typhoid carriers, Ann. Surg., 105: 791, 1937.

Coxon, R. V. and Forbes, J. R.: Agranulocytic angina following administration of M. & B. 693, Lancet, 2: 1412, 1938.

Crimm, P. D. and Short, D. M.: Study of oral typhoid vaccination as measured by blood serum agglutinins, Am. J. M. Sc., 196: 826, 1938.

Dennemark: Quoted by L. C. Havens.

Dennis, E. W. and Berberian, D. A.: Study of production of somatic and flagellar agglutinins in response to anti-typhoid-paratyphoid inoculation, Am. J. Hyg., 20: 469, 1934.

Diefenbach, W. E. and Yuskis, A. S.: Typhoid septicaemia treated with sulfanilamide, California & West. Med., 49: 146, 1938.

Downs, C. M. and Bond, G. C.: Occurrence of O and H agglutinins following subcutaneous and oral administration of typhoid vaccine, Am. J. Pub. Health, 27: 889, 1937.

Editorial: Oral administration of typhoid vaccine, J. Am. M. Ass., 92: 1185, 1929.

——: Vaccination against enteric fever, Brit. M. J., 1: 758, 1937.

Elsom, K. O., Miller, S. G., Forrester, J. S. and Chamberlin, G. W.: Radiation and cholecystectomy as therapeutic procedures for typhoid carriers, Am. J. M. Sc., 194: 466, 1937.

Feemster, R. F. and Anderson, G. W.: Paratyphoid fever in Massachusetts, Am. J. Pub. Health, 29: 881, 1939.

Felix, A.: The qualitative serum diagnosis of enteric fevers, Lancet, 1: 505, 1930.

——: Clinical trials with a new antityphoid serum, Lancet, 1: 799, 1935.

——: Detection of chronic typhoid carriers by agglutination tests, Lancet, 2: 738, 1938.

——: The titration of therapeutic antityphoid serum, J. Hyg., 68: 750, 1938.

—— and Bhatnagar, S. S.: Further observations on the properties of the Vi antigen of B. typhosus and its corresponding antibody, Brit. J. Exper. Path., 16: 422, 1935.

—— and Petrie, G. F.: Preparation of antityphoid serum in horse for therapeutic use in man, J. Hyg., 38: 673, 1938.

—— and Pitt, R. M.: Virulence of B. typhosus and resistance to O antibody, J. Path. & Bact., 38: 409, 1934.

—— and ——: New antigen of B. typhosus; its relation to virulence and to active and passive immunization, Lancet, 2: 186, 1934.

Fenton, J. and Hay, C. P.: Prophylactic use of antityphoid serum in localized outbreak, Brit. M. J., 1: 1090, 1938.

Forsbeck, F. C.: Typhoid Fever Eradication, Lansing, Michigan Department of Health, 1936.

—— and Hollon, H. C.: Standards for determining suitability of bile specimens for detection or release of typhoid carriers, Am. J. Pub. Health, 27: 253, 1937.

Galloway, D. V.: Inoculation and sanitation in control of typhoid fever, New Orleans M. & S. J., 88 : 278, 1935.

Gay, F. P.: Agents of Disease and Host Resistance, Baltimore, Charles C. Thomas, 1935.

Geiger, J. C., Crowley, A. B. and Arnold, C. E.: San Francisco's hotels are examined for cross-connections, Am. J. Pub. Health, 29 : 927, 1939.

Goodpasture, E. W.: Concerning pathogenesis of typhoid fever, Am. J. Path., 13 : 175, 1937.

Gory, M. and Grasset, E.: Sérothérapie antityphoïdique. Méthode de dosage et étude experimentale, Compt. rend. Soc. de biol., 98 : 435, 1928.

Grasset, E.: Concentrated antityphoid serum as specific in treatment of typhoid fevers, J. M. A. South Africa, 4 : 380, 1930.

———: Relations between the toxicity and the antigenic and flocculating power of the endotoxin and endo-anatoxin of the typhoid bacillus, Compt. rend. Soc. de biol., 115 : 1485, 1934.

———: Typhoid endotoxoid vaccine. A review of the results of preventive inoculation in an inoculated population of 400,-000, Brit. M. J., 2 : 58, 1938.

——— and Gory, M.: Vaccination, hyperimmunization et sérothérapie antityphoïdique experimentale. Au moyen des autolysats formales, Compt. rend. Soc. de biol., 97 : 1211, 1927.

———and Lewin, W.: Preparation and comparison of different types of antityphoid sera. Agglutinins—mouse protection and preliminary clinical trials, Brit. J. Exper. Path., 18 : 460, 1937.

Grinnell, F. B.: Study of comparative value of rough and smooth strains of B. typhosus in preparation of typhoid vaccines, J. Immunol., 19 : 457, 1930.

———: Studies on relationship of certain variants of B. typhosus; agglutination and agglutinin absorption, J. Exper. Med., 54 : 577, 1931.

———: Study of dissociation of Rawlins strain of B. typhosum with special reference to its use in production of antityphoid vaccine, J. Exper. Med., 56 : 907, 1932.

Groninger: Bakteriologisches Sektionsergebnis bei zwei chronischen Typhusbacillenträgern, Ztschr. f. Hyg. u. Infektionskr., 107 : 157, 1927.

Gruber, M. and Durham, H. E.: Eine neue Methode zur raschen Erkennung des Choleravibrio und des Typhusbacillus, München. med. Wchnschr., 43 : 285, 1896.

Hac, L. R., Flynn, C. S. and Perry, C. A.: Evaluation of H and O antigens in agglutination tests for typhoid fever, J. Lab. & Clin. Med., 24 : 567, 1939.

Hammer, A. W.: The biliary tract and typhoid infection, Internat. Clin., 3 : 239, 1922.

Hanssen, E. C.: Infection of the Biliary Tract in Typhoid Carriers. "Diagnosis and Management of Diseases of the Biliary Tract," By Carter, R. F., Greene, C. H. and Twiss, J. R., Phila., Lea & Febiger, 1939.

Harkleroad, F. S.: Sulfanilamide in treatment of typhoid fever, West Virginia M. J., 34 : 549, 1938.

Harries, E. H. R., Swyer, R. and Thompson, M.: Sulphanilamide in typhoid fever, Lancet, 1 : 1321, 1939.

Hartzell, J. B.: Personal communication.

Havens, L. C.: The Bacteriology of Typhoid, Salmonella and Dysentery Infections and Carrier States, New York, The Commonwealth Fund, 1935.

Hawley, P. R. and Simmons, J. S.: The effectiveness of vaccines used for the prevention of typhoid fever in the United States Army and Navy, Am. J. Pub. Health, 24 : 689, 1934.

Hegstenberg, H. H.: On the serological response following use of oral typhoid vaccine, J. Med., 19 : 131, 1938.

Henderson, D. W. and Morgan, W. T. G.: Isolation of antigenic substances from strains of Bact. typhosum, Brit. J. Exper. Path., 19 : 82, 1938.

Hoffstadt, R. E. and Thompson, R. L.: Immunological studies of typhoid vaccination by mouth; agglutinins formed in persons treated orally with triple typhoid bacterin, Am. J. Hyg., 9 : 1, 1929.

Holt, R. L. and Hitchens, A. P.: Typhoid vaccine: the technique of its preparation at the Army Medical School, Pub. Health Rep., 52 : 829, 1937.

Horwood, M. P.: The Sanitation of Water Supplies, Baltimore, Charles C. Thomas, 1932.

Huddleson, I. F.: Brucellosis in Man and Animals, New York, The Commonwealth Fund, 1939.

Huggins, C. B. and Roome, N. W.: Typhoid pyonephrosis; its urological and public health significance, J. Urol., 31 : 587, 1934.

Kahle, P. J. and Beacham, H. T.: Typhoid pyonephrosis, with report of case, J. Urol., 30 : 299, 1933.

Kauffmann, F.: Latest results of typhoid serology; their bearing upon the production and testing of typhoid vaccines and therapeutic sera as well as upon typhoid diagnosis, Quart. Bull. Health Organ., League of Nations, 4 : 482, 1935.

———: Studies of the body antigens in the Salmonella group, Ztschr. f. Hyg. u. Infektionskr., 117 : 778, 1936.

Klee, P. and Römer, H.: Prontosil bei Streptokokkenerkrankungen, Deutsche med. Wchnschr., 61 : 253, 1935.

Klinger: Quoted by L. C. Havens.

Kolmer, J. A. and Rule, A. M.: Sulfanilamide and sulfapyridine in the treatment of experimental B. typhosus (Eberthella typhosa) infections of mice, Proc. Soc. Exper. Biol. & Med., 40 : 615, 1939.

Kracke, R. R.: A Text Book of Clinical Pathology, Baltimore, William Wood & Company, 1938.

Kulesza, G.: Treatment of typhoid fever with prontosil, Medycyna, p. 570, August 21, 1937.

Lacy, G. R. and Cohen, M.: Comparison of agglutination tests in individuals treated with typhoid vaccine by subcutaneous and oral methods, Pennsylvania M. J., 40 : 267, 1937.

Lantin, P. T. and Guerrero, F. S.: Blood transfusion in typhoid fever, Am. J. M. Sc., 191 : 850, 1936.

Lewin, W.: Typhoid fever on the Witivatersrand, South African Institute for Medical Research, Johannesburg, 7 : 413, 1938.

Long, P. H. and Bliss, E. A.: Clinical Use of Sulfanilamide and Sulfapyridine and Allied Compounds, New York, Macmillan Company, 1939.

McCollum, E. V., Orent-Keiles, E. and Day, H. G.: The Newer Knowledge of Nutrition, New York, Macmillan Company, 1939.

McSweeney, C. J.: Clinical trials with new antityphoid serum, Lancet, 1 : 1095, 1935.

Malbin, B.: Typhoid fever occurring in immunized persons, J. Am. M. Ass., 115 : 33, 1940.

Myers, G. B.: Sulfanilamide, J. Michigan M. Soc., 38 : 302, 1939.

Perry, R. M.: Comparison of typhoid "O" and "H" agglutinin responses following intracutaneous and subcutaneous inoculation of typhoid, paratyphoid A and B vaccine, Am. J. Hyg., 26 : 388, 1937.

Pijper, A. and Dau, H.: Typhoid agglutination after oral immunization, Brit. J. Exper. Path., 11 : 112, 1930.

Queries and Minor Notes: Oral immunization for typhoid, J. Am. M. Ass., 111 : 1124, 1938.

Rake, G.: Enhancement of pathogenicity of human typhoid organisms by mucin, Proc. Soc. Exper. Biol. & Med., 32 : 1523, 1935.

Sacquépée, E.: Les porteurs de germes (bacilles typhiques et paratyphiques), Bull. Inst. Pasteur, 8 : 49, 1910.

Schottmüller, H.: Die typhosen Erkrankungen, Hab. d. inn. med. Moln und Staehelm. 2 Aufl. Berlin, 1 : Th. 2, 992, 1925.

Senftner, H. F. and Coughlin, F. E.: Typhoid carriers in New York State with special reference to gallbladder operations, Am. J. Hyg., 17 : 711, 1933.

Shattuck, G. C.: Relation of beriberi to polyneuritis from other causes, Am. J. Trop. Med., 8 : 539, 1928.

Shwartzman, G., Baehr, G. and Hollingsworth, W. Y.: Treatment of typhoid with an antitoxic antityphoid serum, Arch. Int. Med., 58 : 799, 1936.

Siler, J. F.: Protective antibodies in the blood serum of individuals after immunization with typhoid vaccine, Am. J. Pub. Health, 27 : 142, 1937.

—— and Dunham, G. C.: Duration of immunity conferred by typhoid vaccine; results of revaccination by intracutaneous injection of typhoid vaccine, Am. J. Pub. Health, 29 : 95, 1939.

—— and others: Protective antibodies in the blood serum of individuals after immunization with typhoid vaccine, Mil. Surgeon, 80 : 91, 1937.

——and Lambie, J. S.: Typhoid and the Paratyphoid Fevers. Communicable and Other Diseases, Vol. 9, p. 15, The Medical Department of the United States Army in the World War, War Department, 1928.

—— and The Laboratory Staff of the Army Medical School: Typhoid vaccine studies; investigation of virulence and antigenic properties of selected strains of typhoid organism, Am. J. Pub. Health, 26 : 219, 1936.

Stebbins, E. L. and Reed, E.: Carrier-borne typhoid fever in New York State, with special reference to attack rates among household contacts, Am. J. Pub. Health, 27 : 233, 1937.

Sturgis, C. C.: Treatment of typhoid fever by sulfapyridine. Personal communication.

Topley, W. W. C. and others: The immunizing potency of antigenic components isolated from different strains of Bact. typhosum, Lancet, 2 : 252, 1937.

——and Wilson, G. S.: The Principles of Bacteriology and Immunity, Baltimore, William Wood and Company, 1938.

Tuft, L.: Active immunization against typhoid fever, with particular reference to intradermal method, J. Lab. & Clin. Med., 16 : 552, 1931.

——, Yagle, E. M. and Rogers, S.: Comparative study of antibody response after various methods of administration of mixed typhoid vaccine, with particular reference to intradermal and oral methods, J. Infect. Dis., 50 : 98, 1932.

Twenty-sixth Annual Report: Typhoid in the large cities of the United States in 1937, J. Am. M. Ass., 111 : 414, 1938.

Valentine, E., Park, Falk, and McGuire: A study of agglutinin response to typhoid vaccine, Am. J. Hyg., 22 : 44, 1935.

Wakeman, F. B.: A specific polysaccharide as the essential immunizing antigen of the typhoid bacillus, Mil. Surgeon, 84 : 318, 452, 1939.

Webb, C. H.: Diagnosis of typhoid fever in infancy and childhood. Study of 75 cases, New Orleans M. & S. J., 87 : 362, 1934.

Weil, A. J., Gall, L. S. and Weider, S.: Progress in the study of the typhoid bacillus, Arch. Path., 28 : 71, 1939.

Weiss, S. and Wilkins, R. W.: The nature of the cardiovascular disturbances in nutritional deficiency states (beriberi), Ann. Int. Med., 11 : 104, 1937.

Welch, H. and Mickle, F. L.: Vi antigen in carrier strains of Eberthella typhosa, Am. J. Pub. Health, 27 : 351, 1937.

Whipple, A. O.: The surgical treatment of bile typhoid carriers, Ann. Surg., 90 : 631, 1929.

There is an intentional break in the continuity of these page numbers. This space will be utilized by future revisions of the text in this volume.

CHAPTER XXXVIII

THE PARATYPHOID INFECTIONS

By C. G. Jennings, M.D.

Definition.—The paratyphoid infections are acute febrile diseases
caused by the invasion of the blood stream by members of the paratyphoid
group of microörganisms, and manifested clinically by either (1) a continued fever closely resembling typhoid fever, or (2) a gastro-enteritis,
frequently of choleraic type.

In this article consideration is given only to the infections produced
by two members of the group: the *Bacillus paratyphosus A* and the
Bacillus paratyphosus B. These two organisms produce the great majority of human paratyphoid bacteriemias.

Etiology.—Predisposing Causes.—In general, the influence of predisposing causes upon the developments of typhoid fever and the paratyphoid infections is the same.

There is one distinction of importance. The *Bacillus paratyphosus B*
causes disease in some domestic animals as well as in man, and is present also in the intestines of certain normal animals. It may live and
multiply in infected meat. From infected meat it may be transmitted
to various other foods. The dietetic habits of a people may thus predispose to paratyphoid B infections. Persons who eat largely of beef,
veal and pork, prepared without adequate cooking, may be infected.
The consumption of sausage, minced and preserved meats predisposes
to infection. In Germany, where foods of this character are largely consumed, infections by the *Bacillus paratyphosus B* have been markedly
prevalent.

Methods of sewage disposal which render possible the contamination

629

of the water supplies of communities or households predispose to the prevalence of paratyphoid fever as they do to typhoid. Both of the paratyphoid infections may be water-borne. Paratyphoid fever A, more closely related to typhoid fever than paratyphoid fever B, is water-borne with the same relative frequency as typhoid fever. An impure water supply is of the same importance as a predisposing factor of paratyphoid fever A as it is of typhoid fever. Water courses or wells, free from the possibility of pollution by human excreta, many be contaminated by animal carriers of the *Bacillus paratyphosus B*. Ingestion of such waters predisposes to infection by this organism.

EXCITING CAUSE: BACTERIOLOGY OF THE ORGANISMS.—The paratyphoid group of microörganisms, in their bacterial reactions and pathogenic properties, lies intermediate between the *Bacillus coli* and the *Bacillus typhosus*.

(*a*) *Morphology: General Characteristics.*—The morphology, general characteristics and group relations of the paratyphoid organisms are considered in the section on the Bacteriology of Typhoid Fever (p. 457).

(*b*) *Distribution inside the Body.*—In their distribution in the body the paratyphoid organisms show the same tendency to localization as the *Bacillus typhosus*. Both para-organisms are uniformly present in the blood stream, but apparently their stay in shorter and blood culture is more uncertain than in typhoid fever.

The organisms exist in great abundance in the intestinal tract and they are readily recovered from the stools very early in the course of the disease. The gall-bladder is always invaded, and their persistence in this viscus is the usual cause of the prolongation of the carrier state. From the relative frequency of jaundice in paratyphoid fever it would appear that the bile ducts are more frequently invaded than in typhoid fever. The bacilli are excreted by the kidneys and in many cases—although not so frequently as in typhoid fever—they may be recovered from the urine. In the outbreaks in the armies in France the cerebral membranes were not infrequently the seat of localization. Localized pus formations occur in about the same relative frequency as in typhoid fever.

(*c*) *Distribution outside the Body.*—With the notable exception that the flesh and intestinal tract of some of the domestic animals frequently harbor the *Bacillus paratyphosus B*, the distribution outside the body of the paratyphoid organisms is the same as that of the bacillus of typhoid fever.

(*d*) *Modes of Conveyance.*—Water and contact, as in typhoid fever, are the most important methods of conveying the infection of paratyphoid A; food is of secondary importance. In sharp contrast, food is the most important medium of conveyance of the infection of paratyphoid B; water and contact are of secondary importance.

Infections by the *Bacillus paratyphosus B* are commonly transmitted by meat foods. The bacilli may be present in the meat of diseased animals, in healthy meat contaminated by contact with diseased meat, or in the intestinal contents of healthy animals or human carriers. Vegetable food of various kinds may be contaminated and become the medium for the transmission of the disease.

Carriers.—From our present knowledge, paratyphoid carriers appear to exist in about the same relative proportion as typhoid carriers. Because of the transmission of the disease by food infection the carrier state is a highly important factor in the etiology of the disease.

Hilgerman estimates that 3.6 per cent. of paratyphoid cases become carriers. Among 157 convalescents from paratyphoid fever in India, 10 were found to be carriers; 9 were acute carriers and recovered before the end of three months; the remaining case recovered in five months.

Krumwiede in 1916 found 4 per cent. of healthy carriers among 786 men of the 14th Infantry, New York State Guard, recently returned from the Mexican border. All these men were exposed to the infection that precipitated an outbreak in which 211 of the 1,000 men of the command had paratyphoid fever. This probably represents an abnormally high percentage of carriers among healthy persons. Berry states that in these groups of men the carrier state did not tend to persist. Under the influence of a more healthy environment many cases spontaneously recovered in a few weeks.

A large majority of paratyphoid carriers are fecal carriers. Urinary carriers are exceptional, and pus carriers rare. As with typhoid carriers, the bacilli live and multiply in the gall-bladder and are excreted with the feces; or they live and multiply in the pelvis of the kidney and are excreted in the urine.

Flies, etc.—Conveyance by flies and other unusual modes occurs with about the same frequency as in typhoid fever.

(*e*) *Types of Infection.*—(*i*) Typical Infection.—The typical infection by the *Bacillus paratyphosus A*, like the typical infection by the *Bacillus typhosus*, is a bacteriemia causing a fever of the continued type, with localization of the bacilli in the gall-bladder, the lymphatic structures of the intestine, the mesenteric glands and the spleen.

The typical infection by the *Bacillus paratyphosus B* is also a bacteriemia with localizations, and the additional characteristic of a tendency to produce gastro-enteritis.

(*ii*) Mild Infections.—The existence of healthy carriers with no history of acute febrile illness recognizable as an attack of paratyphoid fever is evidence that slight infections may occur. It is also reasonable to assume that the organism may enter the gastro-intestinal tract without the development of infection. This is evidenced by the absence of infection in vaccinated individuals as compared with the unvaccinated —both subjected to the same opportunities for the introduction of the organisms into the alimentary canal.

Mixed infections of the paratyphoid bacillus with other water-borne organisms are not uncommon. In many outbreaks of paratyphoid infection due to the ingestion of a highly polluted water, the onset of paratyphoid fever is preceded by an attack of gastro-enteritis, due to the presence in the water of some other infection. Mixed infections of paratyphoid A and dysentery were not infrequent in the British forces at Gallipoli. The two paratyphoid infections may exist in the same subject at the same time; or infection by either of the paratyphoid organisms with typhoid fever may take place. Cases have been reported in which an apparent intercurrent relapse of paratyphoid fever has proven to be the onset of a complicating typhoid infection.

(*iii*) Local Infections.—Local infections by the paratyphoid organisms occur, as in typhoid fever, and with about the same frequency.

PREVALENCE.—The existence of the paratyphoid infections as distinct clinical entities has been known only since 1896. In all probability the disease has coëxisted with typhoid fever from remote times. It has now been identified in practically all parts of the world.

According to Bainbridge, no case of paratyphoid fever had been reported in England previous to 1912; since that time many cases have been recognized. This author states that but two small outbreaks had been reported in France up to the same year. In Germany, previous to the war, the disease was quite prevalent, particularly in the southwestern part. During the war the disease became very prevalent in the Allied armies. French observers believe that the men were infected in the territory re-occupied after the Battle of the Marne, which had been fouled by paratyphoid carriers among the German invaders. The Enteric Fever Commission, in 1906 to 1908, first recognized the disease in India; and since then it has been found to be widely prevalent in the northern half of the country. In the United States, Proescher and Roddy, in 1910, found paratyphoid fever A in eight per cent. of 262 cases presenting the symptoms of typhoid fever. The disease prevailed quite extensively among the troops mobilized along the Mexican border in 1916. It is now occasionally identified whenever bacteriological methods are applied in the differential diagnosis of acute febrile diseases presenting the symptoms of typhoid fever.

Paratyphoid fever is a much less common disease than typhoid fever. It is impossible to state how prevalent it is in this country. It is not often reported and few cases are recognized outside of the large cities. A fair estimate of the actual prevalence of the disease may be made by comparing the number of cases of paratyphoid fever with typhoid fever in epidemics in which the two diseases have prevailed coincidently and have been differentiated.

Kayser, in Strasburg, from 1901 to 1907, examined bacteriologically 505 cases presenting the clinical characteristics of typhoid fever. The typhoid bacillus was recovered from 437 cases and the paratyphoid bacillus A from 5 cases—about 1 per cent. Proescher and Roddy of Pittsburgh found paratyphoid A in 8 per cent. of 262 cases examined. During 1910, in the British Army in India, there were 306 cases of typhoid fever and 44 cases of paratyphoid A—about 15 per cent. German statistics from 1906 to 1909 collected by Uhlenhuth and Hübener show 57,955 cases of typhoid fever and 1,662 cases of paratyphoid—about 3 per cent. Boycott estimates that in England about 3 per cent. of the enteric cases are paratyphoid infections. In 1917 and 1918 there were in the whole United States Army 1,065 cases of typhoid fever and 127 cases of paratyphoid—12 per cent.

In some of the war districts of Europe paratyphoid infections became relatively more frequent than typhoid fever. Unquestionably this condition was due to the fact that in the early period of the war the troops were immunized against typhoid fever but not against paratyphoid. To the end of 1916, 2,534 cases of paratyphoid fever and 1,684 cases of typhoid fever had occurred among the British expeditionary forces in France and Belgium. Among the British troops in Gallipoli and Lemnos 5,700 cases of enteric fever occurred. Of this number, 93 per cent. had paratyphoid fever and 7 per cent. typhoid fever.

Relative Incidence of Paratyphoid Infections A and B.—The relative incidence of paratyphoid infections A and B varies in different localities and at different times in the same locality. In Germany, before the war, about 90 per cent. of the paratyphoid cases were para B infections. In eastern France in the early part of the war para A infections markedly predominated; later the proportion was reversed. Of 735 cases treated by French observers and identified by blood culture, 572— or 84.6 per cent.—were para A infections, and 113—or 15.4 per cent.— were para B infections. Among the British troops in India paratyphoid A infections largely predominated.

Webb-Johnson's analysis of the enteric cases admitted to the largest British isolation hospital in France during the first two years of its operation shows 344 cases of paratyphoid A and 1,038 cases of paratyphoid B. In the Dardanelles campaign in 1915 paratyphoid B was the more prevalent infection during the warm months. About the end of October paratyphoid A infection became more common, and by December it had almost entirely replaced paratyphoid B. Of the 127 cases occurring in the American Army 86 cases were para A and 41 cases para B; approximately two cases of para A to one of para B.

In this country, so far as recorded, the paratyphoid A infections are in large majority. Chamberlain, with the troops on the Mexican border, in 1916 observed 250 cases: 245 cases of para A and only 5 cases of para B. Statistics from the civil population are not available.

Symptomatology.—Infection by organisms of the paratyphoid group may be classified into the following clinical types:

(1) *Paratyphoid bacteriemia,* or *paratyphoid fever,* clinically similar to typhoid fever.

(2) *Gastro-intestinal Inflammations.*

(3) *Local Inflammations.*

The *Bacillus paratyphosus A* causes infections of clinical Types 1 and 3. It rarely if ever causes infections of Type 2. The *Bacillus paratyphosus B* causes infections of all three clinical types. It frequently produces infections of Type 2.

(1) Paratyphoid Fever.—Previous to the isolation of the paratyphoid organisms the paratyphoid bacteriemias were grouped clinically

either with typhoid fever, in the prolonged cases, or with the febrile intestinal derangements of undetermined etiology in the short course cases. Older clinicians will recall their difficulties in attempting to classify the mild enteric infections which were frequently met and which could not conscientiously be called typhoid fever. In our own experience we have vivid recollections of many cases of fever in which the mode of onset and early symptoms seemed to justify a presumptive diagnosis of typhoid fever, only to have them end suddenly and discredit our diagnostic acumen. Present knowledge makes it quite probable that many of these cases were paratyphoid fever.

(a) *Clinical History.*—The clinical history of paratyphoid fever bears a close similarity to that of typhoid fever. Although a few cases run the long and severe course of typical typhoid fever, paratyphoid is, in general, a less severe infection and corresponds more closely in its course to the mild and short duration forms of typhoid. Certain clinical differences are to be noted between the two diseases but, as Gay well says, ''these differences are not any greater than might occur between individual cases of typhoid fever, and could certainly never be used for the purpose of differential diagnosis of the one disease from the other in any given case.'' This close similarity makes a detailed description of the symptomatology of paratyphoid fever unnecessary. The group clinical characteristics of the two diseases will be considered and special features and symptoms compared.

There are practically no clinical differences between the two forms paratyphoid fever A and B. A study of many case records, however, shows that in the fever caused by the *Bacillus paratyphosus B* abdominal symptoms tend to be more in evidence.

Period of Incubation.—The average period of incubation is from ten to fifteen days. It may be as short as five days. Headache and general malaise are occasionally noted during this period. In waterborne outbreaks an afebrile diarrhea is a common symptom.

Period of Invasion.—Symptoms during Progress of Disease.—The onset may be insidious, with gradually increasing intensity of the symptoms, as in typical typhoid fever. A sudden onset, with a rapid evolution of the symptoms, is more frequently seen. There are the same lassitude, headache, shivering, loss of appetite, thirst, nausea and general muscular pain as in typhoid fever. Severe occipital headache and backache are frequent, and abdominal pain, colic and vomiting are apt to be more pronounced than in typhoid. Cramps in the calves of the legs is a common and suggestive symptom. Diarrhea and constipation occur with about equal frequency. In the para A infections which occurred on the Mexican border diarrhea and other abdominal symptoms were very unusual. In Robinson's cases vomiting occurred in twenty-four per cent. Herpes of the lips and face is not uncommon, while in typhoid fever it is quite rare. Sore throat also is frequent.

The temperature rises more abruptly than in typhoid fever, often reaching the maximum for the attack on the second to fourth day, and the fastigium is reached by the end of the third or the beginning of the fourth day. The fastigium is short, lasting four to seven days. During this time the fever continues with remissions or intermissions and the general symptoms are similar to those of the same period of mild typhoid fever.

Defervescence begins about the ninth or tenth day of the illness with wide oscillations in the temperature and a general amelioration of all symptoms. Headache often persists through the period of decline, a condition which is rarely met in typhoid. The disease terminates quite uniformly by lysis. The period of decline is short and is usually complete in four or five days.

Paratyphoid fever curves show great variation in type and may resemble the curves of the continued or remittent malarial fevers.

The total duration of the febrile period is in general much shorter than in typhoid fever, usually being under two weeks. Two-thirds of Robinson's cases were free from fever inside of a week after admission to the hospital. Severe cases may run the long tedious course of typical typhoid fever.

Convalescence.—Convalescence is apt to be slow and attended by persistent muscular debility and an irritable nervous system. While in bed the temperature remains, as a rule, below normal and the pulse slow. Exercise, excitement or a digestive upset easily causes transient rise of temperature or tachycardia.

Relapse.—Relapse occurs about as frequently as in typhoid fever— in about ten per cent. of the cases. Relapse is short in duration, averaging eight or nine days, and, in general, pursues a mild course. A slight evening temperature persisting after defervescence is a frequent prelude to relapse (Fig. 1).

(b) *Special Symptoms.—Temperature.*—The temperature chart shows a curve that is quite distinct from that of the average case of typhoid fever. The temperature rises quickly, with irregular remissions and intermissions, and usually reaches the maximum, 103° to 104° F. (39.4 to 40° C.), by the third or fourth day—often as early as the second day. After a short fastigium, also marked by decided and irregular remissions, the temperature falls with wide daily oscillations and reaches the normal in four to six days. After defervescence a persistent slight evening rise is often seen interrupted by recrudescence and short intercurrent relapses, and extending the febrile period to three or four weeks (Fig. 2).

A course with regular remissions is occasionally met (Fig. 3). Excessive temperatures—above 104° F. (40° C.)—are unusual and a continuous high fever, so often present in typhoid, is very rare.

Pulse.—The pulse rate is slow in relation to the height of the temperature. Robinson found this symptom even more marked than in typhoid fever, a rate of 48 to 60 with temperatures up to 102° F. (38.9° C.). Dicrotism is unusual, although the pulse is soft.

The Rose Rash.—The characteristic rash has been found in about sixty per cent. of the cases. The spots appear, as a rule, late in the febrile period—from the seventh to the nineteenth day; occasionally as early as the fifth day. Wiltshire found spots during the febrile period, usually appearing within a day or two of lysis, in about two-thirds of his cases. In the other third they came during the period of decline or with the recrudescences of the early convalescent period. They are apt to appear in crops at intervals of three to seven days and during intercurrent relapse. Often they do not appear until after

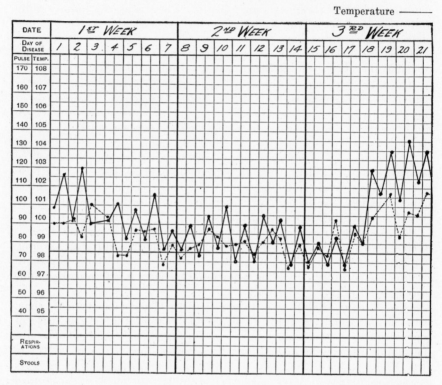

Temperature ———

FIG. 1.—CHART IN
Course prolonged by intercurrent relapse. (Observation

the temperature has reached the normal level and for this reason may be overlooked. The distribution of the rash is usually upon the abdomen and lower chest. In number the spots vary from a half dozen to about a hundred. A very abundant and widely distributed rash is occasionally seen. Writers describe two distinct types of rash which may occur independently or mingled together in the same patient. One type is identical in every respect with the rose rash of typhoid fever. The other, the paratyphoid type, has certain distinctive characteristics. The individual "paratyphoid spot" is larger than the typhoid rose spot, more often elevated, and is lenticular in outline. It is much darker in color, does not completely disappear on pressure and, when it fades, leaves a slight temporarily pigmented and desquamating area. The spot bears a close resemblance to the individual macule of the eruption of measles. These distinctive spots may be few in number or quite numerous. According to Wiltshire, they constitute a distinct diagnostic feature in favor of paratyphoid fever, particularly when they appear as the temperature is falling.

Symptoms of the Respiratory Tract.—The frequence of *epistaxis* and

Pulse ......

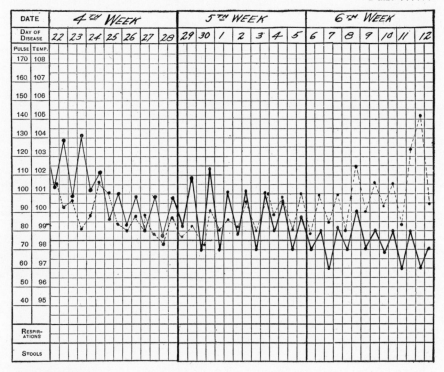

PARATYPHOID A.

at Fort Sam Houston, Col. [now Maj. Gen.] M. W. Ireland.)

of the symptoms of *catarrhal inflammation* of the respiratory tract is about the same as in mild typhoid fever.

Abdominal Symptoms.—*Nausea* and *vomiting* are common early symptoms much more frequently in paratyphoid than in mild typhoid fever. *Diarrhea* is a frequent symptom, occurring in from one-third to two-thirds of the total cases reported. It is a symptom of the first three or four days of the invasion period and frequently marks the day of onset. In water-borne infections it may precede the febrile period by a week or more. It is not often severe and declines with the appearance of lysis. It is a much more constant symptom in paratyphoid B fever than in mild typhoid. Of the cases studied by Vaughan in the American Expeditionary Forces, diarrhea was a symptom in 65.2 per

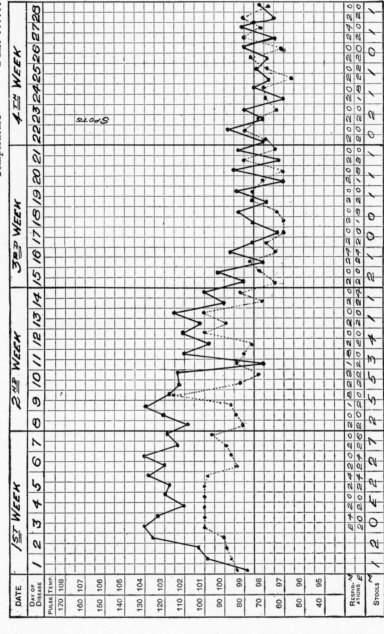

Temperature ——— Pulse ······

FIG. 2.—CHART IN PARATYPHOID B.

Sudden onset; persistent slight evening fever after lysis. (After Wiltshire.)

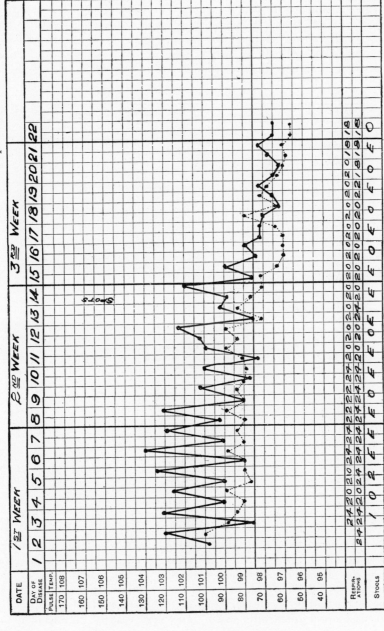

FIG. 3.—CHART IN PARATYPHOID B.

Sudden onset; remittent type of temperature. (After Wiltshire.)

cent. of the cases of paratyphoid B, and in 33.3 per cent. of the cases of paratyphoid A. The stools are composed of loose, unformed fecal material and are brown in color. The light colored "pea soup" stool of typhoid fever is not often seen. As above stated the *Bacillus paratyphosus A* does not cause gastro-enteritis. In the reported American outbreak in which cases of paratyphoid A infection predominated, diarrhea was exceptional. It is reasonable, therefore, to

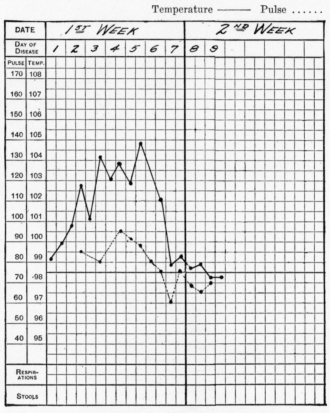

FIG. 4.—CHART IN PARATYPHOID A.
Short course. (After Hurst.)

assume that in outbreaks in which diarrhea affects a large percentage of those attacked the incidence of paratyphoid B infections is relatively high. *Pain* is a frequent symptom of the early days of the disease, perhaps more frequently observed than in typhoid fever. It may be severe and be accompanied by *rigidity* and *tenderness,* especially in the right lower quadrant. Such cases may readily be mistaken for appendicitis. The *spleen* is palpable only in about 25 per cent. of the cases. It rarely shows the marked enlargement so common in typhoid. On the other hand the *liver* is more frequently enlarged in paratyphoid fever. *Jaundice* is a frequent symptom in some outbreaks.

Nervous Symptoms.—There is a marked *absence of nervous symptoms of severity.* Headache is often of longer duration than in typhoid, but not more severe. Mild mental confusion is not uncommon but delirium is very exceptional. The patient is mildly apathetic but rarely shows the stupor so common in typhoid, and rarely develops the typhoid state.

(2) GASTRO-INTESTINAL INFLAMMATIONS.—Gastro-intestinal inflammations of paratyphoidal origin are caused by the *Bacillus paratyphosus B.* The *Bacillus paratyphosus A* rarely, if ever, has been found to be the cause of this clinical type. A clinically identical gastro-enteritis—one of the forms of food poisoning—may also be caused by the *Bacillus enteritidis* of Gärtner, a member of a subgroup of the paratyphoid organisms.

The symptoms are those of a gastro-enteritis of the food poisoning type. *The period of incubation* is short, the symptoms coming suddenly from twelve to thirty-six hours after the ingestion of the infected food. The extreme limits are one hour and four days. The short interval between the ingestion of the poisoned food and the onset of symptoms is probably due to the fact that the gastro-enteritis is a local process excited by the toxins elaborated in the food by the bacillus and is not a manifestation of a bacteriemia.

It is difficult to explain why a bacteriemia with clinical symptoms of the typhoidal type does not more frequently result from such an infection. In Whitman's 52 cases of paratyphoid B infection all recovered as soon as the local inflammation subsided.

Invasion begins with nausea and vomiting, abdominal pain and diarrhea. *Headache* is an initial symptom in about one-half the cases. *A chill or repeated shivering* is usually present. There are often *faintness and dizziness* or, in severe cases, *collapse with small pulse and cold wet skin. Stupor or coma* are occasionally observed. *Abdominal tenderness* may be a marked feature and, as in the paratyphoid fever type, the attack may closely simulate appendicitis. The *temperature* rises quickly to a moderate height and reaches its maximum during the first day or two of the illness. It varies in height from 101° to 104° F. (38.3° to 40° C.). It pursues an irregularly remittent course and falls rather abruptly.

In this type of infection the *rose spots* are present in about the same percentage as in the typhoidal type, although they often do not appear until after defervescence.

Severe attacks may assume the clinical characteristics of cholera nostras.

The disease runs a *short course* and terminates in from three to eight days. In an outbreak reported by Whitman, of 53 cases, the duration of the shortest was three days and the longest seven days.

Convalescence is usually slow and often followed by a long period of muscular weakness and mental depression.

(3) LOCAL INFLAMMATIONS.—Local inflammations may be caused by either of the two paratyphoid organisms. These inflammations occur with about the same frequency as in typhoid fever and tend to invade the

same structures. Meningitis is more often produced by the paratyphoid organisms than by the typhoid bacillus. The gall-bladder is constantly invaded and cholecystitis is not very rare. The rather frequent occurrence of jaundice indicates a greater tendency for the infection to invade the bile ducts than is shown in typhoid fever.

The symptoms of the various local inflammations caused by mem-

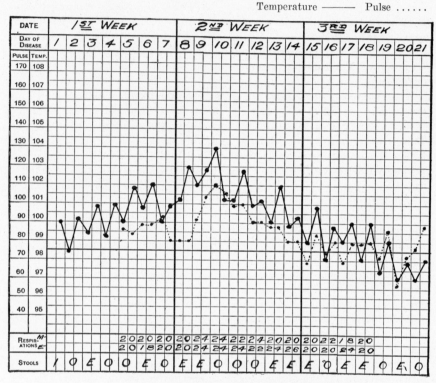

FIG. 5.—CHART IN PARATYPHOID B.
Steplike rise of temperature of invasion period. (After Wiltshire.)

bers of the paratyphoid groups of microörganisms are the same as when they are the result of other infections.

Diagnosis.—CLINICAL DIAGNOSIS.—The problem of the clinical diagnosis of paratyphoid fever requires the analysis of the same symptom-complex that is presented by typhoid fever. Differentiation from other acute febrile diseases is made from the same clinical data that are available in the differentiation of typhoid fever.

In paratyphoid, as in typhoid fever, a presumptive diagnosis only can be made from clinical findings. Laboratory confirmation, by the agglutination reaction or by the recovery from the blood, stools or urine of the specific organism of the disease, is essential to a positive diagnosis.

The frequency of short duration cases of paratyphoid fever in the recent war areas of France and the simultaneous prevalence of *influenza* made the differential diagnosis of these two diseases a question that often came up for consideration. Wiltshire gives the following points in favor of a diagnosis of paratyphoid fever: "The more gradual onset of symptoms and ascent of fever; the absence of coryza; the rarity

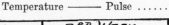

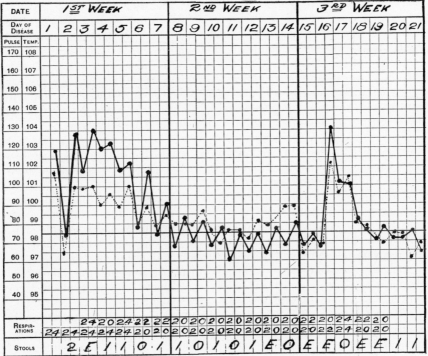

Fig. 6.—Chart in Paratyphoid B.

Sudden onset; short course; recrudescence on 16th day. (After Wiltshire.)

of rigors; the absence of early cough; the gradual onset of prostration, and its mild character compared with the degree of fever; the occurrence of diarrhea; abdominal tumidity; the absence of signs of cardiac embarrassment during the febrile stage; the absence of postfebrile psychoses and affections of special sense."

Is it possible clinically to differentiate between paratyphoid fever and typhoid fever? Before the clinical experience gained in the recent war, checked up by abundant laboratory investigation, writers answered this question with an emphatic negative. With individual and isolated cases this answer still holds good. Wide variations from group characteristics are so frequent in both diseases that individual cases cannot with certainty be distinguished one from the other.

The main clinical differences between paratyphoid and typhoid fever, as presented in large groups of cases, have been brought out with distinctness by observers in the war zones and may serve for making a presumptive diagnosis in outbreaks either of paratyphoid or of typhoid infection, or in epidemics in which both diseases prevail together.

The following points are *in favor of a diagnosis of paratyphoid fever:* the abrupt onset often accompanied by vomiting and chills; the shorter duration of all stages of the febrile period; the early appearance of marked remissions of fever; the very slow pulse and infrequent appearance of dicrotism; the moist and cleaner tongue; the greater frequency of gastro-intestinal symptoms; the darker color of the stools; the frequency of jaundice and enlargement of the liver; the infrequency of a palpable spleen; the different character of the rose spots and their appearance when other symptoms are improving; the greater frequency of herpes; the absence or mild character of the nervous symptoms except headache; the persistence of headache after defervescence; the frequency of occipital pain and of joint and muscle pains.

These clinical characteristics of paratyphoid fever are significant when applied to cases in the aggregate; a positive differential diagnosis from typhoid fever in any given case is not possible, however, without the aid of *laboratory examinations.*

Paratyphoid infections of Type 2—the gastro-intestinal inflammations—can be differentiated from *gastro-enteritis due to other causes* only by the recovery of the paratyphoid organism from the blood or stools. In the local inflammations—Type 3—diagnosis will be made by the recovery of the bacillus from the affected organ or tissue.

LABORATORY DIAGNOSIS.—The technical details for the laboratory diagnosis of paratyphoid fever are identical with those of typhoid fever and may be found in that section. (See page 518.)

Blood Culture.—Recovery from the blood of one of the paratyphoid organisms is conclusive evidence of a paratyphoid bacteriemia, or paratyphoid fever. Figures are not available that give the percentage of positive findings. It is certain that this percentage is lower than for typhoid fever. The paratyphoid bacillus remains in the blood stream for a shorter time than the typhoid bacillus and, for this reason, is more difficult of isolation. Diagnosis by blood culture was the method of choice with the armies in France.

Fecal Culture.—Paratyphoid bacilli are excreted by the feces in abundance and quite continuously during the course of paratyphoid fever. Positive findings are more frequent than in typhoid fever and in much higher percentage in the early stages of the disease. Krumwiede examined the stools of 57 cases of paratyphoid fever occurring among the men of the 14th Infantry, New York National Guard, with the following results: Positive findings: period of incubation, 15 per cent.; 1st week, 83 per cent.; 2nd week, 50 per cent.; 3rd week, 33 per cent.; 4th week, 20 per cent.; 5th week, 15 per cent. and 6th week 20 per cent. The technic of fecal culture is much simpler than that of blood culture and, judged by the excellent results obtained by

Krumwiede, the bacteriological examination of the feces is the most satisfactory method of laboratory diagnosis of paratyphoid fever.

The Agglutination Test.—The value of the Widal reaction in the differential diagnosis of paratyphoid fever is still the subject of controversy. That it is not as reliable a method in paratyphoid as in typhoid fever has been demonstrated, and in recent years the reliability of the test has become further vitiated by the introduction of antiparatyphoid vaccination. Satisfactory conclusions can be drawn from the test only when it is made by an expert and when due consideration is given to all the possibilities of error.

Complications.—The complications of paratyphoid fever are of the same general character and relative incidence as of typhoid fever, but far less frequent. In the outbreaks along the Mexican border complications were rare and unimportant. In civil practice in this country they are also infrequent. Under war conditions in Europe the percentage was higher and in some sections in France paratyphoid fever closely followed typhoid in the incidence and severity of complications.

In Webb-Johnson's series of cases of paratyphoid fever, of the two most important complications, hemorrhage occurred in 17 cases—1.22 per cent., and perforation in 5 cases—.37 per cent. In 1,118 cases of typhoid fever during the same period and under the same conditions, hemorrhage occurred in 50 cases—4.74 per cent., and perforation in 9 cases—.80 per cent.

The influence of prophylactic vaccination in ameliorating the severity of paratyphoid fever is shown by his statistics to be very great. The incidence of all complications is reduced to an insignificant number. In 364 vaccinated cases there was but one instance of perforation. The percentage of complications in the cases of paratyphoid B fever was nearly double the percentage in the cases of paratyphoid A.

Clinical Varieties.—*Mild Forms.*—The recent reports of the disease as it has occurred among troops in this country and Europe show that mild forms of the paratyphoid infections are very common. They bear only a faint resemblance to typhoid fever and, except for the laboratory studies of the medical officers of the army, they would probably have been classified as cases of digestive derangement, influenza or fever of undetermined etiology. It is quite certain that such cases also occur among the civil population but escape identification. They are rarely admitted to the hospitals, but come under the care of physicians in private practice and recover and pass from observation before an opportunity is given for laboratory study.

Treatment.—Paratyphoid and typhoid bacilli escape from infected individuals by the same routes. Transmission also of both infections is by the same channels, with the single conspicuous difference that the *Bacillus paratyphosus B* more frequently gains entry into the human organism through the medium of infected food.

PROPHYLAXIS.—The specific measures for the prevention of typhoid **fever** by the *destruction of the bacillus at its source* and by the *prevention of its transmission from the sick to the well* apply with equal force to the prevention of the paratyphoid infections. The transmission of the paratyphoid organisms by food infection can be prevented by cleanliness in food distribution through sterilization of all food supplies. Unlike the *Bacillus typhosus* the paratyphoid organism multiplies in infected meat which has been imperfectly cooked, or in well cooked meat which has been contaminated after cooking by unclean hands, cooking utensils or flies. Preserved and canned meats, minced meats and sausage are especially liable to act as such culture media and should be given special consideration.

The carrier problem has the same significance here as in the prophylaxis of typhoid fever. Carriers should be sought among those who have to do with the preparation and distribution of food and, when found, treated in the same manner as typhoid carriers. All persons who of necessity must be in contact with carriers should be protected by vaccination.

Antiparatyphoid Vaccination.—This subject has been fully considered in the section on antityphoid vaccination. The evidence available at this date confirms the opinion that vaccination against paratyphoid infections gives an immunity equal to that given by vaccination against typhoid fever. Among over 2,000,000 men of the American Army in the camps and cantonments in this country during the war, paratyphoid as well as typhoid fever was practically unknown. Even under the necessarily defective sanitary conditions at the front in France, and in men subjected to the terrible physical and mental strain of battle conditions, the immunity given by vaccination was broken down in but very few instances. In the whole American Army at home and abroad during the years 1917 and 1918 only 127 cases of paratyphoid fever occurred.

MEDICAL TREATMENT.—The medical treatment of paratyphoid fever is identical in all its details with the medical treatment of typhoid fever. The paratyphoid B infection with the clinical characteristics of gastro-enteritis do not differ in any way from gastro-enteric infections from other organisms and should receive the same treatment. Convalescence should be guarded with the same care as in typhoid fever. Hemorrhage has been observed after convalescence appeared to be well established. **Rest in bed** should be enjoined **for at least a week after defervescence.**

Prognosis.—The mortality of paratyphoid fever under peace conditions is very low. No death occurred in the cases in the American Army on the Mexican border. Sacquepec found only 4 deaths in 2,725 cases—.15 per cent. Under war conditions the mortality is higher. In Webb-Johnson's series of 1,020 cases not protected by vaccination 18 died—1.75 per cent. All of 362 vaccinated cases recovered. In some small groups of cases observed in the French Army the mortality reached 3 per cent.

As a rule the para B infections have a higher mortality than the para A infections. Webb-Johnson recorded a mortality of 2.12 per cent. in para B infections and .45 per cent. in para A infections. Vaughan reported a mortality of 4.3 per cent. in the paratyphoid B infections, and

0 per cent. in the paratyphoid A infections. In an occasional outbreak in France the proportion was reversed.

As in typhoid fever, death usually results from one of the complications—most commonly hemorrhage or perforation. Toxemia alone is rarely fatal.

Pathology.—There is nothing in the morbid anatomy of the paratyphoid infections that distinguishes them from typhoid fever or that distinguishes the two infections A and B from each other. In the few autopsy studies recorded there was found a more extensive ulceration of the colon than is usually found in typhoid fever. The ascending colon is most frequently the seat of ulceration, and in rare cases the process may involve the whole length of the colon. In many cases of para A infection there is no intestinal ulceration and no postmortem evidence of intestinal inflammation.

Historical Summary.—Knowledge of the paratyphoid infections is of recent date. The first of the paratyphoid group of organisms to be discovered was the *Bacillus enteritidis,* isolated by Gärtner in 1888, from the spleen of a patient who died from meat poisoning. In 1896 Achard and Bensaude isolated an organism, distinct from the Eberth bacillus, from two cases of clinical enteric fever, which they named the "paratyphoid bacillus." In one case the bacillus was recovered from the urine and in the other from a complicating purulent arthritis. Gwyn, in 1898, working in Osler's clinic, cultivated a paratyphoid bacillus which he described as the "paracolon bacillus," from the blood of a patient presenting the clinical features of typhoid fever. In 1901 Schottmüller obtained by blood culture, from patients presenting the symptoms of typhoid fever, two bacilli which Brion and Kayser named *Bacillus paratyphosus A* and *Bacillus paratyphosus B.*

The demonstrations of these early workers have been verified by subsequent research. During the recent war the paratyphoid infections have prevailed extensively among the troops at the front, and much has been added to our knowledge of the clinical history of the disease. It has been shown that both the paratyphoid organisms cause a bacteriemia with symptoms similar to those of typhoid fever. The para A bacillus practically always produces this type of the disease; it rarely if ever excites a gastro-enteritis. The relation of the para B bacillus to the typhoid-like cases on the one hand and to the food-poisoning type on the other have been the subject of much difference of opinion. Food poisoning epidemics have been very common in Germany, due either to the *Bacillus enteriditis* or to the *Bacillus paratyphosus B.* Bainbridge, writing in 1912, held that food poisoning is not caused by the *Bacillus paratyphosus B* but by other closely related organisms of the paratyphoid group and that infection by this organism produced only typhoid-like symptoms the same as paratyphoid A. Studies made possible by the recent wide prevalence of the disease in Europe appear to have demonstrated that either type of clinical phenomena—the typhoid type or food-poisoning type—may be the result of infection by the *Bacillus paratyphosus B.*

BIBLIOGRAPHY

ACHARD AND BENSAUDE. Bull. et mém. Soc. méd. d. hôp. de Paris, 1896, xiii, 820.

BAINBRIDGE, F. A. Lancet, London, 1912, pp. 705, 771, 849.

BERRY, CHARLES WHITE. New York Med. Rec., Jan. 27, 1917, p. 136.

BOYCOTT, A. E. Jour. Hyg., 1906, vi, 33. (Cited by Gay.)

CHAMBERLAIN, W. P. Jour. Am. Med. Assn., Nov. 25, 1916, 1573.

GAY, FREDERICK P. Typhoid fever, p. 189.

GWYN, N. Bull. Johns Hopkins Hospital, 1898, ix, 54.

HURST, ARTHUR F. Medical diseases of the war. London, 1917.

KRUMWIEDE, C., JR. Jour. Infect. Dis., 1917, xxi, 141.

PROESCHER, FREDERIC, AND RODDY, JOHN A. Arch. Int. Med., v, 263

ROBINSON, HENRY. Lancet, London, Oct. 16, 1915, 851.

VAUGHAN, V. C., JR. Jour. Am. Med. Assn., April 24, 1920, 1145.

VINCENT AND MURANTET. Medical and surgical therapy. Vol. I, p. 80.

WEBB-JOHNSON, A. E. Surgical aspects of typhoid and paratyphoid fevers. London, 1919.

WHITMAN, J. D. Mil. Surgeon, Nov., 1916, xxxix, 495.

WILTSHIRE, HAROLD. Practitioner, Jan., 1916, xcvi, 91.

CHAPTER XXXIX

COLON BACILLUS INFECTIONS

By C. G. Jennings, M.D. and A. F. Jennings, M.D.

Definition.—Colon bacillus infections are acute or chronic febrile diseases caused by the invasion of the blood stream or tissues by the *Bacillus coli,* and are manifested clinically either by a continued fever somewhat resembling typhoid fever or by local inflammations with pus formation, of which inflammations of the urinary tract, the biliary tract and the peritoneum are the most common.

Etiology.—Predisposing Causes.—*Age, Sex, Social Conditions, etc.*—The disease is common to all *ages.* In adults the disease is more frequent in women in the child-bearing age and in men in the age of prostatic obstruction. *Social condition, hygiene, occupation and environment* have no bearing on the disease. *Individual susceptibility* depends more on associated disease than on a natural lack of immunity. Colon bacillus infection is common in the tropics because of the frequency of gastro-enteritis. Sir James R. Roberts states that it is very common in India, and he advises that surgeons intending to practice there should have special training in urology. The infection is more frequent in infants and children during the summer months.

Other Diseases.—Hirschsprung's disease is frequently complicated by *pyelonephritis of the colon bacillus type,* according to Langstein. *Congenital malformations of the kidney* and ureter and ureteral obstruction predispose to the infection. Renal calculus and hypertrophy of the prostate with obstruction to the urinary flow eventually result in infection of the kidney by this organism. Diseases of the intestine, such as acute enteritis or colitis, typhoid fever, intestinal cancer, or parasitism, may be followed by colon bacillus infection. General infections may result from local inflammation of the gall-bladder, urinary tract, pelvic organs and veins and the appendix. Scarlatina, diphtheria and measles are more often followed by colon bacillus infection than are the other acute febrile diseases. Diseases and injuries of the spinal cord, such as fracture of the vertebrae, tabes, acute anterior poliomyelitis and pernicious anemia, usually result in colon bacillus infection of the urinary tract.

Pyelitis and pyelonephritis occur in about 20 per cent of *pregnant women.* The reason for its occurrence is not well understood. Displacement of the kidney, pressure on the right ureter, especially with the fetus in the dextro-position, edema of the pelvic organs with obstruction of the ureter and increased general susceptibility to infection are reasons advanced.

Trauma.—Colon bacillus infection occasionally occurs in newly married women. It is probably the result of trauma to the bladder or genitalia, or it may be due to the activation of a preëxisting unrecognized infection. The infection may occur after instrumentation or minor operations upon the lower urinary tract.

A previous attack renders the patient more susceptible. Whether this is due to latent infection or to pathological changes in the pelvis and ureter is at present unsettled.

EXCITING CAUSE: BACTERIOLOGY OF THE ORGANISM.—The bacteriological description of the colon bacillus will be found in the section on the Colon-typhoid Group of Organisms in the chapter on Typhoid Fever (p. 457, this volume).

Mode of Infection.—Colon bacillus infection is the result of auto-inoculation by the organisms of the patient's intestinal canal. While cases due to infected water supply or to direct contact with the organism occur, they are too rare to be of clinical interest. The bacilli enter the body through the intestinal wall, through the skin in the region of the external genitalia and through the lower urinary tract. Minute breaks in the continuity of the intestinal mucous membrane are sufficient to cause entrance of the bacilli. C. A. McWilliams states that colon bacilli may be found in the sac of a strangulated hernia ten hours after the onset.

Colon bacilli in the peritoneum may enter both the lymphatics, from which they are carried to the thoracic duct, and the blood stream. David has demonstrated this in dogs and has found the bacilli in both the liver and spleen a few minutes after intraperitoneal injection. If a plastic peritonitis is present the bacilli do not leave the peritoneal cavity.

C. Franke has demonstrated lymphatic communication between the right kidney and the ascending colon. It is improbable that the bacteria reach the kidney by this route, though the greater frequency of right-sided pyelonephritis is at present unexplained.

Colon bacilli are frequently present in the bladder and prostate and upon the external genitalia. From these areas they reach the blood stream and lymphatics and they are eventually excreted by the kidney. Cabot and Crabtree have proven that spread of the infection in this manner often results in infection of the kidney, and they believe that ascending infection through the ureters cannot occur when the urinary flow is unobstructed. It is now believed that the urinary flow is obstructed much more often than was formerly thought possible. This is due to ptosis, rotation and mobility of the kidney as well as to congenital anomalies. Hunner's theory of ureteral obstruction is generally accepted by urologists, though true ureteral stricture is a rare finding. Regurgitation of urine from the bladder may occur when the intravesicular pressure is but little above normal. When the organisms have reached the kidney they pass through the glomeruli to the tubules and from there to the pelvis. They remain in the pelvis and at intervals ascend into the kidney, probably along the lymphatics of the intertubular spaces.

Types of Infection.—The colon bacillus is essentially one of the pyogenic organisms with special tendency to localization in the urinary tract, the pelvic organs, the peritoneum and the biliary tract. Variations in the virulence of the organisms have not been proven. The organism is frequently present in the kidney and probably the gall-bladder without resulting in disease, or mild infections of these organs exist without causing symptoms. It is common for mixed infections to occur, especially with the streptococcus and staphylococcus. Many authorities doubt that the colon bacillus is ever the primary cause of disease, believing that when it is found in pure culture it has been preceded by another organism which has been overgrown. In addition to its usual areas of location the colon bacillus has been demonstrated in inflammation of practically all of the tissues of the body. It is common as a terminal infection in heart disease, nephritis or other chronic conditions.

Symptomatology.—CLINICAL FINDINGS.—Infections by organisms of the colon group may be classified into the following clinical types:

(1) Bacteriemia clinically similar to mild typhoid fever.
(2) Local inflammations.
(3) Bacteriemia with local abscess formation.
(4) Secondary implantation of the bacillus upon a tissue already damaged.
(5) Terminal invasion of the blood and organs.

(1) *Bacteriemia Clinically Similar to Mild Typhoid Fever.*—The onset is gradual, with fever, headache, pains in the epigastrium, abdomen and extremities, loss of appetite, sometimes nausea and vomiting, diarrhea or constipation. Rarely the onset is sudden, with chill. The temperature gradually rises, reaching a height of from 101° to 104° F. (38.3° to 40° C.) in several days, and from then on it falls by lysis to normal from the tenth to fourteenth day.

The disease does not pursue the prolonged course of typhoid fever. Exhaustion and emaciation are less severe. Diarrhea of a severe type is not common. Hemorrhage and perforation do not occur, as Peyer's patches are not ulcerated. Secondary anemia is common. Relapses similar to those of typhoid fever have been reported.

Such cases are generally classified as mild typhoid fever or fever of unknown etiology, wherever laboratory methods of diagnosis are not used. Cases have been studied in detail by Coleman and Hastings, and Cabot and Crabtree, all of whom have determined by blood culture or agglutination reactions that the disease is a separate entity from typhoid fever.

McWilliams has described a form of colon bacillus septicemia with hemorrhagic purpura occurring in infants, which is very fatal. *Bacillus coli* has been found postmortem in some cases of Winckel's disease—a fatal infection in the newly-born. The infection enters by way of the umbilical cord stump.

(2) *Local Inflammations.*—(*a*) Urinary Tract.—Colon bacilli may be excreted in the urine in large numbers without the production of symptoms or of pathological changes in the urinary tract. This was first demonstrated by T. Rovsing and has been confirmed by other investigators. The condition occurs in association with constipation, diarrheal attacks, typhoid fever, scarlatina, measles and diphtheria and after abdominal operations. Colon bacilluria may be the first manifestation of a urinary tract infection. It also occurs almost constantly in colon bacillus bacteriemia with abscess formation in other parts of the body.

Cystitis, pyelitis, pyelonephritis and pyonephrosis are the usual results of colon infection of the urinary tract. More rarely it causes urethritis, epididymo-orchitis, prostatitis and peri-urethral abscess.

In view of the fact that the kidney, the renal pelvis and the bladder are involved simultaneously, it is impossible to separate pyelonephritis, pyelitis and cystitis into definite clinical entities. The symptoms are often confused and frequently misleading. In infants the symptoms are of a general nature, including irregular fever with, at times, chills, pallor, restlessness and loss of weight. In children, delirium, coma and convulsions may occur, or there may be symptoms of meningeal irritation. C. R. Box has observed children who are shy, nervous and dull and suffer from headaches and incontinence of urine. The tongue is coated and the bowels irregular. The symptoms disappear with the cure of the colon bacillus infection. Rapid respiration and pain in the lower thorax may be caused by diaphragmatic irritation. Indigestion, loss of appetite, vomiting and abdominal pain occur in children. The symptoms are chronic or recurring.

Culver, Herrold and Phifer report a careful analysis of the symptoms presented by 116 patients. Pain, chills and fever and frequent painful micturition are the three characteristic symptoms of upper urinary tract infection. Pain occurs in about 90 per cent of the cases. In most instances it is in the lower back on one or both sides, and varies in intensity from a dull ache to an acute pain. It may radiate to the pelvis or thigh or to the neck. It may occur in the abdomen simulating acute appendicitis or renal colic, or it may be in the bladder region only. Chills and fever and frequent painful micturition are found in about one-half of the cases. Constipation, headache, vomiting, hematuria, loss of weight and incontinence of urine are less often observed, but may be the only symptoms of which the patient complains.

Uremia may result from *B. coli* infection if the infection has been preceded by slow and extensive renal destruction, or if it has been superimposed on cases of chronic nephritis or polycystic disease of the kidney. Its occurrence is rare.

Colon bacillus infection of the kidneys and pelvis may show every grade of severity. It may be so mild that the patient goes about his daily occupation without symptoms; or it may be rapidly fulminating, with chills, high fever, abdominal pain, delirium, severe toxemia and prostration. The usual picture, however, is one of moderate or severe sepsis.

The duration of colon infection of the urinary tract is variable. While certain cases promptly recover, the greater number become chronic. Other cases may clear up temporarily both as to symptoms and urinary findings, and later relapse. Others still continue to have symptoms of little or moderate severity associated with occasional periodic exacerbations. Much depends upon the success of local treatment by the urologist.

Acute or chronic urethritis, epididymo-orchitis and prostatitis are caused by the colon bacillus in rare instances. Endometritis and pelvic inflammations due to this organism are occasionally observed.

(b) Appendix.—H. A. Kelly states that the colon bacillus has been found in 86 per cent of the cases operated upon at the Johns Hopkins Hospital, generally associated with other organisms, especially the streptococcus and staphylococcus. He noted that the cases due to the colon bacillus alone were milder and that the disease was limited to tissues of the appendix region, while the cases of mixed infection showed extensive and severe peritonitis. The colon bacillus rapidly overgrows the streptococcus and the staphylococcus, and for this reason may be found alone even when it is a secondary invader. H. C. Low has reported the bacteriology of 100 cases of appendicitis. The colon bacillus was present in pure culture in 8, and with cocci in 74. The streptococcus was present in pure culture in 2. In cases of three days' duration or less the colon bacillus was found in 62 per cent and the streptococcus in 81 per cent. In cases of two or three weeks' duration the colon bacillus was present in 87 per cent and the streptococcus in 55 per cent. The colon bacillus alone was found in only one acute case of less than three days' duration. Low also noted that the colon bacillus alone causes a less severe disease than the streptococcus alone or than a mixed infection. Metastatic abscesses due to the colon bacillus may follow appendicitis.

(c) Biliary Tract.—A. O. J. Kelly, studying in Deaver's clinic, found the colon bacillus alone in 28.33 per cent of 240 cases of cholecystitis, and associated with staphylococcus in 0.85 per cent of the cases. Cholangitis, liver abscess and subphrenic abscess may be due to the colon bacillus.

(d) Peritoneum.—Dudgeon and Sargent conclude that the colon bacillus causes the largest number of fatalities in peritonitis. Its virulence varies, and while it is less virulent than the streptococcus it occurs more frequently. Flexner, in 56 cases of peritonitis due to bowel infection, found the colon bacillus in pure culture in 8, and associated with other organisms in 35—a total of 43 cases. J. C. Briscoe reports three chronic cases in which caseating peritoneal masses due to the colon bacillus were operated upon.

(e) Organs Other Than the Kidney, Liver, Bile Ducts, Appendix and Peritoneum.—In rare instances the colon bacillus invades organs other than the kidney, liver, bile ducts, appendix and peritoneum. Lobular pneumonia, pleuritis, empyema and multiple abscesses of the lung have been observed. Endocarditis and pericarditis are reported. Meningitis may follow acute enteritis or otitis media. Brain abscess and myelitis are sometimes due to the colon bacillus. The organism may be found in otitis media or mastoiditis, tonsillitis or empyema of the nasal accessory sinuses. In the extremities, periostitis, suppurative arthritis and infections in lacerated wounds have been reported. Cutaneous abscesses of infants, herpes of the lips and mucous membrane of the mouth and septic onychia have been due to this organism. It may be found in the wounds of abdominal and other operations, and was first observed outside of the digestive tract by Tavel in the wound of an operation on the thyroid gland.

(3) *Bacteriemia with Local Abscess Formation.*—Blood-stream infection is associated with localized inflammation in many cases. It may precede or follow the local infection. Recognition of this condition has been delayed, owing to the difficulty in isolating the colon bacillus from the blood.

Jacob, studying colon bacillus bacteriemia, found that local abscesses resulted in 22.5 per cent of the reported cases and in 1 of 13 cases of his own. Of the 8 cases taken from the records of the Massachusetts General Hospital, 2 showed evidence of local areas of inflammation. Coleman and Hastings in their 3 cases of colon bacillus septicemia found clinical evidence of acute cholecystitis in 1 of them. Cabot and Crabtree took blood cultures of 32 cases of pyelonephritis during or shortly after a chill and found *B. coli* present in 12. They cite one case in detail— a patient with enlarged prostate and residual urine, who was being treated by inlying catheter. On the eighth day there occurred burning micturition followed in two hours by a rigor. The urine at this time showed no microscopical evidence of infection, although the blood culture was positive. The following day pus and bacilli appeared in the urine. They quote Kowitz, who found that certain infants suffering from diarrhea showed first colon bacilli in the blood and then albumin, bacteria and pus, in sequence, in the urine.

Felty and Keefer have studied in detail 28 cases in which *B. coli* was found by blood culture at the Johns Hopkins Hospital. The portal of entry of the organism was the urinary tract in 16 cases, the female genitalia in 6, the intestinal tract in 2, wound infection in 1. No portal of entry was found in 3 cases, 2 of them being terminal infection. The infection followed cystoscopy or some surgical trauma in 20 and was spontaneous in 8. The organism did not persist in the blood stream over five days, showing its tendency to die rapidly in this medium. The fever was usually of about seven to ten days' duration. Jaundice was observed in 3 cases, petechiae in 2 and hemoglobinuria in 1. Metastasis occurred in 5 cases, the lungs and kidneys being the organs involved. The mortality was 32 per cent, 11 cases. The fatal outcome was due rather to the serious focal lesion than to the dissemination of the organism into the circulation.

Widal and Lemierre report 16 cases in which *B. coli* was recovered from the blood stream. The condition followed gastro-enteritis in 3 cases, typhoid fever in 1 case, cholecystitis or cholangitis in 4, pyelitis in 3, puerperal infection in 2, wound infection in 1, tuberculosis in 1 and was without obvious preceding disease in 1. The duration of the fever was from 5 to 26 days, and the organism was recovered from the blood up to the twenty-second day. Four patients of this series died and 12 recovered.

Sison and Cruz report a fulminating case of colon bacillus sepsis with death following gall-bladder infection.

The onset of the septicopyemic type of the disease is generally with chill followed by high fever. The symptoms are more serious than those of either of the uncomplicated infections already mentioned. The accompanying local disease may be manifest or it may remain obscure for many days. The temperature curve is extremely irregular, with wide daily swing and chills. It may be intermittent, remittent or relapsing in character. The course of this type of the disease is long, extending over many weeks.

(4) *Secondary Implantation of the Colon Bacillus upon a Tissue Already Damaged.*—In appendicitis, peritonitis, cholecystitis and urinary tract infections, the colon bacillus is associated with other organisms in many cases. Even when it is obtained in pure culture it is quite probable that it has overgrown the original organism.

(5) *Terminal Infections.*—Flexner has made a careful investigation of the terminal infections of heart disease and chronic nephritis—patients in whom no infection had existed until shortly before death. There were 222 cases studied. Colon bacillus appeared alone in 2 cases of general infection, and in combination with other organisms in 4. It appeared alone in 24 cases showing local infection of the various organs, and 41 times in combination with other organisms. In all, the colon bacillus invaded the blood stream or tissues in 71 of 222 cases.

The organisms were found by culture or stained section in all of the viscera and also in the peritoneum, pericardium, endocardium and pleura. It was found that they may cause a definite lesion of the tissues in which they lodge or they may be present without local reaction. Flexner believes that the bacillus wanders through the intestinal wall wherever a small lesion such as ecchymosis, erosion or ulcer exists. It is found in distant viscera almost without exception if a serious lesion of the intestine is present.

PHYSICAL FINDINGS.—*Bacteriemia.*—The patient has the appearance of mild typhoid fever. The tongue is coated and tremulous. A rose rash similar to the rash of typhoid fever is present upon the abdomen. Tympanites occurs and the spleen is enlarged.

Local Inflammations and Septicopyemia.—The local inflammations and septicopyemia present the physical signs typical of inflammation of the organs involved.

In urinary tract involvement the patient may appear well or he may present varying degrees of toxemia and prostration. On palpation, moderate or severe tenderness is found, most frequently in either costovertebral angle, also in the flanks, along the course of the ureter or in any part of the abdomen. The infected kidney may be palpable and tender. The liver and spleen may be felt.

Terminal Invasion.—The terminal invasion of the body by the colon bacillus is rarely accompanied by physical signs other than unexplained fever.

Fever.—In colon bacillus infection the fever is high at the onset, falling to normal in from 5 to 10 days. Some cases have a septic or irregular temperature curve of weeks' duration, showing wide daily variations.

The fever may be of an intermittent type. Rare cases show a course of fever similar to that of typhoid. It is rarely as high—it reaches its maximum in three or four days and declines to normal in two or three weeks. Enright and Bahr report cases in which the curve was of the relapsing type with pyrexia of 5 to 7 days, and remissions of 7 to 10 days.

Chills.—Chills are frequently observed at the onset and may occur at irregular intervals. Chills in infants and children are often due to this type of infection.

LABORATORY FINDINGS.—A moderate anemia of the secondary type is common in the prolonged, severe infections.

There is generally leukocytosis if the infection is localized. The septicemias may show leukopenia.

The colon bacillus can always be recovered from the blood in the septicemic type of the disease and frequently in cases of pyemia. Cabot and Crabtree have shown that it can be recovered from the blood in cases of pyelonephritis if the culture is made during or shortly after a chill.

Urine.—Colon bacilluria occurs in a large proportion of the cases of septicemia or pyemia.

In urinary tract infections the urine may appear normal or show only a few bacilli or pus cells during the first forty-eight hours of the disease. This finding is the result if the infected kidney fails to excrete or if the urinary flow is blocked by calculus or other obstruction.

When the infection has become established the urine is obviously turbid, due to pus; or it may show a haze or shimmering, due to bacilli. In the latter case filtration through ordinary filter paper or sedimentation does not affect the haze. The urine is commonly acid, although faint alkaline reactions may occur. Ammoniacal decomposition is never present because the colon bacillus does not decompose urea. The specific gravity is high—a surprising contrast to the pale color of the specimen. Obvious hematuria is not common, being recorded in only 12 per cent of the cases by Culver, Herrold and Phifer. Albumin is generally present. The sediment shows bacilli and pus cells. Red blood cells may be present, and casts indicate renal involvement.

The culture of the urine may be positive for colon bacillus even with a microscopically clear urine. The organism is generally present in turbid urines but it is possible to have a negative culture in these cases.

Tissues, Sputum, Peritoneal Fluid, Pleural Exudate, Cerebrospinal Fluid.—The colon bacillus can be grown from the infected tissues and from sputum, peritoneal fluid, pleural exudate and cerebrospinal fluid.

SPECIAL EXAMINATIONS.—Cystoscopic examination is essential in urinary tract infections. By this means the ureters are catheterized, urograms and pyelograms are made, and the separate functions of the kidneys are determined by either the phenolsulphonephthalein test of Rowntree and Geraghty or the indigo carmine test. The phenolsulphonephthalein test and the determination of the nonprotein nitrogen, urea or creatinin of the blood are valuable in determining the combined function of the kidneys. The dye excretion is especially sensitive in this disease, showing rapid variations from day to day.

Diagnosis.—The diagnosis is established by the recovery of the colon bacillus. The organism may be found in the blood, in exudates, in pus and in the tissues. It is found in the urine in kidney and bladder infections and in many localized infections remote from the urinary tract.

Serum agglutination does not have the important diagnostic significance in colon bacillus infections that it has in typhoid fever. The test is unreliable because of group reactions and the variable reactions given by the different strains. Using the homologous organism, Coleman and Hastings found that the reaction may occur in dilution of 1:100 in septicemia and that it disappears during convalescence. Dudgeon found that a positive reaction with the homologous organism was rare in cases of renal and peritoneal infection. W. J. Stone states that a positive reaction in a dilution of 1:40 is indicative of colon infection.

DIFFERENTIAL DIAGNOSIS.—Colon bacillus bacteriemia is to be differentiated from *typhoid and paratyphoid fevers*. The symptoms of the three diseases are practically the same, and differential diagnosis can be made only by the isolation and identification of the infecting organism from the blood by the methods given in the section on Laboratory Diagnosis in the chapter on Typhoid Fever.

The diagnosis of urinary tract infection presents several features. It is necessary to determine the location and severity of the disease process, to recognize the condition when the characteristic symptoms are absent and to differentiate it from other diseases of the genito-urinary tract and from diseases of the abdomen. Fever, abdominal or renal pain and frequent painful micturition are the leading symptoms, although they may often be absent or vague and refer to the abdominal organs. Tenderness of the costovertebral angle is frequent and pyuria is pathognomonic. In the severer types it is impossible clinically to define the disease as being limited to the bladder, renal pelvis or kidney, since all are more or less involved. *Cystitis* may exist as an entity for a few days, but if persistent, infection elsewhere in the tract is certain. Pyelitis, pyelonephritis and pyonephrosis present much the same clinical picture, although there may be some variation in severity and duration. They are differentiated by means of the pyelogram and the determination of the function of the kidney. The condition of the ureter is determined by the insertion of the ureteral catheter or sound and by the urogram.

In infants and children the characteristic urinary symptoms may be absent, the disease manifesting itself only by fever of a remittent or a continued type, or by fever with gastro-intestinal or nervous symptoms. The detection of pus and bacilli in the urine will clear up the diagnosis.

In the differentiation of colon bacillus infections from *other diseases of the genito-urinary system*, the x-ray, the cystoscope and the chemical and bacteriological examination of the urine from each kidney must be employed. *Renal tuberculosis and urinary calculus* are the conditions most liable to cause error.

The diagnosis of *infections of the urinary tract by organisms other than the colon bacillus* is determined by culture of the urine. Certain clinical differences are observed. Streptococcus and staphylococcus infections follow tonsillitis, carbuncles and osteomyelitis, and they cause *alkaline urine* because of ammoniacal decomposition of urea. Colon infections follow intestinal diseases and cause *acid urine*. In the *coccus infections of the kidney* the pus does not appear until twenty-four to forty-eight hours after the onset, and the phthalein output is normal for several days, while in colon infections the pus is found within the first twenty-four hours and the phthalein output is diminished at once.

Pyelonephritis or suppurative nephritis may simulate acute abdominal inflammation. In the latter the pain is abdominal instead of renal, vomiting is present and tenderness and muscle spasm can be found. Confusion is more liable to arise in the case of children than in adults. The finding of pus or bacilli in the urine should make the diagnosis clear, though it is to be remembered that both conditions may exist.

A large percentage of colon infections accompany or follow *pregnancy* and *confinement*. They are admitted to the hospital, diagnosed as "puerperal fever." Sepsis, particularly puerperal sepsis, should be considered in the differential diagnosis.

The diagnosis of *appendicitis, cholecystitis, peritonitis and other local infections which may be due to the colon bacillus* is considered in the various chapters devoted to the consideration of these diseases.

Tuberculosis, malaria, influenza and relapsing fever are to be differentiated from the pyemic type of colon bacillus infection. *Tuberculosis* is distinguished by the pulmonary findings, the low white blood cell count and the demonstration of tubercle bacilli in the sputum. *Malaria* is differentiated by the presence of the plasmodium in the blood. *Influenza* is a disease of short duration and ends quickly. *Relapsing fever* is diagnosticated by finding the spirillum in the blood stream. None of these diseases are characterized by pyuria or bacilluria, which frequently occur in colon bacillus pyemia. The colon bacillus should be isolated if possible.

The occurrence of the colon bacillus as a secondary invader is determined only by recovery of the organism by culture. It is rarely detected as a terminal invader.

Complications and Sequelæ.—Aside from extension of the infection by the blood stream, by the lymphatics or by continuity, complications do not occur.

Association with Other Diseases.—Colon bacillus infection is almost always associated with certain other diseases. These are enumerated in the section on Etiology.

Treatment.—Prophylaxis.—The colon bacillus is one of the organisms that make up the normal intestinal flora. It becomes pathogenic by auto-infection under conditions either of increased virulence of the organism or of diminished resistance on the part of the host. The duty of the physician in the prophylaxis of colon bacillus infection is restricted to the recognition of the various general and local conditions that predispose to colon infections, and to anticipate and, if possible, guard against them. Unfortunately many cases occur without warning and we have no means of preventing them.

Pathological activity of the colon bacillus should be anticipated: (1) in the prolonged fevers, especially typhoid, and in the acute exanthemata; (2) in acute enterocolitis, constipation, ulceration of the colon, intestinal tumors and parasites, hernia, anal fissure and after operations upon the intestines, rectum or anus; (3) in acute urethritis and cystitis, prostatism, urethral stricture, renal and vesical calculus, malformations, tumors, spinal cord disease and other conditions that may cause retention; (4) in pregnancy and after delivery; (5) following instrumentation of the urinary tract.

Colon invasion of the urinary tract may be prevented in many of these conditions by the administration from time to time of **urinary** antiseptics. **Urinalysis at definite intervals** should be made promptly to detect a bacilluria or a pyuria. *Infection by instruments and through open wounds in the region of the genitalia* may be prevented by **strict asepsis and cleanliness. Soiling of the genitalia with bowel contents is especially to be avoided** in female infants and young girls. **Instrumentation** should be done **only under the strictest aseptic precautions** and should be **followed by a liberal ingestion of fluids and the administration of hexamethylenamine.**

TREATMENT OF BACTERIEMIA.—This is similar to the treatment of typhoid fever and does not require separate consideration.

TREATMENT OF LOCAL INFECTIONS.—(1) *Urinary Tract.*—General Management.—**Rest in bed with competent nursing until the urine is free from pus and bacilli** is essential, although it is difficult to keep the patient at rest after symptoms have disappeared. The **room should be kept warm and drafts and chilling of the patient avoided. Hot sponge baths** may be given daily to aid elimination by the skin. The bowels should be kept free with **appropriate cathartics. Calomel** may irritate the kidney and **should be avoided.** *If diarrhea is present* its cause should be sought and proper therapy applied.

Diet.—The protein intake should be low, as in nephritis, and renal irritants avoided. For the average adult 60 to 70 grams (2.12 to 2.47 ounces) of protein per day should be the maximum. The required daily number of calories—40 per kilogram of body weight—may be built up as in the diet for typhoid fever (p. 583, this volume) by the addition of carbohydrates and fats. Carbohydrates are of especial value as they spare protein loss and inhibit the growth of the colon bacillus in the intestinal tract.

In the absence of marked nitrogen retention milk is a suitable food. A liter contains 35 grams (1.23 ounces) of protein and yields 640 calories. It acts as an efficient diuretic. With from one to three pints of milk as a basis the protein and caloric requirement may be obtained by the selection of articles with low protein percentage from the table of foods (Table 7) in the chapter on Typhoid Fever (p. 585, this volume). Vegetables and fruits may be added to the diet when the acute stage of the disease has passed.

TABLE I

Low PROTEIN DIET (Mosenthal)

Salt, sugar and butter may be used as desired and need not be weighed or measured.

Breakfast: Sherry, 30 c.c.; baked apple or orange; "hominy cornstarch cereal," two-thirds hominy, one-third cornstarch; cream, 15 c.c.

Dinner: Sherry, 30 c.c.; potato, baked or mashed; string beans, cabbage, carrots, lettuce, onions, tomatoes, cucumbers, pickles; fruit cornstarch pudding or fruit tapioca pudding.

Supper: Same as dinner.

TABLE II

NITROGEN CONTENT OF FOODS IN LOW PROTEIN DIET

Nitrogen (per cent)		Nitrogen (per cent)	
Cereal:		*Fruit:*	
"Hominy cornstarch cereal"		Baked apple	0.04
two-thirds hominy, one-		Orange	0.16
third cornstarch	0.13	Stewed prunes	0.14
Cream:	0.41	*Vegetables:*	
		Cabbage	0.16
		Carrots	0.10
Desserts:		Cucumber pickle	0.10
Apple tapioca pudding	0.02	Lettuce	0.24
Blackberry cornstarch pud-		Onions	0.17
ding	0.05	Potato, baked	0.48
Peach tapioca pudding	0.06	Potato, mashed	0.40
Prune cornstarch pudding	0.07	String beans	0.23
		Tomatoes	0.23

Certain foods are renal irritants and should be rigidly excluded. These include preserved meats, beef tea, meat soups and broths, sauces and condiments, radishes, parsley, onions and asparagus. Tea, coffee and cocoa in moderation are not harmful. Alcohol in small quantity is not objectionable. Mosenthal finds that an ounce of sherry with each meal does not irritate the kidneys.

(2) *Local Infections Other Than the Urinary Tract.*—The treatment of the local infections other than those of the urinary tract is surgical in a large proportion of the cases. If the infection has become generalized and beyond the reach of surgical methods, the symptomatic and supportive treatment as described for typhoid fever is to be employed. (*See* p. 599, this volume.) A vaccine may greatly hasten the cure of draining abscesses or sluggish inflammatory conditions not resulting in abscess formation, but will not take the place of surgery when the latter is indicated. Terminal infections are rarely recognized and treatment is of little importance.

LOCAL TREATMENT.—Treatment of urinary tract infections by lavage of the renal pelvis and drainage by the inlying ureteral catheter has been perfected by modern urological technic and is of great importance. The method is as applicable to infants and children as to adults. While a general anesthetic may be necessary in a few cases, the procedure can usually be accomplished without this aid. The solutions used for lavage are **silver nitrate** 0.5 to 5 per cent, **mercurochrome** 1 to 2 per cent, **potassium mercuric iodide** 1:5,000 to 1:10,000, **acriflavine** 1:10,000 and **meroxyl** 1:5,000. The ureteral catheter may be left in place for any time up to thirty days. While the effect of the catheter upon a ureteral stricture is dubious, there is no doubt but that improved drainage of the renal pelvis results, and that the disease subsides much more rapidly under this treatment than by medicinal attack alone. Ureteral catheterization is indicated in cases of long duration or marked severity or in cases that do not rapidly clear up under medical care.

TREATMENT OF SYMPTOMS.—*Pain* of any degree of severity may occur.

When mild, **hot-water bottles or hot compresses** will relieve. **Aspirin or phenacetin** may be given at the same time. *In severe pain* **codeine or morphine by the mouth or hypodermically** will be necessary. *Painful urination and tenesmus*—serious because they may cause retention—should be promptly relieved. **Potassium citrate or acetate** in doses sufficient to alkalinize the urine will give relief: 20 to 40 grains (1.3 to 2.6 grams) every four hours, well diluted with water, may be given. A vesical sedative—**tincture of belladonna or tincture of hyoscyamus**—may be prescribed with the alkali. **A suppository of extract of belladonna leaves or extract of opium** often acts well. **Oil of santal,** 5 to 10 minims (0.3 to 0.6 c.c.), **in capsule** is a useful sedative for more prolonged administration.

Fever rarely requires symptomatic treatment. **Hydrotherapy** gives the best results. **Phenacetin,** 5 grains (0.324 gram), given every hour for two or three doses during the afternoon, will reduce the temperature and ease the discomfort of the pyrexia. *Headache, vomiting, convulsions and other uremic symptoms* are treated as in acute nephritis.

Specific Therapy.—*Vaccines.*—A certain degree of success has resulted from the administration of colon vaccines in urinary infections. Cabot has found that with vaccine treatment the symptoms are improved in about 50 per cent of the cases, and that results are equally good in both upper and lower urinary tract infections. The bacilluria, however, is not relieved, and relapse is frequent. An autogenous vaccine is to be preferred.

The initial dose should not exceed 25 millions of bacilli, succeeding doses to be increased according to the clinical reaction of the patient, until a maximum dose of 600 million to 1,000 million is reached. The injections are given at intervals of from five to seven days.

Medicinal Treatment.—**Hexamethylenamine** is the most efficient urinary antiseptic and is indicated in colon bacillus infections of the urinary tract and as a prophylactic in conditions liable to be followed by infection. The drug is not a urinary sedative and should not be relied upon alone in the presence of infection with bladder irritability and tenesmus. An acid urine is essential to the therapeutic action of the drug.

The average dose of hexamethylenamine is 7½ to 10 grains (0.49 to 0.65 gram) every five hours. It should be given once during the night to maintain its action. It may be administered in quantities up to 30 or 40 grains (1.95 to 2.6 grams). In large doses it may cause frequent and painful micturition and hematuria. If these symptoms should occur the remedy should be discontinued and alkali given. *Acidity of the urine* may be assured by the **simultaneous administration of acid sodium phosphate,** in dosage of from 10 to 20 grains (0.65 to 1.3 grams).

Sodium benzoate is an efficient urinary antiseptic in colon bacillus infections. The dose is 5 to 10 grains (0.324 to 0.65 gram) four to six times a day, given in pill or capsule.

The use of the **alkaline diuretics** has been considered. They **should not be given with hexamethylenamine.** The administration of the **alkalis and hexamethylenamine on alternate weeks** has been advised on the theory that the change in the reaction of the urine inhibits the growth of the bacilli. In our personal experience the plan has not been very satisfactory.

Mercurochrome is sometimes useful in infections of the urinary tract that do not yield readily to other measures. It is used in dilution of one per cent in fifty per cent dextrose solution and should be freshly prepared. Ten cubic centimeters is the usual dose and this may be repeated at two- or three-day intervals. It is essential that a sharp febrile reaction be provoked, and if this does not result from a 10-c.c. dose a larger one—up to 25 c.c.—may be given. Not over five successive doses should be injected.

SURGICAL INDICATIONS.—The acute stage of colon bacillus infection of the kidney rarely demands surgical intervention. In pyonephrosis, nephrectomy is the only recourse. The surgical indication is determined by cystoscopic examination.

MANAGEMENT OF CONVALESCENCE.—Active treatment should be continued until all signs of disease have disappeared. It is not enough to relieve the symptoms; pyuria and bacilluria should disappear before the patient can be discharged as cured. During convalescence the factors predisposing to recurrence of the infection should be corrected.

Prognosis.—MODE OF DEATH.—The disease terminates by sepsis.

MORTALITY.—In Jacob's series of 39 cases of bacteriemia and septicopyemia 15, or 40 per cent, died. In Cabot's series of 8 cases taken from the wards of the Massachusetts General Hospital, 25 per cent died. In the cases of Felty and Keefer the mortality was 32 per cent and in Widal and Fernierre's series, 25 per cent. Bacteriemia and septicopyemia due to the *Bacillus coli* are therefore serious diseases with a high mortality.

The mortality of local infections depends upon the tissue or organ invaded and the virulence of the infection. Primary, uncomplicated colon infection of the urinary tract does not have a high mortality. Appearing as a complication of calculus, prostatic hypertrophy or other pathology, the outlook is serious.

Recovery after infection of the lower urinary tract depends upon the nature of the individual case. Without free drainage of the infected areas the condition tends to become chronic and to persist indefinitely. Reinfections are common. Infections of the pelvis of the kidney are very apt to relapse and become chronic. Renal infections of mild type may recover completely in a few weeks. The more severe lesions, however, heal by scar formation and may leave little renal tissue. Pyonephrosis results in complete destruction of the kidney.

Pathology.—The lesions caused by the colon bacillus vary from a mild inflammatory reaction to abscess formation. Microscopically there is an exudate of lymphocytes or polymorphonuclear leukocytes with serum and eosinophile cells, and the organism can usually be seen in the stained section. The process terminates in sclerosis or scar tissue. According to Mallory, the lesions in general are mild, though acute and intense reactions may occur.

The lesions of the kidney have been fully described by Cabot and Crabtree. In the pelvis the mucous membrane is reddened, granular and dull. Microscopically the mucosa is thickened and the submucosa is infiltrated. Bacilli can be found in the submucosa. Simple pyelonephritis shows a kidney which is slightly enlarged. The capsule is thickened but strips easily and the cut surface is pale. Microscopically the tubules are dilated and hyaline degeneration is present. There is lymphocytic or polymorphonuclear infiltration of the interstitial tissue. The glomeruli are not damaged unless they are situated in the center of an infected area. The process begins in the pyramids and spreads toward the cortex and pelvis. When the infection is more severe the cortex is mottled and the medullary portion shows many yellowish-red or opaque pinhead-sized areas from which bands and streaks extend toward the pyramids. These areas are seen microscopically to be the centers of degeneration and necrosis. True abscess formation in the kidney due to the colon bacillus alone is rarely, if ever, observed. In cases of long duration the pelvis and calices are much dilated and contain dirty purulent urine or, in the case of pyonephrosis, a thick ropy pus. The kidney tissue is diminished in amount and shows areas of scar tissue.

In the liver cholangitis and abscesses result from colon bacillus infection. Microscopically exudation of serum and polymorphonuclear leukocytes with necrosis are seen in the tissues surrounding the ducts. Cirrhosis confined to the periphery of the lobules follows the inflammation.

In the peritoneum the inflammation tends to remain localized and is not of a severe type. Rare cases of chronic peritonitis with dense adhesions and caseating, tubercle-like masses due to the colon bacillus have been observed.

Historical Summary.—The *Bacillus coli* was first cultivated by Emmerich, in 1885, from the feces of cholera patients, and it was cultivated from the feces of healthy infants by Escherich, in 1886. The organism was first observed outside of the intestinal tract by Tavel, who recovered it from the wound of an operation upon the thyroid. During the development of the science of bacteriology the *Bacillus coli* was recovered from various tissues, Rovsing having furnished the most complete early studies on its pathogenicity. The invasion of the blood stream by the *Bacillus coli* was first reported in detail by L. Jacob, in 1909, who observed a series of cases of continued fever and pyemia due to this organism. Except in the case of urinary tract infections, comparatively little study has been devoted to this bacillus as a cause of disease.

BIBLIOGRAPHY

ABT, I. A.: Urinary infection in children. J. Am. M. Ass., 49: 1972–1976, 1907.
ANDREWES, F. W.: A case of malignant endocarditis due to Bacillus coli communis. Tr. Path. Soc. Lond., 53: 39–42, 1902.
AUCHÉ, B.: Abcès intra-dermiques multiples à coli-bacilles chez un nourrison. Compt. rend. Soc. de biol., Par., 63: 130, 1907.
BABLER, E. A.: Colon bacillus infection of operation wound. J. Am. M. Ass., 55: 1519–1520, 1910.
BARBER, W. H. AND DRAPER, J. W.: Renal infection, a further experimental study of its relation to impaired ureteric function. J. Am. M. Ass., 64: 205–210, 1915.
BARNARD, H. L.: Multiple abscesses of the kidney due to acute ascending infection of the normal urinary tract by Bacillus coli communis. Lancet, 2: 1243–1248, 1905.
BASSLER, A.: Innocent colon bacilli in urines. Med. Rec., 82: 20–22, 1912.
BENTLEY, F.: Report of a case of endogenous panophthalmitis due to colon bacillus. Ophth. Rec., 20: 352–354, 1911.
BERNHEIM, A.: Ueber den Befund des Bacterium coli commune in einem Panaritium bei Typhus abdominalis. Centralbl. f. klin. Med., Leipz., 14: 273–276, 1893.
BERNSTEIN, E. P.: Brain abscess due to the Bacillus coli communis. Med. Rec., 85: 249, 1914.
BONNER, W. P.: Acute epididymo-orchitis due to Bacillus coli. Lancet, 2: 996, 1913.
BOX, C. R.: On certain bacterial infections of the urinary tract in childhood. Lancet, 1: 77, 1908.
BOX, C. R., PARDOE, J. AND PARKINSON, J. P.: Discussion on infections of the urinary tract by bacillus coli in infancy and childhood. Brit. M. J., 2: 1128–1135, 1910.
BRISCOE, J. C.: On certain B. coli infections. Lancet, 2: 1269–1273, 1909.
CABOT, H. AND CRABTREE, E. G.: The etiology and pathology of non-tuberculous renal infections. Surg., Gynec. & Obst., 23: 495–537, 1916.
COLEMAN, W. AND HASTINGS, T. W.: Bacillus coli communis: the cause of an infection clinically identical with typhoid fever. Am. J. M. Sc., 137: 199–215, 1909.
CRABTREE, E. G.: A case of thrombophlebitis of the veins of the cord associated with colon bacillus infection of the epididymis. Boston M. & S. J., 173: 705, 1915.

CRABTREE, E. G. : A method of demonstrating bacteria in urine by means of centrifuge, with some observations on the relative value of examinations by culture or stained sediment. Surg., Gynec. & Obst., 22 : 221–224, 1916.

CULVER, H., HERROLD, R. D. AND PHIFER, F. M. : Renal infections; a clinical and bacteriologic study. J. Am. M. Ass., 70 : 1444–1448, 1918.

DAVID, V. C. : Ascending urinary infections; an experimental study. Surg., Gynec. & Obst., 26 : 159–170, 1918.

————: Peritonitis; an experimental study. Surg., Gynec. & Obst., 45 : 287–293, 1927.

DOUGHERTY, D. S.: Colon bacillus infection in middle-ear disease. New York M. J. (etc.), 100 : 1163–1165, 1914.

DRAPER, G. : A case of intrahepatic biliary calculi with fatal colon bacillus pyemia. Proc. Path. Soc. Phila., 13 : 16–20, 1910.

DUDGEON, L. L. AND SARGENT, P. W. G. : The Bacteriology of Peritonitis. A. Constable & Co., London, 1905.

ENRIGHT, J. I. AND BAHR, P. H. : On a pyaemia due to organisms of the Bacillus coli group occurring in Turkish soldiers. Lancet, 2 : 585–587, 1918.

FELTY, A. R. AND KEEFER, C. S. : Bacillus coli sepsis; a clinical study of twenty-eight cases of blood stream infection by the colon bacillus. J. Am. M. Ass., 82 : 1430–1433, 1924.

FLEXNER, S. : A statistical and experimental study of terminal infections. J. Exper. Med., 1 : 559–576, 1896.

GERAGHTY, J. T. : The treatment of chronic pyelitis. J. Am. M. Ass., 63 : 2211–2214, 1914.

HARTWICH, W. : Bacterium coli im Liquor cerebrospinalis. Berl. klin. Wchnschr., 48 : 795, 1911.

HELMHOLZ, H. F. : The production of local renal lesions in rabbits by intravenous injections of certain strains of B. coli. J. Infect. Dis., 41 : 448–456, 1927.

HITSCHMANN, F. AND MICHEL, E. : Eine vom Bacterium coli com. hervorgerufene Endocarditis und Pyämie. Wien. klin. Wchnschr., 9 : 341–347, 1896.

HOUSTON, T. AND THOMSON, W. W. D. : Bacillus coli as a cause of septic onychia. Lancet, 1 : 1461, 1914.

HOWLAND, J. AND HOOBLER, B. R. : The use of bacterial vaccines in children's diseases. Tr. Cong. Am. Phys. & Surg., 18 : 369–375, 1910.

JACKSON, H. : Malignant endocarditis, an analysis of fifty-nine cases. Med. & Surg. Reports, Boston City Hosp., 11 series, 67–82, 1900.

JACOB, L. : Ueber Allgemeininfektion durch Bacterium coli commune. Deutsche Arch. f. klin. Med., Leipz., 97 : 303–347, 1909.

KELLY, A. O. J.: Infections of the biliary tract. In : Modern Medicine, Its Theory and Practice. Edited by William Osler, Lea & Febiger, Philadelphia & New York, 1913–15.

KELLY, H. A. AND HURDON, E. : The Vermiform Appendix and Its Diseases. W. B. Saunders & Co., Philadelphia & London, 1905.

KENDAL, A. I. : Bacteriology, General, Pathological and Intestinal. Lea & Febiger, Philadelphia & New York, 1916 : Bacillus coli, p. 253; Gastro-intestinal bacteriology, p. 580.

KOLL, I. S.: The experimental effect of the colon bacillus on the kidney. J. Am. M. Ass., 64 : 297–299, 1915.

KRETSCHMER, H. L. AND GAARDE, F. W. : The treatment of chronic colon bacillus pyelitis by pelvic lavage. J. Am. M. Ass., 66 : 2052, 1916.

LOW, H. C. : Bacteriological report of one hundred cases of acute appendicitis. Med. & Surg. Reports, Boston City Hosp., 11 series, 173–178, 1900.

MACGOWAN, G. : Hematogenous kidney infections. J. Am. M. Ass., 64 : 226–231, 1915.

MACWATTERS, J. C. : Vaccine therapy in general practice. Practitioner, 83 : 327–333, 1909.

MCPHERSON, R. AND LOSEE, J. R. : Report of a severe case of pyelonephritis with a colon bacillus infection of the blood, complicating pregnancy. Bull. Lying-in Hosp. N. Y., 11 : 100–104, 1917.

MCWILLIAMS, C. A. : Infections by the bacterium coli commune with particular reference to the urinary tract. Med. Rec., 70 : 7–13, 1906.

MILNER, C. E. H. : Acute septic meningitis due to B. coli following skull wound. Brit. M. J., 2 : 254, 1915.

MOSENTHAL, H. O. : The symptoms and treatment of retention of waste products in nephritis. Med. Clin. N. Am., 3 : 353–377, 1919–20.

NEAL, J. B. : Meningitis caused by bacilli of the colon group. Am. J. M. Sc., 172 : 740–748, 1926.

NILES, W. L. AND MEARA, F. S. : Lobar pneumonia of micrococcus catarrhalis and bacillus coli communis origin. Am. J. M. Sc., 142 : 803–810, 1911.

PANTON, P. N. AND TIDY, H. L. : A note on the occurrence of the colon bacillus in the blood. Lancet, 2 : 1500, 1912.

PARK, W. H. AND WILLIAMS, A. W. : Bacillus coli communis. In : Pathogenic Micro-organisms, Including Bacteria and Protozoa. 8 ed., Lea & Febiger, New York & Philadelphia, 1924.

PEARCE, N. O. : Winckel's disease. In : Abt's Pediatrics. W. B. Saunders & Co., Philadelphia & London, 2 : 385, 1925.

PEARCE, R. M. : The bacteriology of lobar and lobular pneumonia; various infections due to the diplococcus lanceolatus. Boston M. & S. J., 137 : 561–564, 1897.

PEARSON, G. H. : A case of meningitis in which the bacillus coli communis was obtained from the cerebrospinal fluid. Lancet, 1 : 722, 1912.

POTTER, A. : A bullous dermatitis caused by the colon bacillus. J. Cutan. Dis. incl. Syph., 33 : 272–278, 1915.

REYNOLDS, W. S. : Epididymitis due to the colon bacillus. Am. J. M. Sc., 146 : 72–77, 1913.

RICHARDS, L. : Abscess of the brain due to colon bacillus with pneumocephalus. Arch. Otolaryng., 6 : 36–42, 1927.

RITCHIE, J. : A case of acute pyelitis in infancy. Scottish M. & S. J., 11 : 1–6, 1902.

ROBERTS, J. R. : Two forms of infection of the kidney. Indian M. Gaz., 62 : 75–76, 1927.

ROLLESTON, H. D. : Discussion on the pathogenic effect of B. coli. Brit. M. J., 2 : 1186–1192, 1911.

ROVSING, T. : Colinfektionen i urinvejene, dens pathogenese kliniske billeder og behandling. trans. in : Cong. internat. (xvi) de med. 1909, Budapest, sect. 14 : 11–24, 1910.

ROVSING, T.: Om vakcinationsbehandling of colinfektion i urinorganerne. Hosp.-Tid., Købonh., 5. R., 2 : 569–583, 1909.

SALLE : Le pseudo-rheumatisme dysénterique et ses déterminations articulaires et abarticulaires ; arthropathies, myalgies et conjunctivites ; leur nature bacillaire. Bull. et mém. Soc. méd. de hôp. de Par., 3. s., 20 : 359–374, 1903.

SCHOLL, A. J.: Cohabitation, colon bacillary, urinary tract infection. J. Am. M. Ass., 87 : 1794–1799, 1926.

VON SCHRÖTTER, H. AND WEINBERGER, M.: Zur Kenntnis der Kolibazillose der Respirationsorgane. Wien. klin. Wchnschr., 21 : 505–510, 1908.

SEVESTRE AND GASTON : Arthritis due to bacillus coli. Tr. M. Soc. Lond., 24 : 26–27, 1901.

SISON, A. B. M. AND CRUZ, P. V.: An unusual case of colibacillemia. J. Philippine Islands M. Ass., 6 : 294–298, 1926.

SITTMANN AND BARLOW: Ueber einen Befund von Bacterium coli commune im lebenden Blute. Deutsches Arch. f. klin. Med., Leipz., 52 : 250–258, 1893–94.

STEINBERG, B. AND GOLDBLATT, H.: Studies on peritonitis ; passage of bacteria from peritoneal cavity into lymph and blood. Arch. Int. Med., 39 : 449–455, 1927.

STONE, W. J.: Bacterial therapy in lesions produced by the bacillus coli communis. In : Forchheimer's Therapeusis of Internal Diseases. D. Appleton & Co., New York & London, 5 : 236, 1914.

SWEET, J. E. AND STEWART, L. F.: The ascending infection of the kidneys. Surg., Gynec. & Obst., 18 : 460–469, 1914.

THOMAS, G. J.: Clinical review of 240 cases of non-surgical infection of the kidneys and ureters. Collected Papers Mayo Clinic, Philadelphia & London, 7 : 336–345, 1915.

THOMSON, J.: On acute pyelitis due to Bacillus coli as it occurs in infancy : with pathological reports on two fatal cases of pyelonephritis, by S. McDonald. Quart. J. Med., 3 : 251–268, 1909–10.

——— : Notes on the symptoms and treatment of acute pyelitis in infants. Scottish M. & S. J., 11 : 7–15, 1902.

THOMSON, W. H.: Acute, subacute, and chronic infection of the kidneys and of other organs by the Bacillus coli. Med. Rec., 77 : 907–910, 1910.

WELCH, W. H.: The bacillus coli communis ; the conditions of its invasion of the human body, and its pathogenic properties. Med. News, 59 : 669–671, 1891.

WHALE, H.: A case of spasmodic rhinorrhea cured by irrigation of the maxillary antra, which was infected by B. coli. Lancet, 2 : 1012, 1912.

WIDAL, F. AND LEMIERRE, A.: Colibacillose. Nouveau Traité de Médecine. Fascicule III, Masson et Cie, Paris, p. 233, 1924.

——— : Septicémies colibacillaires. Gaz. d. hôp., Par., 77 : 801–805, 1904.

WIDAL, F., LEMIERRE, A. AND BRODIN, P.: Quatre cas de septicémie coli-bacillaire. Bull. et mém. Soc. méd. d. hôp. de Par., 3. s., 44 : 963–975, 1920.

FOR further literature upon infection of the urinary tract due to *Bacillus coli* the reader is referred to the following :

THE Journal of Urology. The Williams & Wilkins Co., Baltimore, Vol. X to XX.

CABOT, H.: Modern Urology in Original Contributions by American Authors. 2 ed., Lea & Febiger, Philadelphia & New York, 1924.

LOWSLEY, O. W. AND KIRWIN, T. J.: A Text-book of Urology. Lea & Febiger, Philadelphia & New York, 1926.

YOUNG, H. H. AND DAVIS, D. M.: Young's Practice of Urology. W. B. Saunders & Co., Philadelphia & London, 1926.

CHAPTER FORTY

MEGACOLON

By Henry J. Bartle, B.S., M.D.

Synonyms.—Hirschsprung's disease; Myà's disease; giant colon; congenital enlargement of the colon; idiopathic hypertrophy of the colon; congenital idiopathic dilatation of the colon; dolichocolon; pelvirectal achalasia; megalocolon.

Definition.—A disease beginning in intra-uterine life, or in the first year of life when its symptoms usually manifest themselves, characterized by enlargement (dilatation with hypertrophy) of the pelvic colon, the sigmoid, and possibly the descending colon as well. At times the transverse colon and the ascending colon may show involvement rarely alone or, more commonly, as an extension of the process from the lower bowel.

True megacolon is not to be confused with the *acquired* form of hypertrophy of the colon resulting from such numerous long-standing obstructive processes in and about the lower colon as hypertrophy and fixation of Houston's rectal valves, stenosis and aplasia and segmental spasm of the rectum and lower sigmoid, extra-rectal tumors and inflammatory changes of the pelvic organs leading to the formation of bands and adhesions, and tending to produce a chronic volvulus.

Incidence.—In 1900 Fenwick,[1] reviewing 30,000 necropsies in the London Hospital for Sick Children, found about 1 case in 10,000. With such a vast amount of material at his disposal, it would seem that this incidence should hold even today for British children and be the same for those of other nationalities. Three males are afflicted to each female.

History.—In the seventeenth century one Fredrick Ruysch, as recorded by Jayle,[2] is said to be the first physician describing congenital idiopathic dilatation of the colon in a girl five years of age. Finney,[3] in his excellent review of the literature, notes that Parry reported a case in 1825, Billard one in 1829, Ebers one in 1836, and von Ammon two cases in 1842—one a child who died shortly after birth, the other a fetus of about seven months. In America, Lewitt in 1867 and Jacobi in 1870 each reported a case. Sixteen years later, in May 1886, Hughes[4] recited the autopsy findings of a boy of three years—the colon had a capacity of fourteen pints (7,000 cc.), the gut wall was hypertrophied and the bowel, while dilated throughout, had a diameter of four inches in the sigmoid portion.

Abroad, Hirschsprung[5] in 1888 published his monograph which bears the date of 1886 as the time of writing. He reported two cases which, during life, presented symptoms of constipation and meteorism without signs of stenosis of the gut tract. His first patient died at the age of eleven months of progressive cachexia, his second died at seven months of multiple ulcerations of the colon. Autopsy in each instance revealed dilatation of the colon with hypertrophy of the bowel musculature. Later he added two more cases.

Again in America, Formad[6] in 1891 reported the condition in a man, aged twenty-nine years, in whom the colon was the size of a cow's and contained forty pounds of contents. The colon itself, weighing a little less than seven pounds, showed a progressive enlargement in diameter from the cecum downward with hypertrophy of the musculature throughout. Formad further cited one case of Gruber with a sigmoid four to five inches in diameter; one of Peacock in which the colon had a capacity of fifteen quarts (15,000 cc.) and a sigmoid diameter of six to eight inches; one of Little and Galloway in which the diameter of the transverse colon was six inches and that of the sigmoid varied from twelve to twenty inches; and one remarkable case of Cruveilhier in which the colon was the size of a horse's great gut with an incredible diameter of fourteen inches. When in 1894 Myà[7] added two cases, his review of the literature showed a total of nine cases—quite obviously incorrect, as this short history shows. Less than a decade and a half later, Finney,[3] in 1908, making an exhaustive review of the published cases, found two hundred and six in all.

Following this, the literature rapidly becomes fairly replete with case reports—due no doubt both to the education of the physician with regard to the symptoms of this disease as well as to the x-ray having become utilizable in helping him to make his diagnosis. For example, in 1913, Neugebauer[8] reported a series of one hundred and sixty-nine cases, in seventy-four of which the sigmoid alone was involved. About the same time, Barrington-Ward[9] did necropsies on nineteen patients; Löwenstein[10] had already reported forty-four cases treated surgically, together with fifty-nine treated medically; and Terry[11] had reported one hundred and ten surgically treated cases. It is understood, of course, that many of these case reports in a measure overlapped. That is, each writer cited many of the cases which already had played a part in previous statistical studies. Nonetheless, at the turn of the twentieth century, and with the advent of the x-ray as an aid to diagnosis with the bismuth (now barium) enema, the number of reported cases quickly increased.

For further historical facts see the monographs of both Finney[3] and Bartle.[12]

Etiology.—Quite naturally the cause of this unusual dilatation, lengthening and hypertrophy of the musculature of the colon was obscure when the condition was first studied by the early investigators. And just as naturally many bizarre theories were bound to arise to explain its occurrence in the first year of life, or even during intra-uterine life. It is known, for example, that an acute obstructive process will lead to dilatation and thinning of the colon, and that a chronic obstruction will eventuate in dilatation *with hypertrophy*—the acquired form of megacolon. So, basing their conclusions on these well-established facts, the earlier students tried to fit the pathologic condition to the obstructing theory. As a result we have, today, two opposing schools of thought regarding etiology:

1. MECHANICAL.—Because of extreme mobilization of the sigmoid with an unusual length of mesosigmoid, or because of a too great length of the tube itself, or because of actual blocking of the fecal current (from atresia of the anal canal, rectum or sigmoid, from imperforate anus of the partial type, from hypertrophied Houston's valves or overdevelopment of O'Beirne's sphincter), it was thought that there followed torsion of the sigmoid—that the drag of a sigmoid overladen with meconium acted as a valve at the rectosigmoidal junction to prevent its own emptying. Further, for the sake of textbook completeness of thought, neuromuscular defects producing paralysis of a segment of gut, and reflex spasm due to anal fissure, must be listed as possible causes. So excellent a clinician as Brennemann [13] wonders still, with a certain justification, if idiopathic megacolon (but certainly the acquired form of megacolon) may not be "due to a lack of complete fusion of the mesenteron and the proctodeum" resulting in "a tight fibrous obstruction just a little above the sphincter ani." But, in the light of our present knowledge of both physiology and pathology, it would seem that all these mechanical theories of etiology must give way to the more recent neurogenic theory.

2. NEUROGENIC.—Many physiologists, clinicians and surgeons [12, 14-16] are now agreed that a congenital imbalance exists between the colonic parasympathetic innervation on the one hand and the sympathetic impulses on the other. Developmentally there is either a lessening of the parasympathetic control (the vagopelvic, bulbosacral or autonomic) or else an increase of the sympathetic innervation of both the bowel and internal anal sphincter. Indeed, it is quite possible that improper response of this sphincter to nervous stimulation may be the sole cause initiating the change of colon away from the normal—dilatation, lengthening, hypertrophy.

It must be remembered, first, that the sympathetic impulses cause the bowel to remain in a state of what Sherrington [17] refers to as "plastic tonus" or the "posture of rest"; and that, further, they maintain the normal tonicity of the internal anal sphincter. Opposed to this action, the parasympathetic impulses cause the bowel musculature to contract in an effort at emptying, the while relaxing the sphincter. It follows then, that, if the neurogenic mechanism of this sphincter is out of balance even before birth to the extent that it cannot well relax, we should expect to find the colon undergoing a compensatory hypertrophy—just as it does in acquired megacolon resulting from any kind of obstruction.

Earlier writers, if they mentioned the anus at all, pronounced it "normal at autopsy"; but more recent observers find the *living* internal anal sphincter markedly hypertonic.[12, 18-22] What causes this imbalance, other than dysendocrinism, constitutes one of the problems still facing us. And that this imbalance of nerve control between anus and colon is not confined to the bowel alone, is evidenced by the coincidental finding of dilatation and hypertrophy of both the urinary bladder and the ureters similar to that of the colon in two patients as reported by Adamson [23] and Learmonth.[24]

It would seem that Robertson and Kernohan,[25] in their recent studies of sections of the colon, may have found for us the true nature of this imbalance. Keeping in mind the observation of Lendrum on esophagi in which cardiospasm existed without any evidences of obstruction or spasm at the cardiac sphincter, and in which a study of the plexuses of nerve structures in the esophageal wall revealed definite degenerative phenomena, they suspected that in megacolon the plexuses of Meissner and Auerbach might present similar signs of degeneration accounting for the failure of the propulsive mechanism. Let me quote from their important paper. ''Our microscopic examination of the colon . . . consisting of study of paraffin sections stained with hematoxylin and eosin, Gros-Bielschowsky silver impregnation and cresyl violet, confirmed this suspicion. The ganglion cells and fibers of the plexus of Auerbach were definitely smaller than normal, vacuolated, and the ganglion cells were absent or very imperfectly formed. . . . To test the validity of this hypothesis we studied the walls of the colon in several cases of ulcerative colitis. In this disease there is over-activity and marked hypertrophy of the muscular elements. Theoretically, the nerve plexuses in the walls also should be hypertrophied and the ganglion cells and fibers should be prominent and even increased in number. This proved to be true in the two cases we have studied.'' A valuable contribution, but it is difficult to reconcile the almost immediate recovery of function of the bowel after sympathectomy with the evidences of denervation which they found.

Symptomatology.—There are three cardinal signs and symptoms: (1) a history of constipation from birth, with either a laxative or enema habit; (2) abdominal distention; (3) x-ray evidence with the barium enema of dilatation of the sigmoid or other portions of the colon.

There is a mixed array of concomitant symptoms usually present: (4) muscular atrophy of the abdominal wall, allowing coils of bowel undergoing peristaltic activity to be seen; (5) weakness of the extremities; (6) loss of subcutaneous fat from inanition; (7) toxic manifestations—headache, so-called bilious attacks, nausea, vomiting, chilliness, prostration, stupor and lassitude with irregular fever; (8) anemia more pronounced as the age increases; (9) lack of growth and development; (10) disturbed sleep, restlessness, irritability and general unhappiness; (11) failure to make the necessary effort to defecate—''Will sit for hours on the pot''; (12) stool following an enema may be formed and only thumb-size—indeed, not the massive balls and sausages the textbooks would have us believe; (13) palpation of the left lower quadrant may reveal a large mass, but if the mother has been giving careful attention to the child the bowel may be found relatively empty even by digital examination through the anus; (14) fecal impaction as stressed by the older textbooks is not necessarily present, but always the bowel is distended with gas and is readily compressible without the production of pain; (15) hypertonicity of the anus—a neglected sign in many of the articles on megacolon.

The author wishes to predict that if the anus is examined on the sickbed, rather than on the postmortem table, spasm or spasticity of the anus, and possibly of O'Beirne's sphincter as well, may well become a fourth cardinal sign.

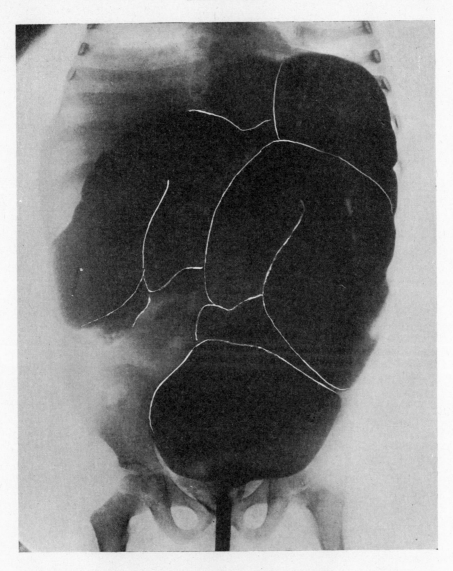

Fig. 1.—Barium enema filling entire colon as far as cecum. Note capacity of gut, refolding, absence of haustra, as well as disproportion in size as compared with the pelvic bones in this child of four years.

Diagnosis.—Today, with the x-ray so readily available on every hand, the doctor should not be long in doubt as to what is wrong with his patient. The barium enema alone is only needed to make the diagnosis glaringly self-evident. However, the trick is to teach the practitioner to call upon his x-ray confrere for help. But, once he has done so, he need consider no further the possibilities of the child's having

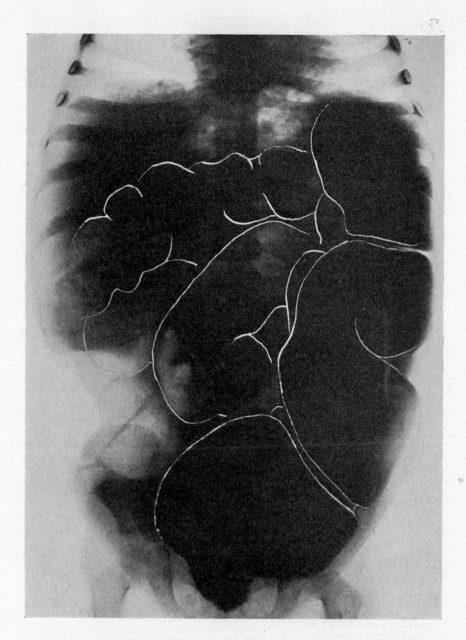

FIG. 2.—Only rectum, sigmoid and ascending portions of the colon are distended by barium enema which did not go beyond splenic flexure. Note refolding, absence of haustral markings, and enormous capacity of gut. Age four years.

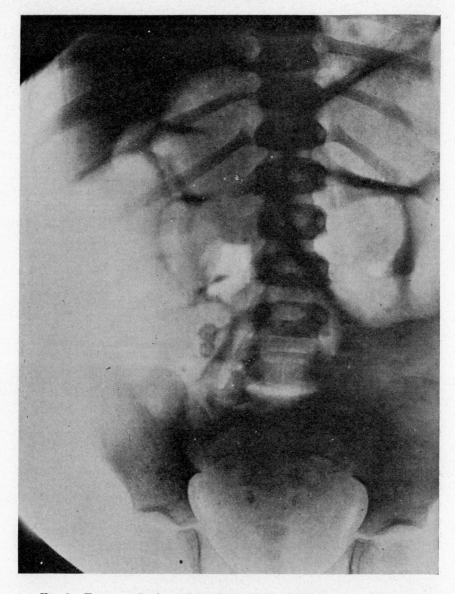

Fig. 3.—Exposure showing colon under natural conditions before barium enema was administered. Note distention of bowel with flatus, absence of haustral markings, and refolding of gut. Age four years.

obstinate constipation and a potbelly from rickets or tuberculous peritonitis. Volvulus, regional ileitis, intra-abdominal cyst, carcinoma, sarcoma and other obstructive lesions are readily ruled out by x-ray.

As to the possibility of sympathectomy or ganglionectomy helping the child, spinal anesthesia, as recommended by Van Buskirk[26] and Cas-

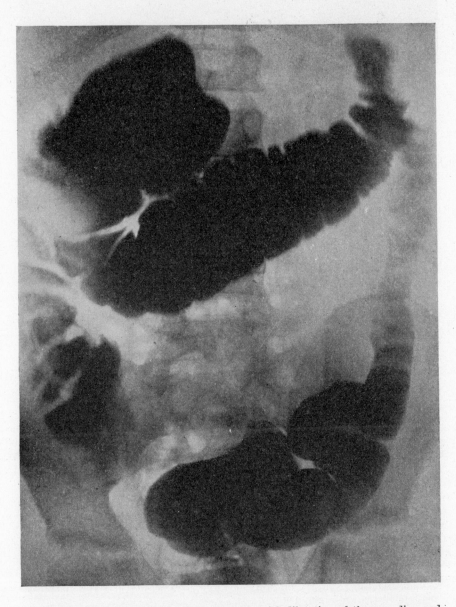

Fig. 4.—From a patient aged twelve years, with dilatation of the ascending and
the right half of the transverse portions of the colon. The descending portion, as
well as the sigmoid and rectum, is normal as to size and tone. Comparison should be
made between the size of this sigmoid in a child of twelve years and that in the
roentgenograms of a patient aged four years.

sidy and Salkin,[27] and others, should be tried. By means of it, having suppressed the action of the sympathetics for a time, a resumption of bowel movements spells success for the operation.

Treatment.—It will have been noted that practically all the early descriptions of megacolon, emanating as they did from the postmortem table, had to do with theorizing as to the cause of the morbid anatomy. Little was said concerning treatment because, for the most part, the patients had already passed through the valley of death. But early in this century, with the coming of the x-ray and later the barium enema, ante-mortem diagnoses began to be made together with attempts at treatment. And, as is common with most little-understood pathologic conditions, the surgeons, seeing an enormous bowel, took up the scalpel and rushed into the belly to remove it—as well as many of their patients for all time. Now, having acquired a comprehensive knowledge of the etiology of megacolon, they mass their attack against the *cause*, disregard the dilated and hypertrophied bowel, and cure or vastly improve the condition, seeing their patients live on. Indeed, because of the study and suggestions made by physiologists and clinicians, together with improvements in surgical technic, the mortality rate has been reduced from fully 50 per cent to almost nil. Without either surgical or medical management the mortality rate is said to be 85 per cent.[28, 29]

There are two plans of treatment—conservative or medical, and radical or surgical. But we should keep in mind, and accept, the premise that nothing short of surgery will ever bring about a complete and permanent cure.

1. CONSERVATIVE OR MEDICAL TREATMENT.—Until the little patient can be brought to such a state of health as to safely withstand the operation, conservative medical measures must be employed. Foremost, the devitalizing intoxication from food decomposition in the colon must be kept at a minimum by removing from the **diet** all foods containing animal protein. The exception to this rule is milk and such products of milk as cheese, butter and cream. Even milk may have to be withdrawn if it causes excessive distention. As long as it remains a part of the dietary it should carry lactose and living acidophilus bacilli into the colon—again provided these do not increase the distention, thereby causing increased discomfort. Although many clinicians warn against an excess of carbohydrates, the author has found sweets and starches to be well borne. They serve best in building up the caloric requirements of these impoverished little patients. On the other hand, fats are not readily tolerated by children. The normal child dislikes them, the sick child loathes them. And it must be remembered that an excess beyond the power of the pancreatic juice to digest them, will only lead to further bowel discomfort because of the formation of irritating fatty acids.

To procure sufficient bowel action **laxatives** must be administered. Sodium sulphate in ½-dram (2 Gm.) doses night and morning is possibly the best saline aperient because of its tonic action on the bowel musculature as contrasted with the relaxing effect of magnesium sulphate. In the author's experience magnesium sulphate is not well borne. Nor are the many preparations of mineral oil. Lubricants are not indicated. Further, the likelihood of their impairing assimilation of the much-needed pabulum from the small bowel is too great. This risk cannot be taken, for these patients are already far below normal in growth and nutrition, weight and strength. They must be built up with sufficient food, with olive and cod liver oil, with vitamins, with calcium and phosphorus, with arsenic and iron.

Sheldon, Kern and Hakansson [30] report encouraging results from parathormone administration. Ballard [31] recommends diathermy, pituitrin, eserine (physostigmine) and dilatation of the anal sphincter. To these Adson [32] adds acetylcholine. Klingman,[33] who has observed seven cases, feels that atropine sulphate is useful but too toxic. Therefore, he tried syntropan for its inhibiting effect on the anal sphincter without lessening peristalsis, and found that five of his patients responded satisfactorily. Also, he found that a physostigmine-like preparation—prostigmin—gave good bowel action on a gradually diminishing dosage. Berger [34] recommends 10-drop doses of pituitrin by oral administration four times a day. Reeves and Harrison [35] have used a pancreatic tissue extract by intramuscular injection, and found it to be of definite value, in that its action is that of epinephrine-antagonist, stimulating the parasympathetics and producing a more normal rhythm of the intestine. The author has observed marked improvement in bowel function from the wearing of an elastic abdominal support and from the use of sinewave electricity with massage. Friedell [18] recommends irrigation of the colon with gallons of hot saline solution (115° F.) for from thirty to ninety minutes each day.

Indeed, the simple enema should be given daily rather than to overload the patient with laxatives. Normal salt solution alone, or with 5 to 10 per cent glucose, or with 5 per cent sodium bicarbonate, or with 1 to 5 per cent sodium sulphate, may be used—but not soapsuds.

Assuming that our conception of a relative overactivity of the sympathetic innervation is correct, then it follows that adrenalin is decidedly contraindicated because of its stimulating effect on the sympathetic side. Conversely, belladonna the gastro-enterologist's sheet anchor in matters of sphincteric spasms, immediately suggests itself as a brake on "the brakes of the gastro-intestinal track." But it has been found useless by all who have given it a fair trial. It seems not to depress the sympathetics in the lower reaches of the gut tube.

Lastly, keeping in mind the fact that the parasympathetics may need to be urged to further activity—if the sympathetics cannot be readily suppressed—the administration of **nux vomica** seems to be a rational form of treatment. And it is, in ascending doses of the tincture to the point of tolerance with each meal. However, if the child's rest is disturbed through night-terrors or restlessness, the evening dose should be reduced to one-half or even one-quarter that of the former doses. Its action seems to be enhanced by the addition of **arsenic,** preferably in the form of Fowler's solution well diluted.

2. RADICAL OR SURGICAL TREATMENT.—In little more than a decade a vast change has occurred in the surgical attack on megacolon. The simplest of all operations—that of anal divulsion and even anal incision —was soon found to be useless. The anus returned to its original state of spasticity within a few months. Also, colostomy, colectomy, colon plication, colopexy, ileosigmoidostomy and appendicostomy have very properly been discarded. They were brutal operations and carried a high mortality—25 to 50 per cent under the best surgeons, and much higher under

the tyro. The patients requiring these devitalizing operations were not only small—from one to six years of age—but also extremely frail. No wonder they succumbed in such large numbers.

Faced with the problem of providing a safe and at the same time a curative surgical measure, provided skilled neurosurgeons would attempt it, the author,[12] in a paper read in May 1925 and published in January 1926, proposed the operation of ramisection—severance of the white rami of the lumbar sympathetic cord. For spastic paralysis of the extremities Royle and Hunter [36] had relieved the spasticity by removing the sympathetic nerve supply of the limb. Therefore, the author conjectured, a similar operation should relieve the spasticity of the bowel.

In just a year later, January 1927, came the report of Wade and Royle [37] from Australia of this operation specifically directed against megacolon. Having severed the first, second, third and fourth white rami, they had gone a step beyond the original proposal by cutting the sympathetic cord below the fourth ramus. The first patient operated upon by the new method—a boy of ten years—made a rapid and complete recovery. Following this, in September 1928, Judd and Adson,[38] having added ganglionectomy to ramisection, reported two cases operated upon in June and December, 1927, with good bowel function resulting. In one of these, who was followed closely with frequent x-ray observations, the capacity of the colon was reduced 50 per cent within six months.

In 1934 Adson,[39] reporting his statistics for ramisection combined with ganglionectomy, unilateral as well as bilateral, cites eleven cases. One, a very poor surgical risk, died of shock on the table, five were 100 per cent cured, the other five were from 50 to 85 per cent improved. Denk,[40] quoting the statistics of Gask and Ross, reported fifty-one cases gathered from the literature in 1936. Of these fifty-one patients, twenty-four were cured and seventeen improved. The fate of the ten others is not recorded, nor is any mention made of even one fatality.

In his 1937 report, Adson [32] divides his thirty megacolon patients into twenty-two with Hirschsprung's disease and eight with dilated colon. All were subjected to either extensive splanchnic and lumbar resection, or to limited sympathectomies. Ages varied from six months to nineteen years. Twenty-five of the patients were under six years. One patient in whom the entire colon was involved failed to obtain relief from bilateral lumbar sympathectomy, ganglionectomy and resection of the presacral nerves, but was helped by colectomy. Children whose descending colon and sigmoid were involved obtained excellent results. Those in whom the disease had extended to include the left half of the transverse colon obtained results from good to fair. No deaths are recorded.

Bates,[41] and Launay and Aubigne [42] report satisfactory results following sympathectomy. De Takáts [16] says: "So far, more than one hundred patients have been operated on for megacolon: of these, two have died. . . . In our own series of cases we have performed lumbar sympathectomy on forty-eight patients and have lost one—a middle-aged man with Buerger's disease, who had coronary thrombosis on the fifth postoperative day."

Prognosis.—Since the inauguration of sympathectomy as the best form of treatment to relieve—in fact, cure—the symptoms of megacolon, the mortality rate may be given as 2 per cent, and the curative rate as well up to 75 per cent. Without any treatment whatsoever, the mortality varies in direct proportion to the age—few patients live to reach manhood or womanhood. With medical treatment alone, the mortality is said to be from 70 to 85 per cent before the twenty-first year. With the old method of approach—colectomy, etc.—the mortality rate was well above 50 per cent, and few of the surviving patients were actually cured. Finney,[3] commenting on the surgical and medical statistics available thirty years ago, concluded that not only was the surgical mortality rate two-thirds that of the medical, but that, as bad as it was, the surgical recovery rate was three times as great as that following the conservative form of treatment.

Granted, then, that the operation of lumbar ramisection combined with ganglionectomy, and possibly with presacral sympathetic cord resection for the extensively involved patient, is a rational procedure insofar as mortality and curative statistics are concerned, what, we should ask, are the by-effects? What happens after not only these colons but other organs as well have been deprived of their sympathetic innervations? In answer to this query Rankin [43] says: "There are certain postoperative changes such as vasodilatation in the lower extremities and in the organs robbed of their sympathetic nerve supply, which have not proved .detrimental and may be disregarded. In the extirpation of the presacral nerve in man there is a paralysis of the mechanism of ejaculation of seminal and prostatic fluid, but no disturbances of libido and potency. There is no effect on the sexual organs of women after resection of the sympathetic nerves." He also points out that either five or six years of age is the optimum time for operation because of the increased safety factors in young individuals and, in addition, because the older patients apparently give less satisfactory end-results after operation. Adson [32] voices the same view in writing of the sequelae of lumbar, intermesenteric or presacral sympathectomies, noting the flushing of the lower abdomen and thighs and legs, increased skin temperature and loss of sweating function. But he stressed the point that, with loss of the ejaculatory power, following presacral resection, sterility of the male when he reaches the age of puberty is bound to result.

However, through this operation, some of these sad little patients may be helped sufficiently to find life a pleasure rather than a burden. As well, a load will have been lifted from the shoulders of their parents. And, although a complete cure be not always effected, at least some improvement has been brought about—the ability of the patient to *live* and to be a useful citizen has been enhanced.

Pathology.—Approximately 33 per cent of all cases show involvement of the sigmoid portion of the colon alone, which may have a diameter many times its normal size and be greatly lengthened so that it folds and refolds upon itself, filling the pelvis and greater part of the abdomen and crowding the small intestines up under the liver, stomach and spleen. In very few cases is the whole colon involved. Rarely are the cecum and rectum enlarged. The external coat of longitudinal fibers which in the normal colon constitute the longitudinal bands are either absent or else poorly defined. The middle coat of circular fibers is overdeveloped—hypertrophied. The inner coat of muscular tissue may be of normal thickness, as may the mucosa; but this latter usually showns signs of chronic inflammatory changes such as hypertrophy, focal necrosis ranging from minute fissures to large ulcerated areas extending down through the muscular layers and even penetrating the serosa. If there is a great deal of fecal material within the bowel when the abdomen is opened, the serosa will be found blanched, due to the pressure on the mesenteric vessels which are long and tortuous within an unusually lengthy mesocolon. The lymph glands may be found hard and cystic in the presence of chronic lymphangitis as is evidenced by the thickened mesocolon.

This whole pathologic process is very probably a progressive one in that, as the patient's age increases, more and more of the proximal colon undergoes changes. Fischer,[44] after total colectomy, has observed the ileum undergoing dilatation and hypertrophy.

Microscopically there are but few enlightening reports other than that of Robertson and Kernohan,[25] to which reference has already been made under Etiology (q.v.).

REFERENCES

1. Fenwick, W. S.: Brit. M. J., 2: 564, 1900.
2. Jayle, F.: Presse méd., 17: 803, 1909.
3. Finney, J. M. I.: Surg., Gynec. & Obst., 6: 6, 1908.
4. Hughes, W. E.: Trans. Philadelphia Path. Soc., 13: 40, 1887.
5. Hirschsprung: Jahrb. f. Kinderh., 27: 1, 1888.
6. Formad, H. F.: Trans. Philadelphia Path. Soc., 16: 23, 1891–1893.
7. Myà, G.: Rev. mens. d. mal. de l'enf., 12: 629, 1894.
8. Neugebauer: Ergebn. d. Chir. u. Orthop., 17: 598, 1913.
9. Barrington-Ward: Brit. J. Surg., 1: 345, 1913–1914.
10. Löwenstein: Centralbl. f. allg. Path. u. path. Anat., 18: 929, 1907.
11. Terry, W. J.: J. Am. M. Ass., 57: 731, 1911.
12. Bartle, H. J.: Am. J. M. Sc., 171: 67, 1926.
13. Brennemann, J.: Am. J. Dis. Child., 55: 1350, 1938.
14. Adson, A. W.: Ann. Int. Med., 6: 1044, 1933. Surgery, 1: 859, 1937.
15. Hershey, J. H. and McCaughan, J. M.: J. Missouri M. A., 13: 413, 1934.
16. de Takáts, G.: Am. J. Dis. Child., 55: 1348, 1938.
17. Sherrington, C. S.: Proc. Roy. Soc. London, 40: 411, 1896. Quart. J. Exper. Physiol., 2: 109, 1909. Brain, 38: 191, 1915.
18. Friedell, A.: Minnesota Med., 21: 175, 1938.
19. Stabins, S. J., Morton, J. J. and Scott, W. J. M.: Am. J. Surg., 27: 107, 1935.
20. Bonar, B. E.: Am. J. Dis. Child., 48: 123, 1934.
21. Rankin, F. W. and Learmonth, J. R.: Am. J. Surg., 15: 219, 1932. Proc. Internat. Assemb. Interstate Postgrad. Med. Assn. North Am. for 1931, 172, 1932.

22. Litchfield, H. R.: M. J. & Rec., 136: 375, 1932.
23. Adamson, W. A. D. and Aird, I.: Brit. J. Surg., 20: 220, 1932.
24. Learmonth, J. R.: Brit. M. J., 2: 154, 1937.
25. Robertson, H. E. and Kernohan, J. W.: Proc. Staff Meet., Mayo Clin., 13: 123, 1938.
26. Van Buskirk, E. M.: Am. J. Roentgenol., 39: 228, 1938.
27. Cassidy, W. J. and Salkin, D.: Am. J. Surg., 12: 299, 1931.
28. Eiss, S.: Am. J. Surg., 34: 272, 1936.
29. Mercer, W.: Edinburgh M. J., 38: 105, 1931.
30. Sheldon, L., Kern, R. A. and Hakansson, E. G.: Am. J. M. Sc., 1: 94, 1932.
31. Ballard, J.: Delaware State M. J., 9: 63, 1937.
32. Adson, A. W.: Surgery, 1: 859, 1937.
33. Klingman, W. O.: J. Pediat., 13: 805, 1938.
34. Berger, H. C.: M. Clin. North America. 7: 1175, 1924.
35. Reeves, R. J. and Harrison, E. K.: Radiology, 28: 731, 1937.
36. Royle, N. D. and Hunter, J. I.: M. J. Australia, 1: 77 and 1: 86, 581, 590, 1924.
37. Wade, R. B. and Royle, N. D.: M. J. Australia, 1: 137, 1927.
38. Judd, E. S. and Adson, A. W.: Ann. Surg., 88: 479, 1928.
39. Adson, A. W.: Northwest Med., 33: 276, 1934.
40. Denk, W.: Wien. klin. Wchnschr., 50: 694, 1937.
41. Bates, W.: Med. World, 56: 453, 1938.
42. Launay, C. and Aubigne, R. M.: Bull. Soc. de pédiat. de Paris, 36: 124, 1938.
43. Rankin, F. W.: Kentucky M. J., 33: 474, 1935.
44. Fischer, A. W.: Zentralbl. f. Chir., 59: 261, 1932.

OROYA FEVER AND VERRUGA PERUANA

By Charles F. Craig, M.D., M.A. (Hon.), F.A.C.P., F.A.C.S., Colonel, U. S. Army Medical Corps (Ret.), D.S.M.

Synonyms.—Carrion's disease.

Definition.—An infection with an organism known as *Bartonella bacilliformis*, and characterized by two definite clinical pictures: one, an acute febrile attack, known as Oroya fever; the other, a more chronic condition, known as verruga peruana. The Oroya fever stage of the infection is characterized by an insidious onset, irregular fever, severe pain in the muscles and bones, a pernicious type of anemia, tender spleen and liver, glandular enlargement and tenderness of the bones upon pressure, while the verruga peruana stage is characterized by a peculiar granulomatous eruption, slight fever, hemorrhages and pain in the articulations. The Oroya fever stage is not always present, the primary symptoms being those of the verruga peruana stage in some cases.

Etiology.—The disease to which the names Oroya fever and verruga peruana have been given has been known for many generations to occur in certain valleys in the Andes in Peru, and until the work of Strong and his colleagues, in 1913, the medical profession considered the two names as indicating different stages of one disease, but the researches of the investigators named appeared to demonstrate that they were distinct, Oroya fever being caused by an organism first described by Barton, in 1909, and named *Bartonella bacilliformis* by Strong, in 1915, while the cause of verruga peruana was supposed to be unknown. Later observations by Noguchi (1926–1928), Mayer and Kikuth (1927), da Cunha and Muniz (1927), Galliard and Robles (1928), Pinkerton and Weinman (1937), and others, have definitely proved that Oroya fever and verruga peruana are but stages in the infection caused by *Bartonella bacilliformis*. The name of Carrion is always associated with this infection and it is often called "Carrion's disease." Carrion, who was a medical student in Lima, in 1885, inoculated himself with blood from a verruga nodule and later developed Oroya fever, from which he died. He thus proved the identity of the two clinical conditions, an identity later confirmed by the several investigators mentioned above.

Bartonella bacilliformis, the causative agent, is usually regarded as belonging to the bacteria, and was first described by Barton as a motile, rodlike body. These organisms occur within the red blood corpuscles in patients suffering from the symptom-complex known as Oroya fever.

4010

Further studies have demonstrated that it is very variable in its morphology, being rodlike, curved or straight; V-, Y- or cross-shaped, or rounded in contour. Motility is sluggish and from one to four flagella may be seen at one extremity in properly stained preparations. The organism stains well with the Wright or Giemsa stain, and in such preparations the cytoplasm stains blue, the ends staining more intensely than the center, while in some of the rods red or purple dots may be present at the center or near one end. The organism is gram-negative.

In endothelial cells and in tissue cells the organism is rounded and each contains a chromatin mass. Such forms are especially numerous in endothelial cells from the enlarged lymphatic glands. In tissue cultures, according to Pinkerton and Weinman (1937), the cells contain clusters of diplobacillary rods.

Bartonella bacilliformis may be cultivated on several culture media. especially upon blood agar, and in tissue cultures. It may be cultivated from the blood, lymph glands, bone marrow and from the nodules in the verruga stage, and the organisms from all of these sources, either from the Oroya fever or verruga stages of the disease, are identical in their cultural characteristics and in their effect upon experimental monkeys.

The recent work of Pinkerton and Weinman (1937) is of special interest as showing the identity of Oroya fever and verruga peruana. They inoculated tissue cultures with blood from a case of Oroya fever; with cultures from the blood of seven cases of this fever; with cultures of the blood and nodules from human cases of verruga; with cultures from the blood of monkeys inoculated from the blood of cases of Oroya fever and verruga, and with cultures from the cutaneous nodules of monkeys inoculated from cases of verruga. In the tissue cultures from all of these sources *Bartonella bacilliformis* was found in large numbers, while in tissue removed from three cases of Oroya fever and the nodules of seven cases of verruga the same organism was found. In addition, it was demonstrated in cutaneous nodules produced in monkeys by inoculation with material obtained from human cases of Oroya fever and verruga peruana. The types of the disease as observed in man were reproduced in monkeys by the inoculation of material from both the Oroya fever and the verruga peruana stages of the infection.

Epidemiology.—The geographic distribution of this disease is apparently confined to certain ravines and valleys in the Andes of Peru, Chile, Ecuador and Bolivia, situated between the 9th and 17th parallels of south latitude. These ravines and valleys are situated on the western slopes of the mountains at elevations varying from 3,000 to 10,000 feet. They are narrow, deep, well-shaded, hot and moist, and, according to Maldonado (1936), the disease is most prevalent in valleys where the vegetation includes various lactiferous plants and shrubs, upon which flies belonging to the genus *Phlebotomus* find nourishment.

There is a distinct seasonal occurrence of this disease, the cases being most numerous between January and April, when there is a high temperature and plentiful rainfall present in the endemic areas. During June, July and August, Strong noted that the Oroya fever stage of the infection was seldom observed but that the verruga peruana stage was frequently seen. This, of course, would be the case if the verruga stage occurred late in the infection, succeeding the Oroya fever, or primary stage, which is observed from January to April as a rule.

While infection with *Bartonella bacilliformis* usually occurs in endemic form, it may occur in epidemics if large numbers of individuals are collected together in the endemic regions. It has been recorded that over seven thousand laborers employed in the construction of the railway between the cities of Oroya and Lima died from this infection and it is among such labor forces that the disease is most prevalent and fatal.

All races and ages, and both sexes, are susceptible to infection with this parasite. Infection occurs most frequently at sundown or shortly afterward, and long residence in the endemic areas does not afford any protection, as the disease occurs more frequently in people who have resided for some time in such localities. While this is true, travelers have become infected who passed but a single night in a region known to harbor the infection.

The natural method of transmission of this disease is probably through the bites of certain sandflies. As long ago as 1913, Townsend claimed to have infected a dog by the subcutaneous injection of the triturated bodies of twenty female *Phlebotomi verrucarum* collected in a ravine where Oroya fever was known to be endemic. In 1928 Noguchi, Shannon, Tilden and Tyler conducted an extensive series of experiments upon the possible transmission of Oroya fever by sandflies and their results have since been confirmed by others. These investigators were successful in transmitting this disease to monkeys by inoculating these animals with the crushed bodies of certain species of sandflies. They were able to recover *Bartonella bacilliformis* from the blood of the inoculated animals in cultures and found that the animals were immune to the infection after recovery, when inoculated with cultures of the organism. They concluded that the species of sandfly known as *Phlebotomus noguchii* was certainly a transmitter of the infection, *Phlebotomus verrucarum* a probable transmitter and *Phlebotomus peruensis* a doubtful transmitter. Battistini in 1931 confirmed these observations and demonstrated the occurrence of *Bartonella bacilliformis* in infected sandflies and produced the disease in monkeys by the bites of such flies and by the inoculation of crushed, naturally infected sandflies. He proved that *Phlebotomus noguchii*, *Phlebotomus verrucarum* and *Phlebotomus peruensis* were all able to transmit the infection to monkeys.

At the present time the evidence appears to be sufficient to prove that Oroya fever and verruga peruana are, in nature, transmitted from man to man by one or more of the sandflies mentioned above. Other insect vectors have been suspected, but experiments with mosquitoes, mites, ticks, lice, midges, fleas, bedbugs and buffalo gnats have all resulted negatively, with the exception of the experiments of Noguchi who claimed to have produced the infection in monkeys by the bites of a tick, *Dermacentor andersoni*.

That human carriers of this infection are present in the endemic regions has been recently demonstrated by Weinman and Pinkerton (1937), who found that apparently healthy inhabitants of a village in the verruga area harbored *Bartonella bacilliformis*, as they were able to obtain cultures of this organism from the blood of five individuals among those examined, three of whom had no history of any sickness, while two had suffered from verruga some time previously. These results prove that not only may the organism be present in apparently healthy individuals but that it may persist in the blood of patients who have

4010

recovered from the symptomatic stages of the infection. Such carriers must be of great importance in the epidemiology of this infection and undoubtedly account for its endemic persistence in the infested regions.

The question of a possible animal reservoir of this infection is still unanswered. Townsend believed that Oroya fever occurred as a natural infection in dogs, but the occurrence in these animals of an infection with another species of *Bartonella*, *Bartonella canis*, has complicated the situation, as this species may have been confused by Townsend and others with *Bartonella bacilliformis* of man. A species, *Bartonella muris*, occurs in rats and other small rodents, and is transmitted from rat to rat by the rat louse and rat flea, while still another species occurs in cattle, *Bartonella bovis*. The exact relationship of these various species to one another is unknown and Pittaluga (1938) believes that a revision of this genus is essential and that this entire group of diseases are provoked by the proliferation of other disease-producing organisms in the organs of man or animals infected with the bartonellae, resulting in the transformation of a latent infection with the latter organisms into a symptomatic one. However this may be, it is evident that much has yet to be learned regarding the subject under discussion.

Symptomatology.—In considering the symptomatology of this infection it should be remembered that the acute stage, usually called Oroya fever, differs markedly in its symptomatology from that of the chronic stage, called verruga peruana, and that these two stages may occur in the same individual, the verruga stage following the Oroya fever stage, or either may occur alone. Thus, two distinct clinical pictures must be described but it should be borne in mind that both are caused by the same organism, *Bartonella bacilliformis*.

THE OROYA FEVER, OR ACUTE STAGE.—The *incubation period* varies from twenty days to three weeks. The symptoms also vary greatly in severity and it has already been stated that infections occur which are asymptomatic. In addition, very mild symptomatic infections also occur, in which the only symptoms consist in a slight degree of fever, malaise and mild muscle and bone pains.

In the majority of cases the onset is rather gradual with general malaise, headache, and pains in the muscles, bones and articulations, followed by chills or chilly feelings and fever. There is frequently marked tenderness upon pressure over the sternum and long bones. The fever ranges between 38.4 and 40° C. (101.1 and 104° F.) but seldom rises above 38.9° C. (102° F.). Nausea and vertigo are common symptoms and constipation or diarrhea may be present. A marked anemia rapidly develops, and in fatal cases marked prostration, insomnia and delirium, followed by coma, precede death. A rapidly fatal form resembling typhus fever in its symptomatology sometimes occurs. In such cases hemorrhages from the gums and nose may be present and death may occur in from five to eight days. In many of these fulminant cases a petechial eruption, most marked upon the trunk, has been noted. The most striking symptoms of this acute stage of the infection are the fever, the anemia, and the tenderness upon pressure over the sternum and long bones.

The *fever* may resemble that of malaria, being intermittent in type and accompanied by distinct chills, but more frequently it is irregular and remittent in type and accompanied by chilly sensations at irregular intervals. As already stated, the fever seldom reaches 40° C. (104° F.) and varies in duration from a few days to several weeks. In the long-continued fever cases the febrile curve frequently resembles that of paratyphoid or typhoid infection.

The *anemia* develops with excessive rapidity as the result of the destruction of the red blood corpuscles by the invading parasites. The red blood cell count may fall to 1,000,000 cells per c.mm. within three or four days and megaloblasts may be present in large numbers. In a case of moderate severity these cells occur only in small numbers, but poikilocytes and normoblasts are present in large numbers. The *pains in the bones* and the tenderness upon pressure over the sternum and long bones are undoubtedly due to pathologic changes in the bone marrow, and these symptoms are always most pronounced in patients presenting severe anemia and their severity increases with the severity of the anemia.

In this stage of the infection there is enlargement of the lymphatic glands, the spleen and the liver. The usual symptoms of a severe anemia may be present, as marked pallor of the skin and mucous membranes, dyspnea, edema of the legs and about the large joints, cardiac murmurs and tachycardia. Albumin may occur in the urine accompanied by hyaline and granular casts.

VERRUGA PERUANA, OR CHRONIC STAGE.—This stage may follow the Oroya fever stage or may occur without any previous symptoms, but in such cases a latent infection with *Bartonella bacilliformis* must have been present.

The *incubation period* of this stage has varied from fourteen to sixty days, the average period in those cases preceded by an attack of Oroya fever being from fourteen to forty days; while in those cases in which the verruga symptoms are the first noted, the incubation period may be as long as sixty days and usually is over forty days.

The *onset* of this stage is initiated by pains in the ankles, wrists, elbows and large joints, and by a fever of short duration, which disappears with the occurrence of the eruption upon the skin. The temperature may reach 40° C. (104° F.) but usually ranges between 37.8 and 39° C. (100 and 102.2° F.). Some cases are afebrile and in others the fever may persist after the eruption appears, although in such cases some complication causing the fever is almost invariably present. In addition to the symptoms mentioned there are headache, backache, muscular pain and tenderness, and considerable prostration. There is no enlargement of the liver, spleen or lymphatic glands as in the initial, or Oroya fever, stage of the infection.

The characteristic symptom in the verruga stage is the skin eruption which appears in successive crops and varies in its morphology, although in rare cases all types of the eruption may appear simultaneously. With the appearance of the eruption the constitutional symptoms mentioned above disappear and the eruption becomes the only evidence of the disease.

The eruption may be discrete or very abundant and the distribution varies somewhat with the type present. It is usually most abundant on the extensor surfaces of the arms and legs, on the shoulders and on the face. It may also occur upon the trunk and on the palms of the hands and the soles of the feet, as well as upon the mucous membranes.

4010

Several distinct types of the verruga eruption have been described but all of these types may occur upon the same patient, at different times, and in different stages of development, as in yaws; in this infection, as in yaws, all varieties of the eruption may be observed at the same time, new lesions occurring as the older lesions are fully developed or are healing. In this infection, unlike yaws, the eruption may occur upon the mucous membranes during the miliary stage.

Two general types of the verruga eruption are generally recognized, the *miliary* and the *nodular* types.

The *miliary* type of the eruption occurs in all cases and may be the only type in the mild infections. It begins as erythematous areas of a delicate pink color in which minute, darker pink macules and papules develop. These gradually enlarge and become nodular and darker in color, but very rarely become larger than a small pea. Some of these lesions may become pustular or hemorrhagic. When fully developed the nodules are a dusky or cherry-red in color and may be flattened or pedunculated. After persisting for some time, some of these lesions dry up and disappear without scar formation, while others continue to grow and develop into larger nodules characteristic of the nodular type of the eruption. The miliary type of eruption is most frequently observed upon the face and the extensor surfaces of the arms and legs but it may occur upon the trunk and upon the mucous membranes of the nose, mouth, pharynx, esophagus, stomach, intestine, bladder, uterus and vagina, and upon the conjunctivae. Hemorrhages may occur from the lesions on the mucous membranes.

The *nodular* type of eruption is of much longer duration than the miliary type, does not invade the mucous membranes, and the individual lesions are larger, sometimes exceeding the size of a pigeon's egg. The nodules appear in successive crops and are most numerous about the flexures of the arms and legs, especially the elbows and knees, and also occur over the thighs, but may occur upon the face and trunk. They are usually discrete but may be grouped together, forming fungating masses.

In morphology the typical verruga nodules are cherry-red in color, firm in consistence and, in uncomplicated cases, are not covered with a crust, as are the nodules of yaws with which they have been confused. They are smooth and shiny in appearance and resemble cherries projecting from the skin. They bleed easily upon pressure or when accidentally injured and may be pedunculated.

The nodules frequently ulcerate, either due to injury, secondary bacterial infections, or to necrosis brought about by strangulation of the pedunculated lesions. Ulcerated nodules may be covered by a crust causing them to resemble those of yaws, and the coalescence of ulcerated nodules results in the formation of fungating masses which are called the miliary type of verruga. Hemorrhage and septicemia sometimes endanger life during the verruga stage of the infection, while healing of such lesions may result in scar formation producing deformity or loss of function of the affected parts. Unless ulceration occurs the nodules eventually dry up and disappear, leaving no evidence of their presence. In some cases the subcutaneous nodules become ulcerated, extensive areas of the skin being involved, and this type of lesion is called the miliary type by some authorities.

The *duration* of the eruption in infection with *Bartonella bacilliformis* varies from a few days to several months. In those cases in which the miliary type occurs alone, the duration varies from a few days to two or three weeks, but if the nodular type of eruption develops, as it usually does, the duration of the eruption varies from two to three months, or even more.

Diagnosis.—The diagnosis of the Oroya fever, or the acute stage of infection with *Bartonella bacilliformis,* must rest upon the demonstration of the organism in the red blood corpuscles of the patient or upon the cultivation of the organism from the blood or enlarged lymphatic glands. A tentative diagnosis is justified in the case of a patient living in, or coming from, an endemic area, presenting an irregular fever, enlargement of the superficial lymphatic glands, and a rapidly developing anemia, and frequently a diagnosis must be made without the assistance of a blood examination; but, if it is possible, the diagnosis should be made by the demonstration of the causative organism.

Blood smears are made as in the examination for the malaria plasmodia and stained with the Wright or Giemsa stain. The careful microscopic examination of such preparations almost invariably results in the demonstration of the parasite within the red blood corpuscles; if negative results are obtained, one should stain and examine smears of gland juice obtained by puncture of one of the enlarged lymphatic glands. In such preparations the organisms occur as round and rod-shaped bodies containing red-stained chromatin dots. If such preparations are negative, cultures of the blood upon blood agar should be made and examined for the organisms.

In the *Oroya fever stage* this infection is most apt to be mistaken for malaria, typhus fever and paratyphoid and typhoid fevers. The differentiation of these conditions depends upon the utilization of the various laboratory methods which are available for the diagnosis of these infections. Tuberculosis and rheumatic fever have also been confused with Oroya fever.

In the verruga stage of this disease the eruption, in uncomplicated cases, is so characteristic that a diagnosis may be made without difficulty by a mere inspection of the patient. However, other conditions sometimes must be differentiated, the most important of which are yaws, molluscum contagiosum, syphilis, multiple warts, and multiple fibromas or lipomas.

Yaws, or frambesia, is most apt to be mistaken for verruga but in yaws there is a primary lesion followed by a secondary eruption. The typical granulomas of yaws, unlike those of verruga, are covered by a lemon-yellow crust which, when removed, shows the typical strawberry-like surface, from which oozes a clear serum in which *Treponema pertenue* can be easily demonstrated. It should be remembered that the verruga lesions are not crusted, are cherry-red in color, and have a smooth, glistening surface. In yaws there is a positive Wassermann reaction, while in verruga the reaction is negative unless syphilis is also present.

Molluscum contagiosum can be easily differentiated by the demonstration of the molluscum bodies and the appearance of the lesion, the molluscum growth being of solid consistence, not bleeding upon pressure, and having a central opening from which may be expressed a whitish cheesy material.

4010

Syphilis, in some of its skin lesions, might possibly be confused with verruga, but the presence of a positive Wassermann reaction together with the response to specific antisyphilitic treatment should serve to differentiate it. In addition, *Treponema pallidum* might be demonstrated in the suspicious lesion.

Multiple warts and *multiple fibromas* or *lipomas* should cause no confusion, owing to their entirely different morphology.

Treatment.—At the present time we have no specific treatment for infection with *Bartonella bacilliformis.* Some authorities have reported favorable results in the *Oroya fever stage* following the administration of the **arsphenamines,** the dose not exceeding 0.3 Gm. (5 grains), intravenously. The same treatment has been tried in the verruga stage but with comparatively little benefit.

Owing to the tendency of the verruga nodules to bleed, care should be taken to avoid injuring them; if bleeding should occur, the use of compresses and styptics is indicated, as hemorrhage may be excessive and may even endanger the life of the patient. If the nodules become infected or ulcerated, it is good practice to excise them in order to prevent the possible occurrence of septicemia.

During the acute febrile stage of the disease the treatment is symptomatic, special attention being paid to the treatment of the anemia, large doses of **ferrous sulfate** being indicated together with **arsenic,** and such treatment should be continued throughout the verruga stage of the infection. **Good nursing and a nutritious, properly balanced diet** are very important in the treatment of Oroya fever.

PROPHYLAXIS.—The prophylaxis of this infection is in a very unsatisfactory condition and but little has been accomplished in its prevention but as the infection is apparently transmitted by sandflies, protection from the bites of these flies and the prevention of their breeding would appear to be essential in any prophylactic plan.

Comparatively little is known of the habits and life cycle of sandflies in general and of those transmitting Oroya fever in particular. These flies breed in the crevices in adobe or rock walls of habitations, in stone fences, in collections of rubbish and stones if shaded and moist and in excavated material where dark, moist breeding places may be available. They do not live within houses under natural conditions but will enter human habitations after sundown in search of blood, provided the rooms be dimly lighted, as they are repelled by bright lights. During the daytime they hide in the localities mentioned above or in rank vegetation, coming out after sundown in search of food. Only the females suck blood and they will feed upon any warm-blooded animal and are not dependent upon man for their nourishment. The inhabitants of the deep narrow canyons of the Andes are especially liable to be bitten by these flies as in these moist, dimly lit canyons the flies breed in very large numbers.

The eggs are deposited in the localities mentioned above and hatch in from four to eight days and complete development occurs in from four to eight weeks, varying with local conditions and the species of fly. Males and unfed females will pass through ordinary mosquito netting (12 to 18 mesh) but the engorged females cannot pass such netting.

The species of sandflies concerned in the transmission of Oroya fever (see Etiology) have been little studied and we are unacquainted with

most of their habits and with their life cycle.   From what has been said
it is evident that protection from the bites of these flies and the prevention of their breeding is most difficult and, so far as the native population of the endemic areas is concerned, practically impossible.   In the
endemic regions travel should be performed during the day and, so far
as is possible, such regions should be avoided.   Known fly bites should
be promptly treated with **tincture of iodine.**

Prognosis.—The prognosis, in the acute stage of this infection, is
always serious.   According to different authorities the mortality has
apparently varied from as low as 30 to as high as 98 per cent.   As we are
ignorant of the actual number of mild and unrecognized cases that may
occur, the exact mortality cannot be accurately stated, but it is probable
that it does not usually exceed 50 per cent in the recognized infections.
After the development of the verruga stage the prognosis is excellent as
death never occurs at this time unless some complication, as septicemia,
occurs.

Most authorities believe that an immunity follows an attack of Oroya
fever but we know very little regarding this phase of the subject.

Pathology.—Patients dying during the acute febrile stage of Oroya
fever present a yellowish-white skin, resembling that of pernicious
anemia; enlarged lymphatic glands; edema of the face and extremities;
and emaciation.   Petechial hemorrhages may be present in the skin in
some cases.

The principal pathologic lesions occur in the blood, liver, spleen and
lymphatic glands.   The changes in the *blood* have already been described
(see Diagnosis), the morphologic picture being that of a rapidly developing pernicious anemia, with the presence within the erythrocytes of
Bartonella bacilliformis.

The *liver* is enlarged, pale in color externally, and decreased in consistence.   Numerous areas of fatty degeneration and central necrosis are
present, especially around the hepatic veins.   Yellowish pigment is present in the necrotic areas and the same pigment is present as grains or
irregular, larger masses, within the endothelial phagocytic cells, or
macrophages.   This pigment does not give the iron reaction.

The *spleen* is considerably enlarged, firmer than normal, and infarcts
are very frequently present.   Numerous areas of degeneration and
necrosis are present, but the malpighian bodies are normal in appearance.   Masses of yellowish pigment, irregular in shape and varying in
size, occur between the cells in the splenic pulp and within the endothelial cells.   Many very large endothelial cells are usually present, the
macrophages, containing *Bartonella bacilliformis,* in the form of rods
and rounded bodies, the latter staining bluish with the Wright or
Giemsa stain, and containing pink or red-stained grains of chromatin.
Many of the splenic veins are thrombosed.

The *lymphatic glands* are enlarged and contain large endothelial
cells filled with rod-shaped and rounded forms of *Bartonella bacilliformis.*

The *heart* may be enlarged and flabby and the muscular tissue appears very anemic.   The *bone marrow* is softer than normal and areas
of necrosis are present, while there is very active proliferation of the
endothelial cells, many of which contain *Bartonella bacilliformis.*   There
is also an increase in the number of neutrophilic myelocytes and normo-

blasts. In the pleura, pericardium, intestine and subcutaneous fat there may be present small hemorrhagic areas, and *ulceration of the intestine* has been described. The endothelial cells of the lymphoid tissue of the intestine may contain the causative organism. The *lungs* may show edema.

Strong (1915) believes that the lesions noted in the viscera in the acute febrile stage of Oroya fever are caused by toxins formed and liberated by *Bartonella bacilliformis,* an opinion amply supported by the prevalence of necrosis apparently of toxic origin.

The pathology of the *verruga stage* of Oroya fever is essentially that of the nodules, although various authorities have described lesions in practically all of the viscera; but Strong (1915) and others have demonstrated that such lesions were actually caused by other infections, especially by tuberculosis.

The verruga nodules, when uncomplicated by secondary infections, are discrete and, when sectioned, present a bright-red, nonlobulated, moist surface in the early stages of growth, but in the larger and older nodules the cut surface is bluish in color and small areas and strands of connective tissue may be present.

Microscopically, the nodules consist at first of newly formed capillary vessels surrounded by connective tissue. Later, as the nodules increase in size, there is marked proliferation of the endothelial cells lining the blood vessels, eventually resulting in the formation of masses of these cells with numerous angioblasts around the blood vessels. In the older nodules, fibroblasts occur among the endothelial-cell collections, and sections of the nodules may resemble a fibrosarcoma, myxosarcoma or an angioma. There is a marked proliferation of the endothelial cells of the lymphatics and the lymph channels may be occluded by plasma cells and fibroblasts.

BIBLIOGRAPHY

Barton, A. L.: Crón. méd., Lima, 26 : 7, 1909.

Battistini, T.: Rev. sud-am. de méd. et de chir., 2 : 719, 1931.

Byam, W.: The Practice of Medicine in the Tropics. London and New York, Oxford Univ. Press, 3 : 2149, 1923.

Craig, C. F.: Oroya Fever and Verruga Peruana, Oxford Medicine, London and New York, Oxford Univ. Press, 1 : 202 (7), 1933.

Cunha da, A. and Muniz, J.: Compt. rend. Soc. de biol., 97 : 1368, 1927.

Hertig, M.: Proc. Soc. Exper. Biol. & Med., 37 : 598, 1937.

Mackchenie, D.: Bull. Inst. Pasteur, 36 : 961, 1938.

Maldonado: Arch. méd. belges, 89 : 631, 1936.

Mayer, M. and Kikuth, W.: Able. Ansldsk., Hamburg Univ., 26 : 319, 1927. (D. Med. and Vet., Vol. II.)

——, Borchardt, W. and Kikuth, W.:

Arch. f. Schiffs- u. Tropen-Hyg., 31 : 295, 1927.

Noguchi, H. and Battistini, T. S.: J. Exper. Med., 43 : 851, 1926.

——: J. Exper. Med., 44; 533, 697, 715, 729, 1926; 45 : 175, 437, 455, 781, 1927; 47 : 165, 219, 235, 1928.

——, Shannon, R. C., Tilden, E. B. and Tyler, J. R.: J. Exper. Med., 49 : 993, 1929.

Pinkerton, H. and Weinman, D.: Proc. Soc. Exper. Biol. & Med., 37 : 587, 590, 1937.

Pittaluga, G.: Riforma méd., Sept. 15, pp. 1–5, 1937.

Strong, R. P., Tyzzer, E. E., Sellards, A. W., Brues, C. T. and Gastiaburu, J. C.: Rep. 1st Expedition South America, Harvard School of Tropical Medicine, Harvard University Press, Boston, Mass., 1915.

Townsend, C. H. T.: Peru Today, 5 : 840, 1913; J. Am. M. Ass., 61 : 1717, 1913.

Weinman, D. and Pinkerton, H.: Proc. Soc. Exper. Biol. & Med., 37 : 594, 1937.

MELIOIDOSIS

By Charles F. Craig, M.D., M.A. (Hon.), F.A.C.P., F.A.C.S., Colonel, U. S. Army Medical Corps (Ret.), D.S.M.

Definition, p. 693—Etiology, p. 693—Epidemiology, p. 693—Symptomatology, p. 694—Diagnosis, p. 694—Treatment, p. 695—Prophylaxis, p. 695—Pathology, p. 695.

Synonyms.—Stanton's disease, Rangoon glanders, pneumo-enteritis.

Definition.—Melioidosis is an infectious disease caused by a bacillus, *Bacillus whitmori*, and is primarily an infection of rats and other rodents, rarely occurring in man. The clinical picture resembles glanders and the characteristic symptoms are a septicemia accompanied by abscess formation in the lungs, liver, spleen, kidneys and other organs.

Etiology.—Melioidosis is caused by a bacillus, isolated from the lesions, in 1913, by A. Whitmore, and called by him, *Bacillus pseudo-mallei;* but this name had been given previously to another organism and was invalid, and in 1921 Stanton and Fletcher renamed it *Bacillus whitmori*, by which it is now known. In morphology it greatly resembles *B. mallei*, the cause of glanders, being a slender rod with rounded ends, easily cultivated upon ordinary culture media, actively motile, nonacid-fast, and gram-negative. With the Giemsa stain the ends of the rod stain more intensely than the center, thus resembling the plague bacillus. It is an obligate aerobe, does not produce gas in carbohydrate media, and is sometimes chromogenic, the colonies varying from yellow to brown in color. Rough and smooth colonies are formed upon glycerin agar.

The following animals have been found to be experimentally susceptible to infection with *B. whitmori*, and in all death follows infection: rats, mice, cats, dogs, guinea pigs, rabbits, goats, sheep and monkeys. The horse appears to be immune although the disease so closely resembles glanders.

Epidemiology.—The geographic distribution of this disease would appear to be remarkably limited. The first cases were described by Whitmore and Krishnaswami (1912) in paupers autopsied in Rangoon. In 1913 Fletcher observed an epidemic of the disease in guinea pigs in his laboratory at Kuala Lumpur, in the Federated Malay States, and in 1917 Stanton observed human infections at the same place. Infections in man have also been observed in Indo-China, by Pons and Advier (1926), and by Vielle, Morin and Massias (1927), while Denny and Nicholls (1927) have described a case of human infection in Ceylon. The close resemblance of this disease to glanders and tularemia may have resulted in confusing it with these diseases in some localities. Even in

4010

the countries in which it has been observed it is a very rare disease, less than 75 cases having been recorded since its discovery as a disease entity.

The causative organism, *B. whitmori*, can live for long periods of time outside the body of man and animals if the temperatures are favorable, but it is easily destroyed by heat and cold. It will remain alive in fecal material for 27 days, in water for 44 days, and in the soil for 27 days under normal temperature conditions in the tropics and subtropics. It is easily destroyed by disinfectants and by high and low temperatures. Experimentally, infections may be produced in animals by scarification, subcutaneous injection, by feeding, and by spraying infectious material into the respiratory passages. The natural method of transmission to man is unknown at present.

Melioidosis is essentially a disease of rodents, especially of rats, and Whitmore (1913) and Stanton and Fletcher (1924) believe that man is infected by eating food soiled by the excreta of infected rats or mice. The disease is transmitted from rodent to rodent by the ingestion of material contaminated by the urine of infected animals, the bacillus being found in large numbers in the urine. Natural infections have also been found in guinea pigs, rabbits, dogs and cats. All attempts to transmit melioidosis to the horse have failed, but Stanton, Fletcher and Symonds (1927) found a transient nasal infection in a horse and *B. whitmori* was demonstrated in the nasal secretion. However, the horse is not a source of infection so far as is known at present.

Although the causative organism is found in the feces, urine, sputum, nasal secretions and in the material discharged from the skin lesions of the disease, there is no instance known of the infection's being transmitted by contact of uninfected with infected individuals, and patients suffering from melioidosis need not be segregated.

Symptomatology.—The symptomatology of this disease is very variable and the cases may resemble plague, cholera, tularemia, glanders, syphilis, malaria and other disease conditions.

The period of incubation is unknown. The onset is usually sudden, in most cases with vomiting and diarrhea, followed quickly by collapse. Such cases simulate cholera in their symptomatology and are fatal in from two to five days. Still other patients have shown the symptoms of a severe septicemia, with high fever, delirium, extreme prostration and other symptoms suggestive of plague. Pulmonary symptoms have frequently occurred, as pain in the chest, cough, dyspnea, and the expectoration of bloodstained sputum rich in the bacilli. Cases have also been described in which the symptoms have developed gradually and the clinical picture has resembled that of typhoid fever. In patients living longer than a week, abscesses may develop in the subcutaneous and muscular tissues and in the bones. A pustular eruption has been observed in some infections in man.

Death almost invariably occurs within fifteen days after the onset of the symptoms. In one patient who recovered, Stanton and Fletcher (1924) reported that two years afterward there was a condition of chronic invalidism and that abscesses and suppuration had been occurring in the bones during that period of time.

Diagnosis.—A diagnosis of melioidosis based upon clinical symptoms alone is impossible and can be made only by the finding of the causative organism in the blood, urine, tissues or exudates of the patient.

Almost all cases of this disease have remained undiagnosed before death, and Fletcher (1930) is authority for the statement that in but 7 of 65 cases was a correct diagnosis made during the life of the patient.

In all suspicious cases an attempt should be made to cultivate *B. whitmori* from the urine, blood, exudates or lesions, and, in addition, guinea pigs should be subcutaneously inoculated with blood, urine, or pus from the abscesses, if such be present. Guinea pigs are very susceptible and infection rapidly develops after inoculation, with a fatal result. While it may be possible to demonstrate the bacilli microscopically in properly stained preparations made from the exudates or pus, a diagnosis should not be considered conclusive when based upon the morphology of the organisms alone, but cultures should be made before a definitive diagnosis is justified.

As already stated, most cases of melioidosis have been diagnosed at autopsy and this is easily accomplished by making cultures from the contents of abscesses or other lesions present in the spleen, liver or other organs. Fortunately, *B. whitmori* grows easily upon ordinary culture media and can be recovered without difficulty from infected material if it be present. Guinea pigs should also be inoculated subcutaneously with suspicious material.

Treatment.—The treatment of melioidosis is purely **symptomatic** as we possess no drug that is specific and attempts to prepare an antitoxin or vaccines have all resulted in failure. As the disease is really a septicemia it would appear that one or more of the sulfonamide group of drugs might prove to be curative.

PROPHYLAXIS.—As this infection is primarily one of rodents, especially of rats, the **destruction and prevention of breeding** of these animals appear to be the most useful prophylactic methods. Next in importance is the **protection of food** from all contact, direct or indirect, with rodents. The causative organism occurs in large numbers in the urine of infected rats and mice, and the protection of food or drink from such contamination is especially important in the prevention of the disease.

Melioidosis is not contagious and patients suffering from it need not be isolated; but as the bacillus causing it may occur in the urine and feces, the disinfection of these should be followed as a preventive measure, to prevent possible contamination of food or drink. Chloride of lime is an efficient disinfectant for this purpose.

Pathology.—There are no characteristic pathologic changes in the blood in melioidosis. In practically all of the organs the characteristic lesions of this infection occur, consisting of caseous nodules, at first invisible to the naked eye but eventually visible as masses of caseous material, varying in size, and surrounded by an area of acute inflammation. Many of these areas suppurate and thus abscesses are produced, the pus of which contains *B. whitmori*.

The *liver* is usually slightly enlarged and contains numerous irregular caseous nodules, many of them of considerable size, due to the coalescence of several nodules. Suppuration of such masses results in abscess formation and such abscesses are often present in this organ. The *spleen* is enlarged, dotted externally with yellowish-white caseous nodules, of varying size, and section of this organ shows numerous such nodules scattered throughout the parenchyma, while abscesses are also

4010

present. Similar lesions are present in the *kidneys*, while the *lungs* present many caseous nodules and larger caseous masses, but abscess formation occurs less frequently in this organ than in the liver, spleen or kidneys. Caseous nodules and abscesses may also be present in the urinary bladder, gallbladder, subcutaneous and muscular tissues, and in the bones. *B. whitmori* can be recovered from all of these lesions and from the blood and urine of fatal cases.

The manner in which this organism produces the lesions noted is unknown as neither an exotoxin or an endotoxin has been isolated from cultures and it does not incite acute inflammatory reactions when injected into the tissues.

BIBLIOGRAPHY

Craig, C. F.: Melioidosis. Oxford Medicine, London and New York, Oxford Univ. Press, 5: 202, 1934.

Denny, C. R. and Nicholls, L.: Ceylon J. Sc., Sec. D, 2: 37, 1927.

Fletcher, W.: Melioidosis. A System of Bacteriology, Med. Research Council, London, 5: 65, 1930.

Pons, R. and Advier, M.: J. Hyg., 26: 28, 1927.

Stanton, A. T.: Studies Inst. Med. Res., Kuala Lumpur, No. 14, 1917.

—— and Fletcher, W.: Bull. Inst. Med. Res., Kuala Lumpur, No. 5, 1924.

Vielle, A., Morin, H. G. S. and Massias, C.: Bull. Soc. Med. Chir., Indo-China, No. 9, 1926.

Whitmore, A.: J. Hyg., 13: 1, 1913.

—— and Krishnaswami, C. S.: Indian M. Gaz., 47: 262, 1912.

TSUTSUGAMUSHI DISEASE

By CHARLES F. CRAIG, M.D., M.A. (HON.), F.A.C.P., F.A.C.S., COLONEL, U. S. ARMY MEDICAL CORPS (RET.), D.S.M.

Synonyms.—Japanese river fever, Japanese flood fever, island fever, kedani disease, akamushi disease, shimamushi disease, shashitsu disease, yochubio.

Definition.—Tsutsugamushi disease is an acute, endemic, febrile infection, having a high mortality, caused by *Rickettsia orientalis,* and transmitted from man to man by the bites of certain species of larval mites. Clinically, it is characterized by an initial sore at the site of the bite, followed by an ulcer, painful enlargement of the regional lymph glands, fever, a characteristic skin eruption, bronchitis, leukopenia and enlargement of the spleen. It is undoubtedly a member of the great typhus-fever group of infections.

Etiology.—The cause of tsutsugamushi disease is a *Rickettsia* discovered by Ogata and Nagayo and named *Rickettsia orientalis* by the latter. The organism is found in the endothelial cells of the spleen and other tissues and in the cells of the lymph nodes and glands, occurring as minute rods and granules within the cytoplasm of the invaded cells. The blood of patients suffering from the disease also contains the organism and is very infective early in the disease. It has also been found in the salivary glands of the mites which transmit the infection from man to man. The organism has been cultured in tissue cultures. Guinea pigs, rabbits and monkeys are susceptible when inoculated experimentally, and the blood of patients and infected animals gives a positive Weil-Felix reaction with Proteus OXK (Kingsbury strain) but is negative with Proteus OX_{19} and OX_2. The organism disappears from the blood during convalescence.

Epidemiology.—Tsutsugamushi disease has been known and studied in Japan for many years and we owe most of our knowledge of the etiology, epidemiology and symptomatology of this infection to Japanese physicians, especially to Miyajima, Ogata, Nagayo, Kanamura and Nishibi. The disease occurs along the banks of certain rivers, following floods, on the west coast of Japan, in the prefectures of Akita, Echigo, Yamagata and Niigata. It has been found more recently to be prevalent in Formosa, Korea, Sumatra, New Guinea and Borneo, and probably also occurs in Queensland, Australia. It is apparently identical with the "scrub-typhus" of Malaya.

4010

The Japanese have always believed that this disease was transmitted to man by the bites of a larval mite found upon the ears of the field vole, *Microtus montebelli,* a belief which has been confirmed by recent observers. This mite is now known to be the hexapod larva of *Trombicula akamushi,* a red mite, which in its adult stage is not parasitic but lives in the grass. Only the larval mite bites warm-blooded animals, and it attacks man, dogs, cats and the buffalo. As the nymphs and adults do not bite man, this infection is transmitted only by the larval mite, although the causative organism, *Rickettsia orientalis,* is found in the adult mite. The Rickettsia has been demonstrated in the salivary glands of the larval mites. In Sumatra and Malaya the disease is transmitted by the larval stage of *Trombicula deliensis* and *Trombicula schüfferi* respectively.

Infection of man occurs when he is working in, or passing through, the endemic areas where these mites are present and leave their natural host, the field vole, or other rodents, to bite man. The disease is not contagious.

Tsutsugamushi disease has a *seasonal occurrence,* depending upon the life history of the transmitting mites. Thus, the disease occurs in the summer as it is only during this season that the larval, or infectious, stage of the transmitting mites is found.

Males and females are alike susceptible but males are more frequently infected than females because they are more frequently exposed in working in the fields in the endemic regions. One attack is not followed by an immunity but there must be some degree of protection afforded because newcomers to an endemic locality are especially susceptible to infection. The relative percentage of mites that become infectious after biting an infected individual has not been ascertained, but many people are bitten by mites in the endemic regions without becoming infected. The incidence of infection in the endemic localities in Japan is unknown but the total incidence is close to 400 persons per annum.

Symptomatology.—The following description of the symptomatology of tsutsugamushi disease is based upon the study of cases observed in endemic regions in Japan by Ashburn and the writer and reported in 1908. The symptomatology of these cases agrees with that described by other observers in other endemic regions except as noted in the description which follows.

The *incubation period* of the disease, i.e., the time from the receipt of the bite to the appearance of symptoms, is from four to twelve days, rarely less than five days. The bite of the mite is usually painless. There may rarely be premonitory symptoms consisting of malaise and slight headache but usually the onset is sudden with a chill, succeeded by fever, severe headache, anorexia, and general prostration. Enlargement of a group of lymphatic glands, usually in the groin or axilla, with pain and tenderness, leads to the discovery of the lesion resulting from the bite of the infected mite, which is usually situated in the inguinal or axillary region, but may be upon any part of the body. The earliest stage of the lesion consists of a small vesicle but this stage in its development is very rarely observed. Usually the lesion, when first seen, consists of a small, circular, very dark brown or black area of necrosis, adherent to the underlying skin, forming an eschar. It usually measures from 2 to 3 mm. in diameter and is surrounded by a slight area of inflammation. After a varying number of days the adherent eschar loosens and becomes detached, leaving a circular, punched-out ulcer with slightly indurated and inflamed edges. In most cases the lesion is not tender or painful, unless there is a secondary infection present. The lymphatics connecting the lesion with the enlarged group of glands are not enlarged, a lymphangitis not being present. A slight enlargement of the lymphatic glands of the body is often present but only the group of glands draining the region occupied by the local lesion is markedly enlarged.

In the early stage of the infection the conjunctivae are injected, the tongue is moist and somewhat coated, a slight cough is often present, the bowels are constipated, and slight or moderate enlargement of the spleen may be noted. Headache is present but, with this exception, the patient does not feel very sick and the appetite may not be lost. The urine may contain albumin and the diazo reaction is usually present. At this time the temperature usually runs from 38.2 to 40° C. (100.8 to 104° F.) and may reach its maximum within 24 hours. The pulse varies between 80 and 100 and is full and strong.

The symptoms noted become more marked as the disease advances and slight general enlargement of the lymphatic glands is noted. The temperature is continuous and reaches 40 to 40.5° C. (104 to 104.9° F.), the pulse varies between 80 and 100 beats per minute and may be weak and dicrotic, but is usually full and strong. The presence of albumin and casts in the urine is more marked and the diazo reaction becomes stronger. The entire surface of the body may be hypersensitive; lacrimation and intense congestion of the conjunctivae occur, and there may be a marked increase in the number of respirations, and an irritating, dry cough is usually present. The tongue becomes dry and is coated with a thick brown fur, while the breath may be very foul. Sordes collect and the gums may become soft, spongy, and may bleed easily. Constipation is the rule, but abdominal tenderness, pain and diarrhea may occur. Deafness often is present and the patient may be delirious.

The eruption usually appears from the fifth to the seventh day, although it may occur earlier or later than these periods. It consists of irregular, rather faint, dusky or pink macules or papules, 2 to 5 mm. in diameter, which may become confluent, especially upon the cheeks, and give an appearance of swelling. The eruption appears first upon the face and later on the chest, the forearms, the legs and the rest of the trunk, and the palate and buccal surfaces may show the eruption. On the relatively dark skin of the Japanese it is often hard to distinguish the eruption and it may so closely resemble fleabites that confusion may result. The lesions fade upon pressure but return at once when pressure is removed, and they never become petechial or hemorrhagic. Itching does not occur and the duration of the eruption is from four to seven days, although it may be shorter or longer in rare instances. With the appearance of the eruption the infection reaches its height and as the eruption fades the patient's symptoms decrease.

The symptoms that have been enumerated are those which are usually observed in a case of medium severity in which recovery occurs. In more severe and usually fatal cases the symptoms are more marked and continuous, the fever is higher, and numerous complications, as cardiac failure, mania, parotitis, coma, and hemorrhage from the stomach or

4010

bowels, may occur. In such cases death may occur from the ninth to the fifteenth day after the onset, but the average duration of the attack is about three weeks. Pregnant women suffering from this infection invariably abort, except in the mildest cases, and frequently die.

Very mild cases are observed in which the fever may be slight and ephemeral and no eruption may be detected. Such patients may not even go to bed and it is probable that carriers of tsutsugamushi disease exist although we have no direct evidence to this effect. In these mild cases the gland enlargement is present and the ulcer following the bite of the infective mite may be well marked.

In this infection we noted a well-marked leukopenia and a slight anemia, but Miyajima states that the anemia may be marked, counts as low as 3,000,000 red cells per c.mm. being sometimes observed.

The complications most often observed are parotitis, mania, cardiac failure, and hemorrhage from the intestine, indicated by melena.

Diagnosis.—DIFFERENTIAL DIAGNOSIS.—Tsutsugamushi disease may be confused with malaria, plague, typhoid, other forms of typhus fever, measles, dengue and pneumonia. The differential diagnosis clinically of some of these conditions is impossible and recourse has to be had to laboratory procedures. *Malaria* should be easily differentiated by the demonstration of the malaria plasmodia in the blood or by the effect of quinine upon the temperature; *pneumonia,* by the presence of the usual physical signs in the lungs and by the effect of the injection of washed sputum into mice, intraperitoneally; the other forms of *typhus* by attention to the geographic location and the fact that the serum of patients suffering from tsutsugamushi disease does not agglutinate Proteus OX_{19} or OX_2, but only OXK, or the Kingsbury strain of proteus; from *plague* by the presence of *Bacillus pestis* in the buboes, viscera or sputum, and the characteristics of the epidemic; from *measles* and *dengue* by the character of the eruption, the geographic location, and the character of the epidemic, as well as the absence of the mite bite lesion in both of these diseases. From *typhoid fever* it may be differentiated by the absence of the Widal test and the negative results of blood and stool cultures. There should be little difficulty in differentiating tsutsugamushi disease because of its limited geographic distribution.

Treatment.—The treatment of tsutsugamushi disease is largely **symptomatic** and no specific has been discovered for this infection. High temperature is controlled by sponging or bathing in lukewarm water and the other symptoms are treated as is usual. **Stabilarsen** has been reported upon favorably, administered in two doses of 0.015 and 0.3 Gm., at four days' interval, and Hayashi and Mukoyama have used **convalescent serum** from experimentally infected cattle and monkeys with good results in the early stage of severe infections.

PREVENTION.—As tsutsugamushi disease is transmitted by the bites of certain larval mites, the prevention of the disease consists in the destruction of the mites and protection from their bites. Little, if anything, can be done as regards the destruction of the mites, owing to their normal habitat upon field voles and other rodents, but the body can be protected from their bites by properly made clothing. Hayashi and Nagayo have devised a suit which is miteproof and which should be worn when working in the fields in the endemic areas. In addition, all clothing worn by workers in the fields should be sterilized upon returning from such work and any areas upon the skin which suggest a bite should be treated with tincture of iodine.

The burning off of land which is known to harbor rodents 'infested with the mites before cultivating it has been suggested as an efficient method of prevention, but this does not prevent subsequent invasion of the land by infected rodents.

Nagayo recommends the excision of the portion of the skin where the mite may be found biting and states that if this is done infection may be prevented.

Prognosis.—The prognosis of the Japanese form of tsutsugamushi disease is much more serious than that of the Sumatran type. In Japan the death rate apparently varies from 15 to 50 per cent but in Sumatra it is less than 1 per cent. Where the mortality is high, as in Japan, the prognosis should always be considered as serious, for the mildest cases may suddenly develop severe symptoms and a fatal result may occur. The real prognosis, even where the disease is most severe, is unknown, as many mild cases are undoubtedly overlooked or wrongly diagnosed. Miyajima stated to the writer that of 567 cases observed by himself and others, the average mortality had been 27 per cent and that the rate of mortality showed a steady increase from 12.5 per cent in the first decade of life to 57 per cent in the seventh decade.

Pathology.—The lesion at the site of the mite bite is a coagulation necrosis taking place in the epidermis and extending to the corium and subcutis in the immediate area of the bite. Sometimes the area of necrosis is not well differentiated from the surrounding tissue but generally there is a well-marked border. The necrotic focus is surrounded by cellular infiltration extending along the hair follicles, sweat glands and blood vessels.

The *spleen* is usually much enlarged, the consistence decreased, the capsule smooth and the cut surface dark red in color. The pulp is soft and friable and the follicles and trabeculae are usually invisible. There is marked proliferation of the cells of the parenchyma and often miliary areas of necrosis are visible. The stained sections of the spleen show many phagocytic cells and histiocytes containing Rickettsia.

The *liver* is somewhat enlarged and the consistence slightly decreased. The cut surface appears cloudy and there may be evidences of a mild degree of fatty degeneration and areas of miliary necrosis. Cloudy swelling and fatty degeneration of the liver cells are usually present.

The *kidneys* may appear swollen and markedly congested. There is marked cloudy swelling of the cells of the parenchyma and the tubules may contain hyaline and epithelial casts in rare instances. Fatty degeneration may be marked in fatal cases.

The *bone marrow* is grayish-red or red and contains many plasma cells and large mononuclear cells, similar to those observed in the spleen.

The enlarged *lymphatic glands* show great proliferation of the lymphocytes and large mononuclear cells, many of which are phagocytic. Macrophages are present which may contain red blood corpuscles and intracellular granular bodies, arranged in masses which are regarded as Rickettsia by most authorities. Multiple necrotic miliary areas are observed in the cortex of the glands, the necrosis being a coagulation necrosis, while the gland capsule is often infiltrated with small round cells.

4010

Further study of the pathology of this infection is desirable, especially of that of the milder types of the disease.

BIBLIOGRAPHY

Ashburn, P. M. and Craig, C. F.: Philippine J. Sc. (B), 3: 1, 1908.
—— and ——: Boston M. & S. J., 158: 749, 1908.
Bessem, N.: Geneesk. tijdschr. v. Nederl.-Indië, 75: 1909, 1935.
Faust, E. C.: China M. J., 37: 979, 1923.
Fletcher, W. and Field, J. W.: Bull. Inst. M. Research Federated Malay States, No. 1, 1927.
——, Lesslar, J. E. and Lewthwaite, R.: Tr. Roy. Soc. Trop. Med. & Hyg., 23: 57, 1929.
Gunther, C. E. M.: M. J. Australia, 2: 202, 1938.
Kitashima, T.: Kitasato Arch. Exper. Med., 2: 91, 1918.

Lewthwaite, R. and Savoor, S. R.: Brit. J. Exper. Path., 17: 448, 1936.
Miyajima, M.: Kitasato Arch. Exper. Med., 1: 1, 1917.
Nagayo, M.: Practice of Medicine in the Tropics, Byam and Archibald, London, 3: 2134, 1923.
Ogata, N.: Arch. f. Schiffs- u. Tropen-Hyg., 39: 491, 1935.
Palm, T. A.: Edinburgh M. J., 24: 128, 1878.
Sellards, A. W.: Am. J. Trop. Med., 2: 529, 1923.
Wolff, J. W. and Kouwenaar, W.: Geneesk. tijdschr. v. Nederl.-Indië, 76: 272, 1936.
Yoshida, S.: Kitasato Arch. Exper. Med., 12: 324, 1935.

YAWS

(*Frambesia*)

By Charles F. Craig, M.D., M.A. (Hon.), F.A.C.P., F.A.C.S., Colonel, U. S. Army Medical Corps (Ret.), D.S.M.

Synonyms.—Pian (French), boubas (Brazil), coco (Fiji), momba (Angola), parangi (Ceylon), dubi (Gold Coast), puru (Malaya), patek (Java), lupani (Samoa), tonga (New Caledonia).

Definition.—Yaws, or frambesia, is an infectious and contagious disease, inoculable and autoinoculable, occurring in the tropics and caused by a spirochete called *Treponema pertenue*, which abounds in the characteristic cutaneous lesions of the disease during the primary and secondary stages of the infection. The disease is characterized by an initial cutaneous granulomatous lesion, known as the "mother yaw"; a secondary granulomatous eruption of the skin, and certain sequelae which are referred to by many writers as the tertiary stage of the disease.

Etiology.—Yaws is caused by a spirochete known as *Treponema pertenue*, first described by Castellani in 1905, which is morphologically indistinguishable from *Treponema pallidum*, the cause of syphilis. In 1907 Ashburn and the writer confirmed Castellani's findings and produced the disease in monkeys in the Philippine Islands. Since that time numerous investigators have studied this organism and have demonstrated beyond question its etiologic relationship to the disease.

Treponema pertenue is a spiral organism having sharply defined, fine spirals which cause it to resemble *Treponema pallidum* so closely that the statement is warranted that the two spirochetes cannot be distinguished morphologically, although it is stated by some writers that they are morphologically distinct. Ashburn and the writer (1907) believed at first that it was possible to distinguish them morphologically, but further study convinced us that the supposed differences we noted were really due to changes produced by the staining methods employed and were not of any diagnostic importance in the differentiation of the species.

Treponema pertenue is always present in the secretions from the initial and secondary granulomatous lesions in the epidermal layer of the skin, and has also been found in the lymphatic glands, spleen and bone marrow, according to some observers. Its presence in the blood has never been demonstrated microscopically, although the blood of yaws patients is infective to monkeys and its presence in the blood is also proved by the occurrence of the generalized secondary granulomatous skin eruption. The organism is killed almost instantly by ex-

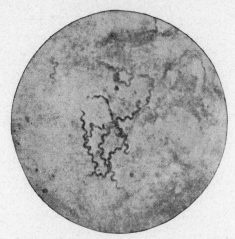
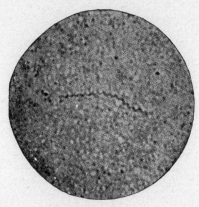

FIG. 1.—Treponema pertenue. Smear from yaws lesion. Levaditi stain. × 1500. (Army Medical School Collection.)

FIG. 2.—Treponema pertenue. Smear from yaws lesion. Levaditi stain. × 1500. (Photo. Ashburn and Craig.)

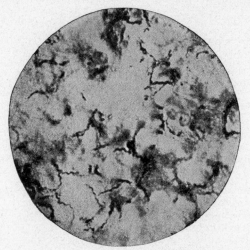

FIG. 3.—Treponema pertenue. Smear of degenerated epithelium from yaws lesion. Levaditi stain. × 1200. (Photo. Ashburn and Craig.)

posure to sunlight and by drying but may live and even multiply if preserved in sealed capillary tubes and kept at room temperature, as first shown by Ashburn and the writer, for periods varying from three to seven days. Upon suitable media it can be cultivated with great difficulty. Noguchi (1911) was the first to cultivate this organism in ascitic fluid containing a small portion of sterile rabbit kidney tissue, the fluid being covered with liquid petrolatum, thus producing an anaerobic condition, which is absolutely essential for cultivation. Others have confirmed his results, although some recent authorities doubt if *Treponema pertenue* has ever been cultivated, as the spirochetes which have been cultivated and which were presumed to belong to this species were not infective to susceptible animals.

The spirochete cannot be stained with the ordinary bacteriologic stains but may be well stained with the Wright, Giemsa, Leishman or Fontana stains and, in tissues, by the silver impregnation methods. In stained preparations the organism usually varies in length from 10 to 12 microns but longer and shorter forms may sometimes be observed. The width is so slight that it often does not appear to be over a line in thickness and 0.25 of a micron may be said to be the usual diameter. The spirals are very regular and close, and measure about 1.5 microns from crest to crest and from 1 to 1.2 microns in depth. In unstained preparations the organisms appear as hyaline, colorless bodies composed of a series of fine and fairly rigid spirals, with pointed extremities. *Treponema pertenue* is best demonstrated by the dark-field apparatus and in such preparations the motility of the organism may be studied as well as the morphology, which is similar to that seen in unstained material, as mentioned above. The India-ink method is also an excellent one for demonstrating this spirochete.

Treponema pertenue does not occur in nature in any of the lower animals, so far as is known, but monkeys and rabbits are susceptible to experimental infection. Castellani (1907) was successful in producing yaws in *Semnopithecus* and *Macacus* monkeys by rubbing material containing the spirochetes into the scarified skin of these animals. Ashburn and the writer (1907), in the Philippine Islands, succeeded in infecting *Cynomolgus* monkeys in the same manner. The most extensive and valuable work along this line has been accomplished by Schöbl (1928), who produced yaws in *Cynomolgus philippinensis*, a common monkey of the Philippine Islands, by the hypodermic injection of emulsified material from yaws lesions. The best results were obtained by inoculation of the skin over the eyebrows and that of the scrotum. Inoculation was followed, after a period of incubation varying from three to five weeks, by the development at the site of inoculation of a typical yaws lesion corresponding to the primary lesion as observed in man. Healing occurred from the center of the lesion and a circinate lesion was eventually produced which healed very slowly. Secondary lesions did not develop, except in one animal, unless superinfection was practiced, when typical secondary lesions appeared distributed over the body of the inoculated monkey. In some of his superinfected animals a condition identical with "gangosa" in man developed, resulting in extensive destruction of the nasal tissues. The observations of Schöbl and others have been of great value in differentiating yaws and syphilis, and his results offer conclusive evidence that the two are not identical.

The rabbit was first experimentally infected with yaws by Nichols (1910) by testicular inoculation of serum from a yaws lesion. After an incubation period of 27 days an orchitis developed, the serum from which contained numerous spirochetes and was infective to monkeys. Sections of the testicle showed numerous spirochetes in and around the tubules and in the connective tissue. Pearce and Brown (1925) confirmed the work of Nichols and produced yaws in rabbits over a period of three years with two strains of the spirochete.

Transmission to mice has been reported by Schlossberger (1927), who used a strain of *Treponema pertenue* furnished by Nichols. Inoculation of mice is not followed by a visible lesion, but the injection of emulsified tissues from the brain, spleen, and glands produced typical yaws lesions in rabbits, according to this investigator. His results have not been confirmed, so far as is known by the writer.

Epidemiology.—Yaws is an infectious, contagious, inoculable and auto-inoculable disease, and all conditions that lead to direct contact and accessibility of the yaws lesions to insects, especially certain species of flies, favor the transmission of the infection.

Yaws is usually acquired by contact with an individual infected with the disease, the secretions from the yaws lesions, which contain multitudes of spirochetes, being deposited in an abrasion or scratch upon the skin of the uninfected individual. Infection cannot occur through the unbroken skin, as proved by many experiments. Direct contact with a yaws lesion is not necessary for infection to occur as the disease may be transmitted by arthropods which have fed upon the secretions from the lesions and then bitten uninfected individuals.

Among native races, in which yaws is commonly present, the chances for transmission by direct contact are very great and, especially in children, who run about naked, the vast majority of cases of this disease are due to contact, but it cannot be denied that arthropods may be a very prolific source of infection under favorable conditions. In Jamaica, where yaws is very prevalent, it is believed by Kumm (1935) that a small fly, *Hippelates pallipes,* transmits the disease. Kumm, Turner and Peat (1935) have shown that this fly feeds in large numbers on yaws lesions, crawling underneath the scabs to obtain their food which consists of the secretions from the lesions which contain multitudes of spirochetes. The spirochetes may remain alive in the stomach contents and proboscis of the flies for several hours, remaining motile for as long as seven hours in the esophageal diverticulum, during all of which time they may be regurgitated if the flies feed upon other individuals, as they frequently do, before the spirochetes have perished. *Treponema pertenue* does not live very long in the proboscis of these flies nor in the stomach, but, as stated, remains motile in the esophageal diverticulum for as long as seven or eight hours after feeding.

In a later series of observations, Kumm and Turner (1936) were successful in producing yaws in rabbits by allowing infected flies of this genus to feed upon the animals, the infection being produced through the regurgitation of spirochetes in the "vomit-drop" deposited when the flies bite, the organisms coming from the esophageal diverticulum. Whether man may be infected in this manner remains to be proved but there is every reason to believe that such a method of infection of man is common in regions where suitable flies are present.

Yaws may be contracted through indirect contact, it not being necessary to come into contact with a yaws lesion. For many years it has been known that certain houses, known as "yaws houses," appear to harbor the virus, and individuals living in them are apt to become infected. Apparently the discharges from the lesions of yaws patients may impregnate the floors and walls of certain houses which are kept in a filthy condition, as often happens among certain natives, and contact with the contaminated surfaces may transmit the infection. It is also possible to contract the disease by an abrasion of the skin coming in contact with any surface recently soiled by the discharges from yaws lesions, and this is probably a common source of infection among natives.

Yaws is an inoculable disease and the natives of yaws regions have utilized this fact in the so-called "vaccination" of their children for the disease. In some regions mothers vaccinate their children by inoculating an abrasion of the skin with a small amount of serum from a lesion, thus producing the disease, which in the very young may be mild and easily handled, whereas in older children and adults the infection may be more severe and much more difficult to control because of the habits of the infected individual. Autoinoculation is also possible during the early stages of a yaw infection and patients suffering from the disease may, by scratching or handling existing lesions, transfer the infection to abrasions elsewhere upon the skin and thus spread the infection. Autoinoculation is most apt to occur in childhood and it is sometimes possible to distinguish clearly the extension of the disease in this manner, numerous yaws nodules developing along definite scratch marks on the skin extending from the primary focus.

Yaws is essentially a nonvenereal disease differing thus from syphilis which is usually of venereal origin. The primary lesion of yaws is almost invariably located upon the skin elsewhere than the genitals, although in rare instances the disease may be acquired through sexual intercourse if a yaws lesion happens to be located upon the genitals. It is estimated that close to 99 per cent of cases of yaws acquire the infection nonvenereally.

Immunity.—Immunity to yaws follows an attack but the immunity develops slowly and is not complete, in most instances, until the disappearance of the secondary lesions, and sometimes not for several years following the disappearance of these lesions. It has been shown by several investigators, especially Turner (1936), who experimented with human volunteers, that one attack of yaws confers an immunity to subsequent infection, and Schöbl (1928), in the Philippines, has conclusively shown that in monkeys a lasting immunity to yaws occurs if the animals are allowed to recover naturally from a generalized infection produced by superinfection of animals after the primary lesion has appeared or healed. In such animals, also, it has been found that an immunity to syphilis has developed, as will be noted later.

A *natural immunity* to yaws undoubtedly exists although we have no very satisfactory experimental evidence demonstrating that this is so. The writer has observed numerous instances in which individuals certainly exposed for long periods of time to infection have remained free from the disease and others in which such long-continued exposure finally resulted in its development. The statement that the white man is immune to yaws and that it is a disease limited to the yellow and black races, continually repeated in our textbooks, is certainly not true. That the white race so seldom is afflicted with this disease is not because of a natural immunity to the infection but because of a different manner of living. Yellow and black native races live very differently from the white race in the endemic areas of yaws and the relatively much greater incidence of the infection in these races is easily explained by their manner of life. In such regions the native children go about naked until nearly adult life and thus contact between the skin of healthy children and those showing the lesions of yaws is almost unavoidable during play and work, while the presence of the disease in nursing mothers is a very frequent cause of transmission to babies. In addition, no precautions are usually taken to protect the yaws lesions from biting-flies or other arthropods, and the sanitary conditions of the native house are such as to favor infection. On the other hand the white child in yaws regions, as in other tropical regions, is fully clothed and contact of the skin with a yaws lesion is almost impossible, while white children are not allowed to play with native children in most regions. Sanitary conditions of the dwelling are infinitely better and flies and other arthropods are controlled and there is little chance of transmission by these arthropods. However, if members of the white race live under the same conditions as the yellow or black native, it will be found that yaws will occur in white children and adults and that there is little, if any, racial immunity. In other words, if a white man or woman "goes native" in yaws regions they will develop yaws if exposed and their children will also suffer from the disease under such circumstances.

The duration of immunity after an attack of yaws has not been accurately ascertained, but the natives of yaws regions believe that they cannot again have the disease if they have previously suffered from it, and this belief is the origin of the practice of producing yaws in the young children by inoculation of yaws secretions subcutaneously or by the scratch method, the latter being largely practiced among some native races.

Climatic Features.—Yaws is essentially a disease of tropical regions and never propagates itself in the temperate zones. Although this infection has been repeatedly introduced into the temperate regions of the earth, there is no good evidence that infections have occurred in such regions. This is the more remarkable as yaws is so readily acquired through contact with the secretions from the lesions. That innumerable opportunities for such contact have occurred in temperate and cold localities is undisputed, but the fact remains that primary cases of yaws in such regions have not been demonstrated to occur.

In the tropics yaws is usually a disease of low-lying, rainy localities, although infections do occur in mountainous regions in the tropics. Even in localities which, because of climate, are favorable for the spread of this infection, the disease often appears to be more or less localized. Thus, in the Philippines, instances were observed by the writer in which the disease was very prevalent in one locality, while, in another, only a few miles distant, it was rare or absent. It is also a well-known fact that yaws is essentially a disease affecting

4210

the population of rural districts, being usually absent from cities, where syphilis is commonly observed. Thus, in Manila, primary cases of yaws were almost unknown, while in rural districts some ten to twenty miles from the city it was a very common infection. The character of the soil has much to do with the prevalence of the disease, limestone formations being unfavorable, while in regions where subsoil drainage is poor, yaws is much more prevalent. Wherever sanitary conditions are poor and yaws is endemic, the infection spreads rapidly and most of the children become infected, sooner or later.

Age Relationship.—Yaws is essentially a disease of childhood, although many adults present the disease in all yaws regions. In Jamaica, Saunders and Muench (1937) found that practically 70 to 80 per cent of the cases of yaws occurred before adult life, while Turner and Saunders (1935) found that 90 per cent of 1,800 persons having the disease contracted it before they were fifteen years of age. In Jamaica, the greatest number of infections occurred before the age of eight years. In the Philippines, in the writer's experience, about 60 per cent of the cases observed by him were in children below the age of seven years and approximately 85 per cent below the age of fifteen years.

Sex Relationship.—Males are more frequently infected than females, in the ratio of 2 to 1, but this is not due to any immunity enjoyed by the females but is probably entirely due to increased chances of infection of the male, because of the more active habits of the latter, and character of play and occupation.

Yaws is not a congenital disease nor is it hereditary, as is syphilis. While nursing children are frequently seen exhibiting the lesions of this infection, the disease has invariably been contracted after birth, in the experience of all who have studied this infection. The milk of a mother suffering from yaws will not convey the disease to her child nor will a nursing child suffering from yaws infect the mother, unless secretions from the yaws lesions contaminate abrasions upon the skin of the latter.

One of the most striking effects of climate upon yaws is the change in the character of the lesions in individuals exposed to hot and cold temperatures in the tropics. In the cooler, mountainous regions of the tropics the lesions of the disease tend to be of the condylomatous type, while in the hot regions condylomatous types are much more rarely observed, and individuals presenting such types and changing from the cooler climate of the mountains to the hot regions develop the typical skin lesions of the disease.

Relationship of Yaws and Syphilis.—It is necessary here to discuss briefly the relationship of yaws and syphilis. For many years a controversy has waged regarding this question, one school of thought regarding the two as identical diseases, while the other regards them as disease entities. Those who favor the identity of yaws and syphilis, ably led by Admiral C. S. Butler, believe that yaws is the primeval form of syphilis and that the modern picture of syphilis, as we see it in temperate regions, is simply yaws modified by climate and other factors. In other words, in the opinion of these observers, yaws is a primitive form of syphilis observed in the tropics, and the two conditions should be regarded as identical and the term "yaws" should be abandoned, as indicating a clinical entity.

In favor of the identity of yaws and syphilis is the fact that *Treponema pertenue* cannot be distinguished from *Treponema pallidum*, the cause of syphilis; that in both infections the Wassermann test is positive; that in both there is a primary and secondary stage, characterized by specific lesions; and that both infections respond to the same specific drugs.

Against the identity of yaws and syphilis the following facts have been stressed: The fact that yaws is a nonvenereal infection; that mucous patches are never observed in this disease; that it is not hereditary, as is syphilis; that it does not produce lesions of the blood vessels or viscera; that it does not cause paresis; that monkeys inoculated with yaws become immune to syphilis but that these animals, when inoculated with syphilis, do not become immune to yaws; that the primary lesion of yaws is not a chancre but a typical granuloma, while the secondary lesions are duplicates, when fully developed, of the primary lesion, only varying in size, which is not true of syphilis; that the primary lesion is extragenital, while that of syphilis is usually situated upon the genitals; that the cerebrospinal fluid in yaws is always Wassermann-negative while in syphilis it is often Wassermann-positive; that the clinical symptoms in yaws are much less severe than in syphilis and differ markedly in character; that the skin lesions of yaws, when uncomplicated, are diagnostic and do not resemble those of syphilis in either the primary or secondary stages of the infection; and that morphologic similarity of the treponema and the presence of a positive Wassermann reaction in the blood do not prove the identity of the two infections any more than does the morphologic identity of *Leishmania donovani, Leishmania tropica* and *Leishmania brasiliensis* prove the identity of kala-azar, oriental sore or espundia. It is also true that mercury has no effect upon yaws.

The writer believes that yaws and syphilis may have originated from a common spirochete but that the two infections today are so clearly differentiated etiologically, epidemiologically, clinically and therapeutically as to be distinct diseases and should be so regarded. The experiments of Schöbl (1928) upon monkeys have, he believes, demonstrated beyond question that yaws is a disease in which the lesions are practically confined to epidermal structures, while syphilis is viscerotrophic in its pathology, and that, whatever the origin of the two infections, today they are clinical entities and should not be included under the term "treponematosis," if by that term is meant that the two are identical. It would appear that little is to be gained by continuing the controversy regarding their identity or nonidentity and that the time and research devoted to this question could be much better devoted to more important medical problems.

Symptomatology.—The description of the symptomatology of yaws is usually divided into that of the primary, secondary and tertiary stages, but some authorities deny the existence of a tertiary stage of this infection, preferring to regard the lesions described as "tertiary" as sequelae. However, in view of the general practice, the writer will retain the usual description, although he personally is inclined to agree with those who regard the lesions observed after the termination of the secondary stage of the disease as sequelae rather than true tertiary lesions.

INCUBATION PERIOD.—The incubation period in man varies considerably and is usually stated as from three to four weeks, but shorter and longer periods of incubation of naturally acquired infection in man have been recorded. The average period of incubation in inoculated yaws in man has been about three to four weeks, while in inoculated yaws in monkeys the incubation period may be several months. The naturally acquired disease apparently has a longer period of incubation than the inoculated disease.

During the period of incubation in natives symptoms may be so slight as not to attract attention, but usually digestive disturbances, malaise, aching in the muscles, rheumatic pains in the joints, headache and irregular rises in the temperature may be noted, especially just before the appearance of the initial lesion. In natives such symptoms are usually ignored and their presence can be ascertained only by careful questioning, but in whites such symptoms are almost invariably complained of before the primary lesion appears.

THE PRIMARY LESION, OR "MOTHER YAW."—The primary lesion of yaws may be single or multiple, consisting of a papule or a collection of papules appearing at the seat of inoculation. With the occurrence of the primary lesion the regional lymphatic glands may be enlarged and tender and there may be a rise in temperature. The location of the primary lesion is almost invariably extragenital and when it does occur on the genitals it is purely accidental and not because this disease is of venereal origin. The site of the lesion is at the point of inoculation of the treponema and may be on any part of the body, but the greatest number of primary lesions are observed upon the lower part of the leg, especially just above the ankle. In the nursing mother the primary lesion may occur upon the breast and in the nursing infant upon the mouth. The Jamaica Yaws Commission observed the primary lesion on the head, face and neck in 1 case, on the upper extremities in 4 cases, on the leg in 12 cases, and on the ankle and foot in 24 cases. In native women, who usually carry their infants astride of the hip, the primary lesion often occurs in that region. It has been noted that the lesion sometimes develops at the site of an old skin ulceration, a pustule, an insect bite, or an abrasion or wound in the skin. The lesion is sometimes so small as to be distinguished with difficulty and its duration varies from a few days to two to four months, or even longer, especially if a secondary infection has developed, as is frequently the case.

Owing to the fact that in yaws regions the natives take the disease as a matter of course, one seldom observes a primary lesion at the time of its appearance, as the native does not consult a doctor at that time; and even after the occurrence of profuse secondary lesions, natives seldom consult a physician regarding the disease unless some complication, as severe secondary infection, develops.

The primary lesion commences as a small papule in the vast majority of cases but may consist of a collection of minute papules. In the course of a few days the papule or collection of papules enlarges until the lesion may attain the size of a large pea. During this time the surface of the papule has gradually become moist and exudes a thick, almost colorless serum which hardens, assumes a yellowish color, and forms a crust covering the papule. If the initial lesion consisted of a minute group of papules the resulting crust covers the entire group, merging it into a single lesion. If the crust is removed at this time the underlying surface is bright red in color, moist, and covered with fine granulations bathed in a serous colorless secretion, which is rich in spirochetes. The surface bleeds upon slight pressure but is not painful. This lesion may heal in a few days, without further progression, but in most cases it continues to enlarge, becomes conical in shape, while the coagulated serum assumes a bright yellow color and forms a rough crust over the granulomatous tumor which may enlarge until it is the size of a large pea or small walnut. Sometimes the crust is streaked with blood due to the cracking of the tissue beneath and the resultant hemorrhage. When fully developed the "mother yaw" is a typical granuloma, projecting from the skin and covered with a thick, rough crust of a yellow or reddish-yellow color. Upon removal of this crust the tubercle beneath resembles somewhat a raspberry, giving the name "frambesia" to the disease, the rounded surface of the granuloma being crossed with delicate trabeculae, the intervening tissue consisting of small granulations. A cloudy, whitish serum oozes from the granulating surface which, upon examination, is found to be filled with spirochetes, and it is this serum which is the principal transmitting agent of the infection.

The primary lesion, or "mother yaw," may heal within a few days but when large and fully developed may not heal for many weeks or months, and, indeed, is sometimes present after the secondary lesions have mostly disappeared. Usually it disappears before the secondary lesions have ceased to occur, leaving a more or less depressed, whitish scar which may afterward become pigmented.

Secondary infection of the primary lesion may occur and result in very atypical pictures which interfere with the clinical diagnosis of the disease. In such cases, extensive ulceration may occur and all resemblance to the typical "yaw" may be lost. In such cases, also, severe destruction of the tissues concerned may occur and resulting deformity due to scar tissue may complicate the condition

In the early stage of the development of the primary lesion an inflammatory areola may surround it and there may be some pain present, but after it is fully developed there is no indication of inflammation of the surrounding skin and the granuloma is not painful, even on pressure, unless secondary infection is present. Itching may be a prominent symptom in the region of the lesion and scratching often leads to autoinoculation and the development of secondary lesions close to the primary one. The scar resulting from the lesion may be small and almost invisible or large and definite, in the Negro often thick and keloid in type. At first the scar is whitish in appearance and unpigmented, but in time pigmentation occurs and, unless ulceration due to secondary bacterial infection has led to the destruction of much tissue, it is often impossible to detect the site of the primary lesion after a few months.

THE SECONDARY LESIONS OF YAWS.—After the appearance of the primary yaw lesion a period of from one to three months may elapse before the appearance of the secondary eruption. During this period, if there have been symptoms associated with the appearance and progress of growth of the primary lesion, they gradually disappear, but just prior to the secondary eruption such symptoms recur, consisting of malaise, headache, pains in the muscles, bones and joints, with slight, irregular fever. The skin feels hot and dry and, if carefully inspected, minute areas of furfuraceous desquamation may be detected. These areas may be so slight as to escape notice or large areas of the skin may present this phenomenon. The furfuraceous areas may be confluent, or widely separate, and round, oval, or irregular in shape. They may form rings encircling a central area of desquamation, the intervening skin appearing normal, or definite patches of desquamated tissue resembling flour scattered over the dark skin of the native may be present. In many cases desquamation appears to be very slight and it often requires the most careful examination to demonstrate its existence, but the writer believes that it is present before the appearance of the secondary lesions in every infection.

A short time after the appearance of the furfuraceous patches it will be noted that minute papules begin to appear within the patches, having a very small yellowish tip, the nodules being surrounded by a slightly reddish areola. Many of these minute papules disappear after a few days but others grow larger and may vary in size from a small pea to a small walnut. The smaller ones tend to occur in groups and in some instances a large papule may be observed surrounded by smaller ones, probably due to autoinoculation, as the papules itch and lead to scratching, thus distributing the infection. As the papules enlarge the surface becomes moist and gradually a crust of a yellowish or reddish-yellow color is formed over the papule, if hemorrhage has been present. These papules are not painful even on pressure and may gradually disappear or develop into the typical "yaw" granuloma or tumor.

The typical granuloma of yaws consists of a tumor, varying in size from a pea to a large walnut covered with an adherent yellow or reddish-yellow crust and either hemispherical or somewhat flattened in shape. The crusted cap of the lesion is generally corrugated and often shows cracks through which slight hemorrhage may occur from the surface of the granuloma. When this crust is carefully removed it will be noted that the rounded surface of the granuloma is red in color, smooth or finely granular, and from it oozes a cloudy, slightly yellowish serum which, upon examination, is seen to contain multitudes of the spirochetes causing the disease. After the original crust is removed a new one is quickly formed by the drying of the serous exudate over the lesion and, in time, a thick crust identical in appearance with the one removed will result. Some authorities describe the exudate from the granuloma as purulent, but this is never true unless a secondary bacterial infection is present, which is frequently the case. The exposed surface of the granuloma bleeds easily but is not painful even when touched with irritating chemicals or with instruments. Itching is often present and leads to the distribution of the lesions through autoinoculation. The fully developed secondary yaws granulomas are exactly like the primary, typical "mother yaw" in their morphology, in uncomplicated infections, except as regards size, but even the smaller secondary lesions are duplications, in miniature, of the primary lesion. This fact distinguishes yaws

4210

from syphilis in which the secondary eruption differs entirely in appearance from the primary lesion, or chancre.

The secondary yaws eruption occurs in crops, one succeeding another, with the result that at one time all variations in size and in development of the lesions may be seen upon the body, from the furfuraceous patches, the small papules and the fully developed granulomas, to healed lesions.

The duration of the secondary stage extends from a few weeks to two or three years, in the cases of longer duration one crop of lesions being followed by others during this period. Usually the secondary lesions disappear after from six months to one year, adults presenting the most persistent infections.

There may be numerous variations in the morphology of the lesions of the secondary stage of yaws and some authorities have described these variations as more or less typical of the infection. As a matter of fact, in the experience of the writer, the typical granulomas, as previously described, are those most frequently encountered and it is rare that the variations to be noted are observed, although, along with the typical lesions which preponderate, atypical lesions may be present at the same time. The following types of secondary eruption have been described by different authorities:

Papular Eruption.—This type of eruption is characterized by the occurrence, on the skin, of numerous small, reddish papules covered with a minute yellowish, moist crust. These papules do not enlarge but gradually dry up and disappear. This type of eruption is very rare, but, along with the typical granulomatous eruption, similar small papules are usually observed scattered between the typical granulomas.

Scaly or Lichenoid Eruption.—This type of eruption resembles the furfuraceous condition of the skin which usually precedes the development of the typical eruption, but in these cases the scaly eruption is not succeeded by the occurrence of granulomatous lesions. It is really identical, in the writer's opinion, with the former and should not be classified as a distinct type of eruption. It is most commonly observed in children and young adults, and it is only in very rare instances that it disappears without the development of the typical granulomatous lesions somewhere upon the body.

Ulcerative Eruption.—This name has been applied to granulomatous lesions which, by reason of secondary bacterial infection, have degenerated and formed ulcers of varying size which heal very slowly. The name should not be retained in the description of this infection, if by it is meant an eruption characterized by ulceration, as uncomplicated granulomatous lesions, characteristic of the secondary eruption of yaws, never suppurate or ulcerate unless a secondary bacterial infection has occurred.

"Crab Yaws."—When the secondary lesions of yaws develop upon the soles of the feet a painful condition ensues owing to the pressure of the yaw tubercles developing in the tough, nonelastic tissue of the epidermis in this region. Eventually the overlying epidermis is cracked and the tubercles emerge and pain largely disappears, although the pressure exercised in walking is painful and gives rise to a peculiar gait resembling that of a crab, hence the name "crab yaws." Secondary infections invariably occur in such patients and the surface of the sole of the foot may present ulcerations and a cracked, scaly or eroded appearance. Such a condition may last for years or even a lifetime, according to some authorities, and a permanent focus of *Treponema pertenue* may be maintained in the sole of the foot. In healing, the corelike center of the granuloma may disappear, leaving an irregular erosion of a chronic type which may seriously interfere with walking.

Sometimes yaws tubercles develop in the palms of the hand and pain is a prominent symptom, especially upon pressure, until the overlying epidermis degenerates and the tubercle emerges. Such lesions are very persistent and disabling, owing to their situation.

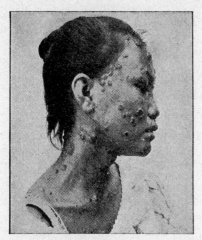

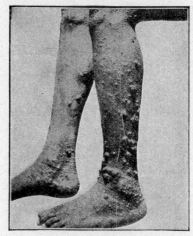

FIG. 4.—Yaws. Secondary lesions. (Photo.   FIG. 5.—Yaws. Secondary lesions. (Photo.
Ashburn and Craig.)   Ashburn and Craig.)

YAWS CONDYLOMA.—The occurrence of yaws granulomas about the anus gives rise to what is known as the condylomatous type of yaws, in which the yaws tubercles resemble the condylomas of syphilis. In this region, due to constant moisture and pressure, the typical crust covering the granulomas upon other portions of the body is missing, the tumors having a smooth, moist, reddish surface, and so closely resembling syphilitic condylomas that, if no other lesions were present, it would be impossible to make a differential diagnosis. Fortunately, such lesions never occur without the simultaneous occurrence of the typical granulomas of yaws upon other regions of the body.

CIRCINATE ERUPTION.—In many infections with yaws, along with the typical solitary yaws tubercles there occur lesions in which the eruption occurs in the form of a circular arrangement of very small papules covered with the typical crust, the latter merging in such a manner as to give the appearance of a circular lesion embracing a small area of normal skin. This arrangement resembles somewhat the circinate type of eruption in syphilis but differs from the latter in the occurrence of the characteristic yellowish or reddish-yellow crust covering the lesion. Another type of circinate lesion often observed in yaws is a circular collection of crusted tubercles enclosing an area of normal skin at the center of which is a typical yaws tubercle, the entire lesion resembling a miniature volcanic crater at the center of which is a minute peak. This type of lesion was frequently observed by the writer in cases of yaws in the Philippine Islands. The circinate type of eruption has been called "ringworm" yaws by some authorities.

MUCOUS MEMBRANE LESIONS.—Yaws differs from syphilis in that the secondary stage of the former is not characterized by the occurrence of mucous patches or other lesions of the mucous membranes. However, in some instances, yaws lesions occurring upon the lips may extend into the mucous membrane of the mouth and produce small granulomatous lesions. Such lesions have also been described by some writers as occurring at the base of the tongue, upon the nasal mucous membrane and upon the vaginal mucous membrane. Whitish areas upon the tongue, resembling syphilitic leukoplakia, have also been noted by some physicians but are very rare and have never been observed by the writer.

SITE OF ERUPTION.—The secondary eruption of yaws may involve any portion of the skin, but the skin of the legs, arms, thighs and face are the areas that usually show the greatest number of yaws tubercles, while the trunk may be relatively free. The writer has observed cases in which the face, arms and legs were thickly covered with granulomas while the trunk showed very few, if any, lesions. The palms of the hands and the soles of the feet are frequently affected. Autoinoculation is frequently observed, the lesions being produced by scratching the papules and thus distributing the virus, and in some instances the extension of the infection may be easily noted following scratch marks. Such lesions are especially apt to occur in the axilla, at the corners of the mouth, on the back, and along the thighs. The forehead is a favorite site of yaw tubercles.

THE BLOOD IN YAWS.—Yaws is frequently attended by a medium degree of anemia, the red blood cell count averaging from 3,000,000 to 4,000,000 cells per c.mm., while the hemoglobin index averages 65 to 75 per cent. The leukocytes are not increased in the absence of a secondary bacterial infection, but as such an infection is a common complication the leukocyte counts are frequently above normal with an increase in the neutrophils. In uncomplicated yaws there is frequently a slight increase in the large mononuclear leukocytes but there is no increase in the lymphocytes as in syphilis. In practically all cases of secondary yaws a positive Wassermann and Kahn reaction develops and in this infection a positive Wassermann and Kahn reaction occurs as frequently and as intensely as in syphilis. The positive reaction often disappears after the secondary eruption is healed and may be negative in the tertiary stage of the infection. The blood of yaws patients is not usually infective unless it is obtained from a lesion and then only if it has been contaminated with material from the lesion. Blood obtained from the general circulation has always been negative for *Treponema pertenue* upon microscopic examination, so far as is known by the writer. This does not mean that the organism does not occur in the blood, as it doubtless does, but simply that it is impossible to demonstrate it therein.

THE TERTIARY LESIONS OF YAWS.—As already stated, some authorities do not recognize a tertiary stage in yaws but regard the various conditions that have been described as tertiary lesions merely as sequelae of the infection. The writer believes that there are excellent grounds for so considering these conditions and has retained the term "tertiary" only because it has become fixed in the literature of the disease. It is also true that in many instances lesions have been described as tertiary that were, in reality, merely secondary lesions complicated by a secondary bacterial infection. This is especially true in those patients still showing a florid secondary yaws eruption and also ulcerative lesions which have been called tertiary by some writers. In the writer's opinion all ulcerative lesions which occur along with typical secondary yaws granulomas are simply granulomas which have broken down because of secondary bacterial infections and the term "tertiary" should never be applied to such lesions but only to ulcerative lesions appearing after the secondary eruption has disappeared.

The so-called "tertiary lesions" of yaws may appear shortly after the disappearance of the secondary lesions or months or years afterward. These lesions vary greatly in character and many of the conditions that have been described as tertiary manifestations of this disease cannot be said to have been definitely proved to be caused by *Treponema pertenue*. This is especially true of the lesions supposed to have been found in the blood vessels, of aneurysms, and of the conditions called goundou and juxta-articular nodules, in all of which the only evidence we have of their connection with yaws is a history of the patient's having suffered from that disease at some time prior to the development of the condition. Of course, such evidence has no scientific value whatever and can only be considered as evidence by those who insist that yaws and syphilis are identical diseases.

We have no definite knowledge of the proportion of patients suffering from yaws who develop the so-called "tertiary" symptoms and lesions, but if one insists in regarding such lesions as "tertiary" as only those which develop after the subsidence of the secondary eruption, it is certainly true that a comparatively small proportion of yaws patients develop "tertiary" lesions.

Sequelae.—ULCERATIVE LESIONS.—Probably the most common of the sequelae of yaws are ulcerations of the skin which may develop at the site of a healed secondary granuloma or, more commonly, may result from the breaking down of gummatous-like tumors, followed by secondary bacterial infection of the degenerated lesion. Such lesions are most apt to be upon the ankle or lower leg or thigh and may be of various size and may involve only the epidermis or dermis or extend into the underlying muscular tissues, sometimes even involving the periosteum of the bones and giving rise to a periostitis. Such lesions may persist for weeks, months or years, causing great deformity, loss of functional activity, and may terminate fatally because of inanition and debility produced through long-continued bacterial infection.

BONE LESIONS.—Among the most common of the sequelae, or so-called "tertiary" lesions of yaws are those affecting the bones. Such lesions occur in from 10 to 20 per cent of cases in which the secondary granulomas have been numerous and of long standing. Painful periosteal nodes, occurring most frequently upon the radius, ulna, tibia and fibula, and which are very painful upon pressure, are frequently encountered. At first, these nodes are exceedingly painful and the skin over them is reddened and swollen, but eventually the pains ceases, the inflammation subsides, and the nodules remain as hard periosteal swellings. Such nodes may also occur upon the forehead and over the ribs but less frequently than upon the long bones. A diffuse periostitis may occur without the formation of nodules and an osteitis may sometimes be observed resulting in deformity of the long bones, as the tibia, where the condition is known as "saber shin." Deformities of the fingers may be present, due to an osteitis or periostitis, and a form of multiple periostitis frequently affects the digital phalanges, causing the multiple dactylitis so often seen in patients suffering from the sequelae of yaws. A rarefying osteitis is more rarely observed in the bones, rendering them very subject to fracture, and the roentgen ray shows that the rarefying process commences early and generally results in deformity of the bone affected. Most of the bone affections that have been mentioned are accompanied by rheumatic pains which may be very severe and exhausting. Secondary bacterial infections occur frequently in patients who present bone lesions and these add greatly to the gravity of whatever condition may be present. When a rarefying osteitis is present the lesions appear as rarefied areas, the long axis of the lesion lying parallel with that of the bone involved, and the vast majority of these lesions appear to originate in the interior of the bone although small, cup-shaped lesions may sometimes be observed upon the surface of the bone. A form of yaws onychia is frequently observed in endemic areas of this disease.

In some cases the inflammatory bone lesions may extend into the overlying skin, resulting in severe ulcerations of a chronic type, with fistulae leading into the periosteum or medulla of the bone. Such lesions are almost invariably secondarily infected with the bacteria of suppuration, and such lesions may last for months or years or even lead to such destruction that amputation may become necessary.

JOINTS.—During the secondary stage of yaws painful articulations are rarely observed, but severe pain in the joints, which may appear swollen, sometimes occurs as a so-called tertiary symptom. Fever may accompany these symptoms and the entire picture is that of acute articular rheumatism. One joint may be involved or several, and the smaller joints are especially apt to become painful and swollen, but involvement of these articulations is not accompanied by fever.

All of the conditions described above may occur at the same time as the secondary lesions and have been called tertiary lesions despite that fact, but it is also true that all of these conditions may occur long after the secondary lesions have disappeared. In such, while it may be allowable to term them tertiary lesions of the disease, the writer believes that it is far preferable to regard these conditions as sequelae, as already stated. In the secondary stage of the infection

4210

such conditions as dactylitis, onychia, paronychia and atrophy and destruction of the nails are not infrequently observed and cannot be considered as tertiary symptoms, although similar conditions occur during the so-called "tertiary" stage of the disease, and most of the "tertiary" symptoms and lesions which have been described as occurring during the secondary stage of yaws were in reality secondary manifestations complicated by a secondary bacterial infection.

GANGOSA, OR RHINOPHARYNGITIS MUTILANS.—This condition is now generally believed to be a sequela or "tertiary" lesion of yaws, although some authorities still think that it may be of syphilitic origin. It occurs in regions where yaws is prevalent and a history of the disease is almost invariably given by patients suffering from this condition. It is characterized by very destructive lesions of the mucous membrane of the throat, pharynx and nasal passages which may involve the bony structures, leading to great deformity and loss of function of the parts affected.

Gangosa was first described by our Navy medical officers who observed it in natives of Guam. At first believed to be of syphilitic origin by them, this opinion was changed when it was noted that syphilis was practically absent in the natives, but that yaws was a very prevalent infection, and further study convinced them that it was a late manifestation of the latter disease. In 1928 a Spanish commission investigated the question, studying the condition as observed in natives of the Ladrone Islands, and regarded it as due to yaws. It has been observed in Guam, the Philippine Islands, the Ladrone Islands, the West Indies, especially Dominica, the Caroline Islands, Fiji, West Africa, the Belgian Congo and British Guiana. It is usually observed in older adults but cases have been observed in young adults and children, although in the latter the condition is very rarely seen.

Patients are seldom observed until the lesions are well advanced but it is said that it usually commences as a small ulcer upon the mucous membrane of the soft palate. However, many cases have been described in which the infection apparently spread to the mucous membrane of the mouth or nose from adjacent yaws lesions upon the skin. The ulcer upon the solt palate is preceded by a whitish membrane which degenerates, resulting in the formation of the typical ulcer which is surrounded by an area of inflammation. From this ulcer the infection spreads from within outward and involves the mucous membrane and bone, destroying both as the condition progresses. It spreads slowly but may eventually destroy the hard palate, the soft parts and bones of the nose and the cartilages of the nasal septum, as well as the tip of the nose, thus producing a funnel-shaped triangular opening which may include the entire nose or there may be remnants of the nostrils left, while the upper lip forms the base of the triangular opening. In rare instances the upper lip may become involved and partially destroyed. Extension of the process may occur through the nasal duct to the eye, which may result in the destruction of the latter or partial or total loss of sight. The extension of the process is very slow, usually covering years, and spontaneous healing of the lesions may occur with more or less scar formation according to the severity of the infection. During the activity of the process a very offensive odor is present, originating from the ulcerated surfaces. The larynx is not usually involved, but speech may be interfered with if the lesions involve the pharynx and tongue.

Owing to the situation of the lesions secondary bacterial infections invariably occur and these will alter their appearance more or less, depending upon the bacteria concerned. Some authorities have considered that Leishmania may be responsible for some of the cases that have been described and it is true that a differential diagnosis between espundia, the mucocutaneous type of leishmaniasis, and gangosa is sometimes impossible unless the respective causative organisms can be demonstrated. As it is very difficult to demonstrate *Leishmania brasiliensis* in the mucosal lesions of espundia and as *Treponema pertenue* has not been demonstrated in those of gangosa, so far as known to the writer, it is obvious that a differential diagnosis between the two must often be impossible. Most authorities regard gangosa as a condition that will develop only when hygienic conditions are very poor or absent and where specific treatment for yaws is not available.

Strong (1942) states that the differentiation of gangosa from syphilis is often impossible and reports the histologic results of a study he made of a case in which the microscopic changes did not "especially suggest syphilis, particularly in the absence of marked vascular changes." So far as the histologic picture was concerned, he states that it evidenced "a chronic inflammatory condition in which there was a tendency to destruction of newly formed tissue" and that neither spirochetes nor fusiform bacilli could be demonstrated in the sections.

The proof of the relationship of yaws to gangosa rests upon its occurrence in yaws regions where syphilis is very rarely observed and the history of a previous attack of this disease. While this evidence is far from satisfactory it is believed that it does indicate that *Treponema pertenue* is the cause of the condition.

GOUNDOU.—This condition, also known by the natives in Africa, as "anakhré," is believed by some authorities to be a late manifestation of yaws but it cannot be said that there is sufficient proof that this is the case. MacAllister in 1882 first described the "horned men of Africa" and later Lamprey gave a more detailed description. For many years every side show in every circus of large size exhibited one or more of these "horned men" and it was not recognized for a long time that the condition was not a natural one but due to some disease process.

Goundou is observed in regions in which yaws is endemic, especially in Central and West Africa, South America and in some of the islands of the West Indies, as Jamaica. The relationship of the condition to yaws is favored by the fact that it often begins in children who have recently suffered from yaws or soon follows an attack of the latter infection in adults, as well as the reported occurrence of an immunity to inoculation with yaws material in those suffering from goundou, but many investigators believe that it is a disease *sui generis* and that its occurrence in individuals who have suffered from yaws is purely coincidental. Many modern observers believe that goundou is really a disturbance of metabolism due to an endocrine disorder and is closely related to *osteitis fibrosa*. Others, as Manson-Bahr (1940), believe that it closely resembles *leontiasis ossea*, and Strong (1942) states that it may be a form of leontiasis ossea which occurs in people who suffer at the same time from yaws, hence its prevalence in endemic yaw regions. It is also true that similar lesions have been observed in individuals in regions where yaws never occurs and who have never suffered from the disease, although Strong believes that the evidence is sufficient to include some cases of the disease among the sequelae of yaws. The writer has included the condition in the description of the sequelae of yaws, not because he considers that it has been proved to be related to the latter infection, but because it is so included in all accounts of the disease.

The essential bony changes in goundou consist in a production of porous bone resulting in a hyperostosis which produces a great overgrowth of the bony tissue, frequently observed in the bones of the ascending or nasal processes of the superior maxilla, but other bones of the skull may be involved in the process. The resultant growth of the nasal bones may resemble a horn projecting from the face, hence the term "horned men of Africa."

The disease usually begins in childhood and the earliest symptoms are severe and prolonged headaches, and general malaise. After these symptoms have lasted for a variable period it will be noticed that a seropurulent discharge occurs from the nostrils, sometimes tinged with blood, while pains develop in the bones of the face and nose. At the same time it will be noted that the nasal bones are apparently somewhat swollen and symmetrical swellings appear about the size of a pea or bean at the side of the nose, the lesions usually being bilateral. These swellings gradually enlarge and eventually, through extension to adjacent bony tissue, form a projecting tumor which varies greatly in size and sometimes becomes as large as a man's fist or even larger. With the gradual growth of the bony tumor the headache and other constitutional symptoms slowly disappear and, aside from the presence of the exostoses, the patient appears normal. The skin over the tumor is not adherent, being freely movable; ulceration never occurs and the exostoses are not painful.

With the growth of the tumor, which projects downward and outward, the vision may be interfered with but the orbits are not invaded by the process, although the nasal passages may be partially or totally obstructed. The shape of the tumor is usually oval and there may be multiple tumors although this is of rare occurrence. The hard palate may become involved and great deformity may result.

The exostoses may not be confined to the nasal bones but may occur upon other portions of the body. Thus Botreau-Roussel states that similar exostoses may occur as sequelae of yaws upon the skull, inferior maxilla, tibia, fibula, femur, radius and clavicle. In Jamaica it has been found that patients suffering from goundou invariably give a positive Wassermann reaction, a fact which still further favors its relationship to yaws.

JUXTA-ARTICULAR NODULES.—Fibrous nodules, frequently found in the vicinity of the joints and bilateral in location, are sometimes observed following an infection with yaws, but similar nodules may be caused by syphilis and by onchocercal infection, and have been observed in other conditions. There are only four reports of the finding of *Treponema pertenue* in the fibrous nodules: those by Clapier, in Africa; Sobernheim, in Berne; Van Hoof, in Africa; and Van Dijke, in the Dutch East Indies. These few observations are more or less invalidated by the impossibility of differentiating *Treponema pertenue* from *Treponema pallidum* and the fact that similar nodules occur in syphilis. Patients suffering from this condition give a positive Wassermann reaction, but as this type of reaction occurs in both yaws and syphilis it is of no value in differentiating the causation of the nodules.

Juxta-articular nodules occur in the subcutaneous tissues especially about the external surfaces of the arms and legs and over the joints. They are very frequently bilateral and the writer has observed a case in which single nodules were present over each elbow and hip joint, and several in which nodules occurred over each elbow joint and each hip joint separately. The nodules are not always bilateral and may be situated over the lower end of the femur, the ankle, along the long bones or distributed over the skin of various parts of the body. They may vary in size from a walnut to a large orange and are painless, even upon deep pressure. Ulceration and suppuration very rarely occur in the nodules. They are of firm consistence and the skin over them may be freely movable or may be attached, usually after the nodule has persisted for weeks or months. They enlarge very slowly and may persist for years and are most apt to develop in locations subject to pressure or irritation, as the elbows, knees or hips.

Pathologically, the nodules are composed of dense fibrous tissue containing very few blood capillaries. Strong (1942) states that in a type which he studied the tumors "consisted especially of a dense fibrous tissue capsule enclosing inflammatory and necrotic areas in which peculiar, large, swollen lipoid cells with multiple inculsions in their protoplasm were situated." In other cases the nodules upon section were composed of strands of fibrous material in which there was little evidence of blood vessel formation and which, in macroscopic sections, appeared of a glistening white color.

Exactly similar lesions have been described by many authorities in patients suffering from tertiary syphilis. Araujo found 60 cases of syphilis showing juxta-articular nodules and was unable to find any such lesions in yaws, while

Jessner, as quoted by Strong, after a study of the literature concluded that in 62 cases of juxta-articular nodules yaws could be excluded as the cause. Hu and Frazier found *Treponema pallidum* to be present in cases studied by them. It is also true that such nodules have been reported in individuals who have never suffered from either yaws or syphilis, so that the exact etiology of juxta-articular nodules cannot be said to have been satisfactorily demonstrated. It is probable that such nodules may be due to a variety of causes and that *Treponema pertenue* may be capable of initiating the process, but this has not been proved. So far, attempts to produce yaws in man or susceptible animals by the inoculation of material from these nodules has not resulted in the production of the disease.

OTHER SEQUELAE.—Among the other sequelae of yaws that have been reported may be mentioned a form of chronic synovitis, ganglion formation in the region of the wrist, and contractures resulting from scars produced by the healing of ulcerations in certain regions. In dark-skinned races the depigmentation following the healing of the yaws lesions may result in depigmented areas scattered over the skin and somewhat resembling the lesions of the disease known as "pinta."

Diagnosis.—In the vast majority of cases of yaws the diagnosis can be easily made by observation of the lesions in the primary and secondary stages of the disease, but in the so-called "tertiary stage" the diagnosis is often very difficult and in many instances it is impossible to differentiate some of the sequelae of yaws from lesions observed in syphilitic infections.

The *primary lesion*, or "mother yaw," can be easily diagnosed, in uncomplicated infections, because of its peculiar morphology. The granulomatous tumor, projecting from the skin and covered with a yellowish or reddish-yellow, rough crust, is typical and does not resemble any other skin lesion observed in man, with the exception, of course, of the secondary lesions of the disease, which are duplicates of the primary lesion. However, if a secondary bacterial infection has occurred the lesion may ulcerate and may somewhat resemble that of oriental sore, but the absence of *Leishmania tropica* and the presence of *Treponema pertenue* will serve to differentiate the two conditions. In such cases, also, the primary lesion of yaws may simulate other ulcerative conditions of the skin but it is usually possible to make a differential diagnosis without much difficulty.

The diagnosis of yaws during the *secondary stage* of the infection is very easily made upon the characteristic clinical picture of the eruption. While some authorities have stressed the difficulty of diagnosing yaws during this stage, the writer is convinced that anyone who has once seen a typical case of yaws during the secondary stage of the disease would never have any difficulty in making a diagnosis by simple inspection of the lesions, and that no lesion ever observed in syphilis could be confused with the typical secondary lesions of yaws by one who has ever seen patients suffering from this disease. The occurrence of crops of granulomatous tumors covered with the characteristic crust, in which *Treponema pertenue* can be easily demonstrated, is diagnostic of yaws during this stage of the disease and it is only in the very rare cases in which few lesions are present and these complicated with a secondary bacterial infection, that it would be at all difficult to make a diagnosis of yaws.

In the so-called *"tertiary stage"* of yaws the differential diagnosis from some other disease conditions is usually difficult and often impossible. This subject will be discussed under the heading Differential Diagnosis, but it may be stated here that many of the sequelae of yaws may be confused with other conditions and that the diagnosis of the disease at this time may be impossible.

DIFFERENTIAL DIAGNOSIS.—The diseases with which yaws has been most often confused are verruga peruana and syphilis.

Verruga peruana, a disease occurring in certain regions in Peru, Ecuador, Bolivia and Chile, caused by *Bartonella bacilliformis,* and characterized during one stage of development by a granulomatous eruption of the skin, might be confused with yaws during the secondary stage; but verruga peruana is preceded usually by a well-defined febrile stage known as Oroya fever, while the granulomas differ greatly in their morphology from those of yaws, being smooth in contour, cherry-red in color, and appearing not only upon the skin but upon the mucous membranes. The Wassermann test is negative in verruga peruana and *Treponema pertenue* cannot be demonstrated in the secretions from the nodules. To one who has observed the two infections there should be no difficulty in differentiating them.

Syphilis and yaws are frequently confused and reference has already been made to the relationship of these two infections. There should be no difficulty in differentiating the lesions of these diseases during the primary and secondary stages of either, but in the so-called "tertiary stage," or sequelae, of yaws, it is frequently impossible to differentiate the various lesions that may occur, as already noted in the discussion of the relationship of the two infections. The essential differences between the two diseases are covered in Table I, but it

TABLE I.—DIFFERENTIAL FEATURES OF YAWS AND SYPHILIS

YAWS	SYPHILIS
Not a venereal disease.	A venereal disease.
Not congenital.	Congenital.
Primary lesion, extragenital.	Primary lesion, genital.
Primary lesion, a nodule.	Primary lesion, an ulcer.
Secondary lesions, duplicates of the primary lesion.	Secondary lesions, unlike primary lesion.
Secondary lesions, when uncomplicated, absolutely characteristic and uniform in general appearance.	Secondary lesions, multiform in appearance.
Mucous patches never present.	Mucous patches usually present.
Itching of lesions a very common symptom.	Itching of lesions very rare.
Alopecia never occurs.	Alopecia common.
Mucous membranes not involved during secondary stage.	Mucous membranes always affected.
Lesions in secondary stage autoinoculable.	Lesions not autoinoculable.
Sequelae, or so-called "tertiary" lesions, do not involve the viscera.	Tertiary lesions involve the viscera.
Paresis or cerebrospinal involvement very rare, if they ever occur.	Paresis and cerebrospinal syphilis very common.
Cerebrospinal fluid gives a negative Wassermann reaction.	Cerebrospinal fluid very frequently gives a positive Wassermann reaction.
Blood vessels not affected.	Blood vessels constantly affected.
Constitutional symptoms in yaws usually slight.	Constitutional symptoms severe.
Mercurial treatment has no effect.	Mercurial treatment curative.
Cardiac disease (aneurysm, etc.) absent.	Cardiac involvement common.

should be remembered that yaws and syphilis may occur in the same individual and that both infections give a positive Wassermann reaction and are caused by spirochetes that are morphologically identical and can only be differentiated by their effects upon susceptible experimental animals.

In considering Table I it will be noted that several conditions are said to be absent in yaws which commonly occur in syphilis, but which some observers claim do occur in yaws. Thus, Choisser, in Haiti, stated that lesions of the blood vessels, as atheroma and aneurysm, were observed in patients giving a history of yaws, but the impossibility of distinguishing between the two infections renders such evidence of very doubtful value, as histories among native populations are notoriously inaccurate. On the other hand, Turner, Saunders and Johnston (1936), as the result of their very thorough study of yaws in Jamaica, reached the conclusion that cardiac disease does not occur in individuals suffering from the disease, as they could find no evidence of such lesions even following radiologic examinations. Williams (1935) states that the evidence that aneurysms ever occur as the result of yaws is unsatisfactory and that in the reported cases syphilis was not certainly excluded. Such evidence has been based upon the history of previous yaws infection, and such evidence is not scientific and is unworthy of confidence, although it is the type of evidence accepted as valid by those who claim that yaws and syphilis are the same disease, and that *Treponema pertenue* causes lesions in the brain, viscera, and blood vessels, and paresis and cerebrospinal disease.

The experiments of Schöbl and his coworkers have conclusively demonstrated that *Treponema pertenue* in monkeys is essentially *epiblastotropic* in its location and production of lesions, while *Treponema pallidum* in monkeys is *panblastotropic* but is essentially *mesoblastotropic* in location and in production of lesions.

Bejel.—In 1936–1938 E. H. Hudson described a form of syphilis occurring in children among the nomad Bedouins of the Syrian Desert and the villagers of the Tigris and Euphrates rivers. This form of syphilis is essentially a disease of children acquired through contact with other children afflicted with the infection, and is not congenital but acquired after birth. Hudson claimed that this disease is generally contracted soon after birth and is not transmitted to the next generation. It is undoubtedly caused by *Treponema pallidum* and the blood serum gives a positive Wassermann and Kahn reaction.

Aside from its evolutionary interest as apparently a clinical condition intermediate between syphilis and yaws, it is of diagnostic importance in that the skin lesions are so like those of the secondary stage of yaws that a differential diagnosis is frequently very difficult. However, in bejel mucocutaneous lesions are always present and mucous patches are present in the pharynx and mucous membranes of the mouth. There should be no difficulty in differentiating the two infections, if it be remembered that in yaws lesions do not occur in the pharynx while in bejel they are almost invariably present.

Tuberculosis of the skin, leprosy, espundia, tropical ulcer and *oriental sore* are among other conditions that have to be differentiated from yaws. All of these may be differentiated by laboratory methods; the first two by the demonstration of the tubercle and leprosy bacilli, espundia by the presence of *Leishmania brasiliensis*, tropical ulcer by the absence of *Treponema pertenue,* and oriental sore by the presence of *Leishmania tropica.*

LABORATORY DIAGNOSIS.—The demonstration of the causative organism of yaws, *Treponema pertenue,* is very simple and, in the primary and secondary stages of the infection the spirochetes are so numerous that they can be easily detected. If a dark-field apparatus is convenient all that is necessary is to place a small drop of the serum which exudes from the surface of a yaw lesion upon a slide, cover with a coverglass and examine with the dark-field. Numerous spirochetes will be seen swimming actively about in the microscopic field, showing the typical morphology of *Treponema pertenue*. If a dark-field apparatus is not available, a small amount of serum from the yaw lesion may be mixed with India ink upon a microscopic slide, covered with a coverglass and examined at once. The spirochetes will be seen as colorless spiral organisms lying in the almost black background furnished by the India ink.

To obtain permanent preparations, smears should be made of the serum from the yaws lesion upon microscopic slides and stained with the Giemsa or Fontana stain, while if permanent sections of the yaws lesion are desired, a yaws tubercle may be removed, sectioned, and stained by the Levaditi silver impregnation method. In routine diagnostic work the dark-field or India-ink methods are most useful or staining smears from the lesions by the Giemsa or Fontana stains may be employed.

In the so-called "tertiary stage" of yaws it is usually impossible to demonstrate the presence of *Treponema pertenue,* and even if a spirochete is demonstrated it is impossible to be sure that one is not dealing with *Treponema pallidum* rather than *Treponema pertenue*. The finding of a spirochete corresponding in morphology with *Treponema pertenue* in the walls of the blood vessels or in the viscera in suspected cases does not prove that it is this spirochete, as it is indistinguishable in morphology from *Treponema pallidum*, the cause of syphilis, and it is impossible to differentiate the two organisms in the tissues.

Serologic reactions are of no value in differentiating yaws and syphilis as both give a positive Wassermann and Kahn reaction, but the presence of such reactions accompanied by suspicious symptoms or lesions in individuals in endemic regions of yaws are of some assistance in diagnosis.

Treatment.—The treatment of yaws is very satisfactory in that we possess drugs which are specific in their action upon *Treponema pertenue*. These drugs are the arsphenamines and the bismuth salts.

TREATMENT WITH THE ARSPHENAMINES.—Strong, in the Philippines, in 1910, was the first to demonstrate the specific action of arsphenamine (salvarsan) in the treatment of yaws during the secondary stage of the infection, and his observations were soon confirmed by numerous investigators. As Strong (1942) well says: "There is no more striking example in medicine of the specificity of a drug than that of arsphenamine (salvarsan) or neoarsphenamine in the treatment of yaws." After a single dose a florid secondary eruption will disappear and the patient will be apparently cured but it has been found best to give from two to three doses in order to obviate any danger of a relapse, and some authorities prefer to give from six to eight injections of the arsphenamines. In the Philippines, Strong states that clinical cures resulted in 94.3 per cent of patients treated with neoarsphenamine, employing 0.1 Gm. (1½ grains) of the drug per kilo weight of the patient.

The drugs that have been most widely used in the treatment of yaws, until comparatively recent times, have been arsphenamine, neoarsphenamine, sulfarsphenamine and novarsphenamine. At the present time neoarsphenamine is probably most largely employed in the treatment of the infection in older children and adults, while sulfarsphenamine is preferred for the treatment of younger children and adults where intramuscular injection is indicated. The dose of the arsphenamines employed in the treatment of yaws is usually stated to be about two-thirds that employed in the treatment of syphilis. If **neoarsphenamine** is used intravenously the adult dose is from 0.6 to 0.9 Gm. (9 to 14 grains) and for children between 2 and 10 years of age, from 0.2 to 0.3 Gm. (3 to 5 grains). Younger children should not be given any of the arsphenamines intravenously but sulfarsphenamine intramuscularly. The dose of **sulfarsphenamine** ranges from 0.1 Gm. (1½ grains) in infants to 0.4 Gm. (6 grains) in adults, and the solution to be employed is prepared by dissolving the required amount of the drug in 1 cc. of freshly distilled water.

TREATMENT WITH BISMUTH PREPARATIONS.—While none of the bismuth preparations are as specific in the treatment of yaws as are the arsphenamines, excellent results are obtained by this form of treatment. In mass treatment the bismuth salts are to be preferred, owing to the much greater cost of the arsphenamines. The bismuth salts most frequently employed in the treatment of yaws are sodium potassium bismuth tartrate and bismuth salicylate.

Sodium potassium bismuth tartrate has probably been more largely used than any of the other bismuth salts and should contain from 50 to 60 per cent of metallic bismuth. It is administered intramuscularly, in an oil suspension, the dose varying from 0.15 to 0.3 Gm. (2¼ to 5 grains). Injections should be given at weekly intervals and usually several injections are necessary before the lesions disappear and the infection is eliminated.

Bismuth salicylate, in a 10 per cent suspension in olive oil, administered intramuscularly, in doses varying between 0.1 and 0.2 Gm. (1½ and 3 grains), has given excellent results in treatment and several proprietary bismuth preparations, as **bismuth arsanilate, bismuth tryparsamide** and **bistovol,** have also been found to be followed by excellent results. There would seem to be some advantage gained by employing a combination of bismuth and arsenic, as in bismuth arsanilate and bismuth tryparsamide, but these preparations are more costly and are not essential in the treatment of this infection.

TREATMENT WITH STOVARSOL (ACETARSONE).—This is an arsenical preparation which has the advantage of oral administration, and has been largely used in mass treatment of yaws in natives and with excellent results, according to Chesterman and Van den Braden. Sometimes as few as three doses have resulted in a cure of the infection. The drug is administered to children in doses varying between 0.5 and 1 Gm. (8 and 15 grains) and to adults in doses varying between 1 and 3 Gm. (15 and 45 grains). In adults it is best to begin with a dose of 1 Gm. (15 grains), increasing on successive days to 1.5 Gm. (23 grains) to 2 or 3 Gm. (30 or 45 grains); in children, to begin with a dose of 0.5 Gm. (8 grains) and increase to 1 Gm. (15 grains), according to age. In adults it has been found that usually after a total amount varying from 8 to 15 Gm. (2 to 3¾ dr.) the Wassermann reaction becomes negative, although the secondary eruption disappears some time before this total amount is administered. The drug is quite expensive and this is the principal objection to it for use in mass treatment.

TOXIC SYMPTOMS FOLLOWING TREATMENT.—Toxic symptoms frequently follow treatment with the arsphenamines and the same precautions should be used in the administration of any of the arsenicals as are employed in the treatment of syphilis. Renal disease is a contraindication to treatment with any arsenical and care should be taken to ascertain if disease of the kidneys is present. Arsenical eruptions sometimes follow the administration of the arsphenamines or acetarsone, and other toxic symptoms may occur in susceptible patients, as diarrhea, colic, and nausea and vomiting. The appearance of such symptoms should be the signal for discontinuing the arsenical and substituting some other form of treatment.

The toxic symptoms that have been noted after treatment with the bismuth preparations are diarrhea, skin rashes, stomatitis and albuminuria. The two latter symptoms are apt to develop in patients having septic mouths, but toxic symptoms following bismuth treatment are much less frequently encountered than after treatment with the arsenicals.

TREATMENT OF SEQUELAE.—The various *contractures* and *deformities* which may result from the healing of ulcerous lesions observed during the so-called "tertiary stage" of yaws require various types of **plastic surgery** for their correction, while the *juxta-articular nodules,* if troublesome because of their location, may be **surgically removed.**

The treatment of *ulcerative lesions,* whether occurring because of secondary bacterial infection during the primary or secondary stage or as the result of the breaking down of gummatous lesions during the so called "tertiary stage," is important and consists in keeping the ulcerated surface clean by bathing in an antiseptic solution, as a solution of **potassium permangate,** and avoiding secondary bacterial infection by proper covering of the ulcers. If the ulcers are located on the legs, **rest** is an important feature of treatment and **daily cleansing** of the ulcers is essential.

The treatment of *periostitis* and *osteomyelitis* occurring as sequelae of yaws follows that usually employed when these conditions are caused by other infections, together with the administration of the **arsphenamines** or **bismuth salts.** In gangosa the administration of the arsphenamines is often followed by marked improvement, but, of course, destroyed tissue cannot be replaced. However, in many such patients plastic surgery will give excellent results, so far as correcting certain deformities is concerned. Many patients in the advanced stage of gangosa do not seem to be much benefited by either the arsphenamines or bismuth salts and in such cases it is probable that secondary bacterial organisms are largely responsible for the lesions that may be present.

Ulcerative lesions of years' duration are most resistant to treatment and do

4210

not respond to either the arsphenamines or bismuth salts and here, again, it is probable that bacterial agents are responsible. In all cases showing a secondary infection with streptococci or staphylococci, the **sulfonamide** group of drugs should be considered in treatment.

For the *chronic headache* and *neuralgic pains* that have sometimes been observed in yaws, **potassium iodide** has been found useful and also in the sequelae of yaws some authorities regard this drug as valuable. Mercurials, so useful in syphilis, are without any effect in yaws and should never be administered.

PROPHYLAXIS.—As yaws is a contagious disease, easily acquired during the primary and secondary stages through direct contact with the lesions, or with the serum which oozes from them, the most important preventive measure consists in avoiding contact with the infected individual. Among native races, owing to living habits, it is impossible to avoid such contact, so that little can be accomplished in prevention of the disease in endemic regions through sanitary precautions alone. Among the more intelligent and well-to-do natives it is possible to prevent infection through contact by isolation of infected individuals and prompt and specific treatment, and in white populations in such regions infection is seldom observed because of the different manner of living and the wearing of clothing protecting the greater portion of the body.

As clothing soiled with secretions from the lesions may be infective, care should be taken to disinfect such clothing as soon as possible and it should not be handled by one having cuts or abrasions upon the hands until it has been disinfected. The fact that yaws may be transmitted by species of flies renders the protection of man from fly bites of much importance, and all cuts and abrasions of the skin should be protected from flies in endemic yaws regions. Thus, the prevention of the breeding of flies and proper screening is a practical preventive measure in such regions.

Mass Treatment in Prophylaxis.—The eradication of yaws in endemic regions has been attempted through segregation and treatment of infected natives and has met with success in certain tropical localities, as Haiti, where an extensive anti-yaws campaign through treatment has been conducted by physicians attached to the United States Navy and public health officers. There is no question that the proper treatment of all yaws cases in endemic regions would eventually result in the practical disappearance of the infection, but if, as seems to be true, yaws confers a more or less degree of immunity to syphilis, it is somewhat questionable whether the end results will be for the best good of the individual and community. It has been shown by Schöbl that animals do not become immune to syphilis after suffering from yaws unless the yaws infection is allowed to persist through the secondary stage of the disease. If the same holds good in man, the indiscriminate treatment of yaws patients before the completion of the secondary stage of the disease would theoretically deprive the patient of the immunity to syphilis that would have been his had he not been given anti-yaws treatment, and certainly one would much rather suffer from yaws than from syphilis. This phase of the subject does not appear to have been considered in the initiation of mass treatment of yaws as a preventive measure, but it would appear to deserve some consideration. It would be interesting to ascertain in regions, where mass preventive treatment has been followed, whether it has resulted in an increase in the amount of syphilis in natives so treated, as would be expected if yaws does really protect native races from syphilis.

In the treatment of yaws, whether as a remedial or preventive measure, the recognition and proper treatment of complicating parasitic infections and of other disease conditions is most important and should not be neglected.

Prognosis.—The prognosis of yaws, so far as life is concerned, is excellent and most observers state that they have never seen a fatal case of this infection, if uncomplicated. The occurrence of sequelae, as gangosa, renders the prognosis more serious, but even in the latter condition death is very rarely, if ever, due to the condition itself but may occur from secondary bacterial infections. The same statement is true of the bone lesions, as periostitis and osteomyelitis, as well as the severe ulcerative lesions that may occur during the so-called "tertiary stage" of the infection. Rarely in such cases, especially in debilitated individuals, a fatal outcome may result but always from secondary infections, usually of streptococcic nature.

While the prognosis of yaws is excellent as regards life it is often serious from the standpoint of general health and economic status. Yaws is a long-continued infection, lasting for many weeks, months, or even years, and greatly depletes the individual's resistance to other infections and renders him less valuable as an economic unit in his community. It is true that most natives in yaws regions do not regard the disease of much importance and seldom consult a physician, chiefly because during the primary and secondary stages of the infection the symptoms are not severe, there being practically no pain connected with the lesions, but it is also true that individuals suffering from moderately severe or severe attacks are much more susceptible to other infectious diseases and their working capacity is considerably reduced. If the disease could be eradicated from a community there is no question but that the general health of the people would be much improved, although the greater susceptibility of the population to syphilis might be the ultimate result.

Pathology.—The general pathology of yaws has already been mentioned in the discussion of the symptomatology and diagnosis. The pathology of the primary and secondary lesions consists essentially in the invasion of the epidermis with resultant degenerative changes in the epithelial cells, thickening of the epidermis, accumulations of leukocytes, elongation of the papillae with vascularization and infiltration with leukocytes, lymphocytes and plasma cells. As the yaws nodule develops there is an accentuation of the downgrowth of the papillae, while the covering epithelium exhibits a marked hyperkeratosis. The perivascular cellular infiltration of the corium, so common in syphilis, is not observed in yaws. In well-stained preparations with the Levaditi stain, *Treponema pertenue* may be observed, usually situated in the rete malpighii. While early in the disease the spirochetes are located in the skin, before the appearance of secondary lesions they have invaded the body and produced a general infection evidenced by the secondary eruption characteristic of the infection.

The pathology of the gummatous ulcerations occurring as sequelae of yaws is often confused by that of secondary bacterial infections, but in uncomplicated cases the histologic picture is that of granulation tissue containing areas rich in cells, increase of connective tissue, and, very rarely, a few giant cells. Coagulation necrosis often occurs if nodular lesions are present. Unlike syphilis, there is no evidence of marked endarteritis and the vessel walls are not thickened.

History.—As is true of leprosy and some other infections, certain authorities believe that yaws is referred to in the Bible; but Oviedo, in the sixteenth century, was the first to describe a disease existing in the West Indies, which was undoubtedly yaws, while Bontius mentioned its presence in the East Indies after the observations of Oviedo. During the days of the slave trade between America and Africa it was noted that yaws was prevalent among the African slaves but quickly disappeared and did not propagate itself after the slaves reached the temperate regions of America. In 1905 Castellani discovered the cause of the disease, *Treponema pertenue*, and Ashburn and Craig in 1907 confirmed his observations and produced the disease in monkeys by the inoculation, into the skin, of serum containing the causative organism obtained from typical yaws lesions. *Treponema pertenue* was first successfully cultivated upon artificial culture media by Noguchi (1917), and Nichols (1910) produced the disease in rabbits with cultures of *Treponema pertenue*.

Geographic Distribution.—Yaws is essentially a tropical disease and is not found in temperate regions or in the tropics at elevations above 1,000 feet, according to most observers. While a few cases of so-called yaws have been described as occurring in the temperate zones, none of them have been conclusively proved to be yaws and it is a perfectly safe assumption that any yaw-like lesion observed in the temperate zones in individuals who have never been in the endemic yaw regions in the tropics cannot be true yaws, for this disease cannot perpetuate itself in a cool climate. This is a useful fact to remember when one is called in consultation in a case of suspected yaws originating in the temperate zones.

Yaws is fairly well distributed in the tropical regions of the world but it does not occur in all tropical regions, and even in regions where it is endemic it has a remarkably local distribution and is essentially a disease of rural as compared with urban communities. In some tropical regions it is so prevalent that practically every native suffers from it during some period of life, usually during childhood, while in others only sporadic infections are encountered. The reasons for this difference in incidence are not entirely clear but probably have to do with certain biologic conditions as well as sanitary conditions favoring or hindering the transmission of the infection.

THE AMERICAS AND WEST INDIES.—Yaws has been observed in Brazil, Venezuela and Colombia but is not very prevalent in these localities. In British Guiana, where it used to be a common infection, it has almost disappeared although syphilis is prevalent. In the West Indies yaws is a common disease, being present in most of the more thickly populated islands, especially in Jamaica and Haiti. In the latter island it was so prevalent that mass treatment was adopted by the authorities, aided by naval physicians, to eradicate the disease, and these measures have met with much success.

AFRICA.—Yaws is apparently rarely seen in Egypt and in most of the countries of North Africa but it is prevalent in Tripoli and in the southern Sudan. The countries upon the west coast of Africa are all endemic centers of the disease and it is very frequently observed in the Congo Free State, Angola and along the Gabon River, and less frequently in Nigeria and the Gold Coast. The islands of Mozambique, Madagascar, and the Comoro Islands all present endemic centers of yaws, and in Uganda and the country about the Great Lakes the disease is not infrequently noted. In South Africa it occurs among the Kaffirs and it has also been observed in natives in other South African localities and in Kenya Colony, Rhodesia and Nyasaland. It may be stated that this infection is pretty generally distributed among the natives of the tropical belt of this continent but it is much more prevalent in some regions than in others, although climatic and sanitary conditions appear to be similar.

ASIA.—Yaws occurs in the Malay Peninsula, Assam, Thailand, Upper Burma, Ceylon, Java, the southern part of China, and rarely in India. Japan is free from the disease but it is prevalent in the Philippine Islands. Until recently yaws was a very common disease in Ceylon but it is said to be decreasing gradually, probably due to treatment and improvement in general sanitation.

OCEANIA.—Most of the islands of the Pacific lying in the tropics are endemic centers of yaws and this is especially true of Samoa, the Solomon Islands, New Caledonia, Fiji and the New Hebrides. New Zealand and Tasmania are free from the infection and this is also true of the Hawaiian Islands.

AUSTRALIA.—Yaws occurs in North Australia but is not observed elsewhere upon this continent and it is not a very common infection even in the regions in which it has been noted.

From this summary of the geographic distribution of yaws it is evident that it is confined to the tropics and is essentially a tropical disease, one of the very few that can be claimed to be truly tropical in distribution.

BIBLIOGRAPHY

Ashburn, P. M. and Craig, C. F.: Philippine J. Sc., 2: 441, 1907.

Butler, C. S.: Syphilis sive Morbus Humanus, 1936.

Castellani, A.: J. Ceylon Br., Brit. M. A., 2: 54, 1905.

Craig, C. F.: Brennemann's Practice of Pediatrics, Hagerstown, Md., W. F. Prior Company, Inc., Vol. 2, Chap. 36, 1942.

Ferris, H. W. and Turner, T. B.: Arch. Path., 24: 703, 1937.

Hudson, E. H.: Am. J. Trop. Med., 18: 675, 1938.

Kumm, H. W.: Report of Jamaica Yaws Commission for 1934. Published, 1935.

————, Turner, T. B. and Peat, A. A.: Am. J. Trop. Med., 15: 209, 1935.

———— and ————: Am. J. Trop. Med., 16: 245, 1936.

Manson-Bahr, P. H.: Manson's Tropical Diseases: A Manual of the Diseases of Warm Climates, Ed. 11, Baltimore, William Wood &

Company; London, Cassell & Co., Ltd., p. 618, 1940.

Nichols, H. J.: J. Exper. Med., 12: 616, 1910.

————: Am. J. Trop. Med., 5: 429, 1925.

Noguchi, H.: München. med. Wchnschr., 58: 1550, 1911.

————: Am. J. Syph., 1: 261, 1917.

Pearce, L. and Brown, W. H.: J. Exper. Med., 41: 673, 1925.

Saunders, G. M.: Am. J. Trop. Med., 17: 335, 1937.

Schöbl, O.: Philippine J. Sc., 35: 209, 1928.

————: Philippine J. Sc., 39: 260, 1928.

———— and Miyao, I.: Philippine J. Sc., 40: 91, 1929.

Strong, R. P.: Philippine J. Sc., 5: 433, 1910.

————: Stitt's Diagnosis, Prevention and Treatment of Tropical Diseases, Ed. 6, 1: 388, 1942.

Turner, T. B.: Am. J. Hyg., 25: 477, 1937.

———— and Saunders, G. M.: Am. J. Hyg., 21: 483, 1935.

INFECTIOUS JAUNDICE

(*Weil's Disease*)

By Charles F. Craig, M.D., M.A. (Hon.), F.A.C.P., F.A.C.S., Colonel, U. S. Army Medical Corps (Ret.), D.S.M.

Synonyms.—Icterus gravis, odan-eki (Japanese), spirochaetosis ictero-haemorrhagica.

Definition.—Infectious jaundice, or Weil's disease, is an acute, infectious disease, characterized by severe fever, marked prostration, jaundice, and enlargement of the liver and, more rarely, of the spleen. It is caused by a spirochete, *Leptospira icterohaemorrhagiae*, and rats and mice serve as natural reservoirs of the infection for man.

Etiology.—The causative organism, *Leptospira icterohaemorrhagiae*, is present in the blood, urine, sputum and cerebrospinal fluid of infected individuals and is identical in its morphology with certain free-living spirochetes. It measures from 5 to 20 microns in length, has very closely wound spirals and one hooklike extremity. It is rapidly motile and is best seen with the dark-field apparatus but stains with the Wright, Giemsa, Leishman or Fontana stains. Smears of the blood or urine so stained will usually show the spirochetes in small numbers. It can be cultivated upon special culture media and the inoculation of cultures into susceptible animals is followed by the symptoms of the disease.

Leptospira icterohaemorrhagiae occurs in small numbers in the peripheral blood during the febrile stage of the disease and rarely after the termination of the fever, and in the urine about eight days following the onset and for as long as 100 days afterward. Rarely it may be found in the blood after the subsidence of the fever.

A lasting immunity follows an attack of this disease as shown by Uhlenhuth and Fromme (1918), who found the blood serum of recovered patients still protective twenty-two years after recovery. Agglutinins, lysins and complement-fixing bodies may be demonstrated in the blood serum beginning after the second week from the first appearance of the symptoms.

Epidemiology.—The rat is the natural reservoir of infection and the spirochete occurs in the feces and urine of these animals. No apparent disease is produced in rats, but these animals cause the infection of man by the contamination of food with the feces and urine, by contamination of water, and by their bites. This spirochete has also been found in slime in mines and sewers, and miners and workers in sewers are often infected, probably through skin abrasions contaminated by slime containing the spirochetes. The water of rivers, ponds and pools may also contain this spirochete, and infection may occur through bathing in such water. Many cases occurred in armies during the first World War, when, because of trench warfare, the soldiers were forced to stand in water for long periods, and rats were numerous in the trenches. The following rodents have been found infected in nature: *Mus decumanus, M. alexandrinus, M. rattus, Microtus montebelloi* and field mice belonging to the genus *Apodemus*. Wild rats are most frequently infected, but the dog has been found infected in some localities.

Laboratory animals are usually resistant to the infection with the exception

4210

of guinea pigs, but these animals are very susceptible and can be infected by rubbing a little infected material into the scarified skin or by subcutaneous, intramuscular or intraperitoneal inoculation. Dogs are susceptible to the infection, while monkeys have been found naturally infected. Wilbert and Delorme (1927) have described an epidemic of this disease among chimpanzees in French Guiana.

Symptomatology.—The *incubation period* varies but usually averages from 6 to 10 days. The symptomatology varies with the severity of the infection, and Martin and Pettit recognize benign catarrhal jaundice, long-continued febrile, pulmonary, nervous, and very grave jaundice types.

The *onset* is sudden with fever, severe aching in the muscles of the back and extremities, prostration and headache. Nausea and vomiting may occur and pain in the abdomen may be present. The face is flushed, the conjunctivae are much congested, and a fine network of congested capillaries may be observed in the cornea and sclerae, a very useful diagnostic sign. As the infection progresses the symptoms increase in severity, the muscular pain and prostration being very marked in the case of usual severity. Jaundice usually begins in about forty-eight hours and occurs in over half of the cases. It may be very slight or severe and accompanied by hemorrhages in the mucous membranes, conjunctivae or skin. In the average case the skin has a lemon hue but in severe cases it may be dark orange or mahogany in color. Pruritus is marked in severe cases but may be absent in those with slight jaundice. Melena and epistaxis may occur and in very severe infections blood may be vomited, simulating the "black vomit" of yellow fever. Hyperesthesia, delirium or somnolence are common symptoms in severe infections.

The fever is remittent in type, rising rapidly and reaching its maximum of from 39 to 40° C. (102.2 to 104° F.) in from 24 to 36 hours, after which it remains remittent in type for from a week to ten days, falling by lysis as a rule. A secondary rise in temperature usually occurs and it is during this rise that the spirochetes are usually found in the urine. Convalescence usually begins during the third week of the fever and is usually uneventful, although a third rise in temperature is rarely observed during convalescence. Mild infections are observed in which the symptoms are very slight and the fever may disappear after from three to five days.

A petechial eruption may occur upon the skin early in the disease and between the fourth and eighth days a measly or urticarial eruption may occur, lasting several days. In very severe and fatal cases purpura may occur and erythematous and papular eruptions have also been noted.

The liver is enlarged and the gallbladder may be painful. The spleen is seldom enlarged, but the inguinal and lymphatic glands are enlarged and tender, especially the axillary glands. In cases showing meningeal symptoms the cerebrospinal fluid is increased in amount and contains numerous spirochetes which may persist in this fluid for several months after recovery.

At first the pulse is rapid but becomes slow with the development of jaundice, at which time the blood pressure also decreases. The urine may be markedly bile-stained and contains albumin, varying in amount with the severity of the infection. Albuminuria lasts for several days and red blood corpuscles and epithelial casts may be present in the urine. *Leptospira icterohaemorrhagiae* appears in the urine toward the end of the fever, usually between the ninth and tenth days, and may persist long after recovery. The blood, at the beginning of the attack, shows an increase in the number of polymorphonuclear neutrophils but later the leukocytosis disappears and there is a relative increase in mononuclear leukocytes. The red blood corpuscles are decreased in number and there is a reduction in the hemoglobin index.

Complications.—Relapses may occur after the third week of convalescence but are very rare. Bronchopneumonia or lobar pneumonia, hematuria, deafness, iritis, iridocyclitis and pharyngitis have been observed as complications.

Sequelae.—These are few, but alopecia is often observed during convalescence, and mental depression, anemia and general debility also may occur.

Diagnosis.—The *clinical diagnosis* of infectious jaundice is not difficult in
cases of average severity but is impossible in very mild infections. The important diagnostic symptoms are the sudden onset, the temperature curve, the congested conjunctivae, jaundice, albuminuria and great prostration, but all of
these may occur in yellow fever and make the differentiation impossible without
aid of laboratory methods. The diagnosis should always be confirmed by the
demonstration of *Leptospira icterohaemorrhagiae,* if possible.

LABORATORY DIAGNOSIS.—The demonstration of *Leptospira icterohaemorrhagiae* in the peripheral blood is possible but as the organism occurs often in
very small numbers, at least 5 cc. of blood should be collected from a vein in the
arm, centrifuged, smears made from the sediment and either examined with
the dark-field or stained with the Wright, Giemsa or Fontana stains. Should
the smears be negative a guinea pig should be inoculated percutaneously, subcutaneously or intraperitoneally with the patient's blood. Usually, within
twenty-four hours, the animal will have a rise in temperature which will persist
until death, which usually occurs within a week to ten days. Before death
marked jaundice is present, albumin and casts appear in the urine, and hemorrhages occur from the nose and anus, and from the genitalia in female animals.
Leptospira icterohaemorrhagiae may be demonstrated in the blood and urine
of the inoculated guinea pig. Necropsy will show the characteristic pathology
of infectious jaundice and smears from the liver and spleen should show the
spirochetes. The preferable method of inoculation is intraperitoneal and from
3 to 5 cc. of the patient's blood should be inoculated.

Blood cultures are often successful as a diagnostic method, if employed during the first week of the disease. Cultures are made by inoculating special
media with about 0.5 cc. of the blood in each tube of the medium, after which
the tubes are kept at a temperature between 28 and 30° C. (82.4 and 86° F.)
and examined at the end of a week by the dark-field microscope or in stained
smears. If negative, the cultures should be kept for three weeks and examined
at weekly intervals, as the spirochetes may be very slow in developing.

The culture media found most useful are the Fletcher; Noguchi and Lindenberg, and the Vervoort media. The Fletcher medium consists of 5 cc. of distilled
water; 0.5 cc. of a melted 2.5 per cent agar; and 1 cc. of fresh rabbit blood
serum, in each tube. The Noguchi and Lindenberg medium consists of 800 parts
normal saline solution; 100 parts fresh rabbit blood serum; 100 parts 2 per cent
agar, pH 7.2, and 10 to 20 parts rabbit hemoglobin solution, made by adding
1 part defibrinated rabbit's blood to 3 parts of distilled water. The Vervoort
medium consists of a solution of 0.1 per cent peptone and 0.05 per cent NaCl in
tap water, which has been buffered by the addition of 5 to 10 per cent of a phosphate solution and adjusted to a final pH of 7.2.

After the first week of the disease cultures of the urine should be made instead of the blood.

From seven to ten days following the onset of the fever stained smears of
the sediment obtained from centrifuged urine should be examined for the spirochete, or unstained preparations examined by the dark-field apparatus. If negative a guinea pig should be inoculated and cultures made from the urine sediment.

Agglutination tests are most useful as affording confirmatory evidence of a
past infection with *Leptospira icterohaemorrhagiae,* as agglutinins persist in the
blood for months and the titers are high, usually between 1 : 500 and 1 : 15,000.

Brown and Davis (1927) have devised a diagnostic test known as the "adhesion test," which is also useful in differentiating *Leptospira icterohaemorrhagiae* from other spirochetes. It consists in mixing the blood serum of the
patient with a solution containing *Leptospira icterohaemorrhagiae* and either
blood platelets or bacteria. If this mixture is examined with the dark-field

4210

microscope several minutes after it is prepared, it will be seen that the bacilli or blood platelets are adherent to the spirochetes, and such a reaction is regarded as positive.

In general practice the examination of the blood and urine microscopically and the inoculation of the guinea pig are the laboratory methods which are most useful and most generally employed.

DIFFERENTIAL DIAGNOSIS.—The diseases with which infectious jaundice is most frequently confused and which are most important from a differential standpoint are yellow fever, the relapsing fevers, and malarial infections in which jaundice is a complicating factor.

Yellow Fever.—Infectious jaundice is more apt to be confused with yellow fever than with any other disease and in many instances it is impossible to differentiate between them unless laboratory methods of diagnosis are employed. In both infections the onset is sudden, jaundice and albuminuria are present, and hemorrhages may occur. The lack of correlation between the pulse and temperature in yellow fever, known as Faget's sign, in which a very slow and receding pulse is present with a rising or stationary temperature, should serve to distinguish the two infections. In infectious jaundice, while a slow pulse may be present after the appearance of jaundice, it is not so pronounced as in yellow fever and the pulse does not become slower and slower as the temperature rises during the secondary fever. In mild cases of both infections a clinical differentiation is generally impossible.

The inoculation of a guinea pig with the blood of the patient is a valuable diagnostic method, as in yellow fever such inoculation is not followed by any apparent symptoms, while in infectious jaundice the animal develops fever and jaundice, and dies and within ten days, as a rule. During convalescence, the mouse protection test for yellow fever will determine whether or not that disease existed, for the blood serum of patients suffering from infectious jaundice does not protect mice from yellow fever infection.

Relapsing Fevers.—Certain of the relapsing fevers may be confused with infectious jaundice, but the occurrence of regular relapses of fever, together with the presence of spirochetes of relapsing fever in the peripheral blood in considerable numbers during the entire febrile periods and their absence between the relapses, should serve to differentiate these infections.

Malarial Fevers.—Jaundice may occur as a complication of the malarial fevers, especially in estivo-autumnal infections in the tropics, but the presence of the malaria plasmodia in the peripheral blood and the absence of *Leptospira icterohaemorrhagiae* will serve to differentiate such infections.

Epidemics of a form of febrile nonspirochetal jaundice have been observed but such infections can be differentiated by the inoculation of guinea pigs as already described.

Treatment.—We possess no drug that is specific in the treatment of infectious jaundice, as the arsphenamines, which are specific in other spirochetal infections, are worthless in the treatment of this disease.

The *specific treatment* consists in the administration of an **antiserum** prepared by immunizing horses with cultures of *Leptospira icterohaemorrhagiae*, but this treatment is valueless unless it is administered early in the disease. The antiserum is administered intravenously, in doses of about 20 cc., and repeated at intervals of several hours, according to the severity of the infection. The total amount for an adult varies between 40 and 60 cc. daily for three to four days. The intramuscular injection of **convalescent serum**, if of a titer of from 1: 15,000 to 1: 20,000, has been found to give good results if an antiserum is not available. The dose is 30 cc. daily for three or more days, according to the results obtained.

The *general treatment* is important and **good nursing** aids greatly in recovery. Symptoms should be treated as they arise. *Severe kidney symptoms* should be treated by the intravenous injection of **normal saline** and **5 per cent**

glucose solution should be injected intravenously if indicated. The patient should not be allowed to leave his bed until convalescence is well established. During the attack the **diet** should be liquid and a full diet gradually adopted during convalescence.

PROPHYLAXIS.—The most important thing in prevention is the destruction of rats and preventing these animals from coming into contact with food, drink, or water used for any purpose. Rat bites should be cauterized and bathing in water known to be contaminated should be forbidden. Miners and sewer workers should avoid coming into contact with slime, and any abrasions on the skin so contaminated should be cleansed and disinfected. As the urine of patients contains large numbers of spirochetes during, and for months after, convalescence, it should be disinfected and the hands should be disinfected after handling such urine. In caring for patients it is safest to wear rubber gloves to prevent infection. **Vaccine** treatment as a preventive measure would appear to be indicated and a vaccine prepared from killed cultures of *Leptospira icterohaemorrhagiae* may prove effective.

Prognosis.—This varies in different localities. In Japan the mortality has been as high as 50 per cent but the usual mortality is between 5 and 10 per cent.

Pathology.—The pathology is characteristic. Jaundice is usually well marked and hemorrhages are present in the fatty tissues, lungs, liver, kidneys, striated muscles and adrenals. The liver is enlarged and covered with small hemorrhagic or necrosed areas, and, microscopically, fatty degeneration and necrosis are present. The kidneys show an acute nephritis; the spleen is soft and hemorrhagic; the stomach and intestines show hemorrhages in the mucosa, and the lungs may show hemorrhagic infarcts. The blood presents a severe anemia. The causative spirochetes may be found in sections of the tissues, especially of the liver, when stained with the silver impregnation methods.

History.—Infectious jaundice was described by Weil in 1886, and the cause of the disease, *Leptospira icterohaemorrhagiae,* was discovered by Inada and Ido in 1915. In 1917 these investigators found the spirochete in rats and field voles and demonstrated that these animals acted as reservoirs of infection for man.

Geographic Distribution.—Infectious jaundice is world-wide in distribution but most common in Japan, where it occurs in September and October. During the first World War cases were numerous in armies operating in Europe, Gallipoli, Salonika and Egypt, and the disease is frequently seen in all of the countries bordering on the Mediterranean. It also occurs in Germany, Holland, Russia, Belgium, England, the United States, Central America, Brazil and Argentina. Sporadic cases have been observed in many other countries, and in the United States epidemics have occurred although the disease is most frequently encountered sporadically.

BIBLIOGRAPHY

Brown, H. G. and Davis, L. J.: Brit. J. Exper. Path., 8: 397, 1927.
Fletcher, W.: Tr. Roy. Soc. Trop. Med. & Hyg., 21: 265, 1928.
Inada, R. and Ido, Y.: Tokyo Ijishnshi, No. 1908, 1915.
Inada, R., Ido, Y., Hoki, R., Ito, H. and Wani, H.: J. Exper. Med., 24: 485, 1916.
Noguchi, H. and Lindenberg, A.: Am. J. Trop. Med., 5: 63, 1925.
Vervoort, H.: Reports Far Eastern Med. Assoc., p. 683, 1923.